OXFORD MEDICAL PUBLICATIONS

## Oxford Handbook of
# Geriatric Medicine

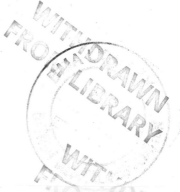

## Published and forthcoming Oxford Handbooks

# Oxford Handbook of
# Geriatric
# Medicine

Third edition

## Lesley K. Bowker
Consultant in Older People's Medicine
Norfolk and Norwich University Foundation Hospital
and
Clinical Skills Director and Honorary Professor
Norwich Medical School
University of East Anglia, UK

## James D. Price
Consultant in Geriatric and Acute General Medicine
Oxford University Hospitals NHS Foundation Trust, UK

## Ku S. Shah
Consultant in Geriatric and Acute General Medicine
Oxford University Hospitals NHS Foundation Trust, UK

## Sarah C. Smith
Consultant in Geriatric and Acute General Medicine
Oxford University Hospitals NHS Foundation Trust, UK

OXFORD
UNIVERSITY PRESS

UNIVERSITY PRESS

Great Clarendon Street, Oxford, OX2 6DP,
United Kingdom

Oxford University Press is a department of the University of Oxford.
It furthers the University's objective of excellence in research, scholarship,
and education by publishing worldwide. Oxford is a registered trade mark of
Oxford University Press in the UK and in certain other countries

First Edition published in 2006
Second Edition published in 2012
Third Edition published in 2018

Impression: 1

Published in the United States of America by Oxford University Press
198 Madison Avenue, New York, NY 10016, United States of America

British Library Cataloguing in Publication Data
Data available

Library of Congress Control Number: 2017952262

ISBN 978–0–19–873838–1

Printed and bound in China by
C&C Offset Printing Co., Ltd.

# Foreword

Geriatrics is medicine of the gaps—such gaps as we see between surgery and social work, and between psychiatry and orthopaedics. It is the medicine of the gaps between what doctors need to know for their everyday work and what they are taught as medical students. Medical curricula are still structured around diseases and technologies, rather than people with diseases and people needing technologies. The majority of such people are old.

Even more importantly, geriatrics has to transcend gaps in 'evidence-based medicine'. This is only partly because older people, and especially frail older people, are left out of clinical trials; there is also a philosophical gap. We start life with different levels of health and function, and we age at different rates. Older people come to differ from each other more than do younger people; logic requires that they are treated as individuals, not as members of the homogeneous groups assumed in the rationale of conventional trial evidence.

Some generalizations are possible. It follows from the biology of ageing that the risk of complications, often preventable or curable, from physically challenging treatments will increase with age. But it follows, too, that the benefits of treatments that are not physically challenging will also increase with age. The n-of-1 trial is the relevant, but sadly under-used, paradigm, its logic (though not its rigour) underlying the better-known 'Let's try it, but stop if it does not work' trial. With the patient as an active and informed partner, even this is better than the unthinking application of the results of a clinical trial of dubious relevance.

Because of the evidence gap, geriatric medicine has to be an art as well as a science—as the authors of this handbook emphasize in their preface. The art of medicine depends, in William Osler's words, on 'a sustaining love for ideals' and, at a practical level, on the ability to recognize similarities and to distinguish significant differences. Good doctors can draw on structured experience and recognize patterns and warning signals that are unrecorded in the cookbook medicine of trialists and managers. The cookbooks are based on what happens on average and our patients expect us to do better than that.

For some of us, its interplay of medicine, biology, and social sciences makes geriatrics a fascinating central interest. But most doctors who meet with ill older people have other responsibilities as well. They will enjoy their work better and be more efficient if they feel able to respond confidently to the commoner problems of their older patients. Not every older person needs a geriatrician any more than every person with heart failure needs a cardiologist. But all doctors need to know what geriatricians and cardiologists have to offer, and all doctors must be able to recognize when they are getting out of their depth.

So here is a *vade mecum* written for the caring and conscientious clinician, but it is not a cookbook. It outlines how to set about analysing complex clinical situations, and the resources that can or should be called on. The authors are worthy guides; they have gained and given of their experience and wisdom in one of the best and busiest of British hospitals. Their aim is not to supplant, but to facilitate thought and good judgement—two qualities that our older patients need, deserve, and expect of us.

John Grimley Evans

# Preface

This pocket-sized text will function as a friendly, experienced, and knowledgeable geriatrician who is available for advice at all times.

This is a handbook, not a textbook. It is not exhaustive—we have focused on common problems, including practical help with common dilemmas which are not well covered by traditional tomes, while excluding the rare and unimportant.

In this third edition, in response to feedback, we have increased the number of 'HOW TO' boxes and updated sections where there have been advances in evidence and practice.

We believe that the practice of geriatric medicine is an art form and aim to provide guidance to complement the algorithms, protocols, and policies found in many textbooks. The evidence-based literature in geriatric medicine is limited, so advice is often opinion- and experience-based.

The satisfaction of good geriatric care is lost to many who become overwhelmed by the breadth and complexity of seemingly insoluble problems. We provide a structured, logical, and flexible approach to problem-solving which we hope will give practical help to improve the care given to older patients in many settings.

Lesley K. Bowker
James D. Price
Ku S. Shah
Sarah C. Smith

# Dedication

We dedicate this book to our families:
Yaw, Kneale, Tineke, Ed, Nina, Jess, Helen, Cassie, Anna, James, Sam, and Harry

# Acknowledgements

We were delighted when the first edition of this handbook was used as the basis of the American *Oxford Handbook of Geriatric Medicine* (2010).

# Contents

# Symbols and abbreviations

| | |
|---|---|
| ๖ | website cross-reference |
| ➍ | cross-reference to other sections of the book or to external material |
| 1° | primary |
| 2° | secondary |
| ↑ | increased |
| ↓ | decreased |
| → | leading to |
| α | alpha |
| β | beta |
| γ | gamma |
| ► | important |
| ►► | don't dawdle |
| ♂ | male |
| ♀ | female |
| ~ | approximately |
| °C | degree Celsius |
| ± | plus or minus |
| > | greater than |
| < | less than |
| ≥ | equal to or greater than |
| ≤ | equal to or less than |
| £ | pound sterling |
| ® | registered |
| ™ | trademark |
| A–a | alveolar–arterial |
| AAMI | age-associated memory impairment |
| AAS | admission avoidance scheme |
| ABG | arterial blood gas |
| ABPI | ankle–brachial pressure index |
| ACE | angiotensin-converting enzyme |
| ACTH | adrenocorticotropic hormone |
| AD | advance directive |
| ADH | antidiuretic hormone |
| ADL | activity of daily living |
| A&E | accident and emergency |

| | |
|---|---|
| AF | atrial fibrillation |
| AIDS | acquired immune deficiency syndrome |
| AKI | acute kidney injury |
| ALP | alkaline phosphatase |
| ALS | amyotrophic lateral sclerosis |
| a.m. | before noon (*ante meridiem*) |
| AMD | age-related macular degeneration |
| AMTS | Abbreviated Mental Test Score |
| ANA | anti-nuclear antibody |
| ANCA | antineutrophil cytoplasmic antibody |
| AND | allow natural death |
| ARB | angiotensin receptor blocker |
| ARDS | adult respiratory distress syndrome |
| ASA | American Society of Anesthesiologists |
| ATN | acute tubular necrosis |
| AV | atrioventricular |
| AXR | abdominal X-ray |
| bADL | basic activity of daily living |
| BCG | bacille Calmette–Guérin |
| bd | twice daily (*bis die*) |
| BGS | British Geriatrics Society |
| BMI | body mass index |
| BNF | British National Formulary |
| BNP | B-type natriuretic peptide |
| BP | blood pressure |
| BPH | benign prostatic hyperplasia |
| bpm | beat per minute |
| BPPV | benign paroxysmal positional vertigo |
| CABG | coronary artery bypass grafting |
| CCG | Clinical Commissioning Group |
| CDAD | *Clostridium difficile*-associated diarrhoea |
| CDT | clock-drawing test |
| CESR | Certificate of Eligibility for Specialist Registration |
| CGA | comprehensive geriatric assessment |
| CH | community hospital |
| CHD | coronary heart disease |
| CJD | Creutzfeldt–Jakob disease |
| CK | creatine kinase |
| CKD | chronic kidney disease |
| CNS | central nervous system |

| | |
|---|---|
| $CO_2$ | carbon dioxide |
| COMT | catechol-$O$-methyltransferase |
| COPD | chronic obstructive pulmonary disease |
| COX-2 | cyclo-oxygenase-2 |
| CPR | cardiopulmonary resuscitation |
| CQC | Care Quality Commission |
| CRP | C-reactive protein |
| CSF | cerebrospinal fluid |
| CSS | carotid sinus syndrome |
| CT | computed tomography |
| CTPA | computed tomography pulmonary angiography |
| CXR | chest radiograph |
| DBP | diastolic blood pressure |
| DEXA | dual-energy X-ray absorptiometry |
| DGM | Diploma in Geriatric Medicine |
| DH | day hospital |
| DIC | disseminated intravascular coagulation |
| DNA | deoxyribonucleic acid |
| DNACPR | do not attempt cardiopulmonary resuscitation |
| DOAC | direct oral anticoagulant |
| DoL | Deprivation of Liberty |
| DoLS | Deprivation of Liberty Safeguards |
| DPP-4 | dipeptidyl peptidase-4 inhibitor |
| DRE | digital rectal examination |
| DToC | delayed transfer of care |
| DV | domiciliary visit |
| DVLA | Driver and Vehicle Licensing Agency |
| DVT | deep vein thrombosis |
| eADL | extended activity of daily living |
| ECG | electrocardiogram/electrocardiography |
| ECT | electroconvulsive therapy |
| ED | emergency department |
| EEG | electroencephalogram |
| EF | ejection fraction |
| eGFR | estimated glomerular filtration rate |
| ELD | external lumbar drainage |
| ELISA | enzyme-linked immunosorbent assay |
| EMD | electromechanical dissociation |
| EMG | electromyography |
| EMI | elderly mentally infirm |

| EMS | Elderly Mobility Scale |
| ENT | ear, nose, and throat |
| ERAS | enhanced recovery after surgery |
| ERCP | endoscopic retrograde cholangiopancreatography |
| ESR | erythrocyte sedimentation rate |
| EU | European Union |
| EWA | early walking aid |
| EWS | early warning score |
| FBC | full blood count |
| FEIBA | factor VIII inhibitor bypass activity |
| $FEV_1$ | forced expiratory volume in 1 second |
| FIM | Function Independence Measure |
| $FiO_2$ | concentration of inspired oxygen |
| FNA | fine-needle aspiration |
| FT3 | free T3 |
| FT4 | free T4 |
| FVC | forced vital capacity |
| g | gram |
| G | gauge |
| GCA | giant cell arteritis |
| GCS | Glasgow Coma Scale |
| GDS | Geriatric Depression Scale |
| GFR | glomerular filtration rate |
| GLP-1 | glucagon-like peptide-1 |
| GORD | gastro-oesophageal reflux disease |
| GP | general practitioner/practice |
| GPSI | general practitioner with a special interest |
| GTN | glyceryl trinitrate |
| h | hour |
| HASU | hyperacute stroke unit |
| Hb | haemoglobin |
| $HbA_{1c}$ | glycosylated haemoglobin |
| HDU | high dependency unit |
| HFPLVF | heart failure with preserved left ventricular function |
| HHS | hyperosmolar hyperglycaemic state |
| HIV | human immunodeficiency virus |
| HRT | hormone replacement therapy |
| HUTT | head-up tilt table testing |
| HV | health visitor |
| iADL | instrumental activity of daily living |

| IC | intermediate care |
|---|---|
| ICD | implantable cardio-defibrillator |
| ICF | International Classification of Functioning, Disability and Health |
| IDDM | insulin-dependent diabetes mellitus |
| IgA | immunoglobulin A |
| IgE | immunoglobulin E |
| IgG | immunoglobulin G |
| IGT | impaired glucose tolerance |
| IHD | ischaemic heart disease |
| im | intramuscular |
| IMCA | independent mental capacity advocate |
| INR | international normalized ratio |
| IOT | intermediate oxygen therapy |
| IP | interphalangeal |
| IPSS | International Prostate Symptom Score |
| IRDM | insulin-requiring diabetes mellitus |
| ITU | intensive therapy/care unit |
| IU | international unit |
| iv | intravenous |
| IVC | inferior vena cava |
| JVP | jugular venous pressure |
| kcal | kilocalorie |
| KDOQI | Kidney Disease Outcomes Quality Initiative |
| kg | kilogram |
| kHz | kilohertz |
| kPa | kilopascal |
| L | litre |
| LABA | long-acting β2-agonist |
| LACI | lacunar infarction |
| LACS | lacunar stroke |
| LAMA | long-acting muscarinic antagonist |
| lb | pound |
| LBBB | left bundle branch block |
| LCP | Liverpool Care Pathway |
| LDH | lactate dehydrogenase |
| L-dopa | levodopa |
| LFT | liver function test |
| LHRH | luteinizing hormone-releasing hormone |
| LKM | liver–kidney microsome (antibodies) |

| LMN | lower motor neuron |
| LPA | lasting power of attorney |
| LTOT | long-term oxygen therapy |
| LUTS | lower urinary tract symptoms |
| LV | left ventricle/ventricular |
| LVEF | left ventricular ejection fraction |
| LVH | left ventricular hypertrophy |
| m | metre |
| MAOI | monoamine oxidase inhibitor |
| MBq | megabecquerel |
| MCA | middle cerebral artery |
| MCCD | medical certificate of cause of death |
| MCI | minimal/mild cognitive impairment |
| MCV | mean corpuscular volume |
| MDT | multidisciplinary team |
| MEAMS | Middlesex Elderly Assessment of Mental State |
| mg | milligram |
| MGUS | monoclonal gammopathy of undetermined significance |
| MI | myocardial infarction |
| min | minute |
| mL | millilitre |
| mm | millimetre |
| MM | multiple myeloma |
| mmHg | millimetre of mercury |
| mmol | millimole |
| MMSE | Mini-Mental State Examination |
| MND | motor neuron disease |
| MoCA | Montreal Cognitive Assessment |
| mol | mole |
| mOsm | milliosmole |
| MPT | melphalan, prednisolone, thalidomide |
| MR | magnetic resonance |
| MRCGP | Membership of the Royal College of General Practitioners |
| MRCP | Membership of the Royal Colleges of Physicians of the United Kingdom |
| MRI | magnetic resonance imaging |
| MRSA | meticillin-resistant *Staphylococcus aureus* |
| MSU | midstream urine |
| MTI | Medical Training Initiative |
| mU | milliunit |

| MUST | Malnutrition Universal Screening Tool |
|---|---|
| Na | sodium |
| NaCl | sodium chloride |
| NCEPOD | National Confidential Enquiry into Patient Outcome and Death |
| NG | nasogastric |
| NGT | nasogastric tube |
| NHS | National Health Service |
| NI | National Insurance |
| NICE | National Institute for Health and Care Excellence |
| NIDDM | non-insulin-dependent diabetes mellitus |
| NIHSS | National Institute of Health Stroke Scale |
| NIV | non-invasive ventilation |
| NMDA | *N*-methyl-D-aspartate |
| nmol | nanomole |
| NOAC | novel/new oral anticoagulant |
| NPH | normal pressure hydrocephalus |
| NSAID | non-steroidal anti-inflammatory drug |
| NSF | National Service Framework |
| NSTEMI | non-ST elevation myocardial infarction |
| OA | osteoarthritis |
| OAB | overactive bladder |
| od | once daily (*omni die*) |
| OGD | oesophagogastroduodenoscopy |
| OT | occupational therapy (or therapist) |
| PACI | partial anterior circulation infarction |
| PACS | partial anterior circulation stroke |
| pADL | personal activity of daily living |
| PAM-aid | post-amputation mobility aid |
| PCC | prothrombin complex concentrate |
| PCI | percutaneous coronary intervention |
| PCR | polymerase chain reaction |
| PDD | predicted date of discharge |
| PE | pulmonary embolism |
| PEFR | peak expiratory flow rate |
| PEG | percutaneous endoscopic gastrostomy |
| PET | positron emission tomography |
| pg | picogram |
| PLAB | Professional and Linguistic Assessments Board |
| p.m. | after noon (*post-meridiem*) |

| PMR | polymyalgia rheumatica |
| po | orally |
| POA | power of attorney |
| POCI | posterior circulation infarction |
| POCS | posterior circulation stroke |
| POP | plaster of Paris |
| POPS | Proactive care of Older People going to have Surgery |
| POSSuM | physiological and operative severity score for the enumeration of mortality and morbidity |
| PPD | purified protein derivative |
| PPI | proton pump inhibitor |
| PPM | permanent pacemaker |
| PPV | pneumococcal polysaccharide vaccine |
| pr | per rectum (anally) |
| PRN | as needed (*pro re nata*) |
| PSA | prostrate-specific antigen |
| PT | physiotherapy (or therapist) |
| PTH | parathyroid hormone |
| PUO | pyrexia of unknown origin |
| qds | four times daily (*quater die sumendum*) |
| RBBB | right bundle branch block |
| RCP | Royal College of Physicians |
| RCSLT | Royal College of Speech and Language Therapists |
| RCT | randomized controlled trial |
| REM | rapid eye movement |
| RIG | radiologically inserted gastrostomy |
| RNCC | Registered Nursing Care Contribution |
| r-tPA | recombinant tissue plasminogen activator |
| SA | sinoatrial |
| SABA | short-acting β2-agonist |
| SALT | speech and language therapy (or therapist) |
| SAMA | short-acting muscarinic antagonist |
| SBP | systolic blood pressure |
| s/c | subcutaneous |
| SGLT-2 | sodium–glucose co-transporter-2 |
| SIADH | syndrome of inappropriate antidiuretic hormone secretion |
| SLE | systemic lupus erythematosus |
| SMA | smooth muscle antibody |
| SNRI | serotonin and noradrenaline reuptake inhibitor |
| SPECT | single-photon emission computed tomography |
| SSRI | selective serotonin reuptake inhibitor |

| STD | sexually transmitted disease |
| STEMI | ST elevation myocardial infarction |
| SVT | supraventricular tachycardia |
| T3 | triiodothyronine |
| T4 | levothyroxine |
| TA | temporal arteritis |
| TAB | temporal artery biopsy |
| TACI | total anterior circulation infarction |
| TACS | total anterior circulation stroke |
| TB | tuberculosis |
| TBG | thyroid-binding globulin |
| tds | three times daily (*ter die sumendum*) |
| TENS | transcutaneous nerve stimulation |
| TFT | thyroid function test |
| TIA | transient ischaemic attack |
| TIBC | total iron-binding capacity |
| TLOC | transient loss of consciousness |
| TMS | Tinetti Mobility Score |
| tPA | tissue plasminogen activator |
| TSH | thyroid-stimulating hormone |
| TTO | to take out (discharge drugs) |
| TUIP | transurethral incision of the prostate |
| TUMT | transurethral microwave thermotherapy |
| TUNA | transurethral needle ablation |
| TURP | transurethral resection of the prostate |
| TVT | tension-free vaginal tape |
| U | unit |
| U, C+E | urea, creatinine, and electrolytes |
| UK | United Kingdom |
| UMN | upper motor neuron |
| UPDRS | Unified Parkinson's Disease Rating Scale |
| USA | United States |
| UTI | urinary tract infection |
| UV | ultraviolet |
| VBI | vertebrobasilar insufficiency |
| VF | ventricular fibrillation |
| V/Q | ventilation–perfusion |
| VT | ventricular tachycardia |
| VTE | venous thromboembolism |
| WBC | white blood cell |
| WHO | World Health Organization |

# Chapter 1

# Ageing

# The ageing person

There are many differences between old and young people. In only some cases are these changes due to true ageing, i.e. due to changes in the characteristic(s) compared with when the person was young.

## Changes not due to ageing

- *Selective survival.* Genetic, psychological, lifestyle, and environmental factors influence survival, and certain characteristics will therefore be over-represented in older people
- *Differential challenge.* Systems and services (health, finance, transport, retail) are often designed and managed in ways that make them more accessible to young people. The greater challenge presented to older people has manifold effects (e.g. impaired access to health services)
- *Cohort effects.* Societies change, and during the twentieth century, change has been rapid in most cases. Young and old have been exposed to very different physical, social, and cultural environments

## Changes due to ageing

- *1° ageing.* Usually due to interactions between genetic (intrinsic, 'nature') and environmental (extrinsic, 'nurture') factors. Examples include lung cancer in susceptible individuals who smoke, hypertension in susceptible individuals with high salt intake, and diabetes in those with a 'thrifty genotype' who adopt a more profligate lifestyle. Additionally there are genes which influence more general cellular ageing processes. Only now are specific genetic disease susceptibilities being identified, offering the potential to intervene early and to modify risk
- *2° ageing.* Adaptation to changes of 1° ageing. These are commonly behavioural, e.g. reduction or cessation of driving as reaction times ↑

## Ageing and senescence

Differences between old and young people are thus heterogeneous, and individual effects may be viewed as:

- Beneficial (e.g. ↑ experiential learning, ↑ peak bone mineral density (reflecting the active youth of older people))
- Neutral (e.g. greying of hair, pastime preferences)
- Disadvantageous (e.g. ↓ reaction time, development of hypertension)

However, the bulk of changes, especially in late middle and older age, are detrimental, especially in meeting pathological and environmental challenges. This loss of adaptability results from homeostatic mechanisms that are less prompt, less precise, and less potent than they once were. The result is death rates that, from a nadir of around 8 years old, ↑ exponentially with age. In very old age (80–100 years), some tailing off of the rate of ↑ is seen, perhaps due to selective survival, but the ↑ continues nonetheless.

# Theories of ageing

With few exceptions, all animals age, manifesting as ↑ mortality and a finite lifespan. Theories of ageing abound, and over 300 diverse theories exist. Few stand up to careful scrutiny, and none has been confirmed as definitely playing a major role. Four examples follow.

## Oxidative damage

Reactive oxygen species fail to be mopped up by antioxidative defences and damage key molecules, including deoxyribonucleic acid (DNA). Damage builds up until key metabolic processes are impaired and cells die.

Despite evidence from *in vitro* and epidemiological studies supporting beneficial effects of antioxidants (e.g. vitamins C and E), clinical trial results have been disappointing.

## Abnormal control of cell mitosis

For most cell lines, the number of times that cell division can occur is limited (the 'Hayflick limit'). Senescent cells may predominate in tissues without significant replicative potential such as cornea and skin. The number of past divisions may be 'memorized' by a functional 'clock'—DNA repeat sequences (telomeres) shorten until further division ceases.

In other cells, division may continue uncontrolled, resulting in hyperplasia and pathologies as diverse as atherosclerosis and prostatic hyperplasia.

## Protein modification

Changes include oxidation, phosphorylation, and glycation (non-enzymatic addition of sugars). Complex glycosylated molecules are the final result of multiple sugar–protein interactions, resulting in a structurally and functionally abnormal protein molecule.

## Wear and tear

There is no doubt that physical damage plays a part in ageing of some structures, especially skin, bone, and teeth, but this is far from a universal explanation of ageing.

## Ageing and evolution

In many cases, theories are consistent with the view that ageing is a by-product of genetic selection—favoured genes are those that enhance reproductive fitness in earlier life but which may have later detrimental effects. For example, a gene that enhances oxidative phosphorylation may ↑ a mammal's speed or stamina, while ↑ the cumulative burden of oxidative damage that usually manifests much later.

Many genes appear to influence ageing; in concert with differential environmental exposures, these result in extreme phenotypic heterogeneity, i.e. people age at different rates and in different ways.

# Demographics: life expectancy

- Life expectancy (average age at death) in the developed world has been rising since accurate records began and continues to rise linearly
- Lifespan (maximum possible attainable age) is thought to be around 120 years. It is determined by human biology and has not changed
- Population ageing is not just a minor statistical observation, but a dramatic change that is easily observed in only a few generations
  - In 2002, life expectancy at birth for women born in the United Kingdom (UK) was 81 years, and 76 years for men
  - This contrasts with 49 and 45 years, respectively, at the end of the nineteenth century
- Although worldwide rises in life expectancy at birth are mainly explained by reductions in perinatal mortality, there is also a clear prolongation of later life
- Between 1980 and 2013, UK life expectancy at age 65 ↑ by 5.3 years for men and 3.9 years for women (see Table 1.1)
  - While projections suggest this trend will continue, it is possible that the modern epidemic of obesity might slow or reverse this

### Individualized life expectancy estimates

UK population statistics (Office for National Statistics) reveal that mean ♂ life expectancy is 78.7 years. However, this is not helpful when counselling an 80-year-old. Table 1.2 demonstrates that as a person gets older, their individual life expectancy actually ↑. This has relevance in deciding on healthcare interventions.

More accurate individualized estimates should take into account sex, previous and current health, longevity of direct relatives, as well as social and ethnic group.

Life expectancy at age 65 is also improving with time, as shown in Table 1.1.

**Table 1.1** Predicted UK life expectancy at age 65

| Period | Women (years to live) | Men (years to live) |
|--------|----------------------|---------------------|
| 1980–82 | 16.9 | 13 |
| 1996–98 | 18.4 | 15 |
| 2011–13 | 20.8 | 18.3 |

Adapted from data from the Office for National Statistics licensed under the Open Government Licence v.3.0.

**Table 1.2** Predicted life expectancy at various ages for men (UK)

| Age at time of estimate | Years left to live | That is, death at age |
|-------------------------|--------------------|-----------------------|
| Birth | 78.7 | 78.7 |
| 65 | 18.2 | 83.2 |
| 85 | 5.8 | 90.8 |
| 95 | 2.8 | 97.8 |

Adapted from data from the Office for National Statistics licensed under the Open Government Licence v.3.0.

# Demographics: population age structure

## Fertility

Fertility is defined as the number of live births per adult ♀. It is currently around 1.9 in the UK. If this rate were maintained, then in the long term, the population would fall unless 'topped up' by net immigration. In contrast, during the 'baby boom' years of the 1950s, fertility rates reached almost 3. This bulge in the population pyramid will reach old age in 2010–2030, ↑ the burden on health and social services.

## Deaths and cause of death

The driver of mortality decline has changed over the twentieth century, from reductions in infant/child mortality to reductions in old age mortality.
- Infant mortality accounted for 25% of deaths in 1901 but had fallen to 4% of deaths by 1950. Currently, over 96% of deaths occur at >45 years
- Deaths at age 75 and over comprised 12% of all deaths in 1901, 39% in 1951, and 65% in 2001

The most common cause of death in people aged 50–64 is cancer; 39% of ♂ and 53% of ♀ deaths are due to cancer. Over the age of 65, circulatory diseases (heart attacks and stroke) are the most common cause of death. Pneumonia as a cause of death also ↑ with age to account for 1 in 10 among those aged 85 and over.

All these statistics rely on the accuracy of death certification (see ➲ Documentation after death, pp. 648–9) which is likely to reduce with ↑ age.

## Population 'pyramids'

These demonstrate the age/sex structure of different populations. The shape is determined by fertility and death rates. 'Pyramids' from developing nations (and the UK in the past) have a wide base (high fertility, but also high death rates, especially in childhood) and triangular tops (very small numbers of older people). In the developed world, the shape has become more squared off, with some countries having an inverted pyramidal shape—people in their middle years outnumber younger people—as fertility declines below replacement values for prolonged periods.

An interactive UK population pyramid can be seen on the Office for National Statistics website (℠ http://www.ons.gov.uk/ons/interactive/uk-population-pyramid---dvc1/index.html).

# Demographics: ageing and illness

### Healthy life expectancy and prevalence of morbidity

Healthy life expectancy is that expected to be spent in good or fairly good health. As total life expectancy rises, it is better for society and the individual to spend as much of this extended life in good health as possible.

It is not known whether 'compression of morbidity'—where illness and disability are squeezed into shorter periods at the end of life—can be achieved. Trends in data from the United States (USA) suggest that compression of morbidity is occurring, but challenges to public health are different in the UK. Obesity and lack of exercise may negate diminishing morbidity from infectious diseases; as more people survive vascular deaths, they might develop dementia (and other old age-associated diseases). The UK Office for National Statistics compared estimates of healthy life expectancy from 2000 to those from a decade later and showed that we are living longer and that more of this time will be in relative health. A 65-year-old in 2011 should expect to live over half their upcoming life free from disability. However, there are significant variations, depending on the region, socio-economic status, and sex.

### Social impact of ageing population

Those >80 are the fastest growing age group in the UK. Currently, around a quarter of the population is >60 years old, but by 2030, this will rise to a third. Governments can encourage migration (economic migrants are mostly young) and extend working lives (e.g. ↑ pensionable age for women), but these will have little effect on the overall shift. The impact of this demographic shift on society's attitudes and economies is huge. Examples include:

- Financing pensions and health services—in most countries, these are financed on a 'pay-as-you-go' system, so they will have to be paid for by a smaller workforce. This will inevitably mean greater levels of taxation for those in work or a reduction in the state pension. Unless private pension investment (which works on an 'insurance' system of personal savings) improves, there is a risk that many pensioners will continue to live in relative poverty
- Healthcare and disability services—the prevalence and degree of disability ↑ with age. American Medicare calculations show that more than a quarter of healthcare expenditure is on the last year of a person's life, with half of that during the last 60 days
- Families are more likely to be supporting older members
- Retired people comprise a growing market and companies/industries that accommodate the needs/wishes of older people will flourish
- Transport, housing, and infrastructure must be built or adapted
- Political power of older people (the 'grey lobby' in America) will grow

## Successful versus unsuccessful ageing

How can success be defined, i.e. towards what aim should public health and clinical medicine be striving? The following definitions are, to some extent, stereotypical and culture-sensitive. More flexible definitions would acknowledge individual preferences.

- *Successful ageing*. Without overt disease, with good physical and cognitive function, a high level of independence, and active engagement with the broader society. Usually ended by a peaceful death without a prolonged dying phase
- *Unsuccessful ageing*. Accelerated by overt disease, leading to frailty, poor functional status, a high level of dependence, social and societal withdrawal, and a more prolonged dying phase where life quality may be judged unacceptable

## Further reading

Office for National Statistics. ℘ http://www.ons.gov.uk.

# Illness in older people

One of the paradoxes of medical care of the older person is that the frequency of some presentations ('off legs', delirium . . . ) and of some diagnoses (infection, dehydration . . . ) encourages the belief that medical management is straightforward and that investigation and treatment may satisfactorily be inexpensive and low-skilled (and thus intellectually unrewarding for the staff involved).

However, the objective reality is the reverse. Diagnosis is frequently more challenging, and the therapeutic pathway less clear and more littered with obstacles. However, choose the right path, and the results (both patient-centred and societal (costs of care, etc.)) are substantial.

## Features of illness in older people

- Present atypically and non-specifically
- Cause greater morbidity and mortality
- May progress much more rapidly—a few hours' delay in diagnosis of a septic syndrome is much more likely to be fatal
- Health, social, and financial sequelae. Failures of treatment may have long-term wide-ranging effects (e.g. nursing home fees >£900/week)
- Co-pathology is common. For example, in the older patient with pneumonia and recent atypical chest pain, make sure myocardial infarction (MI) is excluded (sepsis precipitates a hyperdynamic, hypercoagulable state, ↑ the risk of acute coronary syndromes; and a proportion of atypical pain is cardiac in origin)
- Lack of physiological reserve. If physiological function is 'borderline' (in terms of impacting lifestyle or precipitating symptoms), minor deterioration may lead to significant disability. Therefore, apparently minor improvements may disproportionately improve function. Identification and correction of several minor disorders may yield dramatic benefits

## Investigating older people

- Investigative procedures may be less well tolerated by older people. Thus, the investigative pathway is more complex, with decision-making dependent on clinical presentation, sensitivity and specificity of the test, side effects and discomfort of the test, hazards of 'blind' treatment or 'watchful waiting', and of course the wishes of the patient
- Consider the significance of positive results. Fever of unknown cause is a common presentation, and urinalysis a mandatory investigation. But what proportion of healthy community-dwelling older women have asymptomatic bacteriuria and a positive dipstick? (A: around 30%, depending on sample characteristics). Therefore, in what proportion of older people presenting with fever and a positive dipstick is urinary tract infection (UTI) the significant pathology? (A: much less than 100%)

The practical consequence of this is the under-diagnosis of non-urinary sepsis.

## Treating disease in older people

When treating disease in older people, they:

- May benefit more than younger people from 'invasive' treatments, e.g. percutaneous coronary intervention (PCI). On a superficial level, think 'which is more important—saving 10% of the left ventricle (LV) of a patient with an ejection fraction (EF) of 60% (perhaps a healthy 50-year-old) or of a patient with an EF of 30% (perhaps an 80-year-old with heart failure)?'. Note that the significant criterion here is more the left ventricular ejection fraction (LVEF) than the age, the principle being that infarcting a poor LV may cause long-term distress, morbidity, and mortality, whereas infarcting a part of a healthy myocardium may be without sequelae

- May benefit less than younger people. Life expectancy and the balance of risks and benefits must be considered in decision-making. For example, the priority is unlikely to be control of hypertension in a frail 95-year-old who is prone to falls

- May have more side effects to therapies. In coronary care, β-blockade, aspirin, angiotensin-converting enzyme (ACE) inhibitors, PCI, and heparin may all have a greater life (and quality-of-life)-saving effect in older patients. Studies show these agents are underused in MI patients of all ages, but much more so in the elderly population. The frequency of side effects (bradycardia and heart block, profound hypotension, renal impairment, and bleeding) is greater in older people, although a significant net benefit remains

- May respond to treatment less immediately. Convalescence is slower, and the doctor may not see the eventual outcome of his/her work (the patient having been transferred to rehabilitation, for example)

- The natural history of many acute illnesses is recovery independent of medical intervention, particularly in the young. Beware false attributions and denials of benefit:
  - The older person frequently benefits from therapy, unwitnessed by medical staff
  - The younger person recovers independent of medical efforts, though his/her recovery is falsely attributed to those interventions (by staff and patient)

# Chapter 2

# Organizing geriatric services

# Using geriatric services

Geriatric services are radically different from those developed around the inception of the specialty in the 1950s. Locally, services differ, dependent upon resources, organizational structures, and the drive and vision of local clinical leaders. There are some broader national differences within the UK, e.g. services in Scotland and Northern Ireland lean more towards rehabilitation and long-term care than those in England and Wales.

Services should be configured to deliver the best possible population benefit (patient-centred health and social care outcomes) and patient/carer experience, considering the sustainable financial and human resources. Careful attention must be given to vulnerable, difficult-to-access groups and to the optimal balance of *centralized care* (efficient, resilient, and leveraging high-capital elements such as computed tomography (CT)/magnetic resonance imaging (MRI) scanners) versus *distributed care* closer to home (improved patient experience, greater holism, lower capital costs, and a default enabling approach).

The following is intended as a generic guide, as provision is highly variable.

## Services for acute problems

Urgent assessment of the acutely unwell patient where the disease process is new, severe (e.g. acute MI, stroke, sepsis, delirium), and/or very rapidly progressive.

Service examples:
- 1° care (general practice (GP)) emergency assessment services (see ➐ 'Primary care', p. 44)
- Locality (community)-based emergency multidisciplinary assessment service
- Rapid access ('admission avoidance') services (see ➐ 'Admission avoidance schemes', pp. 20–1)
- Acute medicine assessment service
- Urgent domiciliary visits (DVs) (see ➐ 'HOW TO . . . Do a domiciliary visit', p. 31)
- Emergency departments (EDs; see ➐ 'Acute services for older people', pp. 16–7)

Choosing which is most appropriate will depend on patient clinical characteristics (e.g. if critically unstable, then an ambulance to the ED may be appropriate; if no change is expected imminently, then urgent outpatient assessment may be used), patient preference, local service characteristics (acceptable case mix, hours/days of operation), and operational issues (availability of urgent clinic appointments, transport, etc.). There has been a strong trend towards provision of services 'closer to home'—in 1° care or community health settings such as health centres and community hospitals (CHs), although the evidence of clinical and cost-effectiveness is not good.

### Services for subacute problems

Assessment of a patient with a progressive disease process (e.g. ↑ falls, complex Parkinson's disease), unexplained potentially serious problems (e.g. iron deficiency anaemia, weight loss), or a more refined diagnosis and management plan (e.g. cardiac failure).

Discrete ('single organ') problems can be assessed in more narrowly specialist clinics, less well-defined or 'multi-morbid' problems in a geriatric outpatients, and problems suggesting multidisciplinary need in the day hospital or by a domiciliary multidisciplinary team (MDT).

Local availability, waiting times, and consultant interests affect choice.

There is a strong national drive towards managing patients in an ambulatory (non-admitting) setting. Done well, this improves resource use, may reduce iatrogenic hospital-associated harm, and often improves patient experience.

Service examples:
- Geriatric medicine outpatient clinic
- Specialty clinic (see ➜ 'Specialty clinics', p. 24)
- Day hospital (see ➜ 'Day hospitals', pp. 22–3)
- Intermediate care (IC) facility (see ➜ 'Intermediate care', pp. 26–7)
- DV (see ➜ 'HOW TO . . . Do a domiciliary visit', p. 31)
- Elective (planned) admission (to acute hospital, rehabilitation wards, or CH) is now much less commonly considered appropriate, as the environment may be disabling, iatrogenic harm is common, and resource use disproportionate

### Services for chronic problems

This includes active elective management of slowly progressive conditions by 1° care teams (people aged over 75 in the UK should have a named general practitioner (GP)), community teams, specialist nurses, and 2° care physicians (see ➜ 'Chronic disease management', pp. 42–3) and the provision of care for established need.

Long-term care may be provided in a number of ways:
- Informal carers (see ➜ 'Informal carers', p. 38)
- Home care and care agencies (see ➜ 'Home care', pp. 36–7)
- Day centres (see ➜ 'Other services', p. 40)
- Respite care (in care homes or hospitals) (see Box 2.1)
- Care homes (see ➜ 'Care homes', pp. 32–3)

Allocation of these (usually) long-term services is generally after an assessment of need and financial status by a care manager.

With time, most patients pass through many aspects of the spectrum of geriatric care; a flexible, responsive set of services with good communication between providers is essential (see Fig. 2.1).

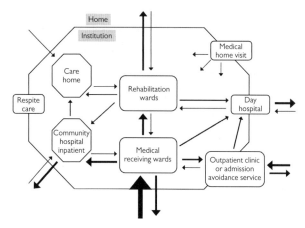

**Fig. 2.1** An example of possible patient flows within a complex system of care for older people.

# Acute services for older people

Since older people present atypically and are at high risk of serious sequelae of illness, high-quality acute services that fully meet their needs are essential. In any setting, older people have special needs and the consequences of not meeting them are amplified in the setting of acute illness. Specific areas meriting attention include the prevention and treatment of delirium, falls, and pressure sores; optimization of nutrition and hydration; and provision of an enabling, individualized setting that maximizes independence and well-being. Accurate, early, and comprehensive diagnosis(es) is (are) essential, alongside careful determination of goals that are valued by the patient and that are realistic.

An acutely unwell older person may present to one of several services, depending on:

• Local service provision
• The individual's understanding of the system
• Advice from others (e.g. relatives, health professionals, NHS 111)

Any service aiming to diagnose acute illness in older people must have access to immediate plain radiography, electrocardiography (ECG), and 'basic' blood tests (including prompt results, often facilitated by 'point of care' testing technology delivering results in non-laboratory settings in minutes). Access to complementary specialist clinical input (e.g. geriatrician, urologist, neurologist, etc.) is essential, through a range of mechanisms including face-to-face assessment, telephone advice, or telemedicine. Cross-sectional imaging (ultrasound, CT, MRI) must be available promptly, although it may be on another site.

## Emergency department (accident and emergency)

Common presentations include falls (with or without injury), 'fits and faints', and a broad range of acute surgical and medical problems traditionally referred directly by 1° care to specialist (non-ED) surgical or medical teams.

Direct presentation of such patients to the ED (rather than following initial assessment by 1° care teams known to the patient) has ↑, due to changes in 1° care services both in and out of hours, advice by agencies such as NHS 111, and changing public expectation and behaviour. Often the acute illness itself is not severe but occurs in the context of frailty, comorbidity, and social vulnerability, leading to reflex escalation of care and a brisk and direct channel to the ED.

The ED is potentially inhospitable and dangerous for older people. The environment may be cold, uncomfortable, disorientating, noisy, and lacking dignity and privacy. There is a risk of pressure sores, delirium, and avoidable immobility and falls. Provision and administration of food and fluid may be neglected or inappropriately prohibited on spurious medical grounds. A medical model of care may presume serious illness and restricted mobility (to allow invasive monitoring and treatments) can occur at the expense of a more holistic, individualized, and enabling approach. Staff are experts in emergency medical management, but their expertise in complexity, frailty, and holistic care is often less developed.

For those patients who do require urgent hospital assessment, there is ↑ focus on offering ambulance clinicians and 111 teams direct access to Acute Medicine, Geriatric Medicine, and other urgent care specialties; done well, this can deliver quicker, more effective care in a more age-appropriate environment. However, it is important that older patients who would benefit from ED capability—such as the critically unwell—are not excluded.

Deadlines and targets that minimize time spent in the ED (e.g. the 4-hour standard) generally benefit older ED users with limited physiological and functional reserve, for whom the best outcomes are often time-sensitive.

Strategies to optimize care for older people in the ED—that must be available for extended hours and 7 days a week—include:

- Close liaison with geriatric medical and nursing specialists
- Medical, nursing, and therapist rotation between ED and geriatric specialist settings
- Focus on optimizing food and fluid provision and pressure-relieving care
- Provision of alternative modes of admission and assessment, e.g. Rapid Access Clinic, direct admission to a geriatric ward
- Provision of specialist geriatric assessment units which may be embedded in or near the ED ('Acute Frailty Units')
- Occupational therapist (OT), physiotherapist (PT), and social worker with expertise in older people based in the ED

There are ↑ calls for the creation of discrete areas in the ED with an environment and clinical capability tailored to the needs of frail, complex patients. This development—akin to that of the 'Children's ED'—is hampered by constraints on human and capital resources and physical space; in practice, immediate pragmatic assessment and 'streaming' to more appropriate settings is a more sustainable and deliverable approach, particularly in smaller departments.

**Further reading**

British Geriatrics Society. *Quality care for older people with urgent and emergency care needs: 'Silver Book'.* ℅ http://www.bgs.org.uk/campaigns/silverb/silver_book_complete.pdf.

# The integration debate

There is a long-standing debate among UK geriatricians about the best model of care for older people in hospital. Historically, age-related care grew out of poor-quality workhouse facilities, and the advent of specialist care provided from mainstream hospital settings with equitable access to services was a major progressive step. Traditionally, care has been divided into either:

• *Age-related*. A separate team of admitting doctors to deal with all patients over a certain age (varies—commonly around 75 years) who then care for these patients on designated geriatric wards
• *Integrated*. In truly integrated care, specialists maintain additional generalist skills. These generalists admit all adult medical patients, regardless of age, and continue looking after them on 'general medical' wards, in parallel with specialist clinical commitments (see Table 2.1)

The debate has not been fuelled by high-quality evidence and has become less febrile as constraints—not least reduction in junior doctors' working hours—have made it less practical to run two entirely separate acute teams. As a result, a range of blended or 'hybrid' systems have been developed, managing patients pragmatically and delivering the best compromise of robust 24–7 generic acute services with selective, complementary specialist in-reach.

A common compromise is that there is integrated acute assessment, with a single admitting team, but rapid dispersal to the most appropriate service. This dispersal occurs at varying points in the patient pathway, depending on local service strengths and constraints. Models include triage of need ('function'-related segregation) by an appropriate person immediately after admission (admitting specialty registrar or consultant, experienced nurse, bed manager, etc.) and dispersal by a ward allocation system after removal from the admitting ward, or over a period of a few days (by inter-specialty referral) as special needs become apparent.

As individual systems evolve, the debate recedes and energies are invested into providing the best possible care for all patients through innovation and flexibility within a certain hospital structure, rather than in drawing boundaries and maintaining rigid definitions. Relentlessly, ↑ median age and the complexity of the inpatient population in most specialties are driving the development of systems that put in place a geriatric capability in *all* relevant settings, ideally integrated with that of the local 'organ or condition specialist' team (e.g. Oncology, Surgery, Neurology). Vigilance against ageism in these evolving systems remains essential.

**Table 2.1** Comparison of age-related and integrated care

*Age-related care*

| Advantages | Potential drawbacks |
| --- | --- |
| All old people seen by doctors with a special interest in their care | Possibility of a two-tier standard of medical care developing, with patients in geriatric medicine settings having lower priority and access to acute investigation and management facilities |
| All old people looked after on wards where there is an MDT | Less specialist knowledge in those doctors providing day-to-day care |
| Even apparently straightforward problems in older patients are likely to have social ramifications that are proactively managed | May be stigmatizing for all patients of a certain age to be defined as 'geriatric' |
| | May be less kudos and respect for geriatric medicine practitioners |

*Integrated care*

| Advantages | Potential drawbacks |
| --- | --- |
| As the majority of patients coming to the hospital are elderly, it maintains an appropriate skill base and joint responsibility for their care | Many generalists will not be skilled in the management of older patients, so those under their care may not fare as well |
| There is equal access to all acute investigative and maintenance facilities, as older patients are not labelled as a separate group | Specialist commitments are likely to take priority over the care of older patients |
| Trainees from all medical specialties will have exposure to, and training in, geriatric medicine assessment | The MDT input is harder to coordinate effectively where the patients are widely dispersed |
| Sharing of specialist knowledge is more collaborative and informal | Management of the social consequences of disease tends to be reactive (to crisis), rather than proactive |

# Admission avoidance schemes

Admission avoidance schemes (AAS) are variable in content and name. Schemes may be divided into those that do and those that do not offer specialist geriatric assessment (provided by a geriatrician, a GP with a special interest (GPSI), or a geriatric specialist nurse).

## Non-medically supported schemes

These may include emergency provision of carers, district nurse, OT, and PT, delivering prompt functional assessment and ↑ care after a fall, acute illness perceived as minor, or carer illness. As specialist medical assessment is not a part of the scheme, treatable illness may be missed. As a minimum, such schemes should incorporate assessments by capable healthcare professionals who can recognize the need for specialist geriatric assessment and can access such services promptly.

## Schemes with a medical assessment

- Variously titled Early Assessment, Rapid Assessment, Emergency or Rapid Access clinics
- All aim to provide a prompt response to medical needs in older people, with acuity falling somewhere between immediate admission and more elective outpatient services
- Some schemes provide same-day assessment; most assess within a day or at most a fortnight (the equivalent of cancer '2-week wait')
- There is an assumption that patients are midway between first symptoms and more severe disease, and that early intervention may prevent decline, permit less aggressive or invasive treatment, and reduce health service resource use (not least inpatient care)
- Services are best accessed via telephoned, faxed, or electronic referral, with prompt 'triage' by an experienced professional

There is a risk that acutely unwell older people who need emergency assessment or treatment are referred to AAS, rather than admitted immediately. If in doubt, arrange immediate assessment by the emergency medical/geriatric medicine team. Delirium is an example of a presentation where admission to hospital from home should be considered carefully, balancing the risks and benefits of both settings; neither setting is risk-free.

- In practice, most schemes admit a modest proportion of patients to hospital following assessment. In some cases, this two-stage pathway represents optimal care, but there is a risk of clinical harm if delay is material
- AAS staffing usually includes senior medical staff (± junior support). Experienced nursing assistance is invaluable; roles are variable but may be very advanced, to include history taking, physical and mental state examination, and prescribing

- Most commonly, AAS are housed in 'general' outpatient facilities. Examples of problems managed here include anaemia or breathlessness
- A more comprehensive geriatric response (see ➔ 'Comprehensive geriatric assessment', p. 68) is facilitated when the AAS is housed in, or adjacent to, outpatient multidisciplinary services, e.g. day hospital (DH)
- AAS should have prompt (ideally same-day) access to OT and PT services, to support the patient at home while the effect of medical interventions become apparent. Patients with complex needs are best managed in this environment, e.g. Parkinson's disease with on/off periods

Increasingly, driven by financial penalties, there is a focus on *readmission* avoidance. Services provide rapid access to specialist assessment and treatment in an ambulatory (non-admission) setting, following recent discharge.

# Complex day services/day hospitals

DHs provide a health intervention and a patient experience quite distinct from that of outpatient or inpatient care. Typically, patients receive an extended intervention (for a half or full day), during which there is a multi-factorial, multidisciplinary assessment and/or treatment.

DHs usually provide a mixture of new patient assessment, rehabilitation, and chronic disease management. Patients may be referred directly from the community, from other hospital outpatient services, or following an inpatient stay. Some units designate sessions for specific patient groups (e.g. movement disorder, admission avoidance).

The case mix and interventions vary widely between units but can include:

- Medical—new patient assessment, e.g. for falls, frailty, immobility, multi-morbidity
- Nursing, e.g. pressure sore, leg ulcer, or continence assessment and treatment
- Physiotherapy and/or occupational therapy, e.g. following stroke, fracture, surgery, or non-specific functional decline
- Diagnostics   facilities for blood tests (including point-of-care testing), urinalysis, ECG, radiology, 'tilt-testing'
- 'Drug' treatments, e.g. blood product transfusion, intravenous (iv) furosemide, iron infusion, levodopa monitoring

A flexible, tailored, holistic approach is usual. Many DH clients benefit from several elements in a 'one-stop-shop' approach.

Multidisciplinary teamwork, comprehensive geriatric assessment (see ➔ 'Comprehensive geriatric assessment', p. 68), and functional goal-setting are important tools.

## History and evolution

The first DHs began in the 1960s. With time, many units attracted a large number of long-term patients who were very frail but had little or no active health needs—the benefits were largely social (respite for carers and social interaction for patients). Unacceptably long waiting lists hindered efficient running in some units. Transport arrangements were often weak, with patients spending lengthy periods of time waiting for, or during, transport.

This monitoring and supportive role has now been largely taken over by day *centres* (see ➔ 'Other services', p. 40). Contemporary DHs have a much higher ratio of 'new to follow-up' patients and rapid patient turnover, and are supportive of the urgent care pathway, including acute admitting functions and the ED.

Strong drivers to ambulatory care have led to the introduction and expansion of 'rapid access' ('admission avoidance') clinics and early supported discharge schemes. These teams, vertically integrated across the hospital and home, often have a base in, or adjacent to, the DH.

## Cost-effectiveness

A number of studies have examined clinical and cost-effectiveness. While this area remains controversial, systematic reviews have shown that a multidisciplinary DH intervention results in less functional deterioration, institutionalization, and hospital admission than control groups receiving no care. However, DHs did not generally prove superior to other comprehensive care approaches such as domiciliary rehabilitation.

DH care is costly, but this is offset by ↓ inpatient bed usage, institutionalization, and home care costs. Insightful clinical leadership with careful 'prescription' of DH intervention is essential in ensuring that the DH team delivers the greatest possible population benefit.

# Specialty clinics

Every region configures resources in different ways, reflecting the local context. All have a portfolio of specialist clinics, supporting the care of patients with a range (narrow or broad) of symptoms or conditions (e.g. Parkinson's disease, falls/syncope, chest pain). Pathways and resources should be configured in a way that optimizes available resources to deliver the best outcomes, including patient experience, with consideration of the need to provide a responsive (sometimes 7-day) service.

The portfolio of clinics for older people may be delivered by geriatricians, by other specialists, or sometimes jointly. Advantages of specialty clinics include:

• Optimized referral protocol and access
• Concentration of expertise
• Improved training quality for juniors
• Specialist nursing and therapy staff
• ↑ patient education and awareness of the condition—through meeting others with the same diagnosis, the work of specialist nurses, and the availability of dedicated information
• Supporting parallel scheduling of relevant diagnostic investigations (e.g. carotid Doppler ultrasound or magnetic resonance angiogram in transient ischaemic attack (TIA) clinics)
• Supporting improved quality through use of agreed care pathways and protocols

Where the same clinic is offered by differing specialties, or where you are unsure if referral to a geriatrician or an 'organ specialist' is the most appropriate, ask the following:

• *Is this a new or urgent problem?* An ↑ number of clinics have a protocol-defined maximum wait for urgent assessment. This may support admission avoidance and effective outpatient management of many conditions (e.g. TIA, chest pain, possible malignancy) but are prone to being overwhelmed with referrals, thereby rendering them less responsive to the needs of truly urgent cases. Non-urgent cases should be referred to routine clinics
• *How well defined is the diagnosis?* A patient with 'cardiac-sounding' chest pain without extensive comorbidity is likely to benefit from a specialist cardiology-delivered service, giving rapid access to the appropriate expertise and investigations. If the source of the pain is less clear, then the patient may be more effectively managed in a generalist clinic (general or geriatric medicine) where multiple options can be considered and explored in parallel
• *Does the patient have a single dominant problem?* If so, then they are likely to benefit from a focused clinic delivered by a narrowly specialist team. If, however, co-morbidities and/or frailty are prominent, then a geriatric clinic is likely to deliver a more comprehensive, holistic, patient-centred assessment and care plan
• *Is this patient already attending a geriatric clinic for follow-up?* If so, most new problems can be addressed by that team, rather than referring to another specialty

# Intermediate care

IC is a generic term referring to a spectrum of services lying between acute hospital inpatient care and 'usual' (unenhanced) 1° care, aiming 'to promote faster recovery from illness, prevent unnecessary acute hospital admission and premature admission to long-term residential care, support timely discharge from hospital, and maximize independent living'.

The term came into widespread use in 2001 as a key element of the UK National Service Framework for older people. Generally, these services were designed to deliver a time-limited, enabling intervention outside hospital. Many were refashioned from existing services and re-branded, but some approaches have been genuinely progressive and innovative and have a strengthening evidence base.

Many geriatricians welcome the emphasis on non-hospital-based care for older people, but others have warned against IC as a vehicle for covert ageist care that allows rationing of acute hospital medicine, substituting less expensive, and perhaps less effective, care.

The emphasis is often not primarily medical, but multidisciplinary and holistic. There are two main bodies of patients:
• 'Step-down' (following admission) care. Following acute admission or planned intervention such as major surgery. For those requiring rehabilitation, reablement, and/or reassessment of care needs in a non-acute setting
• 'Step-up' (admission avoidance) care. For patients at home who require enhanced assessment and treatment following functional deterioration or acute illness. The aim is to minimize functional decline and/or to avoid a hospital stay

Provision has developed locally; models of staffing, facilities, ethos, and access are heterogeneous. Some services concentrate on very specific groups (e.g. 'post-surgical hip fracture in older people'); others are more generic. Most regions have a set of complementary services organized according to geographic and/or clinical rationales.

IC occurs in a range of environments, e.g.:
• The patient's own home (the most common arrangement)
• CH
• Care homes, usually 'care homes with nursing'
• DH (in acute or CH)
• Other community facilities, e.g. day centre

Interventions are often based around a comprehensive geriatric assessment (CGA) (see ➲ 'Comprehensive geriatric assessment (CGA)', p. 68) by an MDT, including appropriate medical support. More focused services may lack important team members (e.g. medical, social work); in those services, care is needed that important interventions (such as treatable illness or unclaimed benefits) are not overlooked.

The variety of different models and quantum of provision results in inequity of access across territories. Research into the clinical and cost-effectiveness of IC is sparse and at times contradictory; the general conclusions are that there are sometimes cost benefits, compared to more traditional 'hospital-centric' approaches, but that these benefits are often marginal; some studies showed ↑ 'whole system' costs. Patient experience is more often a beneficiary. The UK National Audit of Intermediate Care continually identifies weaknesses in governance, the breadth of clinician support, and the quantum of provision at a population level.

Examples of popular approaches include:

- *Crisis care*. Rapid response to 'social care failure' in the home, often following unforeseen carer illness. Carers support the client at home, preventing 'social admission' to hospital
- *Hospital-at-home*. Intensive nursing, medical, and/or therapy input at home delivers effective treatment without hospital admission, or following hospital admission, to minimize length of stay
- *'Rapid response' or 'supported discharge' teams*. Sometimes vertically integrated, providing inputs to hospital and home. The 'front door' intervention is across accident and emergency (A&E) and acute assessment areas, providing a rapid holistic assessment of needs to support immediate enabling home care ('discharge to assess'); domiciliary teams pick up care promptly following hospital assessment or else respond to a patient with an urgent need at home ('assess to determine need for admission'). These approaches contrast with the traditional 'assess to (= before) discharge' and 'admit to assess', which lead to unnecessary hospital care
- *Reablement at home*. A team of trained carers, acting under the supervision of a therapist team, deliver a prescribed enabling care package. Usually a time-limited intervention, with specified functional goals, aiming to reduce long-term social care needs and institutionalization
- *Early supported discharge*. A term most commonly applied to multidisciplinary rehabilitation following a stroke. Evidence for effect is good.
- *'Care home plus'*. 24–7 support in a care home, with additional clinician support from PT, OT, and the care manager. May have specialist medical input beyond that of the home's 'retained' GP

In hospital, *discharge coordination teams* (often comprising nurses experienced in the care of older people and who understand complex care pathways) have an important role in bridging the gap between often complex and disintegrated hospital and community-based services.

# Community hospitals

CHs vary substantially in size, clinical focus, and facilities. Some deliver a substantial contemporary clinical function that supports effective care of older people closer to home. Others have much more limited capability and may not meet contemporary patient needs.

Their origins were commonly as small 'cottage' hospitals, providing very limited services from buildings dating from the first half of the twentieth century. This century, some have undergone substantial change, with reinvention as decentralized foci of inpatient, outpatient, and increasingly day (diagnostic or therapeutic) care.

Often there is substantial community support, both emotional and tangible (volunteers, gifts, legacies). This makes service changes politically sensitive, slow, and difficult, if it is possible at all. In some cases, CH facilities are in desperate need of reconfiguration to reflect current patient needs. Emotive, unevidenced preservation of traditional arrangements risks patient care.

Facilities may include:
- Inpatient beds for between 10 and 60 patients
- PT, OT, and other therapy services (in- and outpatient)
- DH for urgent or planned intervention
- Office/professional base for community-based health and social care
- Outpatient facilities for medical and surgical clinics
- Psychogeriatric services; outpatient and/or inpatient
- Minor injuries unit—often staffed by nurse specialists
- Maternity services—midwife office base ± maternity beds
- Often a GP practice is based on site or close by, with mutual benefits
- GP out-of-hours service base
- Diagnostic testing, e.g. near-patient blood tests, plain radiography. More complex tests (e.g. CT, ultrasound, endoscopy) usually require transport to another hospital, although the most modern facilities may include them
- Local health (e.g. Clinical Commissioning Group (CCG) locality) management base

*Medical cover.* The traditional 'cottage hospital' approach was to admit patients on their own practice list and to visit reactively when called. More contemporary models employ dedicated specialist clinicians (GPSIs, geriatricians, or nurse consultants) to deliver proactive care. Visits should be both regular—identifying potential problems and planning prospectively—and highly responsive to acute problems identified by nursing staff.

*Specialist geriatric medical input* must be available when the need is identified. Other specialists, e.g. surgeons or neurologists, may hold outpatient clinics on site.

*Nurses and therapists* are often very experienced in the care of older people and are able and willing to work more independently from doctors. Nursing staff often lead the discharge planning process, including MDT meetings. Staff turnover is often low, with a high proportion of committed long-term staff.

## Community hospital admissions

Groups of patients being admitted include the following.

### Rehabilitation and discharge planning

Often transferred from acute hospitals following surgery (elective or emergency) or acute medical problems. Timing of transfer must be appropriate—is the patient medically stable? Have relevant investigations been completed? Are ceilings of care clear?

### Palliative care

Where the nature of illness is clear, and cure is not possible, CHs can provide high-quality care and symptom control when things can no longer be managed effectively in the patient's home. A CH setting is preferable to an acute hospital admission. Hospice beds are often limited and focus on those in whom symptom control is especially difficult.

### Acute illness or functional decline

- 'Step-up' (acute) admissions to CHs must be considered carefully, based on local CH capability to offer effective diagnosis and treatment of what may be concealed or an atypical acute severe disease
- Admission to a CH is more likely to be justified in cases of strong informed patient preference, where the diagnosis is clearer, where invasive treatments and advanced monitoring are unlikely to be required, or when logistics dictate (e.g. very long distances). CHs with more advanced clinical capability can accept a more extensive 'step-up' case mix
- Admission may also be appropriate after specialist assessment in a rapid access clinic, DV, or frailty unit
- After accurate diagnosis and completion of invasive (e.g. iv) treatments, transfer to a CH becomes appropriate

### 'Social' admissions

Where staff perceive that the precipitant to admission has been a change in social supports (e.g. death or illness of a carer), not the condition of the patient. These patients are often very frail; high death rates in such admissions have been reported. Beware covert medical factors driving admission—seek and address them proactively.

### Respite care

Usually now performed out of hospital, in care homes. Some especially complex or emergency/unplanned respite care may occur.

## Effectiveness/cost-effectiveness

As with other forms of IC, there is little evidence that CHs provide improved outcomes or cheaper care than alternative systems. Much depends on local arrangements (scale, co-location, integration), governance and leadership arrangements, and the enthusiasm and innovation of local teams striving to deliver the best possible individualized care from available resources.

# Domiciliary (home) visits

A medical assessment in the home, usually by an experienced geriatrician or, in some cases, a consultant nurse. This involves visiting the home of the ill person, sometimes alone, but perhaps with a GP, therapist, nurse, or care manager. Distinguish this 'medical' home visit from the home assessment visit performed by an OT to determine functional capacity and the needs for aids/adaptations.

Historically, DVs were widely used to prioritize patients on the waiting list for admission to hospital, but with the disappearance of such lists for acute medical problems, this is now rarely done.

There are advantages and disadvantages. The disadvantages—and an appreciation of how much elderly people benefit from selective use of modern acute hospital facilities—led to a substantial reduction in the number of visits performed. In many regions, their use atrophied to focus predominantly on those who refused to attend hospital and who appeared seriously or terminally ill.

The frequency of home visits is now ↑ again, as 'care closer to home' strategies intensify. DVs by geriatricians now often occur, whilst working within community-based MDTs supporting admission avoidance or early supported discharge.

### Disadvantages

- Lack of equipment and other hospital facilities
- Lack of nursing support (chaperone, lifting/handling during clinical examination)
- A limited portfolio of tests, although the repertoire is ↑ (e.g. point-of-care haematology and biochemistry technology delivers results in minutes from a device the size of a desk phone)
- An inefficient use of time—as well as travelling time, patients and family often expect longer discussions and they effectively control the duration of the consultation
- Difficulty in coordinating synchronous multidisciplinary assessment, treatment, or discussion

### Advantages

- Brings 'care to the patient' with generally better patient experience
- Function may be rapidly and effectively assessed, e.g. is there evidence of incontinence, is the larder stocked, is the dwelling acceptably clean, what degree of mobility is achieved (through, e.g. 'furniture walking'), are there appropriate aids and adaptations?
- Assessment of mental state may be more accurate in the patient's home
- Assessment of drug compliance (see ➲ 'HOW TO . . . Improve concordance', p. 130)
- Patients appear more frail and vulnerable in a hospital setting and are usually less functionally capable in an unadapted, impersonal setting
- Some patients adamantly refuse hospital assessment. The experience of the visit itself may persuade a reluctant patient to be admitted

- Provides a second opinion for the community care team, which may be struggling to diagnose or treat, or needs reassurance that it is doing all that is possible
- Provides effective learning for predominantly 'hospital-based' clinicians about the imperfect correlation between function assessed in hospital versus the home

---

### HOW TO . . . Do a domiciliary visit

*When?*
- Combine with other trips, if possible
- Not too early or late (patient may rise late and settle early)

*Will you and your property be safe?*
- Danger from patient, relatives/carers, neighbours?
- Tell someone where you are going and when you should be back

*What do you need to know before you go?*
- Name, address, directions (especially in rural areas), satnav
- Do you have a referral letter?
- Review and take any previous medical notes
- Can the patient's family or carer attend? (One or two is useful— discourage excessive numbers of family members)
- Will the patient be in? Telephone in advance, including just before you set off

*What to take?*
- Blood pressure (BP) cuff, stethoscope, tendon hammer, auroscope, ophthalmoscope, 'PR tray' (jelly, gloves, wipes), urinalysis sticks, phlebotomy
- Scoring charts, e.g. the Abbreviated Mental Test Score (AMTS), Barthel, Geriatric Depression Scale (GDS)
- Paper and pen, dictation device

*What will you do?*
- History, examination
- Functional assessment
- Environmental inspection
- Medication (check the drug cabinet or top drawer for over-the-counter and prescription drugs)
- Accepting a cup of tea will inform in several areas!
- Discuss your findings and plan with the patient and family

*What to do afterwards*
- Telephone or email the GP to report findings and discuss plans
- Dictate a letter, copy to the GP and hospital notes

# Care homes

The care home sector is developing rapidly, with changes driven by:
- ↑ in numbers of severely co-morbid older people
- Reduced numbers of informal carers
- Care home legislation, improved mandatory standards, and systematic inspections by the Care Quality Commission (CQC)
- Economics:
  - Many smaller homes have proportionately higher per capita costs, both revenue (salary) and capital (buildings) costs
  - Reductions in social services funding

Until recently, there was a clear division between 'residential homes' (providing hotel-style services and basic personal care) and 'nursing homes' (providing full care to very dependent, often bed-bound patients). This distinction was always arbitrary, and as patients' care needs fluctuated or ↑ with time, they could find themselves inappropriately housed. There is a trend to larger establishments, often in modern, purpose-built accommodation, which provide services for a wider range of dependencies under the generic term 'care homes'.

## Staffing

Most of the care provided in care homes is by staff with limited training, who nonetheless may have extensive experience. In 'care homes with nursing', a trained nurse has to be available on site at all times.

The quality of care is a key factor for clients and their relatives in selecting a home. Care quality is variable, often independent of the quality of the physical fabric of the home, and is difficult to judge. Observations that are useful include the subjective well-being of residents, the extent to which they are cared for outside their rooms, the attitude of staff during routine interactions with residents and their response to calls for assistance, the provision of food, drink, and call bells close to residents, and the reports of patients and family.

Regrettably, high-profile cases illustrate how poorly managed and monitored homes can harbour a very small proportion of staff ranging from uncaring to criminal in their interactions with residents. Continual vigilance by professionals helps identify such cases early.

## Care home medicine

Medical care is usually provided by one or more GPs from a local 'retained' practice (clients are rarely able to keep their own GP), who may be in receipt of an enhanced service contract. Some community geriatricians routinely visit care homes to provide focused support and education; other areas have dedicated in-reaching MDTs. Attention should be paid to optimizing medication, maximizing preventive interventions (e.g. 'flu, falls), and advance care planning (e.g. decisions about future hospitalization, regional 'do not attempt cardiopulmonary resuscitation' (DNACPR) forms). Telemedicine and other advanced clinical support can reduce inappropriate A&E attendances or admissions, particularly outside routine 1° care hours.

**HOW TO . . . Advise a patient about care home placement**

This task is of great importance; there are implications for the patient's independence, quality of life, and finances. Ensure that the patient has a full assessment (ideally CGA; see ➋ 'Comprehensive geriatric assessment', p. 68) at a point of maximized health and functioning and, if indicated, an adequate trial of rehabilitation.

It is unwise to make recommendations based on only your own or family's impression—an OT's or social worker's perspective is complementary. Consider the prognosis and likely functional trajectory.

Some patients (often with normal cognition, living alone) may choose to go into care and are grateful for help with arrangements. They often describe loneliness or fear. If they are functionally independent, ensure that sheltered housing, day centres, or befriending have been considered as alternatives.

Most patients resist care home placement because of:
• Negative 'workhouse' preconceptions
• Emotional attachment to neighbours, spouse, home, pets
• A fear of loss of independence and dignity
• Anxiety over costs and loss of the family's inheritance for family
• Stigmatization and perception that they have failed

Patients with dementia may lack insight into their care needs (see ➋ 'HOW TO . . . Manage a patient insisting on returning home against advice', p. 662). Many of the principles of 'breaking bad news' apply, e.g. 'warning shots' prepare the patient. Explain what factors make it advisable to consider residential care and why other options are not feasible—use factual examples (e.g. you need help during the night and we cannot provide this at home). Clarify the contribution that other professionals have made to this assessment. The following positive points can be persuasive:
• By actively choosing a care home, they are more likely to get one they like. Leaving it until an emergency may remove choice
• Placements are often on a trial basis initially
• Emphasize the positive—company, hot meals, less family anxiety
• Where placement is from home and is not urgent, then a trial stay/ respite period of a week or two can sometimes be arranged
• Reassure there will be help with financial/logistical arrangements
• Some care homes allow well-behaved pets

## Care homes for people with dementia

Elderly mentally infirm (EMI) homes are registered to take patients with significant dementia with behaviour problems such as aggression, antisocial behaviour, or 'wandering'. These homes are in particularly short supply. They have specially trained staff and secure entrances/exits. Some ordinary homes are not registered to take patients with a diagnosis of dementia and decline to do so, although many patients in ordinary homes will have a degree of cognitive impairment.

## Further reading

Age UK. *Care homes.* ✎ http://www.ageuk.org.uk/home-and-care/care-homes/.

# Paying for residential care

- The cost of care in a care home ranges from around £500 to over £1500 a week, depending on client dependency, local costs (e.g. house prices, staff availability), and the quality and variety of facilities provided. Social care 'block contracts' pay homes far less than individual private payers
- Contributions by social services are means-tested and calculated on a sliding scale, dependent upon income and capital (savings and investments, including the home, unless it is occupied by someone else, e.g. a spouse)
- 'NHS Continuing Health Care' is a complete package of ongoing care arranged and funded by the National Health Service (NHS), for people with particularly extensive care needs (intense, complex, and/or unpredictable). Only a small minority of people entering care homes meet the current criteria. Assessment is first by a screening tool, followed by a more extensive assessment by a health professional if the initial screening criteria are met. The provision of continuing care has been inconsistent between health authorities, and the determination of funding is often a process that is challenged by patients or their advocates
- If a nursing home is needed and Continuing Health Care funding criteria are not met, then the NHS (CCG) should pay a sum for nursing care, direct to the care home. This was formerly known as the Registered Nursing Care Contribution (RNCC) and is not means-tested
- Funding issues are addressed by a care manager (usually a social worker; see ➲ 'Social work and care management', p. 96)

For extensive guidance and current information, see: ℅ http://www.ageuk.org.uk/home-and-care/.

### Delayed discharge

While some patients are admitted directly from their home to a care home in a planned move, the majority are admitted following an acute illness. This often occurs via a hospital setting (e.g. a patient who has a major stroke, or a pneumonia on a background of frailty and who does not regain sufficient function to return home after rehabilitation).

Where patients remain in NHS hospitals after they no longer require hospital treatment while awaiting care home beds or for other reasons (such as rehousing or while waiting for home care), they are referred to as being subject to a 'delayed transfer of care (DToC)'. Sometimes the term 'bed blocker' is used, but this is pejorative and stigmatizing—most delayed patients are desperate to leave hospital and cannot because sufficient care 'downstream' of hospital is not available.

Such delays cost hospital services millions of pounds a year and reduce the availability of hospital beds for patients with urgent care needs. Delays in placement are due to one or more of the following:

- Shortage in care home places, especially for EMI homes. Availability varies according to region and generally stems from financial and staffing shortfalls
- Pressurized care systems may prioritize urgent cases from home over patients in hospital (a relative 'place of safety')
- Social services that are short of cash may limit the number of new care home places they fund
- Patients/relatives may oppose discharge because they are unwilling to accept that there is no further prospect of meaningful functional recovery
- Patients/relatives may be reluctant to move from free NHS care to means-tested social care because of financial implications
- Delays in financial or other assessments, e.g. for Continuing Health Care funding

### Role of doctors caring for delayed discharge patients

- Ensure that it is clear to everyone (including the patient and relatives) that the patient no longer requires acute hospital care. Explain the supports available outside the acute hospital. Record 'medically ready for discharge' in the notes. Document follow-up arrangements for outstanding problems
- Continue medical monitoring, but switch to a more holistic, less intensive 'care home medicine' approach. Remember, however, that people living with frailty are highly prone to new or recurrent illnesses, not least hospital-acquired infections. Continue to promote enabling care, and be vigilant for complications such as deep vein thrombosis (DVT), pressure sores, dehydration, or poor nutrition
- Actively drive discharge—continual communication is crucial—with the health and social care MDTs, patient, carers, and other stakeholders. Pick up the phone if relatives do not visit during 'doctor hours'. A walk through the ward in the late afternoon provides opportunities to update relatives and address questions or concerns
- Consider interim options while continuing to plan. For example, the patient may be able to move to an IC facility such as a CH or a 'transitional' bed in a private care home arranged by social services

# Home care

In most countries, the majority of people needing personal care remain at home, rather than moving into an institution (e.g. care home). Their needs are provided by a carer who may be a family member, informal carers, or professional carers (self-employed or employed by a private care agency or public body). In the UK, the care needs of a patient are often specified by a care manager (social services) and then delivered by care agencies operating independently, mostly as private companies, but some with a 'not-for-profit' structure (e.g. social enterprise).

## Needs assessment

In England, this is the process whereby a care manager determines the needs of a person and how they can be met. Assessing needs requires information from the patient and others, often including the relatives, OT, PT, and nurse. Meeting those needs requires agreement between the care manager and the client (patient, or next-of-kin/legal representative if the patient lacks capacity) after considering the options, and financial and other resources (e.g. accommodation).

### Delivery of care

- The bulk of care is delivered by care assistants, who should have training in delivering personal care and lifting/handling
- In specific cases, they may be trained further to deliver care that is more complex, e.g. bowel care, thickening oral fluids, percutaneous endoscopic gastrostomy (PEG) care
- Carers perform important supervision of patients and are often the first to note the possibility of illness

Continuity of care is an important contributor to quality. There is a risk of physical, emotional, or financial abuse by carers (see ➜ 'Elder abuse', p. 674); although this is prominent in the media, such cases are relatively uncommon—most carers are hugely committed to providing the best possible care in often clinically challenging and resource-constrained circumstances.

In the UK, there is a national shortage of carers, worse in some geographical areas. This can delay discharge for days or weeks. It also renders existing care packages vulnerable to unexpected carer absence, e.g. due to sickness. Care packages provided by larger organizations tend to be more robust than those provided by a single small provider operating in isolation.

### Tasks routinely performed by carers

- Washing, bathing, dressing
- Safe moving and handling, including hoists
- Feeding, meal preparation, and housework
- Supervision of self-medication from a monitored dosing system
- Emptying of urinary catheter, fitting of penile sheath catheter
- Bowel care if trained

### Tasks not usually performed by carers

- Dressings
- Administration of medications from individual containers
- Insulin injections
- PEG feeding

## Home care costs

- In the UK, state support for care fees is 'means-tested'—a financial assessment is performed by the care manager. In general, only those with no significant savings have care costs met by the state
- Purchasing personal care is expensive. In the UK, care costs about £15 per hour (but much more in expensive areas). A care package of a total of 2h daily would therefore cost around £210 per week—less expensive than a care home, but a major financial burden for those who meet the fees themselves

*Structuring the care package*

- *Tailor to the individual.* A package usually consists of between one and four visits per day, by one or two carers. A common pattern is for two visits daily, one early (wash, dress, toilet, food preparation) and one late (evening meal, ready for bed). Lunch may consist of a pre-prepared meal, frozen and simply reheated by the patient, removing the need for a midday visit. Two carers are needed for 'double-handed care', e.g. turning or transferring a dependent patient
- *Night-time visits* are rarely needed and difficult to provide reliably. Roles may include toileting, pressure care (turns), or administering medication, but there may be other solutions (e.g. other continence management, changing medication regimens)
- *Continuous ('24h') care* is sometimes requested by patients or the family but is difficult and expensive to provide—sufficient staff are difficult to find, and the care is very expensive; a move into a care home is usually cheaper. Therefore, these packages are usually privately funded. Live-in carers are sometimes employed long-term but cannot be on hand the whole 24h, need holidays, and may go sick unpredictably
- *Access* to the home by carers can be difficult if the patient is immobile and cannot get to the door. Combination locks or a 'key safe' (conventional key locked within a small combination—or key-accessed safe) provide a secure solution
- *Equipment* is often necessary before a patient can be discharged and a care package initiated, e.g. hoist, bed, chair, cushion. OTs usually assess the needs and provide

## Commonly reported problems with care packages

- Timing—unpredictable, too early or late (e.g. 7 p.m. 'bedtime' visit)
- Carers—variable quality, lack of continuity
- Cost—often a significant issue. Discourages some patients from taking an adequate (or any) care package and may result in it being stopped after a period
- Visits—may be brief; carer and patient feel rushed

The CQC ( http://www.cqc.org.uk) inspects and deals with complaints about social care providers. National minimum standards must be met if a care agency is to gain and retain a licence.

# Informal carers

This term describes anyone who provides regular and substantive care to a person on a non-professional basis, usually without financial reward. This is often a family member but may be a friend or neighbour.

• One in ten adults are currently providing informal care in the UK
• A total of 7 million people acted as carers in 2016, projected to rise to over 10 million by 2030
• The carer's allowance in England is worth £62.10 per week, for an average of 35h caring—just £1.77/h (2017)
• Ten per cent of the >80s are carers, the majority providing over 60h of care per week
• The health of carers themselves is often poor—65% of older carers have long-term health problems and nearly 70% say that being a carer has an adverse effect on their mental health

This vital group of people support many older adults at home; the scale of support provided is often under-recognized. For many people, the support of informal carer(s)—often in addition to formal care—makes the difference between enforced institutionalization and remaining in their own home. For example, a mobile patient with cognitive problems may require constant supervision to ensure safety—a level of care that can only be provided by an informal live-in carer (often a spouse). This level of continuous supervision will often exceed that which can be provided in a care home, leading to dissatisfaction when patients are temporarily or permanently admitted to institutional care.

The importance of carers is recognized in a series of government and non-governmental papers and initiatives, which aim to improve information and support to carers and improve the care they themselves receive. This includes the right of a carer to a 'carer's assessment', carried out by social services, which addresses the following points:

• Is the carer getting enough sleep?
• Is the carer in good health?
• Does the carer have time for themselves?
• Are relationships adversely affected by the care-giving?
• Are there concerns about work?
• Is the carer collecting all available benefits?
• Is all available help being provided (services include emotional support, help with household and caring tasks, accessing benefits and local activities, arranging respite care—see Box 2.1)

The informal carer's role can be relentless, unrewarding, solitary, and depressing. Elder abuse is a rare, but possible, consequence (see ➔ 'Elder abuse', p. 674). Support—both proactive and reactive—is essential.

As well as government resources, a number of charity and self-help organizations provide tangible and intangible support.

• Carers UK: ℘ http://www.carersuk.org
• Princess Royal Trust for Carers: ℘ http://www.carers.org
• Crossroads: ℘ http://www.crossroadscare-sc.org
• The Children's Society: ℘ http://www.youngcarer.com/

## Box 2.1 Respite care

Being a carer is often exhausting, both physically and mentally, and often the patient finds accepting extensive help from a loved one difficult.

A successful care package must be sustainable, which includes proactive consideration of periods of relief for the carer(s). Some of the charities listed above (e.g. Crossroads) will offer a carer support worker to take over the caring role for a few hours at a time, but a longer break may be needed.

In such situations, respite care in a residential setting may provide the solution. Many care homes are able to provide flexible respite care packages. These can range from a stay of one or more weeks (e.g. to cover a holiday) to day care or an overnight stay. A regular arrangement can be made, e.g. one week in every eight may be spent in residential care.

Most local authorities operate a discretionary policy when considering funding for respite care in care homes; several weeks a year of respite may be funded if it sustains a home care arrangement where an informal carer is providing intensive support. This is means-tested.

Respite care provision in NHS settings is now very rare. Patients with challenging psychiatric needs will sometimes receive respite care on psychogeriatric wards. Terminal care patients will often be offered respite care in hospices or, less commonly, in CH wards. These services are free to the patient.

# Other services

### Day centres

Day centres differ from DHs (see Table 2.2). Attendance is often longer term and cognitive impairment is more common.

- Traditionally commissioned and provided by social services (sometimes jointly with health services). Now increasingly run by 'not-for-profit' (e.g. British Red Cross, Age UK)
- Accessed via social services (who assess needs) or by self-referral
- Offer regular attendance (e.g. once or twice weekly), with transport if needed
- There is a charge that is likely to be means-tested and varies with provision (e.g. transport, meals)
- Vary enormously but may include:
  - Catering (e.g. coffee, tea, and lunch)
  - Social support network
  - Personal care (e.g. bathing facilities, hairdressing, etc.)
  - Respite for carers
  - Skills development (arts and crafts, adult learning classes)
  - Access to health services (e.g. podiatry, district nurse)
  - Leisure activities (e.g. quizzes, reminiscence, music, gardening, keep fit, trips out)
  - Enables monitoring of progressive conditions (e.g. dementia) and early referral for extra support to prevent crisis
  - Rehabilitation and independent living skills (may occasionally have OT, PT, and speech and language therapy (or therapist) (SALT) input)

### Social clubs

Many different types that vary from county to county. Usually run by voluntary organizations. Information on locally available clubs can be obtained from libraries, the local county council, or Age UK. They include:

- Lunch clubs (often with transport)
- Bingo clubs
- Tea dances
- Keep fit groups
- Special interest groups (e.g. all ♂, all ♀, ethnic groups, hobby groups—gardening, model railways, etc.)

### Befriending

Scheme run primarily by third-sector organizations, e.g. Age UK, providing lonely, isolated older people with a regular volunteer visitor who will sit and chat and help with minor jobs such as fetching library books, etc.

### Pet schemes

Volunteers bring pets to visit people who can no longer keep them, e.g. in care homes.

### Holiday support

Voluntary organizations can provide information on suitable holidays for the disabled, and some will offer financial assistance.

**Table 2.2** Differences between DHs and day centres

|  | DH | Day centre |
|---|---|---|
| Medical input | Yes—patients often clinically unstable | No—medically stable clients |
| Attendance | Usually short term | Longer term |
| Staff:patient ratio | Higher | Lower |
| Functional aim | Greater independence | Usually maintenance and monitoring |
| Activities | Health/rehabilitation bias | Social/well-being bias |
| Relationship with hospital services | Close | More distant |
| Role | Complex geriatric assessment and treatment | Patient support and well-being |
|  | Rehabilitation | Carer relief |

# Chronic disease management

- Around 60% of the adult population has a chronic ('long-term') condition (commonly asthma, diabetes, hypertension, and cardiac failure); older people make up most of this group
- Multiple chronic diseases lead to increasingly complex healthcare needs and provision and are a particular phenomenon among elderly people, who become increasingly frail as chronic problems accumulate and progress
- Most needs are managed in 1° care, although in 2° care, the 10% of the population who have high-level chronic disease account for over 50% of inpatient bed days

There has been a shift in emphasis away from a reactive acute sector response towards the proactive management of chronic disease. Lessons have been learned from 'managed care organizations' in the USA (such as Kaiser Permanente in California) where comprehensive healthcare is provided to a defined population by a single 'unified' provider; there are then built-in incentives to actively manage chronic disease, as this may reduce acute (and total) expenditure.

Severity of chronic disease can be summarized as follows:

- *Level 1*—70–80% of patients who have a single chronic disease (e.g. hypertension). Management is enhanced by ↑ personal responsibility for the condition with education and encouraging active participation in care. Patient experts are developed who take on some of the education of their peers
- *Level 2*—more complex patients, but still with commonly recognized complications of disease (e.g. Parkinson's disease). Management is at a population level, with broad guidelines for care, protocols, and patient pathways. The approach is multidisciplinary with innovative delivery of a standard care set (email, telephone, group meetings, nurse clinics, etc.)
- *Level 3*—highly complex patients with individual needs (e.g. frail elderly patient with multiple interacting pathologies). Active case management by a key worker (often a nurse) promotes early intervention to prevent crisis and facilitates joined-up care

In coordinated proactive care, a competent lead clinician (often a specialist nurse) supports the identification of needs, comprehensive initial assessment, engagement of complementary functions (e.g. social services, voluntary groups, condition-specific teams), creation of a proactive care plan, and communication of that plan to key people/teams (patient, carers, ambulance service, community and acute teams).

The management of older patients who are frail is at the most challenging end of the spectrum of chronic disease management; guidelines and protocols are of less value than insightful, holistic, experienced clinicians who can work flexibly to deliver outcomes important to the individual.

The following are useful ways of managing these patients:
- 'Frailty registers' to identify and risk-stratify patients
- Use of information systems and shared patient records
- Specialist nurses, e.g. community matrons with close medical backup
- Involving community MDTs, district nurses, and health visitors
- Coordinated care—using care managers
- ↑ liaison between 1° and 2° care with free and frequent sharing of information and care goals and easy access to urgent clinical review (e.g. in urgent assessment clinics)
- GPSIs in geriatrics
- Utilization of ambulatory care services to monitor those most at risk of acute deterioration

## Further reading

Goodwin N, Dixon A, Anderson G, Wodchis W; The King's Fund (2014). *Providing integrated care for older people with complex needs.* https://www.kingsfund.org.uk/publications/providing-integrated-care-older-people-complex-needs.

# Primary care

- Ninety per cent of older people see their GP at least once a year
- One-third of GP appointments are for adults over 65 years
- Consultations tend to be more frequent, more complex, and more prolonged than in younger patients
- Consultations in the home are declining, as they are time-consuming, but older people remain the biggest user group. Increasingly, home visits are performed by non-medical clinicians such as nurses or paramedics, liaising as needed with GPs in the team
- GPs tend to be aware of the health problems of their older patients—those that do not attend tend to be healthy. The most common consultations are for respiratory and musculoskeletal problems (whereas 2° care sees more complications of vascular disease such as ischaemic heart disease (IHD) and stroke)
- >70% of those >75 are on three or more medications—treatment is usually prescribed and monitored by the GP
- Most older people live with chronic conditions (such as arthritis, chronic obstructive pulmonary disease (COPD), diabetes); scheduled care is usually by GPs and the extended 1° care team who play a key role in long-term management and 2° prevention
- Input from 2° care may come at a time of crisis (through admission to hospital, rapid referral clinics) or may be planned and more extensive, with regular clinic or day hospital attendance
- Increasingly, teams are integrated across 1° and 2° care—they work closely together, in ways that are patient-centred, rather than service- or team-centred, with sharing of information, proactive care, and advanced expertise 'closer to the patient' in community health settings. GPs act as a vital link between hospital and community services, identifying patients at particular risk of crisis, so allowing preventative action to be taken (a skill that is as much intuitive as systematic)
- Patients with multiple co-morbidities and/or extreme frailty may benefit from proactive identification and a preventative multifactorial intervention, focusing on optimizing chronic disease management, advanced care planning, social care management, and strategies to escalate care rapidly during acute illness. GPs, community nursing, health visitors, and therapists all have a role to play
- GPSIs in geriatrics can act as community specialists, working with other MDT members and liaising with hospital departments. They will often take the Diploma in Geriatric Medicine (DGM) (see ➌ 'Diploma in Geriatric Medicine', p. 48)
- NHS strategy is for rapid development of an extended 1° care and community capability. Key elements include merger of existing smaller practices into 'mega-practices' with much larger clinical teams and a greater specialist capability; 'polyclinics' (sites of extended healthcare, including 1° care, specialist clinics, and advanced diagnostics); outreach of 2° care to community settings; and decision support focused on 'high admission' settings such as care homes

## Further reading

NHS England. *NHS Five Year Forward View*. ♒ https://www.england.nhs.uk/five-year-forward-view/.

# Careers in UK geriatric medicine

## Consultant career pathway

- After qualification, Foundation level 1 and 2 jobs are undertaken; most include some time in geriatric medicine or in a specialty with geriatric team in-reach (e.g. acute orthopaedics). This is followed by competitive entry into Core Medical Training (2 years); most doctors will obtain the MRCP (Membership of the Royal Colleges of Physicians of the United Kingdom) at this stage
- Competitive application for a Specialty Registrar post may follow a period of research, but most commonly is directly after core training
- Specialty training in geriatric medicine takes only 4 years but is almost always paired with another specialty, e.g. general internal medicine, rehabilitation medicine, or stroke medicine. Dual accreditation typically takes 5 years
- Triple accreditation in geriatric medicine, general internal medicine, and stroke medicine is an increasingly popular career path and takes 6 years
- A few 'progressive' trainees combine training in unusual, but innovative and valuable, ways, e.g. emergency medicine (A&E) with geriatric medicine
- The *Shape of Training*' report recognizes complexity and ageing as key challenges and recognizes the need for doctors—such as geriatricians— who can provide 'general care in broad specialties across different settings'

## Non-consultant career grade pathway

- Includes specialty doctors and other locally determined posts
- Responsibilities of the post-holder vary considerably
- The main differences from a consultant post are that roles are often very clinically focused, with modest responsibility for management, administration, and training, and that overall clinical responsibility remains with a consultant
- There is a pathway to convert to consultant grade, but it is time-consuming and expensive ('CESR: Certificate of Eligibility for Specialist Registration')

## Primary care physicians

- GPs may wish to sub-specialize in geriatric medicine
- They may provide clinical leadership and care within a practice, a cluster or federation of practices, or in-locality functions such as a CH or a multidisciplinary acute/crisis team
- GP skills are also very valuable in larger hospital settings, including the ED and acute assessment units (medicine or frailty), and in ward settings (acute or rehabilitation)
- Such GPs often have significant experience in geriatric medicine during their vocational training scheme and may obtain the DGM
- Some GPs have migrated almost completely to an acute 'interface' setting, developing a much expanded acute capability and working at the front foor of hospitals 'shoulder to shoulder' and as peers with hospital colleagues

### Non-European overseas doctors

- Many overseas doctors wish to train in the UK for a period of time. It can be challenging to secure that opportunity; the first post is often the most difficult to obtain
- Many overseas doctors begin with clinical attachments, which are unpaid observer posts that enable the doctor to become familiar with the UK healthcare system
- Following the UK decision to leave the European Union (EU), arrangements are likely to change, but currently (2017):
  - Doctors trained in the EU may apply for any job in the UK
  - Non-EU-trained doctors are only able to take up a training post that cannot be filled by an EU applicant
  - The Royal College of Physicians (RCP) Medical Training Initiative (MTI) supports placement of internationally trained graduates as paid training fellows within UK hospital trusts
  - It is essential for non-EU-trained doctors to take the PLAB (Professional and Linguistic Assessments Board) examination (℞ http://www.gmc-uk.org/doctors/plab.asp)
- Obtaining the MRCP and the DGM helps to define an interest and demonstrates capability

# Diploma in Geriatric Medicine

Qualification awarded by the RCP (UK) to recognize 'competence in the provision of care of older people'.

## Candidates

The qualification is appropriate for any doctor who cares for older people, including GPs, psychiatrists, trainees in internal medicine, and those in specialties, such as orthopaedics or general surgery, where the patient cohort is increasingly complex and frail.

Candidates must be 2 years post-medical qualification and have held a post in geriatric medicine.

Studying towards the Diploma is also of value to junior doctors who are current trainees in geriatric medicine, as it motivates them to study important topics that recur in the MRCGP (Membership of the Royal College of General Practitioners) and MRCP and rewards them with a tangible product following an attachment.

Satisfactory completion of the DGM may contribute to more substantial geriatric qualifications (e.g. Masters), so it may also be pursued by specialist trainees, although it is not primarily designed for this group.

## Examination structure

*Written section*
• 3h—100 'best of five' (multiple choice) questions

*Clinical examination*
• 76min—4 × 14min stations (incorporating history taking, comprehensive geriatric assessment, communication skills and ethics, and clinical examination skills), with 5min prior to each station

## Syllabus

• Demographic and social factors
  • UK demography
  • Social influences on ageing
• Clinical aspects of ageing
  • The ageing process
  • Disease prevention
  • Features of atypical presentation of disease
  • Management of common conditions
  • Domiciliary care for the disabled
  • Legal and ethical considerations
  • Terminal care
• Administrative aspects
  • Knowledge of social services
  • Special geriatric services and facilities such as day centres, nursing homes, etc.
  • Financial considerations
  • Audit

Full details of eligibility, entry, examinations, and syllabus, are at: ℬ https://www.rcplondon.ac.uk/diploma-geriatric-medicine

# Clinical assessment of older people

# Consultation skills

There are certain skills that are key to any consultation, but some are more important with an older patient.

### Arranging an appointment

- For older patients, attending hospital may be more of a physical and an emotional challenge, for which there is a need to feel well. Patients often decide not to attend clinic appointments because they feel ill
- Hospital transport is often used. Morning appointments usually require a patient to be ready by 8.30 a.m.—daunting for someone who takes time to get going in the morning. Offer late morning or afternoon appointments, using early slots for patients who travel independently
- When informing the patient about the appointment, make sure that instructions are clear. Patients with dementia should probably have appointments sent to carers who would ideally attend with them; visually impaired patients may need a large-print letter or a telephone call. Text message or email reminders may be less appropriate
- Remind the patient to bring both medication and prescription lists to their appointment. Muddled medications may indicate self-medication problems. Comparison of drugs and lists helps to assess concordance
- Establish who has requested the consultation—e.g. memory clinic appointments are often in response to family concerns, and the patient may not attend as they do not perceive or wish to face the problem
- DH settings for consultation can be more relaxed, allowing the patient to recover over lunch before facing the trip home again
- Are hospital attendances really necessary? Discuss with the GP, offering to discharge the patient to his/her care, but supported by open telephone access for advice and a hospital review on request
- If all else fails, DVs may be useful

### Rapport

- Good rapport with the patient makes the interview easier, more productive, and more enjoyable
- Smart dress ↑ patient confidence, especially in older patients
- Always introduce yourself—shake hands if it seems appropriate, and address formally (Mr/Mrs/Miss) unless invited to do otherwise
- Be friendly, but not patronizing or over-familiar. Informal chat can break the ice and show that you have time for, and interest in, the person, e.g. asking about their occupation or how they came to live in the locality
- Older patients deserve and expect respect from (inevitably) younger doctors but often have more respect for the medical profession
- Patients are likely to have great faith in a trusted GP than in a young junior met for the first time. When asked what is wrong, they may quote the GP diagnosis ('Dr Brown said I had a stroke'), rather than offering their experiences. Emphasize that you work as part of a team ('Your doctor has asked for our opinion, so we need to go over things again. I will let them know what I think.'). After a hospital admission, explain changes to prescriptions and that you will inform the GP

- Acknowledge and apologize for waiting times and uncomfortable conditions (e.g. during an emergency admission)—it may not be your fault, but apologizing may defuse frustrations that hamper the consultation

## Environment

- Older patients are more likely to feel helpless and vulnerable in hospital if only partially clothed and on a couch. Interviewing a fully dressed patient sitting in a chair gives more dignity and respect
- Good light, quiet, and no interruptions will minimize problems from visual and hearing impairment

## Giving advice

- Advice is taken more often if rapport has been good during the interview. Appearing knowledgeable and professional ↑ the chance of agreement to investigations and medication changes. For example, some patients refuse to take aspirin, having been told years ago by a trusted doctor 'never to take aspirin again' because of an ulcer. Take time to explain that risks and benefits change with evolving disease and as new therapies develop. Gain understanding and agreement (see ➔ 'HOW TO . . . Discuss warfarin for AF', p. 280)
- Multiple conditions require multiple investigations and medications. For example, following a TIA, the patient may be well, yet tests can include bloods, ECG, chest radiograph (CXR), brain scan, and carotid Doppler, and several drugs are often prescribed. Take time to explain the rationale for each, thereby ↑ concordance
- Write a list of planned investigations and medication changes along with their justification. Give the list to the patient. This takes time but ↑ the likelihood that advice will be followed
- Offer to repeat your advice to family members, if not already present (may be sitting in the waiting room), or to telephone someone who is at home. A frail spouse may not be able to attend outpatients, or a busy daughter may not have time to attend, yet both may be vital to the delivery of effective ongoing care, e.g. administering medications or organizing appointment diaries
- It can sometimes be helpful to send a copy of your GP letter to the patient, but providing a second letter with key messages in 'lay' language to the patient is even better

# Multiple pathology and frailty

Most diseases become more common in an older population. Some conditions, such as osteoarthritis, are present in the majority (radiographically 70% of the over 70s). By the age of 80, it is very likely that an individual will have at least one disease. Many will have more than that (*multiple pathology*). As ↑ numbers of medications are advocated in the practice of evidence-based medicine, so polypharmacy and adverse effects become more common too. All of this contributes to frailty (see ➔ 'HOW TO . . . Assess for frailty', p. 53).

## Chronic stable conditions

The patient may have adapted to the limitations imposed by the disease (e.g. not walking as far or as fast because of osteoarthritis knees; reading large-print books because of failing vision) or medicated to aid symptom control (e.g. analgesia in arthritis). However, background multiple pathologies should be noted for two main reasons:
- Cumulative chronic disease will cause decline in physiological reserve:
  - The older patient with multiple stable diseases has *less resilience* to physiological challenge than a fit, young person; a smaller insult is needed to cause illness
  - *Non-specific presentations* reflect the complexity of the pathology—background problems interacting with new (perhaps seemingly minor) insults to cause acute decline without obvious cause
- Many patients adapt to impairments, particularly if the functional decline is gradual
  - Assessment and intervention remain helpful, e.g. failing vision is often accepted as a part of ageing, yet is often amenable to treatment

## Acute presentations

There are several aspects to consider:
- What is the acute precipitant? This may be minor, e.g. medication changes, influenza, constipation
- What are the underlying pathologies making the patient more susceptible to the acute precipitant?
- Note that one acute pathology can lead to another in a vulnerable patient, e.g. a bed-bound patient with pneumonia is at high risk for thromboembolic disease

So, for any single presentation (e.g. fall, confusion), there are likely to be *multiple aetiologies* which need to be unravelled. This can be difficult, but applying a structured, logical approach assists the process:
- Use a *problem list* to help structure the approach (see ➔ 'Problem lists', pp. 58–9)
- Allow *time* for the acute event to settle, physical and psychological adjustments to occur (much slower than in a younger person), stamina and confidence to build up, care arrangements to be put in place, etc.
- Involve an *MDT* to take a holistic look at the patient and evolve the problem list and action plan

## HOW TO . . . Assess for frailty

The British Geriatrics Society (BGS) defines frailty as a distinctive health state related to the ageing process in which multiple body systems gradually lose their in-built reserves. Around 10% of people aged over 65 years have frailty, rising to between a quarter and a half of those aged over 85 years. It appears to be a valid construct correlating well with mortality, hospitalization, and institutionalization.

Frailty is an old term that has new emphasis. It is increasingly being used within medical parlance with varying degrees of accuracy.

Geriatricians have always, and should continue to embrace the concept of a holistic term that describes physical and social functioning. Scientific measurement of frailty is complex and fraught with pitfalls. Repeated studies have shown that assessment by an experienced clinician is as accurate as formalized scoring systems.

Scoring systems vary from simple questionnaires (PRISMA 7), functional assessments (timed get up and go), to those approximating to the CGAs (Edmonton frailty score). These scoring systems have use within research and for triage selection of patients who would/could benefit from a multidisciplinary management approach. In an attempt to standardize this approach, the BGS is promoting FrailSafe and 'Fit for Frailty' campaigns. There is a push to improve identification of those at risk of frailty, with the hope of promoting healthy ageing. There is yet little evidence that this proactive approach works.

Older people may object to being labelled 'frail', whereas relatives will often identify with the concept. Use the term judiciously.

Frailty is sometimes used to justify withholding/withdrawing treatment. Once diagnosed, it should still prompt a comprehensive management plan, rather than inaction.

## Further reading

British Geriatrics Society. *What is frailty?* ✒ http://www.bgs.org.uk/index.php/frailty-explained.

# Taking a history

Histories taken from older people vary as much as the patients themselves, but some common problems make the process more difficult:
- Multiple pathology
- Multiple aetiology
- Atypical presentation of disease
- Cognitive impairment, both acute and chronic
- Complex social situations

Failing to recognize the importance of obtaining an accurate and comprehensive history risks misdiagnosis and mismanagement.

There is often a difficult balance to be struck between being inclusive and being focused and efficient

## The patient interview

The most direct information source but requires patience and skill.
- An elderly person with multiple problems may give a history that is hard to unravel. Someone with chronic back pain will answer positively to the closed question 'Do you have pain?', but it may be no worse than the last 10 years and not at all a part of the new presentation. Ask 'Is this new?' and 'Is it different from usual?'
- Allow time to volunteer symptoms. Avoid interrupting. If a symptom is mentioned in passing, return to it later to enquire about its nature, precipitants, etc. Interrupting may cause the main issue to be lost
- The patient may underplay issues that are emotive (e.g. failing memory, carer abuse, incontinence) or perceived as leading to institutional care. Foster an atmosphere of trust and mutual interest in problem-solving

## Cognitive impairment

Patients with dementia or delirium may not answer clearly or succinctly, and symptoms may need to be teased out. Quantities of seemingly irrelevant information may be interspersed with gems of important history. Do not get frustrated and give up—continue with a combination of open questions and careful listening, punctuated by closed questions that may result in a clear 'yes' or 'no'. General enquiries such as 'Do you feel well?' and 'Does it hurt anywhere?' can be rewarding. A patient who is made to feel silly will often dry up—if you are getting nowhere with specific questions, then broaden the conversation to get dialogue flowing again.

## Sensory impairment

Poor vision and hearing make the whole interview harder and more frightening for the patient. Use a well-lit, quiet room. Guide the patient to where you want them to sit. Ensure hearing aids are in and turned on. Speak clearly into the good ear, and do not shout. Use written questions if all else fails. Facilitate communication, however laborious—patients will worry that they appear stupid and may elect to withdraw completely if obstacles cannot be overcome (see also ➔ 'HOW TO . . . Communicate with a deaf person', p. 551, and ➔ 'HOW TO . . . Optimize vision', p. 572).

## Terms that should be banned and why

(See Table 3.1.)

▶ Patients admitted with the labels 'social admission' or 'acopia' are frail and have a high in-hospital morbidity and mortality. Statistically they are more likely to die in this hospital admission than a patient with MI.[1] Just because they are more challenging to diagnose and often require multidisciplinary assessment does not mean that they should be regarded as time and resource wasters for the system.

**Table 3.1** Terms that should be banned

| | |
|---|---|
| 'No history available' | It is almost always possible to get a history, if not from the patient, then from family, carers, GP, community nurse, or ambulance personnel. Nursing homes are staffed 24h a day and they all have telephones |
| 'Poor historian' | The historian is the person recording the history—this term is a self-criticism. If the patient is unable to give a history, this is important and the reason should be documented, along with evidence, e.g. AMTS, Glasgow Coma Scale (GCS) |
| 'Social admission' | A social admission is one caused solely by a change in the social situation, e.g. a carer who has died suddenly or a hoist that has broken. True social admissions are very rare and should in general be avoided (admit to a non-hospital setting, e.g. care home, or ↑ care at home). If the patient's function has changed, e.g. new incontinence, falls, confusion, and their unchanged social situation cannot cope, then the admission is NOT social. Often there is a combination of altered health and social circumstances. It is true that a younger patient might be able to stay at home with a minor change in health (e.g. Colles' fracture, flu), whereas an older patient needs hospital care, but by blaming only the social care, the doctor is at risk for missing the medicine, stigmatizing the patient, and labelling carers as failures |
| 'Acopia' | Usually a more accurate description of the clerking doctor than the patient. A grammatically incorrect and unhelpful term. Ask yourself why the patient cannot cope. What problem has led to this presentation and can it be treated? |
| 'Bed-blocker' | Pejorative term that implies that the patient is actively hindering discharge. Delayed discharge or delayed transfer of care are acceptable terms, as they remove any hint of blame from the patient |
| 'Failed discharge' | Most readmissions are appropriate and occur when the patient has deteriorated unavoidably at home, usually due to a new illness. The term is unnecessarily critical of the discharging team |

---

[1] Kee YY, Rippingale C. The prevalence and characteristic of patients with 'acopia'. *Age Ageing* 2009; **38**: 103–5.

# Other sources of information

Many patients, especially those with acute illness, are unable to give a full and reliable history. If so, a history must be obtained from other sources.

### The family

Often a rewarding source of information, especially at the initial assessment. Older people may underplay their symptoms, fearful of being thought unable to cope or not wishing to fuss. The family will often have concerns and it is useful to establish these as they may (or may not) be justified; weigh them up as more information is gathered.

Family members often wish to speak away from the patient—this can be useful and is acceptable if the patient gives consent.

▶ Your duty is to the patient and you are their advocate. Family members may have louder voices, but take care to listen to those for whom you are responsible. Elderly people are allowed to take risks (e.g. live at home with a high risk of falling), providing that they are competent.

### Neighbours/friends

Elderly patients with no family nearby may be very well known to their neighbours—perhaps they have been found wandering at night, or unusual behaviour has been noted. The neighbour may not feel obliged to volunteer this information and it may need to be sought. Neighbours may also act as informal carers and may contribute more care than family or formal carers. Common law partners are often heavily involved, yet may not be as prominent in hospital as other family members. Rifts may exist between established family and new partners and these need to be understood when planning care.

### Professional carers

They will know the usual functional and cognitive state of the patient and will often have alerted medical services to a change. They are rarely present at the medical assessment. Contact them and obtain all the information that you can.

### General practitioner and community nurse

They may well know the patient very well and have good insight into the dynamics of the care arrangement and family concerns. They can help clarify the medication and past medical history. If a confused patient arrives during GP practice hours, an initial clerking should always include a telephone call to the GP surgery. Patients who are housebound or who have leg ulcers, urinary catheters, or other nursing needs are usually best known to community nurses.

### Ambulance crew

The ambulance crew may be present during the initial hospital assessment of a sick older patient. Ask them what they know—this is a useful source of information that is under-utilized. If they have left, examine written ambulance team documentation—this includes timing, symptoms, and clinical signs, including vital signs. Paramedics may also hold information about the social situation, e.g. state of housing, informal carers, etc.

### Nursing and residential homes

When patients are admitted from institutional care, a good history can almost always be obtained; information should be sent with the patient (many homes have a transfer of care document), but if not, it can be sought by telephone immediately. Information about the usual functional state, past medical history, medications, and acute illness should be kept on file at the home.

### Old medical notes

Obtain them as quickly as possible, as they will provide essential medical information. A search for any MDT assessments can be fruitful. If the patient is not local, arrange for information (letters, discharge summaries, etc.) to be transferred or to speak to health professionals who know the patient. Increasingly, these may be stored electronically, making access easier.

# Problem lists

Useful tools to help formulate plans for complex elderly patients in any setting. They act as *aides-memoire* for multiple pathology and prompt clinicians to consider interacting problems.

Problem lists should include:
- *Acute problems*
  - May be a symptom (e.g. fall), rather than a diagnosis
  - List possible causes with a plan for investigation
- *Chronic conditions*
  - How stable is the disease?
  - What management is already in place?
  - What else can be done?

Lists can be generated at any stage in an illness—ideally at presentation—but need to be worked on and evolve as time goes on. Involve members of the MDT and make the list part of goal-setting and discharge planning.

### Example

- An 86-year-old woman who lives at home alone with a carer once a day is admitted to the medical assessment unit with confusion following a fall
- She has a past medical history of osteoarthritis, MI, and polymyalgia rheumatic (PMR)
- She has been finding it increasingly difficult to cope at home in the last year or so and getting occasionally confused
- Her daughter who lives abroad is very concerned

An initial problem list is suggested in Table 3.2.

- She is found to have an *Escherichia coli* UTI, which is treated, but she remains much less able than prior to admission
- She is transferred to a rehabilitation ward and the MDT involved

**Table 3.2** An example of an initial problem list

| | |
|---|---|
| Acute problem | Fall and confusion |
| Possible causes | Sepsis |
| | Constipation |
| Action plan | Septic screen (midstream urine (MSU), CXR, blood cultures, C-reactive protein (CRP), erythrocyte sedimentation rate (ESR), white blood cells (WBCs)) |
| | Rectal examination |
| Background problems | Osteoarthritis |
| | Vascular disease |
| | PMR |

A problem list at this stage is shown in Table 3.3.
- The patient makes a slow, but steady, recovery and regains mobility with a Zimmer frame, being independent for activities of daily living (ADLs)
- She is successfully withdrawn from steroids and begins appropriate 2° prevention measures
- Her home is adapted for downstairs living, and she returns there with a twice-daily care package after 5 weeks in hospital

**Table 3.3** An example of a problem list for the next stage

| Problem | Status | Action |
|---|---|---|
| Coliform UTI | Recovering | Complete antibiotic course |
| Osteoarthritis | Particularly affects left hip<br>Pain limits mobility<br>Takes paracetamol as needed (PRN) | Regular analgesia<br>PT for walking aids and to improve muscle strength<br>OT to adapt environment to limitations<br>Look into possible joint replacement |
| Vascular disease | MI in 1980s, no angina for years<br>Progressive mobility and cognitive decline likely due to diffuse cerebrovascular disease<br>Takes aspirin, atenolol, nitrates | Consider stopping nitrates as no angina<br>Consider statins or ACE inhibitors to limit progression of cerebrovascular disease<br>MDT input to adapt to chronic changes |
| PMR | Diagnosed in 1991<br>On prednisolone 5mg and calcium and vitamin D<br>Asymptomatic | Slow steroid withdrawalConsider bisphosphonate |
| Frailty | Likely multifactorial: osteoarthritis, cerebrovascular disease, steroid myopathy, probable steroid-induced osteoporosis | Action as above, this table, for each disease<br>PT to improve stamina and confidence |
| Deafness | Noticed by nurses<br>Progressive and bilateral<br>Patient attributes to 'getting older'<br>Likely presbyacusis | Referral for hearing aid |
| Family concerns | Daughter lives abroad and is unable to help | Meet with daughter (with patient's permission) and explain problems and action plan |

# General physical examination

There are two major ways in which examining an older patient can be more time-consuming and challenging:

- The extent of the examination is *wider*:
  - There are more systems with presenting symptoms
  - You often need to 'screen' (by examining a wide selection of systems) where presenting symptoms are vague
  - The chance of detecting incidental pathology (e.g. asymptomatic aortic stenosis, skin cancers) is much higher
- The procedure itself is *more difficult*:
  - Physical constraints—patients are less agile so undress more slowly and cannot always adopt optimal positions for examination (e.g. lying flat). They may wear many layers of clothing. They are more likely to have pain or to tire during the examination
  - Cognitive constraints—examinations that require complex instructions to be remembered and followed (e.g. visual field examination) may be too much for a confused elderly person

Despite these challenges, there are great rewards:

- There is a much higher prevalence of physical signs
- The examination more often makes the diagnosis, e.g. a patient with a non-specific presentation may have an undiscovered abdominal mass or a lobar consolidation

## General advice

- Given the challenges, it is tempting to take shortcuts leading to a sub-optimal examination, but this must be resisted
  - There are differing degrees of this—it might be reasonable to auscultate a chest through a thin shirt or nightdress, but it is useless to examine an abdomen through a rigid corset or with the patient sitting in a wheelchair
  - Sub-optimal examination is dangerous, especially if inaccurate findings are documented and then acted upon by others. It is better to record that you have not completed an examination and put a note at the end of your history that you, or another doctor, needs to complete or repeat the procedure
  - It is sometimes reasonable for a comprehensive examination to take two or three sessions, but start with the most useful elements
- Make use of nurses, relatives, or other carers to ↓ the physical problems of examination. Use electric beds and lifting and handling aids to make the examination more comfortable, effective, and safe
- Try to examine all aspects of one portion of the body at the same time. If organized, you should not have to sit a patient up, roll them over, or stand them more than once per examination
- Always inspect the patient fully. For example, look under clothing (especially sacrum and breasts), between toes, and under wound dressings, wigs, and prostheses

Table 3.4 provides an overview of the physical examination.

## HOW TO . . . Assess gait in an older person

### When?
- Almost always useful whether inpatient, e.g. acute admission, outpatient, e.g. falls, movement disorder clinics, or rehabilitation settings, e.g. functional progress

### Why?
- Provides vital diagnostic information
- Often appears time-consuming but can be surprisingly efficient—a normal gait is a good screening test, and an abnormal one will focus on further examination, e.g. on a single joint or system

### How?
- Ensure the patient is suitably clothed (bare feet, open hospital gowns, and falling down trousers do not encourage a normal gait!)
- Have a nurse or relative 'stand by' the patient if there is any risk of falls, so that you can concentrate on observing
- If they normally use a walking aid, provide this (but you may also wish to try them without or with different aids)
- Ask them to stand and walk to a specified point in the distance, ideally a few metres away (e.g. sink, end of the room)
- Observe setting off, stride height, length, symmetry, and fluidity, trunk position, and sway
- If safe, encourage them to keep going, turn, and return
- Consider if specific examinations indicated, e.g. tone for Parkinson's, Romberg's test if wide-based gait
- Functional assessments may be timed to quantify changes over time, e.g. 'get up and go test':
  - The patient should sit on a standard chair, placing his/her back against the chair and resting his/her arms on the chair's arms
  - Any assistive device used for walking should be available
  - Walk in a line for 3m, turn around and return to the chair, and sit down
  - Patients should be instructed to use a comfortable and safe walking speed

### Common patterns
- *Leaning back*—common with pseudo-Parkinson's (see ↑ 'Diseases masquerading as Parkinson's disease', p. 162)
- *Leaning forward and grabbing furniture*—common in patients with multiple falls and loss of confidence; no single diagnosis
- *Veering to one side*—consider stroke or balance problems
- *Limping/antalgic*—consider hip or knee or foot problems
- *Unsteady on turning*—consider ear, nose, and throat (ENT) pathology (see ↑ 'Vertigo: assessment', p. 562)
- *Unsteady when first stands*—consider postural hypotension (see ↑ 'Orthostatic (postural) hypotension', pp. 116–17)
- *Difficulty setting off*—consider Parkinson's (see ↑ 'Parkinson's disease: presentation', pp. 156–7)

- *Wide-based*—consider cerebellar and subcortical disease, and normal pressure hydrocephalus (NPH) (see ↑ 'Normal pressure hydrocephalus', p. 214)
- *Freezing/halting*—consider anxiety and fear of falling, Parkinson's disease, or frontal brain lesions
- *Footdrop*—consider stroke or localized anterior tibialis lesion
- *Difficulty rising from chair*—consider proximal muscle weakness

**Table 3.4** Physical examination—systems

| System | Of particular importance | Examples/notes |
|--------|--------------------------|----------------|
| General examination | Body shape and height<br>Nutritional status<br>Hydration<br>Mood, e.g. cooperation, insight, anxiety<br>Hygiene<br>Clothing<br>Intellect/presentation<br>Speech<br>Temperature<br>Looks ill/well? | Comments in this category are powerful in drawing the overall picture, e.g. 'a thin (52kg), anxious lady with stuttering, but clear, speech' is very different from 'an obese, cheerful lady with unkempt clothes and a strong smell of stale urine'<br><br>Hypothermia is more common<br><br>Fever may be absent/minimal on presentation—recheck later<br><br>If the patient looks ill, state this and try to say in what way |
| Cognition | Assess and quantify<br>Conscious level (GCS)<br>Orientation (time, place, and person)<br>Assessment scale, e.g. MoCA, AMTS, or clock-drawing test (CDT) | Should already be partially assessed during history<br><br>If unusual/delusional thoughts, record, e.g. 'thinks I am her mother' or 'repeated agitated shouts of "get off"' |
| Signs of systemic disease | Jaundice, clubbing, lymphadenopathy, cyanosis<br>Thyroid<br>Breasts | Consider examination in all women |
| Skin/nails | Bruising, rashes, purpura | Carefully record bruising positions if any suggestion of abuse or accident |
| | Toenail onychogryphosis | If you do not record it, you will not remember to refer to the podiatrist/chiropodist |
| | Venous disease or ulceration, cellulitis | Always inspect the heels and sacrum of immobile patients |
| | Pressure sores | |
| | Skin tumours | Basal cell and squamous cell carcinomas and even melanomas are common incidental findings |

**Table 3.4** (Contd.)

| System | Of particular importance | Examples/notes |
|---|---|---|
| Cardio-vascular | Check the BP yourself, especially if it has been abnormal<br>Postural BP (see ➜ 'HOW TO . . . Measure postural blood pressure', p. 119) | Consider BP readings in both arms—peripheral arterial disease is common and can cause major discrepancy |
| Respiratory | Respiratory rate is very useful (sensitive marker and part of many early warning scores (EWS))<br>Respiratory pattern | Normal 12–16/min in older people<br><br>You may need to watch for >1min to detect Cheyne–Stokes breathing |
|  | Crepitations only helpful if:<br>• Do not clear with cough<br>• Mid or upper zone<br>• Associated with changes in percussion and air entry | 30% of normal elderly chests will have 'basal crepitations' |
|  | Chest shape and expansion<br><br>Cough | Respiratory impairment due to kyphosis common and important<br>Examine any sputum |
| Abdomen | Bladder | Silent retention common |
|  | Rectal examination is almost always relevant | Constipation as well as bowel and prostate abnormalities |
|  | Mouth | Thrush, ulcers, and teeth |
| Cranial nerves | Note if vision obviously impaired and why | Visual fields tricky, but important in those with new visual loss or stroke |
|  | If hearing poor, check for wax<br>Note hearing aids/glasses | Some loss of upgaze is normal |
| Peripheral nervous system | Look for patterns, e.g.:<br>• Asymmetry of muscle bulk, power, sensation<br>• Sensory levels<br>• Peripheral neuropathy<br>• Global hyperreflexia | Some normal elderly will lose ankle jerks and distal (toe) vibration sense |
|  | If tremor, try to qualify (see ➜ 'Tremor', pp. 152–3)<br>Gait and balance (see ➜ 'HOW TO . . . Assess gait in an older person', pp. 61–62) | See also functional assessment, this table |
| Musculo-skeletal | Restricted range or deformity<br>Hot/painful joints<br>Gouty tophi | |
| Functional | Usually through observation during your examination | Do not help unless they struggle—can they dress (including buttons/socks), get on/off bed, lie to sit, roll over? |

# Investigations

Investigations are often less focused in older patients because:
- Presentation is more frequently non-specific
- Multiple pathology is more common
- Screening for many diseases (e.g. thyroid disease) is appropriate

## Simple investigations

Almost all older people who present with new symptoms should have:
- Full blood count (FBC), ESR
- Urea, creatinine, and electrolytes (U, C+E)
- Glucose
- Liver function tests (LFTs)
- Calcium and phosphate
- CRP
- Thyroid function tests (TFTs)
- CXR
- ECG
- Urinalysis

These tests are inexpensive, well tolerated, and rapidly available, and have a high yield. Coupled with a comprehensive history and examination, they will usually give sufficient information to guide initial management and further investigations. The urgency with which these tests are obtained is often determined more by hospital policy and the need for fast turnaround than by clinical need.
- Do not order repeat tests automatically until you have seen the results of the first set—only abnormal ones need to be repeated the next day
- If you order a test, record that you have done so in the notes (most doctors write a list of suggested investigations and then tick the ones they have themselves arranged)
- Ensure that results are reviewed and record them in the notes

## Further investigations

Although it is often tempting to order further investigations at presentation, it is often not helpful as it may mislead the clinician and lead to unnecessary patient anxiety and to further time-consuming and expensive assessments. Often the correct course of investigation is very different when an experienced clinician reviews with the benefit of initial results and a short period of observation.

Do not request an investigation if it will not alter management, e.g.:
- Carotid Doppler is unnecessary if endarterectomy would be inappropriate (e.g. poor functional status)
- Urgent CT head scan will not alter management for a deeply unconscious patient dying of stroke

## Will it change management?

Sometimes making a diagnosis has value, even where definitive treatment is unsuitable. An investigation may alter management, even if 'aggressive' treatment options are inappropriate. For example, sigmoidoscopy and barium enema may be helpful in a patient with bloody diarrhoea, even if colonic resection is not feasible; pathology such as colitis could be treated, and if advanced cancer were found, then the information would help direct:

• Palliative management, including 'surgical' procedures such as stenting
• Non-medical decisions, e.g. making a will
• Discharge arrangements, e.g. choosing care home placement over home
• The diagnosis itself can be reassuring to patients and relatives

These concepts often have to be explained carefully to patients, family, and medical colleagues who may feel that some investigations are unnecessary or that not enough is being done.

## Tolerating investigations

In general, non-confused older people accept and tolerate investigations as well as younger patients.

There are a few exceptions, which include:
• Colonoscopy (↑ risk of colonic perforation)
• Bowel preparation for colonoscopy or barium enema (more susceptible to dehydration)
• Exercise tolerance tests—arthritis, neurological problems, etc. often mean that the patient cannot walk briskly. Consider bicycle or chemical provocation testing

It is often helpful to discuss the procedure with the person performing the test (often a radiologist)—they might have suggestions for modifying the test or substituting a different procedure to make it safer.

You may need to allow more time for gaining consent or for the procedure itself, especially if the patient is deaf or anxious. Elderly patients are less likely to be aware of what modern medical tests involve than younger patients. Particular problems occur with confused patients, who may benefit from escort by a family member or trusted nurse. The cautious use of sedatives or anxiolytics is sometimes helpful.

In the outpatient setting, it is often the trip to hospital, rather than the test itself, that is traumatic. Minimize visits, e.g. by combining a clinic visit with a test or by arranging two tests on the same day. Try asking the GP or district nurse to remove 24h tapes. Where a series of tests or complex management needs to be accomplished, admission to hospital may be the best option.

# Common blood test abnormalities

A screening series of blood tests in an older person usually yields several that fall outside normal laboratory ranges. The examples that follow are those which are most commonly abnormal in the absence of relevant illness. Unless they are very abnormal or something in the presentation makes them particularly relevant, they can usually be ignored. There are four broad categories.

## Different reference range in older patients

- *ESR* may be as high as 30mm/h for men and 35mm/h for women in normal 70-year-olds (see ➔ 'The ageing haematopoietic system', p. 452)
- *Haemoglobin (Hb)*. Some debate, but the reference range should probably be unchanged (see ➔ 'The ageing haematopoietic system', p. 452)

## Abnormal results but common and rarely imply important new disease

- *Thyroid-stimulating hormone (TSH)*—often low with normal free thyroxine (T4) and triiodothyronine (T3) during acute illness; sick euthyroid syndrome (see ➔ 'The ageing endocrine system', p. 420). Repeat 2–4 weeks after acute illness has resolved
- *Low blood sodium*—very low levels should always be investigated (see ➔ Chapter 14), but some patients run with an asymptomatic, persistently mild hyponatraemia (≥128mmol/L) due to (overall beneficial) drugs or sometimes without obvious cause
- *Alkaline phosphatase (ALP)*—if LFTs are normal, an isolated raised ALP can represent Paget's disease (see ➔ 'Paget's disease', pp. 482–3), which is often asymptomatic. ALP remains high for weeks after fractures, including osteoporotic collapse
- *Normochromic normocytic anaemia*—always check B$_{12}$, folate, and ferritin/iron/iron binding. If these haematinics, as well as an ESR and blood film, are normal, then it is usually fruitless to look for the cause of mild, non-specific anaemia (see ➔ 'Investigating anaemia in older people', p. 453)—there is often chronic kidney disease (CKD) or early myelodysplasia underlying. Acutely unwell patients are often haemoconcentrated, with a temporarily normal Hb that then falls to a pathological level after a few days, when rehydrated
- *Bacteriuria* (see ➔ 'Asymptomatic bacteriuria', p. 620). Bacteriuria is a common finding in older patients and does not always indicate significant urinary infection. As a rule, treat urinary symptoms, rather than the bacterial count. The presence of white cells on urine microscopy and nitrites on dipstick can also guide decisions
- *High creatinine/low estimated glomerular filtration rate (eGFR)* (see ➔ 'The ageing kidney', pp. 382–3). Very common, especially in patients with multiple pathology and drugs. Changes in results over time more useful than absolute levels

**False negative result**

- *Creatinine*—low muscle mass can mask poor renal function (see ➜ Chapter 13). Consider with eGFR, e.g. when judging drug dosage
- *Urea*—as creatinine. In a frail older person, urea levels in the middle or higher range of normal are consistent with severe dehydration

**False positive rates very high**

- *Anti-nuclear antibodies (ANAs)*—figures of up to 1:80 are of doubtful significance in older patients
- *D-dimer*—any form of bruising, infection, or inflammation will increase D-dimer. If it is negative (rarely), it can still be a useful test, but do not expect it to be a useful test to exclude DVT/pulmonary embolism (PE) in a frail elderly patient with falls and a UTI
- *Troponin*—although this test is very specific to cardiac muscle, low-level release can occur with arrhythmias, PE, and heart failure. It is not a useful screening test in older patients with no chest pain and a non-specific presentation

# Comprehensive geriatric assessment

A CGA is the multidimensional evaluation of the patient in his/her environment. It encompasses medical, functional, and psychosocial elements which provide an interdisciplinary assessment and informs a plan for treatment and/or care. The management is goal-orientated, with the aim of restoring or maintaining an older person's function and independence.

### The team

CGA usually involves a team including nurses, therapists, doctors, and social workers who work together with a common form of documentation and/or regular meetings. A holistic assessment can be delivered by a capable individual or a subset of the above staff.

### Settings

- Inpatient—in a designated area or a specialized roaming team
- IC settings
- DH (see ➋ 'Day hospitals', pp. 22–3) and other ambulatory settings
- Community/outpatients—specialized clinics aimed at admission avoidance and early supported discharge, or follow-up of recently discharged patients to optimize functional recovery
- Care homes—advise on suitability of long-term placement, e.g. after urgent placement to avoid hospital admission

### Interventions

CGA usually leads to several recommendations/treatments with clear goal-setting and often regular review of progress. Interventions might include physical therapy, changes in medication, environmental modification, or advice about care home placement. The tool of CGA has been adapted to disease-specific management programmes (e.g. heart failure) and to assessing the suitability of older patients for cancer treatments.

### The patients

CGA is expensive and should be targeted to those most likely to benefit and exclude those whose prognosis is very good or very poor regardless of intervention.

### Evidence

It is difficult to compare data from such diverse interventions and settings, and little is known about the effectiveness of individual components of the 'black box' of CGA. However, there is good evidence that CGA can improve important outcomes such as survival, function, and quality of life, as well as reducing the length of inpatient stay and reducing admissions to hospital and nursing homes. It is not surprising that CGA is more effective when coupled with:

- Control over implementation of advice
- Long-term follow-up/review
- Medical management interventions

### Further reading

Ellis G, Whitehead MA, Robinson D, O'Neill D, Langhorne P. Comprehensive geriatric assessment for older adults admitted to hospital: meta-analysis of randomised controlled trials. *BMJ* 2011; **343**: d6553.

# Rehabilitation

# Introduction

Rehabilitation (rehab) is a process of care aimed at restoring or maximizing physical, mental, and social functioning. Can be used for:
- Acute reversible insults, e.g. sepsis
- Acute non-reversible or partially reversible insults, e.g. amputation, MI
- Chronic or progressive conditions, e.g. Parkinson's disease

Involves both *restoration* of function and *adaptation* to reduced function, depending on how much reversibility there is in the pathology. Rehabilitation is an active process done *by* the patient, not *to* him/her. It is hard work for the patient (akin to training for a marathon)—it is not 'convalescence' (akin to a holiday in the sun).

Rehabilitation is the 'secret weapon' of the geriatrician, poorly understood and little respected by other clinicians. Many geriatricians feel it is what defines their specialty and it can certainly be one of the most rewarding parts of the job. The 'black box' of rehabilitation contains a selection of non-evidence-based, common-sense interventions comprising:
- *Positive attitude*. Good rehabilitationalists are optimists—this is partly because they believe all should be given a chance, and partly because they have seen very frail and disabled older people do well. A positive attitude from the team and other rehabilitating patients also improves the patient's expectations. Rehabilitation wards should harbour an enabling culture where the whole team encourages independence: patients dressed in their own clothes, with no catheter bags on show, and eating meals at a table with other patients
- *MDT coordinated working*. By sharing goals, the team can ensure all team members are consistent in their approach
- *Functionally based treatment*, e.g. the Hb level only matters if it is making the patient breathless while walking to the toilet
- *Individualized holistic outcome goals*. These incorporate social aspects which must not be neglected. The team concentrates on activity and participation restrictions, rather than just impairments (see Box 4.1)

## Settings

Specialized rehabilitation wards are not the only place for rehab. If the considerations outlined are in place, then successful rehabilitation can take place in:
- Acute wards
- Specialist wards (e.g. stroke units, orthopaedic wards)
- CHs
- DHs
- Nursing and residential homes
- The patient's own home

These alternative sites often employ a roving rehabilitation team, which may be based in a hospital or the community.

## Box 4.1 International Classification of Functioning, Disability and Health (ICF) World Health Organization (WHO) classification (2001)

This classification attempts to reconcile the *medical* model of disability (the disability of a person caused by a disease) with the *social* model (the disability caused when society attitudes and structures are not able to accommodate a person). A complex biopsychosocial model is required to adequately represent both contributions to disability.

Disability may be defined at three levels:

1. *Impairments* are 'problems in body function or structure such as a significant deviation or loss', e.g. hemiparesis after stroke
2. *Activity limitations* are 'difficulties an individual may have in executing activities', e.g. problems walking after stroke
3. *Participation restrictions* are 'problems an individual may experience in involvement in life situations', e.g. loses job following stroke

It can be seen that disability at different levels requires a different response. PT and time might improve gait after stroke, but modifications of the environment (e.g. use of a stick) may be better at restoring the activity limitation and social/political change may be required to restore participation.

Despite the attractive logic of such a classification, it is actually rarely used in clinical practice but can be used in research and particularly health economics.

The word 'handicapped' is now avoided due to negative connotations and stigma.

## Further reading

World Health Organization. *International Classification of Functioning, Disability and Health (ICF)*. ℘ http://www.who.int/classifications/icf/en/.

# The process of rehabilitation

### 1. Selection of patients
See ➜ 'Selecting patients for inpatient rehabilitation', p. 78.

### 2. Initial assessment
This is not like a medical clerking; you need to get to know your patient on different levels (e.g. their mood, motivation, and expectations, complex social factors). Remember it is more meaningful to assess the full disability, not just the impairment (see Box 4.1).

### 3. Goal setting
See ➜ 'Aims and objectives of rehabilitation', p. 73.

### 4. Therapy
- Medical—doctor-led (see ➜ 'Doctors in the rehabilitation team', p. 92)
- Physical—mainly PT (see ➜ 'Physiotherapy', pp. 84–5) and nurse-led (see ➜ 'Nurses in the rehabilitation team', p. 93). Mobility, balance, and stamina. Confidence is often a key issue
- Self-care—mainly OT (see ➜ 'Occupational therapy', p. 89) and nurse-led
- Environmental modification—aids and adaptations
- Carer/relative training—it is too late to leave this until just prior to discharge

### 5. Reassessment
Usually at weekly MDT meetings (see ➜ 'HOW TO . . . Conduct an MDT meeting', pp. 82–3). Goals are adjusted and new goals are set. Points 3, 4, and 5 are repeated in a cycle until the patient is ready for discharge.

### 6. Discharge planning
See ➜ 'HOW TO . . . Plan a complex discharge', p. 81—should be started as soon as the patient is admitted, but the efforts escalate towards the end of the inpatient period. A home visit and family meeting are often held to clarify issues.

### 7. Follow-up and maintenance
Post-discharge DVs, outpatients, or DH attendance. Ideally done by the same team, but in reality this function often taken over by community, in which case good communication is vital.

# Aims and objectives of rehabilitation

It is essential that the MDT, ideally in conjunction with the patient, states what it plans to do and to achieve, in clear terms that are shared within the team and can be worked towards. A large part of this is achieved through the agreement and statement of targets at two hierarchical levels: aims and objectives.

## Aims

Best set by the team, in discussion with the patient. One or two patient-centred targets that encompass the broad thrust of the team's work—a team 'mission statement' for that individual, e.g.:
- To achieve discharge home, with the support of spouse, at 6 weeks
- To transfer easily with the assistance of one, thus allowing return to existing residential home place at 4 weeks

## Objectives

Best set by individual team members, in discussion with the patient. More focused targets, usually several, that reflect specific disabilities and help focus the team's specific interventions, e.g.:
- To walk 10m independently, with a single stick, at 3 weeks
- To achieve night-time urinary continence at 4 weeks

Both aims and objectives should have five characteristics, summarized by the acronym 'SMART':
- *Specific*, i.e. focused, unambiguous
- *Measurable*, hard to assess nebulous targets
- *Achievable*, and
- *Realistic*, acknowledging time and/or resource limitations. It is futile and demoralizing to set targets that cannot be achieved. Conversely, the team (and patient) should be 'stretched', i.e. the target should not be inevitably achievable
- *Time-bounded*. Specify when the target should be achieved. Many patients are motivated and cheered by the setting of a specific date (especially for discharge). Setting dates for specific functional achievements prompts further actions, e.g. ordering of equipment for the home

## Predicted date of discharge

Specifying a predicted date of discharge (PDD) from the point of admission is useful for patients, carers, and MDT members.
- Emphasizes to the patient that inpatient care is not indefinite and that a more pleasant home or care home environment is the aim
- Can be intrinsically motivating for patient and team
- Prompts the carers and MDT to think ahead to pre- and post-discharge phases of care

# Measurement tools in rehabilitation

### Principles

The most widely used standardized measurement instruments are structured questionnaires that deliver a quantitative (numerical) output. They vary in precision, simplicity, and applicability (to patient groups or clinical settings). For each domain of assessment, several tools of differing size are usually available, reflecting tensions between brief assessments (speed, easy-to-use, well-tolerated) and a more prolonged evaluation (precision improved, give added layers of information).

Measurement tools are helpful at single points (especially entry and exit to a therapy programme), and also in assessing progress and guiding discussion around a likely discharge destination.

### Advantages

- Quantify
- Widely understood and transferable across boundaries
- Facilitate communication between professionals and settings of care
- Provide a synopsis
- May permit a less biased, more objective view of the patient
- Facilitate a structured approach to assessment and clinical audit

### Disadvantages

- May be time-consuming
- Scores may conceal considerable complexity—patients scoring the same may be very different
- Intra-individual, intra-rater and inter-rater variabilities mean that a score may change while a patient remains static, e.g. 3- or 4-point change in the (20-point) Barthel is needed before a team can be absolutely confident that the patient has changed
- There are many scales available, and some are not in general use, leading to confusion when staff or patients move between units

# Measurement instruments

### Activities of daily living

Personal ADLs (pADLs) or basic ADLs (bADLs). Include key personal tasks, typically transfers, mobility, continence, feeding, washing, and dressing. A single scale is valid for all.

- The most common is the *Barthel* (see ➜ Appendix, 'Barthel Index', pp. 702–3). Score range from 0 (dependent) to 20 (independent). It is quick and apparently simple to use but is not very sensitive to change, as steps within each domain (e.g. transfers) are large. A marked ceiling effect is seen, especially for a range of impaired patients living independently at home, many of whom score 20
- The Function Independence Measure (*FIM*) takes longer to complete but is more sensitive to change during rehabilitation and can be useful in predicting length of stay and discharge destination

### Extended activities of daily living (eADLs)

Also known as instrumental ADLs (iADLs). Include key daily household tasks, e.g. housework, shopping. Useful for the more independent person. Scales are selected according to an individual patient's needs, e.g. Frenchay Activities Index, Nottingham ADL Score.

### Mobility

For example, Elderly Mobility Scale (EMS), Tinetti Mobility Score (TMS), timed get up and go test.

### Cognition

- Several screening and assessment tools are in common use
- The 10-point AMTS (see ➜ Appendix, 'The abbreviated mental test score', p. 704) is brief and useful for screening in both outpatient and inpatient settings
- Clock drawing tests (see ➜ Appendix, 'Clock-drawing and the Mini-Cog™', p. 707) are alternative screening tests
- The 30-point Mini-Mental State Examination (MMSE) provides sufficient precision to be used for serial assessment, e.g. tracking recovery from delirium, or therapeutic response to cholinesterase inhibitors in dementia—but takes <10min to administer
- The Middlesex Elderly Assessment of Mental State assesses systematically the major cognitive domains, using a range of targeted subtests. Time-consuming (15min) but gives more detailed information. Often used by therapists

### Depression

For example, the GDS. Several versions of this are available, but the most commonly used is the 15-point score (see ➜ Appendix, 'Geriatric Depression Scale', p. 701), administered in 5–10min. Superficially distressing questions, but well tolerated by most patients. Sensitive (80%), but only moderately specific (60%).

## Nutrition

The Malnutrition Universal Screening Tool (MUST) (see ➲ Appendix, 'Malnutrition Universal Screening Tool (MUST)', p. 709) is widely used to screen inpatients and is superior at predicting malnutrition than weight alone.

## Pressure area risk

Prompt systematic evaluation of patients at risk, and brisk response in those at risk, is essential. Several scores are available, but the most widely used is the Waterlow Pressure Sore Prevention Score, a summary score derived from easily available clinical data. High score indicates high risk. Note that the score does not take into account the ability of the patient to lessen risk by changing position, the acuity of the medical condition, etc.

## Disease-specific scales

All of the common diseases have dedicated scales, usually developed for use in research and then introduced variably into clinical practice. They are often more complex than used in general clinical practice, with corresponding disadvantages—time-consuming, less easily transferable. For example, the Unified Parkinson's Disease Rating Scale (UPDRS) quantifies all the motor and behavioural aspects of the disease as a single number.

# Selecting patients for rehabilitation

Most hospitals do not have enough rehabilitation services to cater for all patients who could benefit, so places are a valuable resource. This is often not understood by the patients, relatives, or referrers. Be aware that some referrers are motivated to get the patient 'out of their beds'. Patient selection is a time-consuming, important, and complex task.

## Settings

Rehab can be provided in acute hospitals, CHs, care homes, or even at home (e.g. virtual wards), depending on availability and motivation of carers, as well as how services are set up locally.

## Who should select patients?

Review of referrals is often done by geriatricians but can equally well be done by another experienced rehabilitation professional. In some settings, a team assessment is done and discussed in conference.

## Who to choose?

Two factors need to be considered:
- Which patients will benefit most from what is a limited resource?
- What does the MDT need to keep it positive and functioning well?

At first glance, the 'best' rehabilitation patient has had an acute event with good prognosis (e.g. a fracture), who is motivated and cognitively intact—able to participate enthusiastically in therapy and who has clear, easily attainable goals. Rapid results provide turnover, variety, and interest for the team. However, consider whether this patient might actually get better in almost any supported setting with a bit of supported convalescence time.

Contrast this with a frail elderly woman with multiple medical problems, moderate cognitive impairment, barely managing at home alone before a prolonged hospital inpatient stay with repeated complications, who has gone downhill physically and mentally. If asked, she wishes to go home, but this may not appear altogether realistic. Her daughter thinks she should go into a care home for 'her own safety'. It is all too easy to write this patient off, deny them rehabilitation, and arrange placement. This is the kind of complex 'heartsink' patient who has the most to gain personally (and who provides cost-effective utilization) of the expertise of the rehabilitation team. In any other specialty, the most complex cases are dealt with by the specialist; the same applies to rehabilitation. These types of patient sometimes do remarkably well and should be considered for a trial of rehabilitation. Even patients with virtually no recovery potential can benefit, e.g. learning adaptation, teaching skills to carers, or arranging complex discharge packages.

In practice, it is often a balance between the two types of patient where a broad case mix is maintained—some slower-stream complex cases with some more rapidly treated, simpler cases.

▶▶ In general, the harder a problem seems to be, the less likely it is that it will be sorted out in a non-specialist setting and the more likely it is that the patient will benefit from the rehabilitation team.

**Information required for patient selection**

Should be gleaned from all available sources (including nurses, hospital notes—medical, nursing, and therapy, family, carers, 1° care team, specialists, etc.) and may involve telephone calls and/or several visits. Regardless of who does the assessment, the following information should be acquired.

*Premorbid features*

- Physical problems—list of medical conditions, how active they were, and how disabilities impact on life; list of medications
- Functional limitations—assess by conversation (Did you use a stick? Did you ever go out alone? Could you get up and down stairs?, etc.) Quantify with a rating scale
- Social set-up—who do they live with (and how fit and willing to help are they?); where do they live (rural or in town)?; what is the property like (e.g. flat or house, any stairs to access and once inside the property, whether the bedroom and bathroom are up or downstairs)?; does anyone help out (formally, e.g. home carers, or informally, e.g. neighbours, family, friends)?; what did they do on a regular basis (e.g. walk to the pub for lunch, attend day centres or lunch clubs, cycle into town for groceries, etc.)?
- Cognitive state—range from mild memory problems (may predispose to delirium) to significant dementia. Ask about any objective assessments (e.g. MiniCog™) and the difficulties the problem causes in everyday life

*Acute features*

- Nature of acute insult—is it reversible (compare amputation to acute confusional state)
- Interacting comorbidities
- What is the expected recovery curve?—Varies with the disease: a patient with a large stroke may show very slow progress at outset and then steady, but slow, progress after several weeks; a patient with a fractured neck of femur, by contrast, is likely to improve rapidly after the operation and continue to make quick progress; a septic patient is unlikely to improve at all until the acute illness has resolved and is then likely to improve steadily. If the assessor has limited knowledge of the disease, obtain information from the specialist currently caring for the patient

*Patient wishes*

- Do they understand about the problems they face?
- Do they know what they wish to do when they leave hospital (e.g. go home as soon as possible, return to their residential home, not go home unless they are able to function as before, etc.)?

# Patients unlikely to benefit from rehabilitation

- Patients in a steady state who are awaiting placement
- Patients for whom the process of waiting for a rehabilitation bed will delay discharge (e.g. where expected recovery to discharge fitness is under a week)
- Patients with a single requirement for discharge (e.g. provision of commode)
- Patients who are still medically unstable, requiring frequent medical review, investigation, or treatment
- Patients with pure nursing needs (e.g. unconscious patient)
- Probably inappropriate for terminal care patients (palliative care teams likely to be able to support discharge planning when needed)

### Dementia and rehabilitation

This can be frustrating and difficult (but also very rewarding). Therapists will often prefer patients with 'carry over'—who are able to recall the last session and build on it. Nurses may find patients with behavioural problems disruptive to the ward. Safety issues are more difficult, as awareness of danger and the ability to make an informed decision about risk-taking are less. Relatives' anxiety is likely to be high. However, there is still a lot that can be done.

Repeated exercise can build stamina and some learning may occur. Rehabilitation settings allow more time for spontaneous recovery to occur. The more complex the discharge, the less likely it is that this can be managed in a non-specialist setting and the greater the need for the MDT expertise. Patients with dementia are most at need of an advocate for their rights and wishes, and the expert team assessment of feasibility and risk is the best way to ensure they are respected.

▶ In general, dementia alone is not a reason for refusing rehabilitation.

## HOW TO . . . Plan a complex discharge

- There is no such thing as a *safe discharge*—only a safer one. There is widespread misapprehension that hospitals and nursing homes are 'safe', while home is dangerous, but this is the wrong way round, e.g. rate of falls in institutions is higher (there is just someone there to pick you up) and the ↑ exposure to infection (e.g. meticillin-resistant *Staphylococcus aureus* (MRSA), 'flu) can be life-threatening
- The *timing of discharge* is sometimes obvious (e.g. when the patient returns to premorbid functioning) but can be controversial. Some patients want to go before the MDT feels they are ready and others (or their families) wish to stay longer (usually due to unrealistic aspirations or dislike of the chosen discharge destination)—communication is the key to avoiding this. Patients should understand that discharge is not necessarily the end of recovery following an illness
- Start to *plan discharge* from day 1, e.g. by obtaining background social history and patient aspirations. Set a target that patient and team are aware of—it is better to revise a PDD or destination than to have none at all, because it helps to focus goal-planning
- *Involve relatives early*—family meetings will ensure effective two-way communication. It will also reduce the chance of 'the daughter from America syndrome' where a relative comes out of the woodwork just before a carefully planned discharge to challenge or block existing plans

The MDT members should anticipate and pre-empt, but the following are common pitfalls which can cause a discharge to fail:

- Care availability (especially night-times)—check well in advance with the care manager that the care package you plan is available
- Modifications and equipment—ideally any environmental modifications should be in place before your patient is ready for discharge; otherwise there can be lengthy delays. It is amazing how long it can take for simple measures such as a bed to be moved downstairs. For more complex interventions (e.g. stairlifts, walk-in showers, deep cleaning), get a realistic estimate of time—sometimes the patient may need alternative accommodation while these works are completed
- Appropriate transport available (relative, ambulance)—remember not just for the patient, but also for their equipment
- Keys—who has got them? Who needs keys/door entry codes?
- Night-times—discharge plans often fail because the patient who looks good by day has unanticipated needs at night. Check with the nurses that they are not incontinent, immobile, or confused at night

### HOW TO . . . Conduct an MDT meeting

This is a ward- or team-based meeting with the $1°$ functions of communication, goal-setting, reviewing progress, and discharge planning.

There are also wider aims of:
- Team building. There is usually a chance for discussion over tea and biscuits. This is not time-wasting, it is vital for team bonding
- Education. Sharing knowledge and insight into each other's jobs

Usually weekly for inpatient settings but can be less frequent in community or outpatients. Most commonly, the team meets in a room away from patients/relatives—sometimes involving the patient by bringing them into the room.

Any member of the team can 'run'/chair the meeting, but in practice, where a doctor attends, they usually take this role. The chair is responsible for:
- *Timing*—the last few patients discussed should not be rushed. Some patients take a lot longer than others, but this should be a function of need, not just where they happen to appear on the list. Do not use the same order each week
- *Involving all team members*—ensure each member has an unimpeded opportunity to comment on each patient—some may need prompting. Do not allow assumptions that everyone knows certain information or that it is unimportant. A well-established team may automatically take turns—others may need you to force an order. Ask members to clarify jargon or code that may not be universally understood
- *Ensuring decisions are made/goals are set.* Without good leadership, a long discussion can occur without a positive action plan. Prompt with 'So what are we going to do about this?', 'Who is going to take that on?', 'When will that actually happen?'. If discussion is going in circles or there is dispute, it can be helpful to summarize what has been said so far to allow things to move on. Where there is agreement on goals, make sure they are SMART (see ➲ 'Objectives', p. 73)
- *Maintaining morale*—remember case conferences can be stressful. Keep discussions professional and good-humoured. Careful use of humour and frequent reminders that individuals, and the team, have done well are very important
- *Encourage feedback*—it is interesting and educational to hear follow-up on discharged patients. Ensure thank-you letters, etc. are shared, as well as news on deaths, readmissions, etc.

The conventional order of presentation is:

1. Doctor—diagnosis, current management and changes planned, prognosis—particularly if symptoms are limiting therapy
2. Nurse—nursing requirements, mood and behaviour, continence, sleeping, relatives/visitors comments
3. PT—mobility, equipment, progress, and potential
4. OT—functional assessments (e.g. dressing, kitchen), cognition, and DVs
5. Social worker/care manager—background, discharge discussions, external liaison (e.g. with council, funding panels, etc.)

This order allows discussions to flow naturally from medical background to current function (therapists) to goal planning and discharge plans (social worker). There is no reason why the order should not be different, but beware one person dominating and avoid discussing endpoints (e.g. discharge) before going through the logical steps, or you will become inefficient or miss something.

Notes of the meeting are vital—ideally they should be written only once, somewhere that all team members have access to. As a minimum, record the date, current status, notes about the content of discussion (even if solutions not found), goals, and plans. You have failed if you summarize a 20min important discussion as 'continue' or 'aim home next week'.

# Physiotherapy

### Training

BSc (Hons) Physiotherapy is a 3–4 years' full-time course. MSc Physiotherapy can be done as a 2-year accelerated postgraduate course. After 1° training, PTs usually sub-specialize in one area such as care of the elderly. See the UK Chartered Society of Physiotherapy website ℘ http://www.csp.org.uk.

### The role of the physiotherapist

- Aimed at improving physical functioning by exercise, reducing pain, and providing appropriate aids
- May be for recovery, adaptation, or prevention, e.g. falls
- Patient needs sufficient motivation, muscle strength, and energy to participate—it is *not* a passive process
- Duration of therapy may be short initially but ↑ as the patient tolerates more
- Cognitive impairment may limit learning and 'carry-over' of skills from session to session, but stamina may be improved with repeated sessions; dementia is not a reason to withhold PT
- PTs are the experts who plan and supervise physical therapy, but rehearsal of skills is often delivered by other members of the MDT or patients are given exercises to do alone (often with written instructions). PT assistants, nursing staff, and relatives can all assist in this rehearsal process
- Involved in training others to move dependent patients safely (e.g. carers)

### Range of interventions

*Increasing range of movement*
- Active or passive exercises
- Use after stroke or prolonged bed rest to ↑ joint mobility and prevent pain and contractures

*Increasing strength of muscles*
- Usually general strengthening to improve stamina
- Can be targeted at specific areas of weakness and enhanced by the use of resistance and weights
- Important part of falls prevention

*Improve coordination*
- Usually after stroke
- Repeated movements rehearse skills and improve coordination
- Improve sitting balance

*Transfers (i.e. the ability to get from one place (bed) to another (chair))*
- Strategy depends on patient ability
- Totally dependent patients are hoisted
- Once there is sitting balance, then transfers with assistance of two people and a sliding board can be attempted
- Once there is standing ability, then standing transfers with one person, then a frame can be worked on

*Ambulation*
- Exercises aimed at improving independence in mobilizing
- Realistic goals should be set—ideally premorbid state should be achieved, but 10m may be adequate for discharge home if this is the distance from chair to kitchen
- Balance aided by bars, then walking aids

*Heat treatment*
Using packs, hydrotherapy pools, ultrasound, etc. to treat pain and improve joint mobility.

*Other treatments*
For example, cold treatments, electrical stimulation for pain relief (e.g. transcutaneous nerve stimulation (TENS) machine).

*Provision of aids*
Usually ambulatory aids.

# Walking aids

These ↑ stability, leading to improved confidence and function, and ↓ falls. In general, identifying the need for an aid should prompt consideration of: the cause of functional decline (is it reversible?); provision of a PT assessment for prescription (correct aid, correct size); education (use of the aid, how to get up after falls); and treatment (strength/balance training).

All walking aids without wheels should be fitted with rubber ferrules to optimize grip and then checked for wear regularly (see Fig. 4.1).

## Stick (or cane (USA))

- May be single-ended ('straight'), double-ended ('hemi-' or 'bipod'), three-ended ('tripod'), or four-ended (delta-, quadrupod). The latter offers modest additional stability, compared to the straight stick
- Held in the hand *opposite* the most impaired leg, thus unweighting the impaired limb
- The level of hand placement should be at the greater trochanter, permitting 20–30° of elbow flexion—the most efficient elbow muscular function
- The choice of handle is important, e.g.:
  - *Contoured*: improves grip, reduces pressure, in permanent users or those with deformities
  - *Swan neck*: weight is centred over the base of the stick, providing a little more stability
  - *Right-angled*: more comfortable, but not easily secured when not in use
  - *Crook handle*: hooked over the arm when not in use

## Frame

- A structure of lightweight alloy metal that is self-stabilizing (usually based around four points in contact with the floor), providing unweighting of the lower limbs and greater stability than a stick
- Various heights, depths, and widths are available
- Bulky and difficult to transport. Some folding versions (often only three legs) are available
- May be used indoors or out
- The handgrips should be at wrist level, with the elbows slightly (15°) flexed. Shorter frames are used in patients who fall backwards
- To use a *non-wheeled frame*, lift it and move it 10–30cm in front of the body; then lean forwards a little, taking some weight through the arms before taking two equal steps towards the centre of the frame
- A *weighted frame* has weights low on the frame structure to provide additional counter-balance against falls
- A *wheeled frame* has wheels at the front, permitting faster walking and an improved gait pattern, but it provides a slightly less stable base. Small-wheeled frames are suitable only for smooth surfaces
- A *gutter frame* has forearm rests, enabling weight-bearing through the forearms, rather than the hands alone, providing additional support in the early stages of mobilization or when hands/wrists are impaired

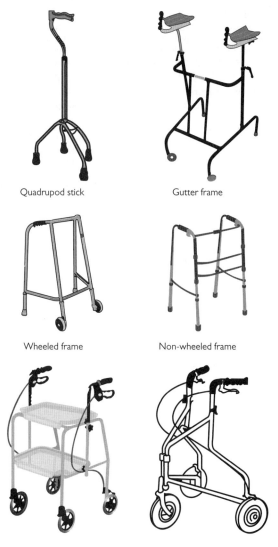

Quadrupod stick    Gutter frame

Wheeled frame    Non-wheeled frame

Wheeled trolley (indoors)    Three-wheeled rollator (in and outdoors)

Fig. 4.1 Different types of walking aid.

### Crutches

A full assessment by a therapist is needed before selecting crutches. Crutches may be of the axilla- or elbow-type. Both are available with various features that should be individually prescribed, e.g. closed elbow cuffs provide added security and enable the user to let go of the handgrip to open a door without the crutch falling to the floor.

### Walkers or rollators

- A frame that has three or four wheels and often hand-operated brakes (for added stability while static)
- Three-wheeled versions usually fold, permitting stowage in a car
- Rollators with additional features, such as bigger wheels (for uneven ground), a seat, or an attached basket for shopping or other house/ garden tasks, are larger than most standard frames and are usually used outdoors
- A trolley walker combines walking support with a means of transporting items from room to room. One or two shelves. The lower shelf is recessed at the back, so that it does not interfere with walking

### Early walking aids (EWAs)

For example, post-amputation mobility aid (PAM-aid). Used early (usually from ~day 7) following amputation, in patients in whom a permanent prosthesis is planned or being considered.

# Occupational therapy

### Training

BSc Occupational Therapy is a 3–4 years' full-time course or can be done as a 2-year accelerated postgraduate course. The courses are 2/3 academic and 1/3 field work. After 1° training, OTs usually sub-specialize in one area such as care of the elderly. See (for the UK) the British Association of Occupational Therapists and Royal College of Occupational Therapists website ℘ http://www.cot.org.uk.

### Role of the occupational therapist

The College of Occupational Therapy definition:

> 'OT enables people to achieve health, well-being and life satisfaction through participation in occupation (i.e. daily activities that reflect cultural values, provide structure to living and meaning to individuals; these activities meet human needs for self-care, enjoyment and participation in society)'.

OTs achieve this by assessing both functional status and the environment, then advising how to adapt.

### Skills versus habits

- A *skill* is having the ability to start, carry out, and complete a task effectively (e.g. making a cup of tea)
- A *habit* is those tasks that are actually carried out (e.g. a person may be able to make a meal but does not do so when alone as they do not feel hungry)

### Components of personal ability

Assessed by direct observation during tasks, formal testing, and information taken from carers, relatives, and other professionals.

- *Cognition*—to understand the task and why it needs doing. May be limited by dementia, poor concentration span, poor problem-solving skills, etc. Assessed with cognitive tests such as Middlesex Elderly Assessment of Mental State (MEAMS)
- *Psychology*—wanting to do and complete the task. Limited by depression, apathy, impaired coping skills, etc.
- *Sensorimotor ability*—especially in the upper limb

# Occupational therapy assessments and interventions

## Assessments

- *Washing and dressing*—aim to be done in the morning, when the patient would normally be carrying out these tasks
- *Kitchen*—looking at competence and safety for required tasks (depending on circumstances, e.g. may need to make a meal on a gas stove, or just pour a drink from a prepared Thermos™)
- *Access visits*—are done without the patient, to study the layout and potential problems of a patient's own home

*Home assessment visits*

- A visit done with the patient, to see them in their own environment
- Can be done by the OT alone, or with another member of the MDT (e.g. PT, care manager)
- May be useful to include intended carers (family or professional), as concerns can be addressed during the visit
- Can be done in the community while the patient is still at home, from a hospital ward prior to discharge to ensure that it is feasible and that all possible problems and dangers have been minimized, or after discharge as a follow-up
- Sometimes surprising—patients may either perform considerably better than expected (as they are in a familiar environment to which they have been adapting for years) or considerably worse (especially when a new physical limitation has occurred, such as stroke, as being at home emphasizes how different life will now be)
- Standard format for assessing all aspects of the property
- Followed by a report containing observations on client performance and a list of recommendations regarding reorganization of furniture (e.g. bring bed downstairs), equipment provision, and care required
- Often typed and circulated to all MDT members

## Interventions

Teaching new skills (e.g. putting on a jumper with an arthritic shoulder) and habits (e.g. heating up microwave meals every lunchtime). Looking at how much can be done by the patient themselves and how much help is needed (family or professional carers). Assessing need for equipment and advising about suitability, as well as training carers in its use. Commonly used equipment includes aids to:

- *Access*—ramps, rails, banisters, stairlifts, perching stools (high stools to enable seated access to a kitchen work surface), etc.
- *Transfers*—'banana boards' (curved boards that the patient slides across from one horizontal surface to another), swivel mats (two circles that twist to allow easier turning of an immobile patient, usually in a car seat)
- *Mobility*—wheelchairs, scooters, etc.

- *Bathing and dressing*—bath boards, accessible baths and showers, long shoehorns, grab handles (to allow picking things up without bending), etc.
- *Toileting and continence*—seat raises, commodes, non-return urine bottles (for use when lying flat), etc.
- *Eating and drinking*—cutlery and cups with easy-grip handles, aids to improve safety with hot water (kettle holders, full-cup alarms), tap turners, etc.
- *Splints*—for wrists (prevent pain) and ankles (foot drop)
- *Sensory aids*—enhanced signals, e.g. large dials on a clock or altered signals, such as flashing light, instead of a bell for the deaf

# Doctors in the rehabilitation team

Doctors are commonly part of hospital rehabilitation teams but may be missing from community rehabilitation teams where a nominated doctor (e.g. GP or community geriatrician) can be consulted about specific issues.

When present, doctors often chair MDT meetings—this may be partly historical and partly because they are 'professional risk-takers' who are more confident at coaxing a shared decision from a team, sometimes in very uncertain circumstances.

Medical ward rounds are often less frequent than on acute wards (a weekly round would be usual), and since the patient is usually medically stable, communication with patient and family may predominate over medical management.

In a rehabilitation setting, the doctor's main duties to the patient are:
• Selecting patients and maintaining a waiting list
• Optimizing and stabilizing medical treatments (e.g. ensure adequate analgesia)
• Rationalizing drug therapy (e.g. stop night sedation)
• Anticipating and treating complications (e.g. pressure sores, *Clostridium difficile*-associated diarrhoea (CDAD), DVT)
• Diagnosing and treating depression
• Identifying and managing co-morbid conditions (e.g. incontinence, skin tumours)
• Initiating $2°$ prevention (e.g. aspirin for stroke, bisphosphonates following osteoporotic fractures, influenza vaccination)
• Organizing $2°$ referral to other specialists (e.g. dermatology, orthopaedics)

Additional duties to the team include:
• Education
• Team-building
• Context-setting—doctors often cross health sector boundaries, whereas therapists and nurses can be fixed in teams or wards. They should share information about the patients on the waiting list and about those who do not reach the rehabilitation unit and why. This overview can help the team understand pressure on beds, etc.

# Nurses in the rehabilitation team

The role of rehabilitation nurses in the recovery of a patient is often under-estimated. They spend the longest time, and often have the most intimate relationship, with patients and their relatives.

Their wide role encompasses:

- Rehabilitation helper—particularly rehearsal of new tasks learned with therapists (e.g. transfers, dressing). It takes longer and more skill to encourage a patient to wash/dress themselves than simply to provide personal care—this is the fundamental difference between rehabilitation and normal ward nursing
- Overall performance assessors versus snapshot—they can detect any differential performance between what a patient 'can do' with the therapist and what he/she 'does do' when on their own, when tired, or when relatives are visiting
- Communication and liaison—first port of call between members of the team and patient and relatives. Emotive information sometimes more readily revealed in such non-threatening discussions
- Nocturnal assessment—they are the only professionals able to monitor sleep, nocturnal confusion/wandering, and nocturnal continence/toileting
- Continence management
- Pressure and wound care management
- Medication administering and monitoring self-medication
- Ward or unit management

Some senior specialist nurses have roles that overlap with the doctor's, e.g. in selecting patients for rehabilitation, chairing MDT and family meetings, nurse prescribing, etc. This is especially true in some CHs which can be exclusively run by nurse consultants.

# Other members of the rehabilitation team

### Speech and language therapy
Trained to degree level (3–4 years) or postgraduate diploma. See the Royal College of Speech and Language Therapists (RCSLT) website ℘ http://www.rcslt.org.

*Assessment and treatment of swallowing disorders* forms the bulk of inpatient work. Careful bedside evaluation of the patient is central to this, complemented, if necessary, by videofluoroscopy, the assessment 'gold standard'.

Useful interventions include patient positioning, changes in the texture or consistency of food/fluid, and carer supervision or prompting with food boluses. A period of 'nil by mouth' may be necessary until possible recovery of a safer swallow, during which artificial feeding should be considered.

*Assessment and treatment of speech disorders* forms the remainder of their work, commonly following stroke or head/neck surgery. Therapists are experts in communication disorders, and their assessments are useful in distinguishing between severe dysarthria and dysphasia, for example. They provide: advice to patient, carers, and staff; and alternatives to speech, including communication boards, non-verbal strategies, and electronic communicators.

### Dieticians
Trained to degree level (3/4 years) or postgraduate diploma. See the British Dietetic Association website ℘ http://www.bda.uk.com.

- Malnutrition in older people is common, underdiagnosed, and undertreated. Prevalence and severity are especially high with (acute or chronic) comorbidity and in inpatients
- Community-dwelling older people may have an unvaried diet, depleted in fruit and vegetables ('tea and toast')
- Dieticians are experts in the assessment and treatment of nutritional problems, but other members of the MDT must be alert to the possibility of malnutrition and initiate interventions and dietician referral. Screening tools are useful (see ➜ Appendix, 'Malnutrition Universal Screening Tool (MUST)', p. 709)
- Effective interventions include offering attractive food tailored to the individual, asking the family to bring in food, offering food frequently, and providing a dedicated assistant by the bedside to assist with feeding (this could be a staff member, family, or an informal carer). Modern packaging (prepacked margarine, snack boxes) can be obstructive
- Where 'normal' feeding is impossible, e.g. after acute stroke, the dietician can provide assessment, monitoring, and advice to the patient (and family) regarding artificial feeding (see ➜ 'Nutrition', pp. 354–5)

## Pharmacists

Pharmacists train for at least 4 years, leading to the MPharm degree. See the Royal Pharmaceutical Society website ℘ http://www.rpharms.com.
- Pharmacists are involved in preparation, prescribing, packaging, and dispensing of medicines. They are key to the system delivering quality drug use to outpatients and inpatients, to older people
- Gatekeepers of many health community formularies (limited drug lists optimizing costs and effectiveness). They advise on all aspects of prescribing, especially interactions and dosing

Issues where pharmacists may help:
- High frequency of adverse drug reactions (up to 17% of hospital admissions)
- Underuse of medications, e.g. preventatives in asthma
- Poor concordance/compliance/adherence
- Poor administration technique, e.g. inhalers
- Frequent and complex changes in medication
- Poor communication with 1° care on discharge
- Absence of full medication history on admission

The National Service Framework (NSF) for older people states that all patients >75 should have their medicines reviewed at least annually, and those taking four or more medicines 6-monthly. Every area must have schemes for older people to access help from pharmacists in using their medicines.

# Social work and care management

Social workers are trained to degree level (3/4 years) or postgraduate diploma. See the British Association of Social Workers website ℘ http://www.basw.co.uk. Care managers may have less formal training.

- Care managers are based in both community and hospital settings and may work with patients of all ages
- The quality of support that they provide to a geriatric medicine service is a key determinant of patient throughput and quality of care
- Any inpatient clinical area managing the needs of older people should have significant input from a social worker with experience in working with older people
- Many EDs in UK hospitals now have a dedicated social worker, aiming to avoid admissions by optimizing access to social care
- To function effectively, social workers must have a detailed understanding of local services and facilities, how those services are accessed, as well as about supporting information such as transport, costs, and waiting lists

Elements of their role include:
- Assessment of client needs, often informed by the MDT in hospital settings
- Translation of care needs into a package of care
- Monitoring delivery of care and modifying its content or providers, if necessary
- Providing patients and families with details of care homes that can meet the patient's needs, in the desired geographical area
- Providing advice about finances and financial support, care homes, and home care
- Performing financial assessments to determine who will fund their own care and who will receive assistance
- Counselling and support to patients and families
- Crisis management. For example, if a carer becomes ill or dies, a care package may be ↑ urgently or emergency admission to a care home arranged. 'Social admission' to hospital should be a last resort, unless the condition of the patient has also changed, in which case urgent medical assessment, perhaps in a hospital, is essential
- Arranging short breaks (for the carer) or respite care (for the patient)

# Community nurses and health visitors

Both are trained nurses with further postgraduate training and experience that enable them to work more independently in community settings. Their precise role and professional relationships vary greatly between districts.

## Community nurses

Usually work for one or more GP practices, providing domiciliary nursing services in excess of those provided by non-nurse carers. A district nurse is a community nurse who has undergone further training.

Specialist skills include:
- Wound care—assessment and treatment
- Insulin injections and diabetes monitoring
- Continence management
- Bowel management
- Chronic disease management
- Education of patients and carers (e.g. PEG feed, catheter care)

Although caring for adults of all ages, much of their work involves older people, especially the frail elderly. They are often an excellent source of information about older people admitted to hospital, often having frequent contacts with frail elderly people who are unable to leave the home and are therefore seen only rarely by GPs.

*Community matrons* are experienced senior nurses who are responsible for identifying and care-coordinating high-intensity users of healthcare. They coordinate agencies for complex, frail, and often elderly patients to promote well-being and try to obtain maximum efficiency from 1° care and 2° care providers. Often this involves trying to reduce emergency admissions to hospital and/or calls to out-of-hours GPs.

## Health visitors

Again, health visitors (HVs) usually work with one or more GP practice, but the dominant focus is on health promotion. Most work with mothers and babies/children, but they can work with any age group. Some HVs specialize in working with older people and carers. They may help older people maintain independence by:
- Providing information about local activities
- Advising on benefits
- Advising on help available from social services to support them in their homes
- Visiting people at home
- Arranging respite care

# Falls and funny turns

# Falls and fallers

▶ A fall is often a symptom of an underlying serious problem and is not a part of normal ageing.

A fall is an event that results in a person non-intentionally coming to rest at a lower level (usually the floor) with or without loss of consciousness. Falls are common and important, affecting one-third of older people living in their own homes each year. They result in fear, injury, dependency, institutionalization, and death. Many can be prevented and their consequences minimized.

## Factors influencing fall frequency

- *Intrinsic factors*. Maintaining balance—and avoiding a fall—is a complex, demanding multisystem skill. It requires muscle strength (power:weight ratio), stable but flexible joints, multiple sensory modalities (e.g. proprioception, vision, hearing), and a functional peripheral and central nervous system. Higher-level cognitive function permits risk assessment, giving insight into the danger that a planned activity may pose
- *Extrinsic factors*. These include environmental factors, e.g. lighting, obstacles, the presence of grab rails, and the height of steps and furniture, as well as the softness and grip of the floor
- *Magnitude of 'stressor'*. All people have the susceptibility to fall, and the likelihood of a fall depends on how close to a 'fall threshold' a person sits. Older people, especially with disease, sit closer to the threshold and are more easily and more often pushed over it by stressors. These can be internal (e.g. transient dizziness due to orthostatic hypotension) or external (e.g. a gust of wind or a nudge in a crowded shop); they may be minor or major (no one can avoid 'falling' during syncope)

If insight is preserved, the older person can, to some extent, reduce risk by limiting hazardous behaviours and minimizing stressors (e.g. walking only inside, avoiding stairs or uneven surfaces, using walking aids, or asking for supervision).

## Factors influencing fall severity

In older people, the adverse consequences of falling are greater, due to:
- Multiple system impairments which lead to *less effective saving mechanisms*. Falls are more frightening and injury rates per fall are higher
- Osteoporosis and ↑ fracture rates
- 2° injury due to post-fall immobility, including pressure sores, burns, dehydration, and hypostatic pneumonia. Half of older people cannot get up again after a fall
- *Psychological adverse effects*, including loss of confidence

Falls are almost always multifactorial. Think:
- '*Why today?*' Often because the fall is a manifestation of acute or subacute illness, e.g. sepsis, dehydration, or drug adverse effect
- '*Why this person?*' Usually because of a combination of intrinsic and extrinsic factors that ↑ vulnerability to stressors

### Banned terms

The terms *simple fall* and *mechanical fall* are used commonly, but they are facile, imprecise, and unhelpful. 'Simple' usually refers to the approach adopted by the assessing doctor.

- For every fall, identify the intrinsic factors, extrinsic factors, and acute stressors that have led to it
- Within each of these categories, think how their influence on the likelihood of future falls can be reduced

# Assessment following a fall

Think of fall(s) if a patient presents:
- Having 'tripped'
- With a fracture or non-fracture injury
- Having been found on the floor
- With 2° consequences of falling (e.g. hypothermia, pneumonia)

Patients who present having fallen are often mislabelled as having 'collapsed', discouraging the necessary search for multiple causal factors.

Practise opportunistic screening—ask all older people who attend 1° or 2° care whether they have fallen recently.

## History

Obtain a corroborative history, if possible. May often need to use very specific, detailed, and directed questions. In many cases, a careful history differentiates between falls due to:
- Frailty and unsteadiness
- Syncope or near-syncope
- Acute neurological problems (e.g. seizures, vertebrobasilar insufficiency (VBI))

Gather information about:
- Fall circumstances (e.g. timing, physical environment)
- Symptoms before and after the fall
- Clarification of symptoms, e.g. 'dizzy' may be vertigo or presyncope
- Drugs, including alcohol
- Previous falls, fractures, and syncope ('faints'), even as a young adult
- Previous 'near-misses'
- Comorbidity (cardiac, stroke, Parkinson's disease, seizures, cognitive impairment, diabetes, incontinence)
- Functional performance (difficulties bathing, dressing, toileting)

## Drugs associated with falls

Falls may be caused by any drug that either is directly psychoactive or may lead to systemic hypotension and cerebral hypoperfusion. Polypharmacy (>4 drugs, any type) is an independent risk factor.

The most common drug causes are:
- Benzodiazepines and other hypnotics
- Antidepressants (tricyclics and selective serotonin reuptake inhibitors (SSRIs)
- Antipsychotics
- Opiates
- Diuretics
- Antihypertensives, especially ACE inhibitors and $\alpha$-blockers
- Antiarrhythmics
- Anticonvulsants
- Skeletal muscle relaxants, e.g. baclofen, tizanidine
- Hypoglycaemics, especially long-acting oral drugs and insulin

## Examination

This can sometimes be focused if the history is highly suggestive of a particular pathology; perform at least a brief screening examination of each system.

- Functional. Ask the patient to stand from a chair, walk, turn around, walk back, and sit back down ('get up and go' test). Assess gait, use of walking aids, and hazard appreciation
- Cardiovascular. Always check lying and standing BP. Check pulse rate and rhythm. Listen for murmurs (especially of aortic stenosis)
- Musculoskeletal. Assess footwear (stability and grip). Remove footwear and examine the feet. Examine the major joints for deformity, instability, or stiffness
- Neurological. To identify stroke, peripheral neuropathy, Parkinson's disease, vestibular disease, myelopathy, cerebellar degeneration, and cognitive impairment
- Vision

## Tests

The following are considered routine:

- ECG
- FBC, $B_{12}$, folate, U, C+E, glycosylated Hb ($HbA_{1c}$), calcium, phosphate, TFT
- Vitamin D—deficiency is common in older adults, and evidence suggests that replacing may reduce falls/harm from falls

If a specific cause is suspected, then test for it, e.g.:

- 24h ECG in a patient with frequent near-syncope and a resting ECG suggesting conducting system disease
- Echocardiogram in a patient with systolic murmur and other features suggesting aortic stenosis (e.g. slow-rising pulse, left ventricular hypertrophy (LVH) on ECG)
- Head-up tilt table testing (HUTT) in patients with unexplained syncope, normal resting ECG, and no structural heart disease
- Carotid sinus massage (see ➜ 'HOW TO . . . Perform carotid sinus massage', p. 121)

However, all tests have false positive rates, and even a 'true positive' finding may have no bearing on the patient's presentation. For example, a patient falling due to osteoarthritis and physical frailty will not benefit from an echocardiogram that reveals asymptomatic mild aortic stenosis.

▶ Use tests selectively, based on your judgement (following careful history and examination) of the likely factors contributing to falls.

## Further reading

National Institute for Health and Care Excellence (2013). *Falls in older people: assessing risk and prevention*. Clinical guideline CG161. ⅋ http://www.nice.uk/CG161.

# Interventions to prevent falls

The complexity of treatment reflects the complexity of aetiology:
- Older people who fall more often have remediable medical causes
- Do not expect to make only one diagnosis or intervention—making minor changes to multiple factors is more powerful
- Tailor the intervention to the patient. Assess for relevant risk factors and work to modify each one
- A multidisciplinary approach is key

### Reducing fall frequency

- *Drug review*. Try to reduce the overall number of medications. For each drug, weigh the benefits of continuing with the benefits of reduction or stopping. Stop if risk is greater than benefit. Reduce if benefit is likely from the drug class, but the dose is excessive for that patient. Taper to a stop if withdrawal effect likely, e.g. benzodiazepine
- *Treatment of orthostatic hypotension* (see ➡ 'Orthostatic (postural) hypotension', pp. 116–17)
- *Strength and balance training*. In the frail older person, by a PT, exercise classes, or disciplines such as t'ai chi
- *Walking aids*. Provide an appropriate aid and teach the patient how to use it (see ➡ 'Walking aids', pp. 86–8)
- *Environmental assessment and modification* (a simple checklist can help the family minimize risk; in some cases, a more detailed assessment by an OT is beneficial)
- *Vision*. Ensure glasses are appropriate (avoid vari- or bifocal lenses)
- *Reducing stressors*. This involves decision-making by the patient or carers. The cognitively able patient can judge risk/benefit and usually modifies risk appropriately, e.g. limiting walking to indoors, using a walking aid properly and reliably, and asking for help if a task (e.g. getting dressed) is particularly demanding. However:
  - Risk can never be abolished
  - Enforced relative immobility has a cost to health
  - Patient choice is paramount. Most will have clear views about risk and how much lifestyle should change
  - Institutionalization does not usually reduce risk

### Preventing adverse consequences of falls

Despite risk reduction, falls may remain likely. In this case, consider:
- *Osteoporosis detection and treatment*
- *Teaching patients how to get up*. Usually by a PT
- *Alarms*, e.g. pullcords in each room or a pendant alarm (worn around the neck/wrist). Often these alert a distant call centre, which summons more local help (home warden, relative, or ambulance)
- *Supervision*. Continual visits to the home (by carers, neighbours, family, and/or voluntary agencies) reduce the duration of a 'lie' post-fall
- *Change of accommodation*. This sometimes reduces risk but is not a panacea. A move from home to a care home may provide a more suitable physical environment, but it will be unfamiliar and staff cannot provide continuous supervision

## Preventing falls in hospital

Falls in hospital are common, a product of admitting acutely unwell older people with chronic comorbidity into an unfamiliar environment.

Multifactorial interventions (such as FallSafe) have the best chance of reducing falls:

- Treat infection, dehydration, and delirium actively
- Stop incriminated drugs and avoid starting them
- Provide good-quality footwear and an accessible walking aid
- Provide good lighting and a bedside commode for those with urinary or faecal urgency or frequency
- Keep a call bell close to hand
- Care for the highest-risk patients in a bay under continuous staff supervision

### Interventions that are rarely effective and may be harmful

- Bedrails (cotsides). Injury risk is substantial—limbs snag on unprotected metal bars and patients clamber over the rails, falling even greater distances onto the floor below
- Restraints. These ↑ the risk of physical injury, including fractures, pressure sores, and death. Also ↑ agitation
- Hip protectors are impact-absorptive pads stitched into undergarments. Evidence of efficacy is limited to care home residents and they cause more falls in community-dwelling trials

## Further reading

Royal College of Physicians. *FallSafe resources*. ℘ http://www.rcplondon.ac.uk/guidelines-policy/fallsafe-resources-original.

# Syncope and presyncope

*Syncope* is a sudden, transient loss of consciousness due to reduced cerebral perfusion. The patient is unresponsive with a loss of postural control (i.e. slumps or falls). *Presyncope* is a feeling of light-headedness that would lead to syncope if corrective measures were not taken (usually sitting or lying down).

These conditions:

- Are a major cause of morbidity (occurring in a quarter of institutionalized older people), recurrent in one-third. Risk of syncope ↑ with advancing age and in the presence of cardiovascular disease
- Accounts for up to 5% of hospital attendances and many serious injuries (e.g. hip fracture)
- Cause considerable anxiety and can cause social isolation as sufferers limit activities in fear of further episodes

## Causes

These are many. Older people with ↓ physiological reserve are more susceptible to most. They can be subdivided as follows:

- *Peripheral factors*. Hypotension may be caused by an upright posture, eating, straining, or coughing, and may be exacerbated by low circulating volume (dehydration), hypotensive drugs, or intercurrent sepsis. Orthostatic hypotension is the most common cause of syncope
- *Vasovagal syncope ('simple faint')*. Common in young and old people. Vagal stimulation (pain, fright, emotion, etc.) leads to hypotension and syncope. Usually, an autonomic prodrome (pale, clammy, light-headed) is followed by nausea or abdominal pain, then syncope. Benign, with no implications for driving. Diagnose with caution in older people with vascular disease where other causes are more common
- *Carotid sinus hypersensitivity syndrome*
- *Pump problem*. MI or ischaemia, arrhythmia (tachy- or bradycardia, e.g. ventricular tachycardia (VT), supraventricular tachycardia (SVT), fast atrial fibrillation (AF), complete heart block, etc.)
- *Outflow obstruction*, e.g. aortic stenosis. PE is also a type of outflow obstruction.

The main differential is seizure disorder where loss of consciousness is due to altered electrical activity in the brain (see ➲ 'Epilepsy', pp. 164–5).

▶ Stroke and TIA very rarely cause syncope, as they cause a focal, not global, deficit. Brainstem ischaemia is the rare exception.

▶ A significant proportion of patients referred to specialist clinics for assessment of 'syncope' or 'blackout' are found not to have lost consciousness, but to have had a fall 2° to gait or balance abnormalities.

## History

The history often yields the diagnosis, but accuracy can be difficult to achieve—the patient often remembers little. Witness accounts are valuable and should be sought.

Ensure that the following points are covered:

- *Situation*—was the patient standing (orthostatic hypotension), exercising (ischaemia or arrhythmia), sitting, or lying down (likely seizure), eating (postprandial hypotension), on the toilet (defecation or micturition syncope), coughing (cough syncope), or in pain or frightened (vasovagal syncope)?

- *Prodrome*—was there any warning? Palpitations suggest arrhythmia; sweating with palpitations suggests vasovagal syndrome; chest pain suggests ischaemia; light-headedness suggests any cause of hypotension. Gustatory or olfactory aura suggests seizures. However, associations are not absolute, e.g. arrhythmias often do not cause palpitations
- *Was there loss of consciousness?*—there is much terminology (fall, blackout, 'funny turn', collapse, etc.), and different patients mean different things by each term. Syncope has occurred if there is loss of consciousness with loss of awareness due to cerebral hypoperfusion; however, many (~30%) patients will have amnesia for the loss of consciousness and simply describe a fall
- *Description of attack*—ideally from an eyewitness. Was the patient deathly pale and clammy (likely systemic and cerebral hypoperfusion)? Were there ictal features (tongue-biting, incontinence, twitching)? Prolonged loss of consciousness makes syncope unlikely. A brain deprived of oxygen from any cause is susceptible to seizure; a fit does not necessarily indicate that a seizure disorder is the 1° problem. Assess carefully before initiating anticonvulsant therapy
- Recovery period—ideally reported by an eyewitness. Rapid recovery often indicates a cardiac cause. Prolonged drowsiness and confusion often follow a seizure

## Examination
Full general examination is required. Ensure that the pulse is examined, murmurs sought, and a postural BP obtained.

## Investigation
- Bloods—check for anaemia, sepsis, renal disease, myocardial ischaemia
- *ECG*—for all older patients with loss of consciousness or presyncope. Look specifically at PR interval, QT interval, trifascicular block (prolonged PR, right bundle branch block (RBBB), and left anterior fascicular block), ischaemic changes, and LVH
- *Other tests* depend on clinical suspicion, e.g. tilt test if symptoms sound orthostatic, but diagnosis is proving difficult (lying and standing BPs will usually suffice; tilt testing is a very labour-intensive test and should not be requested routinely); brain scan and electroencephalogram (EEG) if seizures suspected; prolonged ambulatory ECG monitoring or an implantable loop recorder if looking for arrhythmias

## Treatment
- Treat the cause
- Often not found or multifactorial, so treat all reversible factors
- Review medication (e.g. diuretics, vasodilators, cholinesterase inhibitors, tricyclic antidepressants)
- Education about prevention and measures to abort an attack if there is a prodrome. Advise against swimming or bathing alone, and inform about driving restrictions. (Varies from no restriction to a 6-month ban, depending on the type of syncope; see details at ℘ http://www.dft. gov.uk/dvla/medical/ataglance.aspx)

▶ Transient loss of consciousness (TLOC) may be caused by syncope or seizure.

---

### HOW TO . . . Distinguish syncope and seizures

This is difficult; consider investigation for both. Remember that hypoxia 2°
to syncope can present as fits. Table 5.1 summarizes the key differences.

Table 5.1 Differences between syncope and seizures

|  | Syncope | Seizures |
|---|---|---|
| Risk factors | Past history (heart disease, syncope), cardioactive drugs | Past history (stroke, advanced dementia, seizures), electrolyte disturbance |
| Situation | Heat, prolonged standing, meals, etc. | No associations |
| Onset | Nausea, sweating, light-headedness. Occasionally palpitations, chest pain (indicating dysrhythmia or critical myocardial perfusion) | An aura may occur. A focal seizure may later become generalized |
| During event | Often pale, sweaty, absent, or very weak carotid pulse; low muscle tone. There may be brief (few seconds) seizure activity | Muscle tone may be raised without prominent movement; muscular activity and movement may become very prominent |
| After event | Recovery is usually brisk (few minutes); a brief (minutes) period of confusion may occur. There may be more prolonged (hours) fatigue | Slow recovery to full consciousness, with typically prolonged (minutes to hours) confusion |
| Other | Tongue-biting possible; incontinence possible | Tongue-biting common; lateral bites are more specific; incontinence is common |
| Tests | Abnormal ECG (inappropriate bradycardia, prolonged PR interval, or higher orders of atrioventricular (AV) block; intraventricular conduction delay) | Abnormal CT brain; abnormal EEG |

# Balance and disequilibrium

Balancing is a complex activity, involving many systems.

## Input

There must be awareness of the position of the body in space, which comes from:

- *Peripheral input*—information about body position comes from peripheral nerves (proprioception) and mechanoreceptors in the joints. This information is relayed via the posterior column of the spinal cord to the central nervous system (CNS)
- *Eyes*—provide visual cues as to position
- *Ears*—provide input at several levels. The otolithic organs (utricle and saccule) provide information about static head position. The semicircular canals inform about head movement. Auditory cues localize a person with reference to the environment

## Assimilation

Information is gathered and assessed in the brainstem and cerebellum.

## Output

Messages are then relayed to the eyes, to allow a steady gaze during head movements (the vestibulo-ocular reflex), and to the cortex and the cord to control postural (antigravity) muscles.

When all this functions well, balance is effortless. A defect(s) in any one contributing system can cause balance problems or disequilibrium:

- *Peripheral nerves*—neuropathy is more common. Specifically, it is believed that there is a significant age-related loss of proprioceptive function
- *Eyes*—age-related changes ↓ visual acuity. Disease (cataracts, glaucoma, etc.) is more common
- *Ears*—age-related changes ↓ hearing and lead to reduced vestibular function. The older vestibular system is more vulnerable to damage from drugs, trauma, infection, and ischaemia
- *Joint receptors*—degenerative joint disease (arthritis) is more common in older people
- *CNS*—age-related changes can slow processing. Disease processes (ischaemia, hypertensive damage, dementia, etc.) are more common with age
- *Postural muscles*—sarcopenia (a syndrome of reduced muscle mass with weakness) due to inactivity, disease, medication (e.g. steroids), or intrinsic ageing

In the older person, one or more of these defects will occur commonly. In addition, skeletal changes may alter the centre of gravity, and cardiovascular changes may lead to arrhythmias or postural change in BP, exacerbated further by medications.

## An approach to disequilibrium

- Aetiology is usually multifactorial
- Consider each system separately, and optimize its function
- Look at provoking factors (medication, cardiovascular conditions, environmental hazards, etc.) and minimize them
- Work on prevention:
  - Alter the environment (e.g. improve lighting)
  - Develop safer ways to mobilize, and ↑ strength, stamina, and balance
- Small adjustments to multiple problems can make a big difference, e.g. when appropriate, combine cataract extraction, a walking aid, vascular 2° prevention, a second stair rail, brighter lighting, and a course of PT

▶ If falls persist, despite simple (but multiple) interventions, refer to a falls clinic.

# Dizziness

A brain that has insufficient information to be confident of where it is in space generates a sensation of dizziness. This can be due to reduced sensory inputs or impairment of their integration. Dizziness is common, occurring in up to 30% of older people.

However, the term dizziness can be used by patients and doctors to mean many different things, including:
- Movement (spinning) of the patient or the room—vertigo (see ➜ 'Vertigo', p. 560)
- Disequilibrium or unsteadiness (see ➜ 'Balance and disequilibrium', pp. 110–11)
- Light-headedness—syncope and presyncope (see ➜ 'Syncope and presyncope', pp. 106–8)
- Mixed—a combination of these sensations
- Other, e.g. malaise, general weakness, headache

Distinguishing these is the first step in management, as it will indicate possible causal conditions. This relies largely on the history. Discriminatory questions include:
- 'Please try to describe exactly what you feel when you are dizzy'
- 'Does the room spin, as if you are on a roundabout?' (vertigo)
- 'Do you feel light-headed, as if you are about to faint?' (presyncope)
- 'Does it occur when you are lying down?' (if so, presyncope is unlikely)
- 'Does it come on when you move your head?' (vertigo more likely)
- 'Does it come and go?' (chronic, constant symptoms are more likely to be mixed or psychiatric in origin)

## Causes

The individual conditions most commonly diagnosed when a patient complains of dizziness are:
- Benign paroxysmal positional vertigo (BPPV) (see ➜ 'Vertigo', p. 560)
- Labyrinthitis (see ➜ 'Vertigo', p. 560)
- Posterior circulation stroke (see ➜ 'Vertigo', p. 560)
- Orthostatic hypotension (see ➜ 'Orthostatic (postural) hypotension', pp. 116–7)
- Carotid sinus hypersensitivity
- VBI
- Cervical spondylosis (see ➜ 'Cervical spondylosis and myelopathy', pp. 488–9)
- Anxiety and depression

In reality, much dizziness is multifactorial, with dysfunction in several systems. This means that precise diagnosis is more difficult (and often not done) and treatment is more complex.

▶ Making small improvements to each contributing problem can add up to a big overall improvement (perhaps making the difference between independent living or institutional care).

## HOW TO . . . Manage multifactorial dizziness—clinical example

*History*

Mrs A is 85 and has fallen several times. She complains of dizziness; specifically, she feels 'muzzy in the head', usually when standing. When this occurs, if she sits down promptly, it will pass, but often she does not make it and her legs 'just give way'. She also feels 'muzzy' in bed sometimes when turning over. Past medical history includes hypertension (she takes atenolol 100mg) and osteoarthritis. She lives alone in unmodernized accommodation.

*Examination*

She is thin and has a kyphotic spine. Pulse is 50/min; supine BP is 130/80, falling to 100/70 on standing. There is limited movement at the hips and cervical spine. Neck movement causes unsteadiness.

*Investigations*

Blood tests are normal. ECG shows sinus bradycardia; X-rays show severe degenerative changes of the hip joints and cervical spine, with some vertebral wedge fractures.

*Diagnosis and treatment plan*

This is a multifactorial problem. Some of the relevant factors include:
- Postural instability: caused by arthritis, kyphosis, and low muscle mass
- Presyncope: caused by bradycardia and mild postural drop
- Possibly BPPV
- Extrinsic factors (e.g. poor lighting) are almost certainly contributing

Approach this problem by listing each contributing factor and identifying what can be done to improve it. For example, see Table 5.2.

Table 5.2 Management of dizziness

| Contributing factor | Management |
| --- | --- |
| Osteoarthritis | Optimize analgesia |
| | Consider referral for joint replacement |
| | PT (provision of walking aids; strength and balance training) |
| Kyphosis | Consider bisphosphonate, calcium, and vitamin D to prevent progression |
| | Walking aids will improve balance |
| Low muscle mass | Take a dietary history |
| | Consider nutritional supplements |
| | PT; encourage exercise |
| Bradycardia and postural drop | Consider stopping (or reducing) atenolol |
| | Monitor BP |
| BPPV | Epley's manoeuvre (see ➲ 'HOW TO . . . Perform Epley's manoeuvre', p. 564) |
| Environment | OT review to: |
| | • Provide grab rails and perching stool |
| | • Improve lighting and flooring |
| | • 'De-clutter' the home |

# Drop attacks

This term refers to unexplained falls with no prodrome, no (or very brief) loss of consciousness, and rapid recovery. The proportion of falls due to 'drop attack' ↑ with age.

There are several causes, including:

• Cardiac arrhythmia
• Carotid sinus syndrome (CSS)
• Orthostatic hypotension
• Vasovagal syndrome
• VBI (see Box 5.1)
• Weak legs (e.g. cauda equina syndrome)

The first four causes listed usually lead to syncope or presyncope, with identifiable prior symptoms (e.g. dizziness, pallor); those episodes would not be termed 'drop attacks'. However, such prior symptoms are not universal and may not be recollected, leading to a 'drop attack' presentation.

In most cases, following appropriate assessment, the cause(s) can be identified and effective treatment(s) begun.

▶ Making a diagnosis of 'drop attack' alone is not satisfactory; assess more completely and, where possible, determine the likely underlying cause(s).

## Box 5.1 Vertebrobasilar insufficiency

A collection of symptoms attributed to transient compromise of the vertebrobasilar circulation. There is often associated compromise of the anterior cerebral circulation.

### Symptoms

These arise from functional impairment of the midbrain, cerebellum, or occipital cortex and can include:

- Abrupt-onset, recurrent dizziness or vertigo
- Nausea and/or vomiting
- Ataxia
- Visual disruption (diplopia, nystagmus)
- Dysarthria
- Limb paraesthesiae

### Causes

Impairment of the posterior cerebral circulation leads to VBI:

- Atherosclerosis of vertebral or basilar arteries
- Vertebral artery compression by cervical spine osteophytes (due to degenerative joint disease), at times triggered by neck movement
- Obstructing tumour

### Diagnosis

This is based mainly on the history, supported, if necessary, by investigations. Invasive tests, such as angiography, are very rarely indicated.

- Check for vascular risk factors (see ➔ 'Predisposing factors', p. 180)
- Cervical spine X-ray may show osteophytes, although these are common and very non-specific
- CT brain may demonstrate a tumour or ischaemic change. MRI is more sensitive for posterior circulation ischaemic change
- CT angiography may reveal occlusive vertebral artery disease
- Doppler ultrasound (rarely) to examine vertebral artery flow

### Treatment

- Vascular 2° prevention measures (see ➔ 'Vascular secondary prevention', p. 310)
- Where there is demonstrated posterior circulation stenosis, vessel stenting may be performed in some centres
- Limiting neck movements, if these are a precipitant for symptoms, can be useful. Soft collars can be worn and act mainly as a reminder to the patient to avoid rapid head turns
- There is no evidence that anticoagulants are effective

# Orthostatic (postural) hypotension

Orthostatic hypotension is common. About 20% of community-dwelling and 50% of institutionalized older people are affected.

- An important, treatable cause of dizziness, syncope, near-syncope, immobility, falls, and fracture. Less frequently leads to visual disruption, lethargy, neck ache, or backache
- Often most marked after meals, exercise, at night, and in a warm environment, and abruptly precipitated by ↑ intrathoracic pressure (cough, defecation, or micturition)
- Often episodic (coincidence of precipitants) and covert (ask direct questions; walk or stand the patient and look for it). May occur several minutes after standing

**Diagnosis**

Thresholds are arbitrary. A fall in BP of ≥20mmHg systolic or 10mmHg diastolic on standing from supine is said to be significant. Severity of symptoms often does not correlate well with objective BP change.

**Causes**

- *Drugs* (including vasodilators, diuretics, negative inotropes or chronotropes (e.g. β-blockers, calcium channel blockers), antidepressants, antipsychotics, opiates, levodopa, alcohol)
- *Chronic hypertension* (↓ baroreflex sensitivity and LV compliance)
- *Volume depletion* (dehydration, acute haemorrhage)
- *Sepsis* (vasodilation)
- *Autonomic failure* (pure, diabetes, Parkinson's disease, etc.)
- *Prolonged bed rest*
- *Adrenal insufficiency*
- *Raised intrathoracic pressure* (bowel or bladder evacuation, cough)

**Treatment**

- Treat the cause. Stop, reduce, or substitute drugs incrementally
- Reduce consequences of falls (e.g. pendant alarms)
- Modify behaviour—stand slowly and stepwise; lie down at prodrome
- If still salt- or water-deplete, supplement with:
  - Sodium (liberal salting at table or sodium chloride (NaCl) tablets)
  - Water (oral or intravenous fluids)
- Consider starting drugs if non-drug measures fail:
  - Fludrocortisone (0.1–0.2mg/day)
  - α-agonists, e.g. midodrine (2.5mg three times daily (tds), titrated to a maximum of 40mg/day); unlicensed in the UK; contraindicated in vascular disease
  - Desmopressin 5–20 micrograms nocte, intranasal (used rarely in older patients as causes electrolyte imbalances)
  - In all cases, monitor electrolytes and for heart failure and supine hypertension. Caution if supine BP rises >180mmHg systolic. Dependent oedema alone is not a reason to stop treatment

- The following may help:
  - Full-length compression stockings
  - Head-up tilt to bed (↓ nocturnal natriuresis)
  - Caffeine (strong coffee with meals) or non-steroidal anti-inflammatory drugs (NSAIDs) with extreme caution (→ fluid retention)
  - Erythropoietin or octreotide

# Situational hypotension

### Postprandial hypotension

- Significant when associated with symptoms and fall in BP ≥20mmHg within 75min of meals. A modest fall is normal (and usually asymptomatic) in older people
- Often more severe and symptomatic in hypertensive people with orthostatic hypotension or autonomic failure
- Measure BP before meals and at 30min and 60min after meal. Symptoms and causes overlap with orthostatic hypotension

*Treatment*

- Avoid hypotensive drugs and alcohol with meals
- Lie down or sit after meals
- Reduce osmotic load of meals (small frequent meals, low simple carbohydrates, high fibre/water content)
- Caffeine, fludrocortisone, NSAIDs, and octreotide are used rarely

### Others

- Collapse at initiation or during defecation or micturition are commonly due to hypotension, and a similar management approach should be adopted
- Hypotension in response to cough can also occur—direct management towards reducing cough and optimizing BP

## HOW TO . . . Measure postural blood pressure

1. Lay the patient flat for ≥5min
2. Measure lying BP with a manual sphygmomanometer
3. Stand the patient upright rapidly, if necessary with assistance
4. Check BP promptly (within 30s of standing)
5. While standing, repeat systolic BP measurement continually—at least every 30s for >3min or confirmation of a significant drop
6. Record:
   • Supine BP
   • Nadir of systolic and diastolic BP
   • Symptoms

Note that:

• Lying-to-standing measurements are more sensitive than sitting-to-standing or lying-to-sitting. The latter are sometimes all that is possible for less mobile patients, even with assistance, but sensitivity can be improved by hanging the legs over the side of the bed
• Consider repeat assessment at different times of the day—orthostatic hypotension is more common after a meal and when relatively fluid-depleted (early morning)
• Automatic BP devices should not be used—they cannot repeat measurements rapidly nor track a rapidly changing BP
• Consider referral to a falls clinic for prolonged tilt table testing if symptoms suggest syncope or near-syncope after more prolonged standing

# Carotid sinus syndrome

CSS is episodic, symptomatic bradycardia and/or hypotension due to a hypersensitive carotid baroreceptor reflex, resulting in syncope or near-syncope. It is an important and potentially treatable cause of falls.

CSS is common in older patients and rarely occurs under 50 years. Series report a prevalence of 2% in healthy older people, and up to 35% of fallers >80 years. It is a condition that has been identified recently, and not all physicians are convinced that we fully understand the normal responses of older people to carotid sinus massage or the significance of the spectrum of abnormal results.

Normally, in response to ↑ arterial BP, baroreceptors in the carotid sinus act via the sympathetic nervous system to slow and weaken the pulse, lowering the BP. This reflex typically blunts with age, but in CSS, it is exaggerated, probably centrally. This hypersensitivity is associated with ↑ age, atheroma, and the use of drugs that affect the sinoatrial node (e.g. β-blockers, digoxin, and calcium channel blockers).

## Typical triggers
- Neck turning (looking up or around)
- Tight collars
- Straining (including cough, micturition, and defecation)
- Prolonged standing

Often, however, no trigger is identified.

## Subtypes
- Cardioinhibitory (sinus pause of >3s)
- Vasodepressor (BP fall of >50mmHg)
- Mixed (both sinus pause and BP fall)

## Diagnosis
The diagnosis is made when all three of the following factors are present:
- Unexplained attributable symptoms
- A sinus pause of >3s and/or systolic BP fall of >50mmHg in response to 5s of carotid sinus massage (see ➔ 'HOW TO . . . Perform carotid sinus massage', p. 121)
- Symptoms are reproduced by carotid sinus massage

CSS is often associated with other disorders (vasovagal syndrome and orthostatic hypotension), probably due to shared pathogenesis (autonomic dysfunction). This makes management more challenging.

## Treatment
- Stop aggravating drugs where possible
- Pure cardioinhibitory carotid sinus hypersensitivity responds well to AV sequential pacing, resolving symptoms in up to 80%
- Vasodepressor-related symptoms are harder to treat (pathogenesis is less well understood) but may respond to ↑ circulating volume with fludrocortisone or midodrine (not licensed), as for orthostatic hypotension

## HOW TO . . . Perform carotid sinus massage

1. As this is a potentially hazardous procedure:
   - Perform it in conditions that optimize test sensitivity, e.g. on a tilt table, at a 70–80° tilt, massaging on the right-hand side
   - Ensure that resuscitation facilities are available
2. Check for contraindications—do not perform after recent MI (↑ sensitivity). Concerns about carotid atheroma are probably overplayed; large studies have shown carotid sinus massage to be safe and well tolerated
3. Advise the patient about possible side effects—arrhythmias (most common if taking digoxin) and neurological symptoms (usually transient, occurring in about 0.1% of tests)
4. The patient should be relaxed, with the head turned to the left, lying on a couch with the body resting at 45° (or on a tilt table at 70–80°)
5. Attach the patient to a cardiac monitor with printing facility (to provide documentary evidence of asystole). The fall in BP is usually too brief to be detected by conventional (sphygmomanometric) methods, but continuous ('beat-to-beat') BP monitoring enables the detection of pure vasodepressor CSS
6. Identify the carotid sinus—the point of maximal carotid pulsation in the neck
7. Massage with steady pressure in a circular motion for 5–10s
8. Look for asystole and/or hypotension during massage or shortly (seconds) afterwards
9. If clinical suspicion is high, and the result of right-sided massage is negative, repeat on the left side

# Falls services

The assessment and 2° prevention of falls are multifactorial processes requiring a systematic approach. This is frequently appropriate in 1° and 2° care settings and can be delivered effectively by any trained member of the MDT. More complex cases may benefit from assessment within a specialist setting such as a geriatric or falls clinic.

### Referral criteria

Falls are so common that health services would be swamped if all who had fallen were referred. Instead, refer those with more sinister features suggesting a likelihood of recurrent falls, injury, or an underlying remediable cause. Referral criteria might include:

- Recurrent (≥2) falls
- Loss of consciousness, syncope, or near-syncope
- Injury, especially fracture or facial injury (the latter suggesting poor saving mechanisms or loss of consciousness)
- Polypharmacy (≥4 drugs)

Sources of patients include:

- ED (assess most people with non-operatively managed fractures)
- Acute orthopaedic units (hip and other operatively managed fractures)
- GP or community nurse
- Medical wards
- Self-presenting. Some services advertise directly, via posters and other media

### Service structure

The team structure, diagnostic approach, and delivery of care vary enormously. Falls clinics are often led and delivered by non-physician health professionals such as experienced nurses, OTs, and PTs.

A systematic review of possible contributing factors is essential and will usually include:

- Cardiovascular examination (including postural BP)
- Neurological examination
- Cognitive assessment
- Gait assessment
- Frailty assessment
- Environmental assessment
- Medication review
- Routine bloods (including FBC, U, C+E, haematinics, vitamin D)

Screening for modifiable medical factors should be a routine part of all assessments, with referral to a medical specialist (e.g. GPSI or geriatrician) if such factors are identified.

# Drugs

# Pharmacology in older patients

Perhaps the most common intervention performed by physicians is to write a prescription. Older patients will have more conditions requiring medication; polypharmacy is common.

In the developed world:
- The over 65s typically make up around 14% of the population yet consume 40% of the drug budget
- 66% of the over 65s and 87% of the over 75s are on regular medication
- 34% of the over 75s are on three or more drugs
- Care home patients are on an average of eight medications

Good prescribing habits are essential for any medical practitioner, but especially for the geriatrician.

## Administration challenges include
- Packaging may make tablets hard to access—childproof bottles and tablets in blister packets can be impossible to open with arthritic hands or poor vision
- Labels may be too small to read with failing vision
- Tablets may be large and difficult to swallow (e.g. co-amoxiclav) or have an unpleasant taste (e.g. potassium supplements)
- Liquid formulations can be useful, but accurate dosage becomes harder (especially where manual dexterity is compromised)
- Any tablet needs around 60mL of water to wash it down and prevent adherence to the oesophageal mucosa—a large volume for a frail older person. Some tablets (e.g. bisphosphonates) require even larger volumes
- Multiple tablets, with different instructions (e.g. before/after food) are easily muddled up or taken in a suboptimal way
- Some routes (e.g. topical to back) may be impossible without assistance

## Absorption
- Many factors are different in older patients (↑ gastric pH, delayed gastric emptying, reduced intestinal motility and blood flow, etc.)
- Despite this, absorption of drugs is largely unchanged with age— exceptions include iron and calcium, which are absorbed more slowly

## Distribution
- Some older people have a very low lean body mass, so if the therapeutic index for a drug is narrow (e.g. digoxin), the dose should be adjusted
- There is often an ↑ proportion of fat, compared with water. This reduces the volume of distribution for water-soluble drugs, giving a higher initial concentration (e.g. digoxin). It also leads to accumulation of fat-soluble drugs, prolonging elimination and effect (e.g. diazepam)
- There is reduced plasma protein binding of drugs with age, which ↑ the free fraction of protein-bound drugs such as warfarin and furosemide

## Hepatic metabolism

- Specific hepatic metabolic pathways (e.g. conjugation) are unaffected by age
- Reducing hepatic mass and blood flow can impact on overall function which slows metabolism of drugs (e.g. theophylline, paracetamol, diazepam, nifedipine)
- Drugs that undergo extensive first-pass metabolism (e.g. propranolol, nitrates) are the most affected by the reduced hepatic function
- Many factors interact with liver metabolism (e.g. nutritional state, acute illness, smoking, other medications, etc.)

## Renal excretion

- Renal function declines with age (see ➲ 'The ageing kidney', pp. 382–3), which has a profound impact on the handling of drugs that are predominantly handled renally
- Drugs, or drugs with active metabolites, that are mainly excreted in the urine include digoxin, gentamicin, lithium, furosemide, and tetracyclines
- Where there is a narrow therapeutic index (e.g. digoxin, aminoglycosides), then dose adjustment for renal impairment is required (see Appendix 3 in UK *British National Formulary* (*BNF*))
- Impaired renal function is exacerbated by dehydration and urinary sepsis—both common in older patients

# Prescribing 'rules'

## 1. Is it indicated?

*Treatment of new symptom*

Some symptoms trigger a reflex prescription (e.g. constipation—laxatives; dizziness—prochlorperazine). Before starting a medication, consider:
- What is the diagnosis? (e.g. dizziness due to postural drop)
- Can something be stopped? (e.g. opioid analgesia causing constipation)
- Are there any non-drug measures? (e.g. ↑ fibre for constipation)

*Optimizing disease management*

For example: a diagnosis of cardiac failure should trigger consideration of loop diuretics, spironolactone, ACE inhibitors, and β-blockers.
- Ensure the diagnosis is secure before committing the patient to multiple drugs
- Do not deny older patients disease-modifying treatments simply to avoid polypharmacy
- Do not deny treatment because of potential side effects—while these may impact on functional ability or cause significant morbidity (e.g. low BP with β-blockade in cardiac failure) and need to be discontinued, this should usually be after a trial of treatment with careful monitoring
- Conversely, do not start treatment to improve mortality from a disease if the patient has limited life span for other reasons

*Preventative medication*

For example: BP and cholesterol lowering.
- Limited evidence base in older patients—be guided by biological fitness
- Ensure the patient understands the rationale for treatment

## 2. Are there any contraindications?

- Review past medical history (drug–disease interactions common)
- Contraindications often relative, so a trial of treatment may be indicated, but warn the patient, document risk, and review impact (e.g. ACE inhibitors when there is renal impairment)

## 3. Are there any likely interactions?

- Review the medication list
- Computer prescribing assists with drug–drug interactions, automatically flagging up potential problems

## 4. What is the best drug?

Choose the broad category of drug (e.g. which antihypertensive) by considering which will work best in this patient according to local and national guidelines, which is least likely to cause side effects (e.g. calcium channel blockers may worsen cardiac failure), and if there is any potential for dual action (e.g. a patient with angina could have a β-blocker for both angina and BP control).

Within each category of medication, there are many choices:
- Develop a personal portfolio of drugs with which you are very familiar
- Guidelines and formularies will often dictate choices within hospital

- Cost should be a consideration
- Pharmaceutical companies will try to convince you of the benefits of a new brand. Unless this is a novel class of drug, it is likely that existing brands have a greater proven safety record with similar benefit. Older patients have greater potential to suffer harm from new drugs and are unlikely to have been included in clinical trials. Time will tell if there are real advantages—in general, stick to what you know

▶ Never be the first (or last) of your peers to use a new drug.

## 5. What dose should be started?

- 'Start low and go slow'
- In most cases, benefit is seen with drug initiation, further increments of benefit occurring with dose optimization (e.g. ACE inhibitors for cardiac failure where 1.25mg ramipril is better than 10mg with a postural drop)
- However, do not undertreat—use enough to achieve the therapeutic goal (e.g. for angina prophylaxis, a β-blocker dose should be adequate to induce a mild bradycardia)

## 6. How will the impact be assessed?

Schedule follow-up, looking for:

- Efficacy of the drug (e.g. has bradykinesia improved with a dopamine agonist?). Medication for less objective conditions (e.g. pain, cognition) requires careful questioning of the patient and family/carers
- Any adverse events—reported by the patient spontaneously, elicited by direct questioning (e.g. headache with dipyridamole) or by checking blood tests where necessary (e.g. thyroid function on amiodarone)
- Any capacity to ↑ the dose to improve the effect (e.g. ACE inhibitors in cardiac failure)

## 7. What is the time frame?

- Many older patients remain on medication for a long time; 88% of all prescriptions in the over 65s are repeats; 60% of prescriptions are active for over 2 years, 30% over 5 years, and 6% over 10 years
- This may be appropriate (e.g. with antihypertensives) and if so, the patient should be aware of this and seek an ongoing supply from the GP
- Some drugs should never be prescribed long-term (e.g. prochlorperazine, night sedation)
- Medication should be regularly reviewed and discontinued if ineffective or no longer indicated, e.g. some psychotropic medications (e.g. lithium, depot antipsychotics) were intended for long-term use at initiation, but the patient may have had no psychiatric symptoms for years (or even decades). They can contribute to falls, and cautious withdrawal may be indicated
- An evidence-based comprehensive approach to medication review (e.g. STOPP START v2 criteria) can be useful[1]

---

[1] O'Mahony D, O'Sullivan D, Byrne S, *et al*. STOPP/START criteria for potentially inappropriate prescribing in older people: version 2. *Age Ageing* 2015; **44**: 213–18.

# Taking a drug history

An accurate drug history includes the name, dose, timing, route, duration, and indication for all medication. Studies have suggested that patients will report their drug history accurately around half of the time, and this figure falls with ↑ age.

## Reasons for problems arising
- Inadequate information to the patient at the time of prescribing
- Multiple medications
- Multiple changes if side effects develop
- Use of both generic and brand names
- Variable doses over time (e.g. dopa agonists, ACE inhibitors)
- Cognitive and visual impairment
- Over-the-counter drugs

## Useful sources of information
- The patient's actual drugs—they will often bring them along in a bag to outpatients or when admitted
- Many seasoned patients will carry a list of their current medication—written either by them or a healthcare professional
- Computer-generated printouts of current medications from the GP. Increasingly available via shared electronic networks
- Dosette® and Nomad® systems will incorporate information about the medication they contain
- A telephone call to the GP surgery will yield a list of active prescriptions (but not over-the-counter medication)
- Family members will often know about medication, especially if they help administer them
- Medical notes will often contain a list of medication at the last hospital attendance

These can be extremely useful but have limitations. A prescription issued does not mean that it was necessarily dispensed or that the medication is being taken correctly and consistently. Previously prescribed medications may still be taken and patients may occasionally use another patient's medication (e.g. a spouse).

## Good habits
- Every time a patient is seen (in clinic, day hospital, admission, etc.), take time to review the medication and make an up-to-date list
- Begin correspondence with a list of current medications
- If changes are made, or a new medication tried and not tolerated, document the reason for this, and communicate this to all people involved in care (especially the GP)
- Always include allergies and intolerances in the drug history

## Solutions

- Take the drug history with meticulous care—ask directly about:
  - Inhalers
  - Topical medication (creams, eye drops, patches, etc.)
  - Occasional-use medication
  - Intermittent-use medication (e.g. 3-monthly $B_{12}$ injections, depot antipsychotics, weekly bisphosphonates, etc.)
  - Over-the-counter (non-prescription) medication—a growing number of drugs are available (in the UK, including proton pump inhibitors (PPIs) and statins)
  - Herbal and traditional remedies
- Clarify how often occasional-use medication is taken—analgesia may be used very regularly or not at all
- Be non-judgemental. If you suspect poor concordance (e.g. BP failing to settle despite multiple prescriptions), then the following questions can be useful to elicit an accurate response:
  - 'Have you managed to take all those tablets I suggested?'
  - 'Which tablets do you find useful?'
  - 'Do any of the tablets disagree with you?'—if yes, then 'How often do you manage to take it?'
  - 'What triggers you to remember?' (e.g. take with each meal, leave by toothbrush, etc.)
- Scrutinize computer-generated lists carefully. Remember to look at when the prescription was last issued and estimate when they would be due to run out (e.g. 28 tablets to be taken once a day, last issued 3 months ago means that the drug has either run out or not been taken regularly)
- Pharmacists play an invaluable and ↑ role in 'medicines reconciliation', especially at transitions of care
- The gold standard is to ask the patient to bring in all of the medications that they have at home—both old and new. Go through each medication, and ask them to explain which they take and how often. This allows:
  - Comparison with a list of medications that they are supposed to be taking
  - Old drugs to be discarded (if necessary, retain them and return to pharmacy)
  - Concordance to be estimated (by looking at the date of dispensing and the number of tablets left)
  - Clarification of doses, timings, and rationale for treatment. In a less-pressured setting (e.g. DH), it is useful to generate a list for the patient to carry with them (see Table 6.1, for example)
  - Education of the patient and family where needed (e.g. reason for taking)

**HOW TO . . . Improve concordance/adherence**

*Simplify prescription regimens*
- Convert to once-a-day dosing where possible
- Try to prescribe medications to be taken at the same time of the day—this may challenge firmly held views (e.g. that warfarin must be taken at night)
- Try to use medications that have dual indications for the patient (e.g. β-blockade for both hypertension and angina)
- Consider a daily-dose reminder system (e.g. Dosette® box) or a monitored dosage system (e.g. Nomad®)

*Educate the patient and family*
- Do they understand the reason for taking the medication and how to take it correctly? Are there any problems the patient is attributing to the medication (perhaps incorrectly)?
- Medication summaries (see Table 6.1) can assist with this
- Warn of predictable side effects that are likely to pass (e.g. nausea with citalopram, headache with dipyridamole)
- Promote personal responsibility for medication—this should not be something that the patient feels has been imposed
- Enlist the support of family and carers in monitoring

*Monitor*
- Check tablet boxes and see if they are gone
- Look at how often a repeat prescription has been requested
- Some medications can have serum levels checked (e.g. phenytoin, lithium)

Some medications will produce changes detectable at physical examination (e.g. bradycardia with β-blockade, black stool with iron therapy).

**Table 6.1** Example of a patient drug summary sheet

| Medication | Brand name | Reason | Dose | Morning | Lunch | Evening | Duration |
|---|---|---|---|---|---|---|---|
| Aspirin | | Thins blood, prevents heart attack | 75mg | √ | | | Lifelong |
| Simvastatin | Zocor® | Lowers cholesterol; prevents heart attack | 40mg | | | √ | Lifelong |
| Ramipril | Tritace® | Lowers BP Prevents heart attack | 5mg | | | √ | Lifelong |
| Atenolol | Tenormin® | Lowers BP Prevents angina attacks | 50mg | √ | | | Lifelong |
| Isosorbide mononitrate | ISMO® | Prevents angina attacks | 20mg | √ | √ | | Lifelong |
| Glyceryl trinitrate (GTN) spray | | Treats angina | 1 puff | | | | As needed |
| Amoxicillin | Amoxil® | Antibiotic for chest infection | 500mg | √ | √ | √ | 7 days |

# Drug sensitivity

### Altered sensitivity

Many older patients will have altered sensitivity to some drugs, e.g.:

- Receptor responses may vary with age. Alterations in the function of the cellular sodium/potassium pumps may account for the ↑ sensitivity to digoxin seen in older people. ↓ β-adrenoceptor sensitivity means that older patients mount less of a tachycardia when given agonists (e.g. salbutamol) and may become less bradycardic with β-blockers
- Altered coagulation factor synthesis with age leads to an ↑ sensitivity to the effects of warfarin
- The ageing CNS shows ↑ susceptibility to the effects of many centrally acting drugs (e.g. hypnotics, sedatives, antidepressants, opioid analgesia, antiparkinsonian drugs, and antipsychotics)

### Adverse reactions

Certain adverse reactions are more likely in older people, because of this altered sensitivity:

- Baroreceptor responses are less sensitive, making symptomatic hypotension more likely with antihypertensives
- Thirst responses are blunted, making hypovolaemia due to diuretics more common
- Thermoregulation is blunted, making hypothermia more likely with prolonged sedation

---

#### Drugs that may require dose adjustment in older patients

Despite the variations in drug handling, most drugs have a wide therapeutic index, and there is no clinical impact.

Only drugs with a narrow therapeutic index or where older patients may show very marked ↑ sensitivity may require dose alteration:

- ACE inhibitors
- Aminoglycosides (dose determined by weight, and reduced if impaired renal function)
- Diazepam (start with 2mg dose)
- Digoxin (low-body-weight older patients rarely require >62.5 micrograms maintenance dose)
- Opiates (start with 1.25–2.5mg morphine to assess impact on CNS)
- Oral hypoglycaemics (↑ sensitivity to hypoglycaemia with ↓ awareness—avoid long-acting preparations such as glibenclamide, and start with lower doses of shorter-acting drugs, e.g. gliclazide 40mg)
- Warfarin (load more cautiously)

# Adverse drug reactions

More common and complex with ↑ age—up to three times more frequent in the over 80s. Drug reactions account for considerable morbidity, mortality, and hospital admissions (1 in 25 hospital admissions may result from *avoidable* drug adverse reactions).

Older people are not a homogeneous group, and many will tolerate medications as well as younger ones, but a number of factors contribute to the ↑ frequency:

- *Altered drug handling* and sensitivity occur with age, made worse by poor appetite, nutrition, and fluid intake
- Frailty and multiple diseases make *drug–disease interactions* more common, e.g.:
  - Anticholinergics may precipitate urine retention in a patient with prostatic hypertrophy
  - Benzodiazepines may precipitate delirium in a patient with dementia
- These relationships become even more complex when the *large numbers of drugs* that are prescribed for multiple conditions interact with the diseases, as well as with each other, e.g. an osteoporotic patient is prescribed a bisphosphonate, then sustains a vertebral crush fracture and is given a non-steroidal which exacerbates gastric irritation and causes a gastrointestinal bleed
- *Errors in drug taking* make adverse reactions more likely. Mistakes ↑ with:
  - ↑ age
  - ↑ numbers of prescribed drugs (20% of patients taking three drugs will make errors, rising to 95% when ten or more drugs are taken)
  - Cognitive impairment
  - Living alone

## Strategies to minimize adverse drug reactions

- Consider possible drug–drug and drug–disease interactions whenever a new drug is started
- Some drugs are associated with high rates of drug–drug interactions, e.g. warfarin, amiodarone, SSRIs, antifungals, digoxin, phenytoin, and erythromycin
- For every new problem, consider if an existing medication could be the cause. Try to avoid the so-called *prescribing cascade* where side effects are treated with a new prescription, rather than discontinuing the offending drug. If multiple medications are possible culprits, then stop one at a time and watch for improvement
- Optimize concordance/adherence
- Use extreme caution at times of care transfer—medicines reconciliation is important

# ACE inhibitors

Common indications include BP control, vascular risk reduction, heart failure, and diabetic nephropathy.

## Cautions

*Renal disease*
- Use ACE inhibitors with extreme caution if there is a known history of renal artery stenosis, as renal failure can be precipitated. If the clinical suspicion of this is high (renal bruit, uncontrolled hypertension that is unexplained), then consider investigating for renal asymmetry with an ultrasound before starting treatment
- Renal impairment per se is not a reason to withhold ACE inhibitors (indeed they are effective treatment for some types), although the dose may need to be reduced
- Monitor renal function before and after treatment. Sudden deterioration may indicate renal artery stenosis, and the ACE inhibitor should be stopped pending investigation
- If a patient becomes unwell (dehydrated, septic, etc.), they may need temporary withdrawal of the ACE inhibitor—provide your patient with 'sick day rules'

*Hypotension*
- Older patients are more prone to postural hypotension. Check BP lying and standing, and ask about postural symptoms (e.g. light-headedness)
- The risk of hypotension is greater with volume-depleted patients, e.g. those on high-dose diuretics, on renal dialysis, dehydrated from intercurrent illness, or in severe cardiac failure. Correct dehydration before initiation, where possible
- ACE inhibitor-induced hypotension is common in patients with severe aortic stenosis and, although beneficial in this condition, should be started slowly
- 'Start low and go slow.' Monitor carefully

*Cough*
- Many ACE inhibitors cause a persistent dry cough. Always warn the patient about this, as it can cause considerable distress. Forewarned is forearmed, and many patients will be prepared to accept this side effect if the ACE inhibitor is the best choice for them
- Changing to an angiotensin receptor blocker (ARB) removes the cough in most cases

*Hyperkalaemia*
- There is a risk of hyperkalaemia when ACE inhibitors are used with potassium-sparing diuretics, e.g. spironolactone
- Be aware, and monitor electrolytes. Most tolerate a potassium level of up to 5.5mmol/L
- The tendency to hyperkalaemia can be useful in patients who are also on potassium-losing diuretics (e.g. furosemide), as the two may balance each other out—overall hypokalaemia is more common in patients with heart failure

## HOW TO . . . Start ACE inhibitors

- Screen for contraindications
- Check baseline renal function and electrolytes
- Warn the patient about possible cough and postural symptoms

*An example of initiation/titration is as follows*

*Week 1*

Start ramipril 1.25mg daily.

*Week 2*

Check renal function and BP (lying and standing), and check for postural symptoms. ↑ ramipril to 2.5mg.

*Week 4*

Check renal function and BP (lying and standing) and check for postural symptoms. ↑ ramipril to 5mg at night.

Continue titrating the dose upwards, as tolerated, but most older patients will develop postural symptoms at higher doses, ↑ the risk of falls. The goal should be for safe optimization.

Once established on an ACE inhibitor, periodic renal monitoring is sensible (perhaps annually).

*If a patient becomes acutely unwell*

- Dehydration ↑ susceptibility to ACE inhibitor-induced renal failure and hypotension
- Correct the dehydration first—treat the cause, give fluid supplementation, and stop diuretics
- Temporary cessation of the ACE inhibitor may be needed if dehydration prolonged (>24h)—'sick day rules'
- Monitor renal function daily
- Remember to restart the ACE inhibitor after recovery

# Analgesia

Older patients are more likely to suffer chronic pain than younger ones, owing to the ↑ frequency of conditions such as osteoarthritis, osteoporosis, etc.

Pain management is more challenging, and a standard 'pain ladder' approach is not always useful because of the altered sensitivity of the older patient to certain classes of analgesic medication.

## Non-steroidal anti-inflammatory drugs

Includes aspirin (especially at analgesic doses).

*Potential problems*
- Fluid retention causing worsening hypertension, cardiac failure, and ankle swelling
- Renal toxicity—risk of acute tubular necrosis (ATN), exacerbated by intercurrent infection or dehydration
- Peptic ulceration and gastrointestinal bleeding—there is an ↑ risk with ↑ age, and the bleeds tend to be more significant

▶ The number of older patients requiring hospitalization because of NSAID-induced deterioration in renal or cardiac function actually exceeds the number with gastrointestinal bleeds.
- Age itself is probably not an independent risk factor for most complications of NSAID treatment, but factors such as comorbidities, co-medications, hydration, nutritional status, and frailty are linked to an ↑ risk, all of which are more common with advancing age

*Guidance for use in older patients*
- NSAIDs should be used with extreme caution in older patients and avoided altogether in the very frail
- Should be given for a short period only
- Use low-dose moderate potency NSAIDs (e.g. ibuprofen 0.6g/day)
- Avoid using two NSAIDs together (this includes low-dose aspirin)
- Consider co-prescription of a gastric-protective agent (e.g. omeprazole) for the duration of the therapy
- Avoid using ACE inhibitors and NSAIDs together—they have opposing effects on fluid handling and are likely to cause renal toxicity in combination

## Opioid analgesia

- Wide range of drugs sharing many common features, but with qualitative and quantitative differences
- *Potential problems* include constipation, nausea and vomiting, anorexia, confusion, drowsiness, and respiratory depression

*Guidance for use in older patients*
- Most of these are dose-dependent, and careful up-titration will obtain the right balance of analgesic effect and adverse effects
- Constipation is common (worse in older people) but can be managed with good bowel care
- Most adverse effects are reversible once the medication is reduced or discontinued

## HOW TO . . . Manage pain in older patients

*Diagnose the cause*

Chronic abdominal pain may be due to constipation that will respond to bowel care, rather than analgesia.

*Consider non-drug measures*

- Weight loss and physical activity help with many pains (e.g. arthritis)
- Temperature treatments (e.g. hot/cold packs applied to painful joints)
- TENS machines
- Alternative therapies (e.g. acupuncture, aromatherapy) can help
- Avoidance of (non-essential) activity that provokes pain, if possible

*Consider targeted therapy*

For example: topical capsaicin for post-herpetic neuralgia, local nerve blocks for regional pain, massage for musculoskeletal pain, joint replacement for arthritic pain, or radiotherapy for pain from bony metastases

*Regular paracetamol*

- Well tolerated and with few side effects
- Before moving from this, ensure that the maximum dose is being taken regularly (i.e. 1g taken four times a day (qds)) for optimal analgesic effect. Many patients will find taking an occasional paracetamol ineffective—explain that regular dosing ↑ the analgesic effect

*Opioid analgesia*

- Second-line therapy in most older patients
- Options to deal with mild (e.g. codeine), moderate (e.g. tramadol), and severe pain (e.g. morphine)
- Compound preparations are useful when adding an opioid to regular paracetamol, as it limits the number of tablets taken. Co-codamol (codeine and paracetamol) has variable doses of codeine (8mg, 15mg, or 30mg per tablet), allowing up-titration of the opioid component
- All affect the same receptors, so use as a continuum—if the regular maximum dose of codeine is not working, then step up to the next level of opioid strength
- Various formulations for the delivery of strong opiates. Liquids are useful if there are swallowing problems. Slow-release tablets and transdermal patches provide constant analgesic effect for continuous pain. Be mindful of slow onset of action/accumulation with patch formulation
- Parenteral opiates are used in terminal care (subcutaneous (s/c) injections of morphine and diamorphine for intermittent pain; 24h infusion pumps for constant pain)
- Monitor for side effects—active bowel care with initiation

*Other drug options*

- Very fit older patients can be given short courses of NSAIDs
- Neuromodulators have role in neuropathic pain

*Psychological factors*

- Depression is often coexistent (consequent or causal). Treatment can help with overall pain management
- Informal ('positive mental attitude') and formal psychotherapeutic approaches may be preferable to side effects of analgesic medication

# Steroids

Oral steroids (usually prednisolone) are given for many conditions in older patients, commonly COPD exacerbation, PMR, rheumatoid arthritis, and colitis. Treatment may be long-term. Although the benefits of treatment usually outweigh the risks, awareness of these can minimize harm. Discuss likely side effects with patients and carers.

## Cautions

- *Osteoporosis*—this is most marked in the early stages of treatment. Older people will have diminishing bone reserves anyhow, and all steroid-treated older patients should be offered bone protection at the outset, unless the course is certain to be very short (e.g. <2 weeks). This should consist of daily calcium and vitamin D, along with a bisphosphonate (weekly preparations, e.g. alendronate 70mg, improve concordance)
- Steroids can precipitate *impaired glucose tolerance or frank diabetes*. Monitor sugar levels periodically (e.g. weekly capillary blood sugar or urinalysis) in all steroid users. Steroids worsen control in known diabetics, necessitating more frequent monitoring
- *Hypertension* may develop because of the mineralocorticoid effect of prednisolone, and this should be checked for regularly
- *Skin changes* occur and are particularly noticeable in older patients with less resilient skin. Purpura, bruising, thinning, and ↑ fragility are common
- *Muscle weakness* occurs with prolonged use, predominantly proximal in distribution. This leads to problems rising from chairs, climbing stairs, etc. and may be the final straw for a frail older person with limited physical reserve (see ⊃ 'Muscle symptoms', pp. 480–1)
- There is an ↑ *susceptibility to infections* on steroids, and the presentation may be less acute, making diagnosis more difficult. Candidiasis (oral and genital) is particularly common and should be treated promptly
- High doses (as used in the treatment of giant cell arteritis (GCA)) can cause *acute confusion and sleep disturbance*, and older people are particularly prone. Give steroids in the morning, if possible
- *Cataracts* may develop with long-term steroid use. If vision declines, look for cataracts with an ophthalmoscope and consider specialist referral
- *Peritonitis may be masked* by steroid use—the signs being less evident clinically. Have a higher index of suspicion of occult perforation in a steroid-treated older patient with abdominal pain. There is also an association between steroid use and peptic ulceration, particularly in hospitalized patients
- Adrenocortical suppression means that the *stress response will be diminished* in chronic steroid users. If such a patient becomes acutely unwell (e.g. septic), the exogenous steroid dose will need to be temporarily ↑ (e.g. double the usual oral dose, replace with intramuscular (im) hydrocortisone if unable to take by mouth). Counsel the patient with 'sick day rules'. Suppression can continue for months after stopping chronic steroids; have a low threshold for 'covering' acute illness

## Stopping treatment

Many patients are on fairly low doses of steroids for a long period. It can be difficult to completely tail the dose, as steroid withdrawal effects (fevers, myalgia, etc.) can often be mistaken for disease recurrence, and this often needs to be done very slowly (perhaps reducing by as little as 1mg a month). There is no such thing as a 'safe' dose of steroid so, for every patient you see on steroids, ask the following:

- Can the dose be reduced?
- Could a steroid-sparing agent (e.g. azathioprine) be used instead?
- Is the patient taking adequate bone protection?
- What is the BP and blood glucose?

# Warfarin

Common indications range from absolute (PE, DVT, artificial heart valve replacement) to relative (stroke prophylaxis in AF). Increasingly direct oral anticoagulants (DOACs) are being used instead, but warfarin remains in common use.

## Cautions
- Risk is ↑ if the patient is unable to take medications reliably, so it is not suitable without supervision for cognitively impaired patients or those who self-neglect. If there is an absolute indication, then consider supervised therapy (by spouse, family, or carers via a dispensing system) or (rarely) a course of low-molecular-weight heparin instead
- Risk is higher if there is a high probability of trauma, e.g. recurrent falls
- Excess alcohol consumption is associated with poor concordance and falls. Liver enzymes are induced, making control of anticoagulation more difficult. Highly variable intake is especially problematic
- Comorbidity may ↑ sensitivity to warfarin (e.g. abnormal liver function, congestive cardiac failure) and should be screened for
- GPs will often be good judges of risk—consider discussing borderline cases

## Side effects
- Bleeding is the major adverse event, ranging from an ↑ tendency to bruise to major life-threatening bleeds. The most significant include intracerebral haemorrhage and gastrointestinal blood loss.
  - Warfarin does not cause gastric irritation but may accelerate blood loss from pre-existing bleeding sources. Ask carefully about history of non-steroidal use (including aspirin) and gastrointestinal symptoms (upper and lower). If any are present, then quantify the risk with further testing—FBC and iron studies might indicate occult blood loss. If warfarin is not essential, then a full gastrointestinal work-up may be appropriate before starting in fitter patients
  - Nosebleeds are common in older patients and may become more significant on warfarin. Often due to friable nasal vessels that are amenable to treatment by ENT surgeons, so reducing the risk of epistaxis on warfarin

### Reassessment of risk/benefit balance
- Patients often take warfarin for many years
- During that time, there is usually a change in both the risk (serious bleeding) and the benefit (reduced thromboembolism) of anticoagulation. The most common scenario is that the antithrombotic benefit of anticoagulation remains but that the bleeding risk ↑ and cannot be reduced, e.g. a patient falls frequently despite intervention or has a major bleed that could recur (e.g. diverticular)
- Any drug must be stopped, unless there is a net benefit to the individual patient. In conjunction with the patient (and carer), the indication for warfarin should be reviewed periodically, perhaps annually in frail older people and after any significant event, e.g. hip fracture

## Usual target international normalized ratio

(See Table 6.2.)

**Table 6.2** Target international normalized ratios (INRs)

| Indication | Target INR | Duration |
|---|---|---|
| AF | 2.5 | Lifelong |
| Venous thromboembolism (VTE) | 2.5 | Varies. Usually 6 months. Lifelong if recurrent or with ongoing precipitant (e.g. malignancy). Shorter duration if identifiable precipitant and high bleeding risk |
| Recurrent VTE while on warfarin | 3.5 | Lifelong |
| Mechanical prosthetic heart valves | 3.5 | Lifelong |

## What to do when the INR is too high

- Always look for the reason why the INR became elevated, and correct this factor
- If there is no sign of bleeding, then stop warfarin and monitor the INR as it falls
- If the INR >8 but there is no bleeding, a small dose of vitamin K (0.5–2.5mg) can be given to partially reverse the INR
- Do not give vitamin K routinely, as control of anticoagulation will be made more difficult for weeks afterwards
- If there is bleeding, then warfarin needs reversing with vitamin K and fresh frozen plasma
- For life-threatening bleeds (e.g. intracerebral haemorrhage), prothrombin complex concentrate can be used for rapid reversal

▶ If a patient bleeds at target INR, always consider the possibility of an underlying serious disease, e.g. bladder or gastrointestinal malignancy.

## Further reading

*British National Formulary.* Oral anticoagulants section. ℘ http://ww.bnf.org.

### HOW TO . . . Initiate warfarin

Discuss the risks and benefits of treatment with the patient—the indication is rarely absolute.

*Ensure the patient is told*
- There will be frequent blood tests and monitoring
- Many medications interact with warfarin, so before taking any new medication (including over-the-counter), always check compatibility with the doctor, dentist, or pharmacist
- Use paracetamol or codeine-based analgesia (never NSAIDs)
- Alcohol interacts with warfarin metabolism and should be taken in moderation and on a regular basis (avoid binge drinking)
- Vitamin K-containing foods (e.g. spinach) should not have variable intake
- If trauma occurs, bleeding may last longer. Apply pressure to wounds, and seek medical help if it does not stop
- Give the patient an anticoagulant treatment book that will hold details of their treatment schedule and reinforce the information that you give them

*Induction*
- Check baseline clotting
- Prescribe warfarin to be taken at 6 p.m.
- Medical notes should state the indication, target INR, and duration of therapy
- The normal adult induction dose (10mg day 1, 10mg day 2, then an INR) is rarely appropriate in older patients who are more sensitive to its effects
- Reduce the dose if the patient is frail, has a low body weight, has multiple comorbidities, or has deranged baseline clotting
- For most older patients, 5mg/5mg/INR is a safer approach
- If there are multiple factors causing concern, then 5mg/INR is better

▶ There is no rush. If the indication is absolute, then the patient should also be on therapeutic heparin until the INR is in range. It is much easier to ↑ the dose of warfarin than to deal with bleeding from an overdose.
- The INR will then need checking daily, then on alternate days until a pattern becomes clear
- Many haematology departments will offer automatic dosing with a schedule for retesting
- The INR testing can gradually be done less frequently, stretching to 12-weekly in long-term users
- Induction in hospital is now often done by anticoagulation teams

# Direct oral anticoagulants

This class of drugs (DOACs) is also known as novel/new oral anticoagulants (NOACs) and is increasingly being used in place of warfarin as evidence of non-inferiority emerges.

## Compared to warfarin, the main advantages are

- Immediate onset of action
- No need for INR monitoring
- Reduced rates of bleeding (especially intracerebral)
- No food or alcohol interactions

## The main disadvantages include

- Harder to reverse—although short duration of action means that the drug clears from the system quickly, and reversal agents are in development
- Dose needs adjustment for renal impairment
- Some agents require twice-daily dosing
- Short duration of action means that any missed doses render the patient unanticoagulated
- Less familiar medications, and prescribers should note numerous drug interactions with commonly used drugs (e.g. tramadol, clarithromycin)
- Limited long-term outcome data, particularly in the older patient
- Not licensed for metallic heart valve thromboprophylaxis
- Higher cost

## When to use?

- Patients who have been stable on warfarin should not be changed
- Patients in whom it is unacceptable/very difficult to monitor INR, or who have an unstable INR, would be good candidates for a DOAC
- When initiating anticoagulation, discuss options with patients and be guided by local policy

▶ If a patient is not a candidate for warfarin, it is unlikely they will be 'safe' on a DOAC, and careful risk/benefit analysis is always needed (e.g. a frequent faller will be no safer on a DOAC than on warfarin).

# Proton pump inhibitors

PPIs (e.g. omeprazole, lansoprazole) are very effective in reducing gastric acid secretion and therefore in treating peptic ulcers and gastro-oesophageal reflux disease (GORD). They are perceived as very safe drugs but are not without problems. The combination of effectiveness and safety has led to them being one of the most commonly prescribed drug classes. However, PPIs are often prescribed without an appropriate indication, or are initiated appropriately but not discontinued after a treatment course. Overall, over 50% of PPI use is unnecessary.

## Side effects

- Common side effects are headache, nausea, diarrhoea, and constipation
- Infrequent idiosyncratic reactions include acute interstitial nephritis, erythema multiforme, pancreatitis, and microscopic colitis
- Hyponatraemia and hypomagnesaemia can occur—consider checking in non-specific presentations
- Hydrochloric acid aids protein digestion and absorption of vitamin $B_{12}$ and calcium and is active against pathogens. PPI use is associated with:
  - Community and hospital incidence of CDAD and ↑ likelihood of recurrence
  - Enteric bacterial infections (e.g. *Salmonella, Campylobacter*)
  - Community- and hospital-acquired pneumonia
- Long-term use is associated with higher rates of hip fracture, possibly caused by altered calcium absorption

## Interactions

There are a few important interactions:
- The effects of phenytoin and warfarin are enhanced
- The effects of clopidogrel are reduced
- Plasma concentrations of digoxin are ↑ slightly

## Appropriate prescribing

- Always specify the indication for treatment and its intended duration
- In GORD, always first address non-drug factors (obesity, alcohol), and consider the use of less potent acid suppression (e.g. H2 antagonists such as ranitidine)
- Transient dyspepsia or occasional heartburn are inadequate indications for long-term PPI treatment
- In 1° care, review the need for the drug periodically
- In 2° care, be careful not to extend an initial appropriate PPI prescription for prophylaxis against gastrointestinal bleeding
- When antibiotics are prescribed in hospital, suspend the PPI prescription to reduce the risk of CDAD
- In (confirmed or possible) CDAD, stop PPIs

### HOW TO . . . Manage drug-induced skin rashes

Common side effect in older patients—thought to be due to altered immune function. Rarely life-threatening but cause considerable distress.

*Make the diagnosis*

- Variable in appearance, but most commonly toxic erythema— symmetrical, erythematous, itchy rash, trunk > extremities, lesions may be measles-like or urticarial, or resemble erythema multiforme
- Certain drugs may produce predictable eruptions:
  - Acneiform rash with lithium
  - Bullous lesions with furosemide
  - Target lesions with penicillins and phenytoin
  - Psoriasis-like rash with β-blockers
  - Urticaria with penicillin, opiates, and aspirin
  - Fixed drug eruption (round, purple plaques recurring in the same spot) with paracetamol, laxatives, sulfonamides, and tetracyclines
- Toxic epidermal necrolysis is a rare, serious reaction to drugs such as non-steroidals, allopurinol, and phenytoin. The skin appears scalded, and large areas of the epidermis may shear off, causing problems with fluid and electrolyte balance, thermoregulation, and infection
- Take a careful drug history to elicit a temporal relationship to medication administration, e.g. within 3 days of starting a new drug (may be as long as 3 weeks) or becoming worse every morning after a regular drug is given

*Stop the drug*

- Stop multiple medications one at a time (stop drugs started closest to the onset of the rash first), and watch for clinical improvement
- May get slightly worse before improving
- Usually clears within 2 weeks
- Advise the patient to avoid the drug in the future

*Soothe the skin*

- Emollients, cooling agents (e.g. calamine), and weak topical steroids may help
- Oral antihistamines are often given, with variable success. Sedating antihistamines (e.g. hydroxyzine) may help sleep

*Treat the complications*

- More likely if extensive and prolonged
- Risks include:
  - Hypothermia
  - Hypovolaemia
  - 2° infection

▶ Consider dermatology referral if not improving after 2 weeks off the suspected drug.

# Herbal medicines

Use of herbal supplements by older adults is common (some studies estimate 30–50%). Most patients do not discuss this with their doctors, so remember to ask. Herbal medicines are not regulated like drugs, contain variable quantities of active ingredients, and may contain impurities. Herbal medicines have adverse effects and drug interactions (see Table 6.3).

Table 6.3 Overview of herbal medicines

| Name | Use | Adverse effects | Drug interactions |
|------|-----|-----------------|-------------------|
| Garlic | Hypertension High cholesterol Antiplatelet | Bleeding Gastrointestinal upset Hypoglycaemia | NSAIDs Antiplatelets Anticoagulants |
| Ginkgo | Memory problems | Seizures Bleeding Headaches Dizziness Gastrointestinal upset | NSAIDs Antiplatelets Anticoagulants Monoamine oxidase inhibitors (MAOIs) Trazodone |
| Ginseng | Performance enhancer | Hypertension Tachycardia | NSAIDs Antiplatelets Anticoagulants |
| Glucosamine/ chondroitin | Osteoarthritis | Nausea Diarrhoea Heartburn | Hypoglycaemic agents (reduced efficacy) |
| St John's Wort | Antidepressant Anxiolytic | Nausea Allergy Dizziness Headache Photosensitivity | Cytochrome P450 drugs Anticoagulants Antivirals SSRIs Statins |
| Echinacea | Immune stimulant | Allergy Hepatitis Asthma Vertigo | Immunosuppressants |
| Valerian | Anxiety Insomnia | Sedation | CNS depressants |
| Saw palmetto | Prostatic symptoms | Constipation Diarrhoea ↓ libido Hypertension Urinary retention | Finasteride |

# Breaking the rules

A great deal of prescribing in geriatric practice relies on individually tailored assessment and pragmatic decision-making, as inter-individual variation ↑ with age. In addition, trials often exclude older subjects, making the evidence base an extrapolation. While what is described in the preceding pages is appropriate for many, there are times when 'rules must be broken' in the best interests of the individual patient. This requires careful consideration of risks and benefits; the patient should usually be reviewed to assess the impact of the decision.

Polypharmacy can cause problems but is sometimes appropriate—depriving patients of beneficial treatments because they are old, or already on multiple other medications, can also be wrong. In a recent study of medication changes during a geriatric admission, the total number of drugs was the same at admission and discharge, but they had often been changed. In other words, there was active evaluation of medications going on—the goal being not just to limit the number of drugs, but also to optimize and individually tailor treatment.

Where side effects are very likely, but the drug is definitely indicated, then it may be appropriate to co-prescribe something to treat the expected adverse effect, e.g.:
- Steroids and bisphosphonates
- Opiates and laxatives
- Furosemide and a potassium-sparing diuretic (or an ACE inhibitor)
- Non-steroidals and a gastric protection agent

While certain disease–drug interactions are very likely and should be avoided, others may be an acceptable risk. For example:
- β-blockers:
  - Are to be used with caution with asthma, yet they have such a good impact on cardiovascular risk reduction that these cautions are not absolute. Often 'asthma' is, in fact, COPD with little β-receptor reactivity, so cautious β-blockade initiated in hospital while monitoring the lung function may be appropriate
  - In patients with peripheral vascular disease, they can cause a small reduction in walking distance, but this risk is usually outweighed by the reduction in the risk of cardiac death
- Fludrocortisone (for postural hypotension) will worsen supine hypertension and cause ankle swelling. But if postural symptoms are severe, then it may be appropriate to accept hypertension and the associated risk
- Amlodipine may worsen ankle swelling in a patient with chronic venous insufficiency, but if this is the best way of controlling hypertension, it may be appropriate to accept a cosmetic problem

# Neurology

# The ageing brain and nervous system

As in other systems, intrinsic ageing (occurs in all) is often hard to distinguish from extrinsic ageing mechanisms (caused by disease processes). See → 'Cognitive ageing', p. 202 for discussion of cognitive ageing.

Histological changes in the brain include:
• Each neuron has fewer connecting arms (dendrites)
• Around 20% of brain volume and weight are lost by the age of 85
• There is deposition of pigment (lipofuscin) in the cells and oxidative damage in mitochondria
• The presence of senile plaques and neurofibrillary tangles ↑ with age, but they are not diagnostic of dementia (see Table 7.1)

Table 7.1 Age-related changes to the nervous system

| Age-related change | Consequence |
| --- | --- |
| Loss of neurons (cannot be regenerated)<br>↓ in brain weight (by around 20% at age 85) | Cerebral atrophy common on brain scans (although this does not correlate well with cognitive function) |
| Some neurons become demyelinated and have slowed nerve conduction speed and ↑ latency (time taken to recover before transmitting next impulse) | Reflexes which have long nerve tracts, e.g. ankle jerks, can be diminished or lost<br>Minor sensory loss, e.g. fine touch/vibration sense, may be lost distally |
| Neurotransmitter systems alter, e.g. cholinergic receptors ↓ | ↑ susceptibility to some neuromodulating drugs |
| ↑ frequency of periventricular white matter changes seen on cerebral imaging | Probably not a normal finding.<br>Significance unclear—assumed to be representative of small-vessel vascular disease, but poor post-mortem correlation |

# Tremor

Tremor is more common with ↑ age. It can be disabling and/or socially embarrassing. It is important to try to make a diagnosis, as treatment is available in some cases.

Examine the patient first at rest and distracted (relaxed with arms supported on the lap, count backwards from 10), then with outstretched hands, and finally during movement (pointing or picking up a small object). Tremors fall roughly into three categories:

1. *Rest tremor*—disappears on movement and is exaggerated by movement of the contralateral side of the body. Most common cause—Parkinson's disease. It is usually associated with ↑ tone
2. *Postural tremor*—present in outstretched limbs, may continue during action but disappears at rest. Most common cause—benign essential tremor
3. *Action tremor*—exaggerated with movement. When the tremor is maximal at extreme point of movement, it is called an intention tremor. Most common cause—cerebellar dysfunction

## Benign essential tremor

- The classic postural tremor of old age, worse on action (e.g. static at rest but spills tea from teacup), may have head nodding (titubation) or jaw/vocal tremor, legs rarely affected. May be asymmetrical
- About half of the cases have a family history (autosomal dominant)
- Presents in middle age, occasionally earlier, and worsens gradually
- Often more socially embarrassing than physically impairing
- Improved by alcohol, gabapentin, primidone, and β-blockers, but these are often unacceptable treatments in the long term. Worth considering β-blockers as the first choice in treatment with coexistent hypertension
- Weighted wristbands can reduce tremor and improve function

## Parkinson's disease

See ➲ 'Parkinson's disease: presentation', pp. 156–7.

## Cerebellar dysfunction

The typical intention tremor is associated with ataxia.
- *Acute* onset is usually vascular in older patients
- *Subacute* presentations occur with tumours (including paraneoplastic syndrome), abscesses, hydrocephalus, drugs (e.g. anticonvulsants), hypothyroidism, or toxins
- *Chronic* progressive course is seen with:
  - Alcoholism (due to thiamine deficiency—always give thiamine 100mg once daily (od) orally (po) or iv preparation if in doubt; it might be reversible)
  - Anticonvulsant (e.g. phenytoin—may be irreversible if severe, more common with high plasma levels but can occur with long-term use at therapeutic levels)
  - Paraneoplastic syndromes (anti-cerebellar antibodies can be found, e.g. anti-Yo and anti-Hu found in cancer of the ovary and bronchus)
  - Multiple sclerosis
  - Idiopathic cerebellar atrophy
  - Many cases defy specific diagnosis. Consider multisystem atrophy

## Other causes of tremor

(See Table 7.2.)

Table 7.2 Other causes of tremor

| Diagnosis | Recognition and characteristics | Management |
|---|---|---|
| Thyrotoxicosis | Fine resting tremor<br>This is actually more common in younger patients | See ➲ 'Hyperthyroidism: drug treatment', pp. 442–3 |
| Rigors | Sudden-onset coarse tremor with associated malaise and fever | Diagnose and treat underlying cause |
| Asterixis (tremor and incoordination) with hepatic, renal, or respiratory failure | Coarse postural tremor in a sick patient with physiological disturbance<br>A less dramatic, often fine, tremor can occur with metabolic disturbance such as hypoglycaemia or hypocalcaemia | Diagnose and treat underlying condition |
| Drug withdrawal, e.g. benzodiazepines, SSRIs, barbiturates | Always consider when patient develops tremor ± confusion soon after admission | For therapeutic drugs, recommence and consider gradual controlled withdrawal at later date |
| Alcohol withdrawal | Always take an alcohol history. Tremor ± confusion develops soon after admission | Consider treatment with, e.g. chlordiazepoxide and thiamine |
| Drug side effects, e.g. lithium, anticonvulsants | | Check serum levels are in therapeutic range. Consider a different agent |
| Anxiety/stress—↑ sympathomimetic activity | Fine tremor | Rarely necessary to consider β-blockers |
| Orthostatic tremor—rare, benign postural tremor of legs | Fine tremor of legs on standing, diminished by walking/sitting. Can palpate muscle tremor in legs. Patient feels unsteady but rarely falls | Provide perching stools, etc. to avoid standing for long |

# Neuropathic pain/neuralgia

This describes pain originating from nerve damage/inflammation. It is often very severe and debilitating and seems to be more common in older people. The pain is usually sharp/stabbing and is often intermittent, being precipitated by things like movement and cold.

## Post-herpetic neuralgia

- Severe burning and stabbing pain in a division of nerve previously affected by shingles
- Shingles and subsequent persisting neuralgia is much more common in older patients
- Pain may be triggered by touch or temperature change
- May go on for years, be difficult to treat, and have major impact on quality of life
- Prevent by vaccination to reduce risk/severity of shingles
- If shingles develops, starting antivirals within 72h reduces neuralgia incidence

See ➔ 'HOW TO . . . Treat neuralgia', p. 155 for treatment.

## Trigeminal neuralgia

- Severe unilateral stabbing facial pain, usually V2 and V3, rather than V1
- Triggers include movement, temperature change, etc.
- Time course—years with relapse/remission
- Depression and weight loss can result
- Differential diagnoses include temporal arteritis (TA), toothache, parotitis, and temporomandibular joint arthritis
- Consider neuroimaging, especially if bilateral or if there are physical signs, i.e. sensory loss or other cranial nerve abnormality suggestive of 2° trigeminal neuralgia

See ➔ 'HOW TO . . . Treat neuralgia', p. 155 for treatment.

## Neuralgia can also occur with

- Malignancy
- Cord compression
- Neuropathy

## HOW TO . . . Treat neuralgia

This can be very debilitating, and treatment is difficult. There is often coexistent depression, so always think of this and treat appropriately.

*Simple measures include*
- Distraction
- Relaxation techniques
- Allaying fears (usually about a serious underlying pathology)
- Acupuncture
- Heat/cold treatment
- Osteopathy/massage (to reduce associated muscle spasm)
- Use of TENS machines
- Support groups, e.g. ✍ http://www.tna.org.uk

*Medications*
- Topical treatments, e.g. lidocaine, capsaicin
- Traditional analgesics (paracetamol, NSAIDs, opiates), although these are usually not very effective
- Anti-spasticity drugs, e.g. baclofen. Used especially in trigeminal neuralgia, they treat any muscle spasm that exacerbates the pain

*Mainstay of treatment* is the neuromodulating drugs which may give superior pain control but often have important side effects.
   Examples include:
- Antidepressants with neuroadrenergic modulating abilities, e.g. amitriptyline, duloxetine. Start with a low dose and titrate up slowly. Eventual doses may be similar to those used in younger patients
- Anticonvulsants, e.g. gabapentin, pregabalin (post-herpetic neuralgia) or carbamazepine, oxcarbazepine, valproate (trigeminal neuralgia). Start with a low dose and titrate up slowly

The main side effects from these drugs are sedation and confusion, and reaching a therapeutic dose may be limited by this problem.

*Other options*
- Nerve blocks or spinal stimulation, which can usually be accessed via a specialist pain clinic
- Surgery, e.g. nerve decompression, or treatment with heat or lasers. May provide relief but can result in scarring and numbness

# Parkinson's disease: presentation

A common idiopathic disease (prevalence 150/100 000) associated with inadequate dopamine neurotransmitter in the brainstem. There is loss of neurons and Lewy body formation in the substantia nigra. The clinical syndrome is distinct from Lewy body dementia (see ➲ 'Dementia and parkinsonism', pp. 212–13 for treatment), but they are extremes of a clinical spectrum of disease.

## Presentation

The clinical diagnosis of Parkinson's disease is based on the UK Parkinson's disease brain bank criteria and should include:
• *Bradykinesia* (slow to initiate and carry out movements, expressionless face, fatigability of repetitive movement)

Plus at least one of the following:
• *Rigidity* (cogwheeling = tremor superimposed on rigidity)
• *Tremor* ('pin-rolling' of hands—worse at rest)
• *Postural instability*

Other clinical features:
• Gait disorder (small steps)
• Usually an asymmetrical disease
• No pyramidal or cerebellar signs, but reflexes are sometimes brisk
• Non-motor symptoms are common and should be asked about (see ➲ 'Non-motor symptoms of Parkinson's disease', p. 156)

## Non-motor symptoms of Parkinson's disease

• Depression (treat appropriately)
• Anosmia (may be an early pre-motor feature)
• Psychosis (may relate to medications; avoid typical antipsychotics, as they may worsen the motor features; atypicals such as quetiapine can be tried)
• Dementia and hallucinations can occur in late stages, but drug side effects can cause similar problems. If features suggest Lewy body dementia, a trial of anticholinesterases may be warranted
• Sleep disturbance (treat restless legs; review medications; advise about driving if sudden-onset sleep; daytime hypersomnolence may be treated with modafinil)
• Falls (usually multifactorial; see ➲ 'Assessment following a fall', pp. 102–3)
• Autonomic features are common in older patients. They should be sought and actively managed:
  • Weight loss
  • Dysphagia
  • Constipation
  • Erectile dysfunction
  • Orthostatic hypotension
  • Excessive sweating
  • Drooling

**Investigations**

- Diagnosis is clinical and, once suspected, should be reviewed by a Parkinson's disease specialist
- Trials of treatment may be done, with review of the diagnosis if there is no improvement, but single-dose levodopa 'challenge' tests are no longer performed
- Brain imaging (e.g. CT) can be used to illustrate other conditions that may mimic Parkinson's disease (e.g. vascular disease)
- Specialist scans are becoming more widely used to assist diagnosis (e.g. consider $^{123}$I-FP-CIT single-photon emission computed tomography (SPECT), commonly known as DatSCAN™ after the radiolabelled solution used). Patients with essential tremor, Alzheimer's disease, or drug-induced Parkinsonism have normal scans

# Parkinson's disease: management

Should be overseen by a Parkinson's disease specialist clinic.

## Drugs

It is not possible to identify a universal first-choice drug therapy for either early Parkinson's disease or adjuvant drug therapy for later stages.

Consider the short- and long-term benefits and risks of each treatment, along with lifestyle and clinical factors. Discussion with the patient is key.

*Initiation treatment* is started with one of the following:

- *Levodopa plus a decarboxylase inhibitor* (prevents peripheral breakdown of drug) (co-beneldopa/co-careldopa). Start low and titrate to symptoms
- *Dopamine agonists* (ropinirole, pramipexole, rotigotine). Psychiatric side effects, postural hypotension, and nausea may limit therapy
- *MAOI* (selegiline, rasagiline). These drugs have many interactions with antidepressants and should be used with care by a specialist

*Adjuvant treatment* may be needed as the disease progresses. Firstly, ↑ doses or add a second agent from the list already given; then consider:

- *Catechol-O-methyltransferase (COMT) inhibitor* (entacapone). Will smoothe fluctuations in plasma levodopa concentrations. Must be given with levodopa. Stains urine orange
- *Amantadine*—weak dopamine agonist which can reduce dyskinetic problems
- *Apomorphine*—s/c injections. Specialist treatment—rarely useful in older patients

*Anticholinergics* (trihexyphenidyl, orphenadrine) are mild antiparkinsonian drugs, rarely useful in elderly patients due to severe psychiatric side effects. They do have a beneficial effect on tremor and are possibly the drug of choice where tremor is more of a problem than bradykinesia.

## Surgery

Ablation (e.g. pallidotomy) and stimulation (electrode implants) used in highly selected populations. Older patients often excluded due to high operative risk and rigorous exclusion criteria (e.g. cognitive impairment).

## Other therapeutic options

- Patients and carers benefit from regular review by a specialist doctor or nurse. Many services now have specialist Parkinson's disease nurses
- A course of PT can be helpful to boost mobility and reduce falls
- OT plays a vital role in aids and adaptations for disability
- SALTs, along with dieticians, can help when swallowing becomes a problem
- Inpatient assessment is rarely helpful, as hospital routines can rarely match home treatment and some patients deteriorate in hospital
- Parkinson's UK (⌂ http://www.parkinsons.org.uk) has plenty of information and advice for patients and carers

**HOW TO . . . Manage a patient with Parkinson's disease who cannot take oral medication**

This situation arises quite commonly in advanced disease during a hospital admission.

A patient with advanced disease admitted for another reason (e.g. sepsis) may miss an oral dose of medication (e.g. because they are unwell or because the drug is not immediately available). In some, this will be well tolerated; in others, there will be a rapid decline in function and loss of swallow, with a downward spiral unless promptly managed.

Other situations in which oral medication may not be possible:
- Perioperatively when the patient is nil by mouth
- When an ileus or other cause makes poor drug absorption likely
- After a stroke

▶ Omission of medication will (for most patients with Parkinson's disease) lead to a decline in function, so continuation of treatment is key.

*Reducing the risk*
- Plan ahead—patients should be educated about the importance of taking medication on time and to always bring their own medication with them if they come into hospital and be encouraged to self-medicate where possible
- If surgery is elective, then get specialist advice about medication as part of the pre-operative assessment. Aim for local or regional anaesthesia, if possible
- Have protocols in place for the urgent care of Parkinson's disease patients
- Ensure that wards have Parkinson's disease drugs readily available; involve pharmacy colleagues

*Early action*
- Use nasogastric tubes (NGTs) early if swallow is impaired
- Relax nil by mouth rules pre-operatively for Parkinson's disease drugs
- Use antiemetics (not metoclopramide) when vomiting

*Medication*
- Use a different preparation, e.g. levodopa dispersible down an NGT, buccal selegiline
- Use an enteral preparation, e.g. apomorphine (s/c delivery) or rotigotine (patch delivery). Advice will be needed from a specialist about doses that are equivalent to their usual medication, but a rough rule of thumb is that 100mg levodopa daily is replaced by a 2mg/24h rotigotine patch

## HOW TO . . . Treat challenging symptoms in Parkinson's disease

See Table 7.3.

Table 7.3 Treatment of challenging symptoms in Parkinson's disease

| Problem | Solutions |
|---|---|
| *Wearing off*—improvement gained from a dose of medication does not last until the next dose begins to take effect | Due to disease progression. Patients require higher or more frequent dosing to produce the same effect; use drugs from different classes; try COMT inhibitors |
| *Dyskinesias* | Reduce dopaminergic drug dose if possible. Add amantadine |
| *Motor fluctuations* with choreodystonic 'on' phases and freezing 'off' phases. These worsen with duration of treatment | Reduced levodopa dose more frequently (dose fractionation); controlled-release preparations; add entacapone; add dopamine agonist |
| Other drug *side effects* (confusion and hallucinations, constipation, urinary retention, and nausea and vomiting) are a particular problem in elderly patients and often limit treatment to sub-ideal levels | Treat hallucinations by reducing PD medications if possible, or adding rivastigmine or quetiapine<br><br>Domperidone is the best antiemetic, but use has been restricted due to concerns about arrhythmia |
| In general, *patients prefer dyskinetic side effects* than 'off spells'—relatives/carers may find the opposite easier to cope with, especially if patient confused or falling when 'on' | Ensure you talk to the patient as well, even if it is easier to talk to the carer. Compromise may be necessary |
| *Quantifying response* to treatment is very difficult | Get patients/carers to fill in a 24h chart. A formal quantified drug trial by therapists can be very helpful |
| *Morning stiffness* | Use a rapid-acting drug (e.g. Madopar® dispersible) in bed on waking, or try a long-acting drug last thing at night |
| *End-stage disease* | Ultimately drug responsiveness so poor and side effects so marked that ↓ and withdrawing therapy may be appropriate. Palliative treatment and social support important |
| *Drooling* | Use anticholinergic inhalers, atropine eye drops, or botulinum toxin injections. Hyoscine patches may cause hallucinations |

## Impulse control disorders

- Defined as failure to resist an impulse, drive, or temptation to perform an act that is harmful to the person or others
- Tend to occur after the initiation of dopaminergic therapy in those who are susceptible, and abate with dose reduction

Examples include:
- Hypersexuality (see ➲ 'Sexual function', pp. 530–1)
- Pathological gambling
- Compulsive buying
- Aimless wandering
- Repetitive activities (e.g. arranging objects)
- Dopamine dysregulation syndrome (addictive use of dopaminergic drugs in a Parkinson's disease patient with other impulse control behaviours)

## Further reading

Brennan KA, Genever RW. Managing Parkinson's disease during surgery. *BMJ* 2010; **341**: 990–3.
National Institute for Health and Care Excellence (2006). *Parkinson's disease in over 20s: diagnosis and management*. Clinical guideline CG35. ℗ http://www.nice.org.uk/cg35.

# Diseases masquerading as Parkinson's disease

The majority of slow, stiff, or shaky older patients on geriatric wards do not have true Parkinson's disease (see Table 7.4). As many as one in two diagnoses of Parkinson's disease made by non-specialists are incorrect. It is important to get the diagnosis right or you will subject patients needlessly to the harmful side effects of medications. Coexistence of more than one syndrome can further complicate the diagnosis.

- *Atherosclerotic pseudo-parkinsonism/multi-infarct dementia*: due to neurovascular damage—consider in those with stroke/TIA or with atherosclerotic risk factors, e.g. hypertension. Short-stepping, wide-based unstable gait with relative preservation of arm and facial movements (lower body parkinsonism). Head scan may show lacunae or white matter change
- *Benign essential tremor*: often inherited (autosomal dominant), worse on action (spills tea from teacup), improved by alcohol and β-blockers, may have head nodding or vocal tremor
- *Lewy body dementia*: Lewy bodies are widely present throughout the cortex, not predominantly in the substantia nigra as with true Parkinson's disease. Psychiatric symptoms, e.g. visual hallucinations, tend to precede physical ones
- *Drug-induced parkinsonism*: neuroleptics are the most common cause, but remember that prochlorperazine for dizziness and metoclopramide for nausea are also causes. Some irritable bowel treatments contain neuroleptics
- *Other causes*: Alzheimer's disease, hydrocephalus, and even severe polyarthritis can sometimes cause diagnostic confusion. Rare differential diagnoses include Wilson's disease, Pick's disease, carbon monoxide poisoning, multiple head injuries (ex-boxers), and post-encephalitis or anoxic brain injury

## Parkinson's plus syndromes

This is a confusing array of rare disorders, including:

- *Multisystem atrophy* (aka Shy–Drager syndrome, olivopontocerebellar atrophy) with early autonomic failure (incontinence and postural instability), ataxia, parkinsonism, and pyramidal signs. Cognition intact
- *Progressive supranuclear palsy* (aka Steele–Richardson–Olszewski disease) with up- and downgaze palsy, axial rigidity and falls, dysarthria and dysphagia, and frontal lobe dementia
- *Corticobasilar degeneration* with asymmetrical ataxia, dementia, and speech/swallow disturbance

**Table 7.4** Clues to distinguish Parkinson's disease clinically

|  | True Parkinson's disease | Pseudo-parkinsonism (especially atherosclerotic) |
|---|---|---|
| Response to levodopa | Good<br>Develop dopa dyskinesias | Poor or transient<br>Dopa dyskinesias unusual |
| Age of onset | 40–70 | 70+ |
| Tremor | Unilateral or asymmetrical<br>Resting tremor prominent | Absent or mild |
| Progression | Slow progression/long history | Rapid progression |
| Dementia | Only at late stage | Prominent or early |
| Instability/falls | Late | Early and prominent |
| Dysphonia, dysarthria, or dysphagia | Late | Early and prominent |
| Other neurology (pyramidal signs, downgaze palsy, cerebellar signs) | Rare | Common |

# Epilepsy

1° epilepsy most commonly presents at around the time of puberty, but the incidence of new fits is actually higher in the over 70s (>100 per 100 000) because of the ↑ amount of 2° epilepsy (caused by, e.g. brain ischaemia, subdural haematomas, brain tumours).

In addition, fits can be precipitated by:
- Metabolic disturbance (e.g. hyponatraemia, hypoglycaemia)
- Drugs (e.g. ciprofloxacin)
- Infection (at any site, but particularly meningitis/encephalitis)
- Withdrawal from alcohol or drugs such as benzodiazepines
- Wernicke's encephalopathy (due to thiamine deficiency in malnourished, e.g. alcoholics)

Many of these conditions are more common in older patients who also have a lower fit threshold for any given level of stimulus.

## Diagnosis

(See also ➲ 'Syncope and presyncope', pp. 106–8.)
- An eyewitness account is the most useful diagnostic tool
- Look particularly for post-event confusion/drowsiness which is rare in cardiac syncope
- The classic features of prodrome, tongue-biting, and incontinence are not so useful in distinguishing cardiac from neurological syncope in older patients
- Remember that cerebral hypoperfusion from any cause (e.g. bradycardia) can cause fits, so epilepsy can coexist with other causes of syncope. In these cases, treatment of the 1° syncope/hypoperfusion is more effective than antiepileptics (see ➲ 'HOW TO . . . Distinguish syncope and seizures', p. 108)

## Investigations

- Routine blood screening, CXR, and ECG to look for precipitants and differential diagnoses
- Lactate and creatine kinase (CK) are often elevated after a generalized seizure
- CT scan is vital to exclude a structural lesion
- EEGs can be helpful when positive but very commonly have non-specific changes and low sensitivity, i.e. a normal EEG does not rule out epilepsy

## General management

- Ensure the patient is not taking medication that lowers the fit threshold (check the *BNF*—common examples include tricyclics, ciprofloxacin, tramadol, and phenothiazines. Think about over-the-counter drugs, e.g. Ginkgo biloba, St John's Wort)
- Correct any metabolic derangement (e.g. glucose, sodium, sepsis)
- Advise about driving restrictions—do not assume they do not drive
- Detect and treat complications, e.g. aspiration, trauma, pressure injuries

## Driving regulations and epilepsy

You have a duty to ensure that the patient informs the Driver and Vehicle Licensing Agency (DVLA). If you have reason to believe that the patient has not done so, then your duty to inform the DVLA yourself (after informing the patient of your intention) outweighs confidentiality concerns.

Patients have at least a 6-month ban on driving for a first fit (unless a 'provoked fit', e.g. following brain surgery or stroke, when it may be a shorter period—individual decision). They can then reapply for a licence as long as they remain fit-free. Patients must also refrain from driving for 6 months after withdrawing epilepsy medication.

Further information is available at ℘ https://www.gov.uk/government/organisations/driver-and-vehicle-licensing-agency.

### Epilepsy and stroke

*Onset seizures* (within a week, most commonly within 24h) occur in 2–5% of strokes. More common with haemorrhages, large cortical strokes, and venous infarction. Consider also alcohol/drug (especially benzodiazepine) withdrawal for early fits. Long-term anticonvulsants not usually prescribed unless fits recur.

*After the first week*, stroke remains a risk factor for new epilepsy—first year 5% fit, subsequently 1.5% annual incidence. Many such patients develop transient neurological worsening (Todd's paresis) or permanent worsening without CT evidence of new stroke—in these patients, it is usually worth considering long-term anticonvulsants.

Epilepsy may occur 2° to clinically 'silent' cerebral ischaemia, and 3% of patients with stroke have a past history of fits, most occurring in the preceding year. Some epilepsy experts suggest that aspirin is prescribed for new-onset seizures in an elderly patient once structural lesions have been excluded.

# Epilepsy: drug treatment

## Acute treatment

- Start with benzodiazepines (5–10mg rectal or 2–10mg iv diazepam, or 0.5–2mg lorazepam iv or im)
- If fits continue, consider setting up a loading-dose infusion of phenytoin (use a cardiac monitor) or iv levetiracetam until oral medication can be taken
- Rarely the patient may need intubating and paralysing to stabilize them or to allow an urgent CT scan

## Chronic treatment

- Because of side effects and long duration of treatment, most doctors will resist starting anticonvulsants until after a second fit, especially if the diagnosis is unclear or if there is a reversible precipitant. Presence of an underlying structural abnormality or wishing to return to driving may tip the balance in favour of treatment
- The choice of agent shows regional and personal variation
- Most commonly used agents are similarly effective
- Older agents include phenytoin, carbamazepine (both effective but may be sedative), and valproate (better tolerated, but plasma levels are unhelpful in monitoring compliance or side effects)
- Newer agents such as lamotrigine and levetiracetam are 'cleaner' and increasingly used as first line
- All anticonvulsants have significant side effects, e.g. sedation, confusion, rash, tremor, and ataxia. Serious liver, blood, and pulmonary side effects can also occur—ongoing monitoring to optimize dose and minimize side effects is necessary
- Many anticonvulsants interact with each other, as well as other drugs, and can ↑ toxicity or reduce effectiveness—if in doubt, consult a pharmacist. Gabapentin and pregabalin are less likely to interact with other medications and can be useful alternatives, especially if their pain-relieving properties are also desirable
- If a known epileptic presents with fits in the context of a new precipitant (e.g. sepsis), then short-term use of clobazam can aid control until the precipitant has been treated
- Avoid abrupt withdrawal of antiepileptics—fits may be provoked
- Partial seizures (e.g. face/arm twitching) are rarely dangerous and often distress bystanders more than the patient, but they can progress to 2° generalized seizures. The same drugs can be employed. Partial seizures often indicate structural lesions and an early CT scan is advisable
- Sometimes a trial of anticonvulsants in patients with recurrent unexplained collapse can be revealing
- Refer to an epilepsy specialist if control is proving difficult and multiple drugs are required

# Neuroleptic malignant syndrome

A rare, but important, syndrome in patients taking neuroleptics (e.g. haloperidol, chlorpromazine, risperidone) with a triad of:
- Fever
- Rigidity and tremor
- Rhabdomyolysis with 2° renal failure (see ➲ 'Rhabdomyolysis', p. 507)

▶ Can be fatal (up to 30%), so early recognition is important.

## Diagnosis

May arise at any time during treatment, i.e. the patient may have recently:
- Started (most common) or stopped neuroleptics
- ↑ the dose or been stable on them for a long time
- Added a second drug, e.g. tricyclic antidepressant, lithium

Reintroduction of the offending drug at a later date may not reproduce symptoms. Contributing factors such as intercurrent illness and metabolic derangement may be important in the aetiology.

## Clinical features

- The patient looks unwell with fever, severe lead-pipe rigidity, bradykinesia, occasionally tremor, and ↓ conscious level
- Time course: onset usually over 1–3 days, starts with rigidity/altered mental state
- Seizures and abnormal neurological signs can occur
- Autonomic dysfunction causes sweating, tachycardia, and hypertension
- Multiorgan failure can occur; there is leucocytosis, and CK levels may be over 1000IU/L
- Lumbar puncture, CT scan, and EEG are often required to exclude other diagnoses such as CNS infection

▶ The most common cause of a similar presentation is sepsis in a patient with pre-existing cerebrovascular disease; CK measurement will aid the diagnosis.

## Management

Stop all neuroleptics. Cooling using paracetamol, fans, and damp sponging. iv fluids with careful monitoring of electrolytes and renal function. Dantrolene (direct muscle relaxant) can speed recovery. Short-term dialysis is sometimes required. Bromocriptine is used in some cases, although there is limited evidence for efficacy.

Early transfer to the intensive care unit may be wise—death most commonly occurs by hypoventilation/pneumonia or renal failure. There are sometimes persisting neurological sequelae.

## Serotonin syndrome

A similar syndrome to neuroleptic malignant syndrome in patients taking serotonin reuptake inhibitors, especially if combined with tramadol, a tricyclic, or an MAOI. Patients tend to be agitated and delirious, rather than unconscious. Gastrointestinal symptoms (diarrhoea/vomiting) occur. Onset may be within 2h; resolution is usually quicker than neuroleptic malignant syndrome.

# Motor neuron disease

A progressive idiopathic disease with selective degeneration of motor neurons causing weakness and wasting. There is a variety of manifestations, depending on the site of damage; the most common site for lesions is in the anterior horn cells of the spinal cord (lower motor neuron (LMN)), but the descending motor pathway (upper motor neuron (UMN)) may be affected in the corticospinal tracts, brainstem, and motor cranial nuclei.

▶ The combination of weakness and fasciculations should always prompt consideration of motor neuron disease (MND).

- Onset rises steeply with age, with a peak incidence in late 50s/early 60s. Very rare before age 40. Overall prevalence of 7 per 100 000, but incidence of 1 per 10 000 at age 65–85
- Underdiagnosed in older patients (confused with cerebrovascular disease, myasthenia, cervical myelopathy, motor neuropathy, syringomyelia, and paraneoplastic syndromes)
- Slightly more common in ♂
- 5% will have a family history (autosomal dominant is the most common but can be recessive or X-linked)

## History

- Weakness, cramps, and fatigue in limbs. Weakness usually begins in a focal area and spreads to contiguous muscles; onset in the upper limbs is the most common
- Palatal and vocal cord paralysis can cause stridor, dysarthria, dysphagia, and aspiration pneumonia
- Paresis of respiratory muscles can cause respiratory failure (may present to chest physicians/intensive therapy unit (ITU))
- Intellect, sensation, and continence are usually retained. Some forms associated with frontotemporal dementia (<5%); depression common

## Examination

- Look for wasting with fasciculations (LMN), especially in the tongue, shoulders, and legs. ▶ Fasciculations may be a normal finding in the hands and calves of older people
- Head drop/droop can occur
- Brisk reflexes, clonus, and upgoing plantars (UMN). This is one condition that can cause absent ankle jerks and upgoing plantars
- Atrophy and weakness are less specific signs
- 'Donald Duck' speech
- Sensory changes should make you question the diagnosis

## Investigations

- CK may be elevated
- CT, MRI, and muscle biopsy are usually normal
- Electromyography (EMG) shows denervation of muscles caused by anterior horn cell degeneration and is diagnostic

## Clinical pictures

Diverse presentations and rate of progression, including:

- Amyotrophic lateral sclerosis (ALS) is the most common form—classical picture of mixed UMN and LMN. Term used commonly in the USA
- Progressive pseudobulbar or bulbar palsy—speech and swallow predominantly affected
- 1° lateral sclerosis—UMNs predominantly affected
- Progressive muscular atrophy—LMNs predominantly affected

## Treatment

- *Riluzole* (sodium channel blocker) 50mg twice daily (bd). Prolongs survival by a few months, but not function. Licensed and endorsed by National Institute for Health and Care Excellence (NICE) for ALS only. Expensive and should be initiated by a specialist. Monitor liver function, and check for neutropenia if febrile illness

*Supportive*

- Chest—antibiotics and PT, tracheostomy, and non-invasive nocturnal ventilation (for diaphragmatic palsy and sleep apnoea)
- Speech—early referral to speech therapy for communication aids
- Nutrition—initially pureed food and thickened fluids. Malnutrition and aspiration are indications to consider artificial feeding (see ➋ 'Nutrition', pp. 354–5)
- Muscle spasm—baclofen, PT
- Mobility/independence—OT for wheelchairs and adaptations
- Pain/distress—opiates or benzodiazepines (but beware respiratory suppression)

*Other*

- This is a devastating diagnosis to give to a patient—the mean life expectancy is 2–5 years. Matters are often worse because there is often a considerable delay between symptoms and a concrete diagnosis being made (sometimes the initial diagnosis may have been incorrect). Emphasize the retention of cognition and aspects of supportive care available. Offer regular follow-up appointments
- Specialist neurology/MND nurses are available in some areas
- Refer to Motor Neurone Disease Association for support
- Consider enduring power of attorney and advance directives (ADs)

## Further reading

Motor Neurone Disease Association. ⌘ http://www.mndassociation.org.

# Peripheral neuropathies

Some minor degree of sensory loss in the feet and reduced or absent ankle jerks is so common in older patients (up to 50% of over 85 year olds) that some class this as a normal ageing change, but remember:

- Even mild, asymptomatic neuropathies can contribute to postural instability and falls
- The diagnosis is often missed because of non-specific symptoms and insidious onset with slow progression

## Clinical features

- There may be signs of LMN weakness with wasting and loss of reflexes
- Sensory loss often with joint position and vibration loss before touch and pain. This is classically in a 'glove and stocking' distribution, rather than dermatomal (see ➔ Appendix, 'Dermatomes', p. 700)
- Neuralgia-type pain may be present (especially diabetes and alcohol) (see ➔ 'HOW TO . . . Treat neuralgia', p. 155)
- Autonomic failure and cranial nerve involvement can also occur
- Severe cases may affect respiration

## Classification

Try to determine if the signs are focal or generalized and whether they are predominantly sensory or motor because this can help identify the likely underlying pathology. Further classification by pathology (axonal or demyelinating) requires nerve conduction studies or biopsy.

The most common pattern produces widespread symmetrical sensory loss (typically glove and stocking). This may be combined with distal muscle weakness (mixed motor and sensory neuropathy) or sometimes there is a pure motor neuropathy. Where signs are focal, consider mononeuritis multiplex.

## Causes

The causes are legion and often multiple in older patients. Idiopathic neuropathies are very common (25% defy diagnosis in most studies). The following list is not exhaustive:

- Diabetes
- Paraneoplastic syndromes (e.g. small cell lung cancer)
- Alcoholism (often combined with vitamin deficiency)
- Renal failure
- $B_{12}$ or folate deficiency
- Guillain–Barré syndrome (the most common acute onset)
- Chronic inflammatory demyelinating polyradiculoneuropathy (rare autoimmune motor neuropathy, considered the chronic counterpart of Guillain–Barré)
- Hypothyroidism
- Carpel tunnel syndrome
- Vasculitides (e.g. Wegener's granulomatosis)
- Drugs (e.g. isoniazid, nitrofurantoin, amiodarone, colchicine)
- Paraproteinaemias and amyloid

## Investigations

- Always check B$_{12}$, glucose, TFTs, serum and urine immunoglobulins, ESR, and CRP before labelling a neuropathy idiopathic
- Look carefully for an occult tumour (e.g. breast examination, iron studies, CXR)
- Family history
- Nerve conduction studies will confirm nerve damage and distinguish demyelination from axonal damage (which sometimes helps with the differential diagnosis), but they are not always required in straightforward cases
- Further specialist tests include immunology, tumour markers, lumbar puncture, molecular genetics tests, and nerve biopsy

## Treatment

The important thing is to identify reversible causes quickly, but even treatable causes rarely respond dramatically—the aim is usually prevention of further deterioration. Chronic inflammatory polyradiculoneuropathy is treated by steroids, plasma exchange, and iv immunoglobulins, but most other chronic neuropathies have no specific treatment. Supportive and symptomatic treatment (e.g. appropriate footwear, analgesia, environmental adaptation) is important.

### Guillain–Barré syndrome

This is an acute inflammatory demyelinating polyneuropathy.
- Causes *ascending paralysis*, weakness beginning in the feet and hands and migrating towards the trunk
- It can cause life-threatening complications, particularly if the *respiratory muscles* are affected or if there is *dysfunction of the autonomic nervous system*
- The disease is usually triggered by an acute infection

This is a medical emergency which responds to iv immunoglobulins or plasmapheresis. These patients can deteriorate rapidly and should be managed in conjunction with specialist neurology units. Even patients who look well should have their vital capacity measured daily to warn of impending respiratory failure.
▶ The main hurdle is recognizing the diagnosis.

# Subdural haematoma

A condition which is much more common in old age because as the brain shrinks, the veins which lie between it and the skull are much more likely to get torn following trauma (even minor injury). Older people are also more likely to have falls/head injuries and are more frequently on predisposing drugs (e.g. aspirin, warfarin, NOACs). Other risk factors include alcoholism, epilepsy, and haemodialysis.

## Features

▶ Subdurals frequently present with very non-specific symptoms in frail confused patients. A high index of suspicion is required.

- Subdurals can occur acutely (and present within hours of an accident) or more slowly as the classical 'chronic subdural haematoma', although this distinction does not help guide management
- A history of head injury occurs in only about half
- Common features include drowsiness and confusion (rarely fluctuating), postural instability, progressive focal neurology (e.g. hemiparesis, unequal pupils), headache, and blurred vision
- Rarely transient neurology (mimicking TIA) or parkinsonism can occur
- Some patients are asymptomatic and large collections can be incidental findings
- Examine for papilloedema, focal neurology, and long tract signs

## Diagnosis

- CT head scan—look for crescent-shaped haematoma compressing the sulci (hypodense/black is old blood; hyperdense/white indicates recent bleeding) and midline shift
- All patients who have new UMN signs with confusion and/or drowsiness should be scanned
- It is harder to decide when to scan a confused patient without such signs—most agree it is reasonable to look for other causes of acute confusion before asking for a head scan, as long as the patient is being observed for any change in neurological signs or conscious level
- Have a lower threshold for scanning patients on antiplatelets/anticoagulants and for those who have evidence of falls, particularly facial bruising. MRI can be useful when CT changes are subtle (an isodense phase occurs on CT in transition between hyperdense and hypodense changes) or very small haematomas are suspected

## Management

Decisions are usually made in conjunction with the local neurosurgical team (although in practice, only about one-third of patients will end up having surgery).

Stop antiplatelet agents/NOACs, and reverse warfarin therapy if possible.

Observation and supportive care are frequently used in:

- Asymptomatic patients
- Those with small bleeds who are stable/improving
- Those not fit for transfer/surgery

When conservative management is adopted, record the conscious level (GCS; see ⮱ Appendix, 'Glasgow Coma Scale', p. 710) and any focal neurology at least daily or if there is any change. Any deterioration should prompt a repeat CT scan and reconsideration of surgery.

Burr hole surgery is not complex and is done under local anaesthetic. Recovery after surgery can be dramatic. Complications include re-bleeding and seizures. Use symptoms (especially conscious level), not CT appearance, to decide on surgery. Mortality is around 10%—highest with a depressed conscious level and bilateral haematomas. Those left with residual neurology should receive rehabilitation as in stroke.

# Sleep and insomnia

With ↑ age, less sleep is needed (~1h less than young adults); the circadian rhythm is less marked, and sleep becomes more fragmented with greater difficulty getting to sleep. Deep (stages 3 and 4) sleep is reduced, but dreaming sleep/rapid eye movement (REM) is preserved.

Insomnia is a symptom which correlates poorly with observed actual sleep time (i.e. patients who complain of poor sleep may be observed by nurses/family to sleep well, while those who sleep very little do not necessarily complain). It can be very distressing and is associated with ↑ morbidity and mortality. Around 25% of elderly people have chronic insomnia—even higher rates with psychiatric and medical conditions. Insomnia is a particular problem in an unfamiliar noisy ward environment, and doctors are often under considerable pressure to prescribe hypnotics.

## Treatment of insomnia

First ensure that *underlying causes* are looked for and treated:
- Pain at night—consider using analgesics with sedative side effects, e.g. opiates
- Nocturnal urinary frequency, e.g. due to polyuria, peripheral oedema, prostatism
- Comorbidities, e.g. orthopnoea, oesophageal reflux, Parkinson's disease
- Depression/anxiety—very common and use of an antidepressant will improve sleep much better than a hypnotic
- Alcohol dependence
- Drugs—corticosteroids, omeprazole, phenytoin, amiodarone, sulfasalazine, atorvastatin, ramipril, as well as psychiatric drugs, e.g. paroxetine, haloperidol, and chlorpromazine, can cause insomnia. β-blockers and levodopa cause nightmares

The following *non-pharmacological interventions* (sleep hygiene) can be tried:
- Reduce or stop daytime 'catnapping'
- Avoid caffeine, heavy meals, and alcohol in the evening (alcohol helps to fall asleep but reduces sleep quality)
- Use a bedtime routine
- Ensure the environment is dark, quiet, and comfortable
- Relaxation and cognitive behavioural techniques can be useful
- Try warm milky drinks
- Manage expectations—older people will rarely sleep as much or well as younger people

*Drugs*

- Benzodiazepines (e.g. temazepam 10mg) are licensed for short-term (<4 weeks) management of insomnia and anxiety. They do work well when used correctly (see ➜ 'HOW TO . . . Use benzodiazepines for insomnia', p. 175)
- The newer Z-drugs (e.g. zopiclone, zolpidem) are only for insomnia. They have shorter half-lives and fewer side effects (although zopiclone is still a cause of daytime drowsiness). Overall they are probably slightly superior to benzodiazepines, but the same cautions about dependence apply
- Other hypnotics (e.g. chloral hydrate, clomethiazole, antihistamines) can be toxic, especially in overdose, and provide no major advantages
- A new class of drugs that act on melatonin pathways may be beneficial

---

### HOW TO . . . Use benzodiazepines for insomnia

Tolerance develops after only 4 weeks (i.e. benzodiazepines fail to produce a useful sedative effect). However, it takes only this long for dependence to occur. Dependence may be physical (with rebound insomnia, anxiety, or even delirium) and/or psychological (the patient believes they will not be able to sleep without tablets). The shorter the half-life, the greater the withdrawal effects. Benzodiazepine use has been associated with ↑ falls, reduced functional status, road traffic collisions, depression, and memory impairment.

Although awareness of these problems has reduced the number of long-term benzodiazepine users, there is still over-prescribing.

*Prevention of dependence*

- Do not use benzodiazepines for mild or non-distressing insomnia—try non-pharmacological measures first
- Never prescribe benzodiazepines for >4 weeks
- Never prescribe benzodiazepine medication at discharge from hospital
- All patients/carers should receive warnings about benzodiazepine side effects (especially dependence) and the reason for limiting the course length at the outset
- GPs should limit repeat prescriptions and audit their practice

*Treatment of dependence*

- Explain and motivate the patient/carers
- Gradual reduction regimen
- In difficult cases, switch to an equivalent dose of diazepam first—long half-life produces milder withdrawal symptoms
- Continuing support
- Occasionally acute withdrawal is undertaken by mistake (e.g. drug accidentally not prescribed for a couple of weeks during acute admission with a fractured neck of femur). In these cases, do not automatically restart the benzodiazepines and do explain why to the patient or they will just restart it when they return home

# Other sleep disorders

### Hypersomnolence

This is excessive daytime sleepiness despite a normal night of sleep. Causes include brain disease (e.g. dementia, stroke), cardiopulmonary disease (e.g. cardiac failure, COPD), obstructive sleep apnoea, hypothyroidism, narcolepsy, and sedative drugs.

### Restless legs syndrome

A common (10% older people) unpleasant sensation in the limbs which ↑ with drowsiness and is eradicated by movement. Can be associated with limb jerking during sleep with sleep disturbance. Both symptoms respond to benzodiazepines. Check they are not iron-deficient (replacement can be curative). Treat with dopamine agonists.

### Circadian rhythm disorders

Jet lag is the best known, but advanced sleep phase syndrome (sleepiness occurs too early in the evening, but there is early morning wakening) and delayed sleep phase (sleepiness comes too late at night) can occur without such a precipitant. Treat by gradually altering bedtime and bright light therapy when wakefulness is desired.

### Sleep apnoea in older patients

Obstructive sleep apnoea and central sleep apnoea are very common in older patients and can contribute to daytime sleepiness, accidents, and heart failure. Unfortunately, periods of apnoea are less likely to be symptomatic than in the young and where symptoms do exist, they are often multifactorial, so diagnosis and compliance with therapy (non-invasive positive pressure ventilation) can be problematic.

### REM sleep behaviour disorder

Dream-enacting behaviour during REM sleep, occurring because of a lack of muscle atonia that usually accompanies REM sleep. About half will go on to develop neurological pathology, e.g. Parkinson's disease, Lewy body disease. Treatment with benzodiazepines may be successful.

**Further reading**

Harbison J. Sleep disorder in older people. Age Ageing 2002; **31**: 6–9.

# Stroke

# Definition and classification

## Definition

*Stroke* is the sudden onset of a focal neurological deficit, lasting >24h or leading to death, caused by a vascular pathology.
- Infarction: emboli, in situ thrombosis, or low flow
- Haemorrhage: spontaneous (not associated with trauma). Excludes subdural and extradural haematomas but includes spontaneous subarachnoid haemorrhage

*Transient ischaemic attacks* (TIAs) are focal neurological deficits (including monocular visual loss) due to inadequate blood supply that last <24h (in reality, most TIAs last just minutes).

Infarction and TIAs have the same pathogenesis, and the distinction is likely to become less helpful with time. Both stroke and TIA need urgent treatment, as it is impossible to distinguish TIA from stroke in the first few minutes and hours. Waiting to see if the focal neurology resolves causes neuronal loss at a rate of 1.9 million per minute. It is useful to think of a spectrum of disease severity from TIA to fatal stroke where early intervention to save brain tissue has parallels with approaches to myocardial salvage in coronary syndromes.

## Stroke burden

- Incidence of first stroke is about 200 per 100 000 per year
- Prevalence is around 5–12 per 1000 population, depending on the age of the sample
- It is a disease of older people (over two-thirds of cases occur in the over 65s; <15% occur in under 45s)
- Globally it is the second most common cause of death
- In England and Wales, it accounts for 12% of all deaths and is the most common cause of severe disability among community dwellers

## Classification

Various methods including:
- *Infarct or haemorrhage*
- *Pathogenesis*—large vessel, small vessel, cardioembolic (AF or LV mural thrombus), valve disease, infective endocarditis, non-atheromatous arterial disease (vasculitis, dissection), blood disorders
- *Vessel affected*—anterior circulation (mainly middle cerebral artery (MCA)), lacunar (deep small subcortical vessels), posterior circulation (vertebral and basilar arteries)

Classification systems include:
- *Bamford's classification*—clinical features to define likely stroke territory. Used in major trials and gives prognostic information about each group (see Table 8.1)
- *TOAST classification*—for subtypes of ischaemic stroke: large artery atherosclerosis, cardioembolism, small vessel occlusion, stroke of other determined aetiology, stroke of other undetermined aetiology

**Table 8.1** Bamford classification

| Total anterior circulation stroke (TACS) | | |
|---|---|---|
| Features | Hemiparesis and hemisensory loss | |
| | Homonymous hemianopia | |
| | Cortical dysfunction (dysphasia, visuo-spatial or perceptual problems) | |
| Infarction (TACI) | 85% | |
| Haemorrhage | 15% | |
| Causes | Occlusion of the internal carotid artery or proximal MCA | |
| | Emboli from heart, aortic arch, or carotids, *in situ* thrombosis | |
| Prognosis at 1 year | Dead | 60% |
| | Dependent | 35% |
| | Independent | 5% |

| Partial anterior circulation stroke (PACS) | | |
|---|---|---|
| Features | Two of the three listed in this table above OR cortical dysfunction alone | |
| Infarction (PACI) | 85% | |
| Haemorrhage | 15% | |
| Causes | Occlusion of the anterior or middle cerebral artery | |
| Prognosis at 1 year | Dead | 15% |
| | Dependent | 30% |
| | Independent | 55% |

| Lacunar stroke (LACS) | | |
|---|---|---|
| Features | Hemiparesis OR | |
| | Hemisensory loss OR | |
| | Hemisensorimotor loss OR | |
| | Ataxic hemiparesis OR | |
| | Dysarthria/clumsy hand | |
| | (with NO cortical dysfunction) | |
| Infarction (LACI) | 95% | |
| Haemorrhage | 5% | |
| Causes | Small perforating arteries microatheroma | |
| | Hypertensive small vessel disease | |
| Prognosis at 1 year | Dead | 10% |
| | Dependent | 30% |
| | Independent | 60% |

| Posterior circulation stroke (POCS) | | |
|---|---|---|
| Features | Brainstem symptoms and signs (diplopia, vertigo, ataxia, bilateral limb problems, hemianopia, cortical blindness, etc.) | |
| Infarction (POCI) | 85% | |
| Haemorrhage | 15% | |
| Causes | Occlusion of vertebral, basilar, or posterior cerebral artery | |
| | Emboli from heart, aortic arch, or vertebrobasilar artery | |
| Prognosis at 1 year | Dead | 20% |
| | Dependent | 20% |
| | Independent | 60% |

# Predisposing factors

### Fixed

- *Age*: stroke risk ↑ with age (this is the strongest risk factor)
- *Sex*: ♂ > ♀
- *Ethnicity*: higher risk in people of African and South Asian origin than those of European origin. Probably due to ↑ obesity, hypertension, and diabetes
- *Family history*: positive family history ↑ risk. Not simple inheritance—complex genetic/environmental interaction
- *Previous stroke/TIA*: risk of recurrence is about 10–16% in the first year, highest in the acute phase
- *Other vascular disease*: presence of any atheromatous disease (coronary, peripheral arterial, etc.) ↑ risk of stroke

### Modifiable by lifestyle change

- *Smoking*: causal and dose related. Risk diminishes 5 years after quitting
- *Alcohol*: heavy drinking is a risk factor
- *Obesity*: ↑ risk of all vascular events in obesity—confounded by ↑ in other risk factors (hypertension, diabetes), but probably weak independent factor, especially central obesity
- *Physical inactivity*: ↑ stroke in less active—again confounded by presence of other risk factors in the inactive
- *Diet*: healthy eaters have lower risk but may have healthier lifestyles in general. Low-salt, high-fruit and vegetable, high-fish, and antioxidant diets are likely to be protective, but trials have failed to show an effect from dietary interventions
- *Oestrogens*: the oral contraceptive confers a slightly ↑ risk of stroke and should be avoided in the presence of other risk factors. Post-menopausal hormone replacement therapy (HRT) has been shown to ↑ risk of ischaemic stroke, but not TIA or haemorrhagic stroke

### Medically modifiable

- *Hypertension*: clear association between ↑ BP and ↑ stroke risk across all population groups. Risk doubles with each 5–7mmHg ↑ in diastolic BP. Also ↑ with isolated systolic hypertension
- *AF*: risk of stroke significantly ↑ in AF (see ➜ 'Atrial fibrillation', p. 274)
- *Diabetes*: risk factor independent of hypertension
- *High cholesterol*: weaker risk factor than in heart disease—likely due to diversity of stroke aetiologies
- *Carotid stenosis*: risk ↑ with ↑ stenosis and with the occurrence of symptoms attributable to the stenosis
- *Other comorbidity*: ↑ risk in some conditions such as obstructive sleep apnoea, sickle-cell anaemia, blood diseases causing hyperviscosity and vasculitides

# Acute assessment

A medical emergency increasingly recognized by the general public (helped by UK public health initiatives such as the FAST campaign). Prompt assessment and treatment improves outcomes.

## History

- Is it a focal neurological deficit?
- Did it come on 'at a stroke' or is there a hint of progression (simple stroke may worsen over several days, but think of alternative diagnoses, e.g. tumour)
- Is there headache or drowsiness? (haemorrhage more likely)
- Was there a fall or other head trauma?

▶ Think subdural and request an urgent scan.

- What are the vascular risk factors?
- What was the premorbid state?
- What are the comorbidities? (↑ chance of poor outcome)
- What are the medications?
- Where do they live, and with whom? Who are the significant family members?

## Examination

- *GCS* (see ➜ 'Appendix', 'Glasgow coma scale', p. 710). A standardized measure to assess neurological deterioration. Unconsciousness or deteriorating GCS suggests haemorrhage, a large infarct with oedema, or a brainstem event.
- *National Institutes of Health Stroke Scale (NIHSS)*. Clinical evaluation instrument with documented reliability and validity. Used to assess severity of initial stroke (when making a thrombolysis decision), outcome, and degree of recovery in stroke. Grades the following areas: consciousness, orientation, obeying commands, gaze, visual fields, facial weakness, motor function in the arm and leg, limb ataxia, sensory, language, dysarthria, and inattention.

### General examination

- *General inspection* (head trauma, signs of fitting—incontinence or tongue biting, frailty/general condition, skin, hydration)
- *Temperature* (especially after a long lie)
- *Cardiovascular examination* (pulse rate and rhythm, BP, cardiac examination for source of cardiac emboli, carotid bruits)
- *Respiratory examination* (aspiration pneumonia or pre-existing respiratory conditions)
- *Abdominal examination* (palpable bladder)
- *Neurological examination* (may need to be adapted if patient drowsy):
  - *Cranial nerves*: especially visual fields and visual inattention (if difficulty with compliance, test blink response to threat, and look for a gaze preference which may occur with hemianopia or neglect); assess swallow (see ➜ 'HOW TO . . . Manage swallow after stroke', p. 187)

- *Limbs*: tone (may be diminished acutely), any weakness (grade power for later comparison). Is the distribution pyramidal—arm flexors stronger than extensors, leg extensors stronger than flexors? If weakness subtle, assess for pyramidal/pronator drift and fine movements of both hands—(dominant should be better), coordination (limited if power is diminished), sensation (gross testing by touching both sides with eyes closed), also sensory inattention, reflexes (initially may be absent, then become brisker with time). Plantars extensor on affected side
- *Gait*: assess in less severe stroke—is it safe? If not safe, can the patient sit unaided?
- *Speech*: dysarthria (trouble enunciating because of, e.g. facial weakness or posterior circulation stroke) or dysphasia (cortical disruption of speech—may be receptive or expressive):
  —*Receptive dysphasia* is an inability to understand language—test with one-stage commands—'close your eyes' and progress to more complex tasks 'put your left hand on your right ear'. Do not do the action yourself or the patient will copy you—a test of mimicry, rather than dysphasia. If comprehension intact, reassure the patient that you know they can understand but are having difficulty finding the right words
  —*Expressive dysphasia*—problems producing speech. May be fluent (lots of words that make no sense) or non-fluent (unrecognizable words). Nominal dysphasia is part of an expressive dysphasia and is tested by asking the patient to name increasingly rare objects, e.g. watch, hand, second hand)

---

### HOW TO . . . Assess for inattention

Occurs with parietal cortex damage where there are errors in awareness of self—the patient's 'automatic pilot' has gone wrong.

In extreme cases (neglect), the patient will not recognize their own arm and only wash half of their body. Lesser degrees (inattention) are more common and complicate the rehabilitation process, as the patient must constantly be reminded of the existence of the affected side. Can affect vision or the whole of one side of the body—most commonly non-dominant hemispheric (i.e. right hemisphere, left inattention).

To test:
1. Establish that sensory input is present bilaterally, i.e. check that the patient can feel a touch to each hand individually and does not have a hemianopia (may be hard to establish where extreme gaze preference exists)
2. Provide two stimuli at once (touch both hands together, or move fingers in both sides of the visual field) and see if the patient preferentially notices the sensory input on the good side. If so, there is inattention of the bad side

Even if formal testing does not reveal inattention, sometimes it will become apparent during rehabilitation, often noted by therapists.

# Investigations

(See Table 8.2.)

**Table 8.2** The rationale for investigations in acute stroke

| Test | Rationale |
|------|-----------|
| FBC | Anaemic or polycythaemic<br>Elevated white count suggestive of infection<br>High or low platelet count |
| Urea and electrolytes | Look for evidence of dehydration, and assess fluid replacement |
| CK | Evidence of muscle breakdown (if prolonged lie on floor) |
| Glucose/HBA$_{1c}$ | Diabetic—old or new diagnosis (elevated sugars initially may represent hyperglycaemic stress response)<br>Hypoglycaemia ▶ may mimic stroke |
| Cholesterol | Vascular risk factor |
| ESR | Elevation in vasculitis or sepsis (including endocarditis) |
| CRP | Any evidence of sepsis (e.g. aspiration pneumonia) |
| Blood cultures | Consider if sepsis or new heart murmur heard (endocarditis) |
| Urinalysis | Diabetic, vasculitis, urinary infection |
| ECG | Assess rhythm (look for AF)<br>Evidence of IHD/MI or previous hypertension |
| CXR | Often useful screening test—look for any sign of aspiration, what the heart size is, etc. |
| CT brain | Guidelines advise scan within 24h for all strokes, or sooner (<1h) if:<br>• Thrombolysis candidate<br>• GCS <13 or fluctuating neurology<br>• Severe headache at onset<br>• On warfarin/DOAC<br>• Papilloedema, neck stiffness, or fever<br>CT will distinguish stroke from non-stroke, e.g. tumour, identify whether bleed or an infarct, the likely cause of the event—carotid territory infarcts from stenosis, multiple infarcts from cardiac emboli<br>Blood appears white on early CT; infarcts may not show acutely (first few hours), develop into low-density areas after hours–days<br>Small infarcts may never be seen, and the diagnosis is made clinically or on magnetic resonance (MR) scan<br>▶ A normal CT does not exclude a stroke |
| Carotid Doppler | Request in carotid territory events where the patient has a good recovery and is a candidate for endarterectomy |
| Echocardiogram | Consider where multiple (? cardioembolic) infarcts, after a recent MI (looking for thrombus), or where there is a murmur |

# Acute management

Guidelines for acute care are published by the Royal College of Physicians (% http://www.rcplondon.ac.uk). See also NICE Stroke guidelines (2014). Overall care should occur on an acute stroke unit.

## Diagnosis

Diagnosis should be made clinically (including assessment of the likely cerebral area affected) and reviewed by a clinician with expertise in stroke. CT scan should be performed unless there is good clinical reason for not doing so (e.g. dying patient for terminal care)

## Medical interventions

- *Thrombolysis* with, e.g. tissue plasminogen activator (tPA) should be given promptly where indicated (see ➔ 'Thrombolysis', p. 190)
- *Intra-arterial clot retrieval* has evidence of benefit (up to 6h of onset) where expertise exists either in combination with thrombolysis or where thrombolysis is contraindicated
- *Aspirin (300mg)* should be given as soon as possible after the onset of stroke symptoms if haemorrhage is excluded (can be given nasogastrically (NG) or per rectum (PR)) and not a potential hemicraniectomy case
- *BP*—debate about the optimal BP in the acute phase—high BP is harmful long term but may be required to provide perfusion pressure with altered cerebral autoregulation acutely—trials ongoing. Guidelines advise that BP should not be lowered acutely in general, but existing antihypertensives continued
- *Oxygen supplementation* should be given to hypoxic patients only
- *Hydration* should be maintained to ensure normovolaemia and biochemical normality, and monitored closely
- *Glucose* should be measured and, if >11mmol/L, controlled using iv variable-dose insulin
- *Pyrexia* should be lowered with treatment of the underlying cause, fan, paracetamol, and sponging. High temperatures are associated with poorer outcomes, but the causal nature of this association is unknown
- *DVT prevention* is done with early mobilization. Compression stockings should not be used and the timing of low-dose low-molecular-weight heparin depends on individual risk/benefit analysis. Intermittent pneumatic compression devices are safe and effective in early disabling stroke.
- *Neurosurgical opinion* should be sought for hydrocephalus, posterior fossa haemorrhages/large infarcts, large haemorrhages with midline shift, and large MCA infarcts with malignant MCA syndrome
- *Seizures* should be treated (see ➔ 'Epilepsy and stroke', p. 165)

## Multidisciplinary acute input

Protocols should be developed for early management (<24h), including monitoring consciousness level, assessing swallow (not gag), risk assessment for pressure sores, nutritional status, cognitive impairment, bowel and bladder care (avoiding catheterization if possible), and moving and handling requirements. Early SALT assessment should be done for all with swallow or language difficulties; early mobilization with a PT having expertise in stroke rehabilitation.

---

### HOW TO . . . Manage swallow after stroke

Aspiration of saliva or food is one of the most common complications of stroke and a major cause of morbidity and mortality. Patients who are drowsy and dysarthric and those with dysphasia are most at risk of aspiration.

*Assessment*—ideally all patients should have their swallow assessed promptly by a professional with specific stroke dysphagia training. If the patient is low risk and you wish to do a bedside assessment:

1. Sit the patient upright, and listen to the chest to establish baseline
2. Ask the patient to cough, and note the strength and effectiveness
3. Give the patient a teaspoon of water, and ask them not to swallow
4. Look for leakage of water from the closed mouth
5. Ask the patient to swallow the water
6. Check for prompt, coordinated swallow with elevation of the tracheal cartilage
7. Watch for signs of aspiration—coughing and spluttering. These may not occur for several minutes, so do not leave immediately
8. If no problems, then try a half-glass of water (slowly) or a small amount of yogurt
9. Ask the patient to say name/address, and listen for a 'wet' voice

*Management*—if the patient is high risk, there are concerns during the bedside test, or if there are problems encountered during feeding:

1. Make the patient 'nil by mouth'
2. Provide alternative means of hydration at once with an iv infusion or an NGT
3. Refer for early SALT assessment, to stratify the impairment and make a plan for safe oral intake, reviewing at regular intervals
4. Early nutrition by NGT improves outcomes and allows medication to be given, in addition to feeding. Looped/bridle NGTs are much less likely to be dislodged but are harder to insert. Consider insertion on the inattentive side if recurrent NGT removal is a problem

*Medium/longer-term management*—if the patient continues to have swallowing problems, then a PEG or a radiologically inserted gastrostomy (RIG) tube can be inserted. Patients on long-term feeding should be reviewed regularly, as swallow can return many months later and oral feeding can gradually be introduced and sometimes tubes can be removed.

▶ It is important to understand that artificial feeding by any method does not prevent aspiration and, in some cases, can aggravate it. See ⊅ 'The ethics of clinically assisted feeding', pp. 358–9, for discussion of the ethics of feeding.

# Stroke units

### Definition

Geographically defined unit staffed by a coordinated MDT with expertise in stroke. The gold standard is to admit stroke patients directly and continue care through to discharge—known as a comprehensive stroke unit. Some units deal with the emergency management (including thrombolysis and hemicraniectomy) and are termed Hyperacute Stroke Units (HASU). Others provide ongoing acute care or deal with the post-acute rehabilitation phase only. Regions may organize a 'hub and spoke' model where a single HASU admits all stroke patients for the first 72h of care, transferring rapidly to other local units. There is evidence for stroke-specific early supported discharge schemes reducing death or dependency as part of the overall pathway.

### Benefits

Stroke units, when compared with general ward care, result in lower rates of death, dependency, and institutional care, without lengthening hospital stay. The number needed to treat in a stroke unit to prevent one death or dependency is 18.

### Rationale

The majority of improvement seems to occur in the first 4 weeks, and the mechanism is unclear.

Key components of stroke units include:

• Meticulous attention to physiological homeostasis
• Attention to prevention of complications (such as thromboembolic disease and pressure sores)
• Early mobilization
• Coordinated MDT care
• Interest, expertise, and motivation of staff

## HOW TO . . . Estimate prognosis after stroke

After first-ever stroke, death occurs in 12% by a week, in 31% at 1 year, and in 60% at 5 years. Indicators of a poor prognosis include:

- Impaired consciousness
- Gaze preference
- Dense weakness
- Cardiac comorbidity
- Urinary incontinence
- Pupillary abnormalities

The risk of recurrent stroke among survivors is 10–16% at 1 year, thereafter falling to about 4–5% per annum. The risk is higher with ↑ number of risk factors. Risk can also be estimated using the Bamford classification (see ➲ 'Stroke', 'Definition and classification', p. 179)

Recovery is usually slow, and a clear time frame established early on in the disease with the patient and relatives is helpful. Recovery is most rapid in the first 3 months, and this tends to be 'front-loaded', so the most dramatic improvements occur in the early weeks. Recovery then tends to slow but may continue for years.

▶ Each patient is different—recovery may be delayed by infections, depression, etc., and this time frame should be a guide only.

The risk of not returning to independence varies with stroke type. Overall, about 20–30% of survivors are dependent at a year, and 40–50% are independent.

## Further reading

Stroke Unit Trialists' Collaboration. Organised inpatient (stroke unit) care for stroke. *Cochrane Database Syst Rev* 2013; 9: CD000197. ℘ http://www.cochrane.org/reviews/en/ab000197. html.

# Thrombolysis

### Rationale

In acute ischaemic stroke, an artery becomes occluded by a thrombus *in situ* or an embolus, and blood supply is compromised. Death of surrounding brain tissue results in deficits in function associated with that part of the brain. Early recanalization of the vessel by lysing the thrombus may limit the extent of brain injury.

### Risks

Treatment with thrombolysis leads to an excess in death due to intracranial haemorrhage (a fivefold ↑, compared with placebo).

### Benefits

Despite early excess of deaths due to haemorrhage, treatment with thrombolysis leads to 44 fewer dead or dependent patients per 1000 treated with recombinant tPA (r-tPA) within 6h, and 126 fewer dead or dependent patients per 1000 treated with r-tPA within 3h.

### Imaging

This must be done prior to giving thrombolysis to exclude haemorrhage. Perfusion- and diffusion-weighted MR scans may give more information than CT. All need to be interpreted by someone with the appropriate experience prior to thrombolysis. Plain axial CT remains the mainstay of imaging prior to thrombolysis.

### Use

Thrombolysis is recommended in centres with sufficient expertise in stroke and with facilities to deal with complications. In these centres, treatment is considered in all patients with definite ischaemic stroke who present within 4.5h of the onset of symptoms. Where this expertise does not exist, the service may still be provided via telemedicine links with stroke 'hubs'.

### Exclusion criteria

There is a very long list of exclusions, but the following are the most common reasons to withhold treatment:
- Previous haemorrhage or active bleeding site
- Seizure at onset
- Impaired coagulation
- Caution with very severe stroke
- Uncontrolled hypertension (>180/110mmHg)

# Intra-arterial therapies

### Rationale

Ischaemic stroke patients may present where there is a bleeding risk to sys-temic thrombolysis, and more localized therapy is safer. This can either be localized intra-arterial tPA or, more commonly, clot retrieval. This has been proven to be superior to iv thrombolysis alone and is now being offered in more and more centres. In the UK, this service is provided by interventional neuroradiologists, but elsewhere trained cardiologists or stroke physicians are taking the lead.

# Ongoing management

Should involve all of the MDT.

### Dieticians

Calculate food and fluid requirements for each individual patient; adapt the diet for specific needs (e.g. diabetic, weight loss); develop regimens for NG or PEG feeds; advise on provision of modified diets for stages of swallow recovery (thickened, pureed, etc.); review nutrition as recovery alters needs.

### Doctors

Diagnosis; manage medical complications; establish therapies.

### Nurses

Monitor patient continuously; assist with basic care (physiological and physical); ongoing bowel and bladder management; ongoing skin care; facilitate practice of skills acquired in therapy; promote functional independence; first point of call for relatives.

### Occupational therapist

Optimize functional ability (usually begin with upper limb work, coordinating with the PT); specific assessments of certain tasks (washing and dressing, kitchen safety, occupational tasks, etc.) as recovery continues; adaptation to home environment by a series of home visits, with and without the patient, and the supply of aids (rails, bed levers, toilet raises, bath boards, etc.); provision of wheelchairs where needed.

### Pharmacists

Review charts; promote safe prescribing.

### Physiotherapists

Assess muscle tone, movement, and mobility; maximize functional independence by education and exercise; monitor respiratory function; initial bed mobility, then work on sitting balance, then transfers, and finally standing and stepping; help prevent complications such as shoulder pain, contractures, and immobility-associated problems (pressure sores, DVT/PE).

### Psychologists

Assess the psychological impact of stroke on the patient and family; allow the patient to talk about the impact of the illness; monitor for depression and other mood disorder, highlighting the need for medication; document cognitive impairment; assist in retraining where neglect is prominent.

### Social workers

Psychosocial assessment of the patient and family; support with financial matters (accessing pension, arranging power of attorney (POA), financing placement, etc.); advice and support for the patient and family on accommodation needs, especially finding a care home placement; link to community services (care package, community rehabilitation, day centres, etc.)

## Speech and language therapists

Assess swallow and establish plan for safe oral intake; reassess, and plan nutritional route during recovery; language screening (dysarthria, dysphasia, and dyspraxia) with intervention to improve deficits.

---

**HOW TO . . . Protect your patient from another stroke**

Ensure that the following are addressed:

- *Lifestyle issues*—smoking, diet, and exercise
- *Antiplatelet therapy*:
  - Current advice is aspirin 300mg for 2 weeks, followed by clopidogrel 75mg thereafter. Adding clopidogrel to aspirin ↑ antiplatelet activity but has been shown to ↑ the risk of cerebral haemorrhage, but may be considered for monotherapy failure
- *Lower BP*—choice of agent debated. The important thing is just to lower the BP. If there are no contraindications, lowering BP per se is likely to be beneficial, but aim for <130/85
- *Lower cholesterol*—the Heart Protection Study clarified benefit post-stroke, including in older patients. The cut-off for treatment in this trial was 3.5
- *Anticoagulation for AF*—(see ➲ 'Atrial fibrillation', p. 274). In infarction, likely to be safe to start warfarin/DOAC after 2 weeks. With haemorrhage, judge each case individually. Haemorrhage due to thrombolysis is *not* a reason to withhold anticoagulation. In 1° haemorrhage, anticoagulation may never be justified
- *Carotid endarterectomy*—>70% symptomatic stenosis carries a stroke risk of about 15% per year and is an indication for endarterectomy where there is good recovery and the patient is fit for surgery (which can be done with local anaesthesia). Perform early for greater benefit See also ➲ 'Vascular secondary prevention', p. 310.

---

# Complications

### Contractures
Longer-term complication (see ⮞ 'Contractures', p. 487).

### Faecal incontinence
May be due to immobility, cognitive problems, or neurological impairment. Regulate bowel habit, where possible, with high-fibre diet and good fluid intake, and toilet regularly. If all else fails, then deliberately constipating the patient with codeine and using regular enemas can work. See ⮞ 'Faecal incontinence: management', p. 546.

### Infection
Commonly chest or urine. Think of it early if a patient becomes drowsy or confused or appears to deteriorate neurologically. Prompt screening for sepsis and treatment with antibiotics, oxygen, and hydration are indicated in the majority of patients in the acute phase (stroke outcome very unclear initially) but may be withheld in a more established stroke where the prognosis can be assessed more confidently as dismal (decision made with the family).

### Muscle spasm
Very common on the affected side. Arthritic joints are exacerbated by spasm, and antispasmodics may need to be used, alongside analgesia, for effective pain relief. Try baclofen or tizanidine. ↑ the dose slowly after a few days, if needed, but watch out for drowsiness and loss of tone in the affected side that can hinder therapy. Resistant spasm may benefit from a course of botulinum toxin injections.

### Pain
Commonly shoulder pain in a paralysed arm. Usually multifactorial, e.g. joint subluxation (treat with PT to strengthen muscles and arm support) interacting with muscle spasm and shoulder arthritis. Central post-stroke pain tends to affect all of the affected side and can be treated with neuromodulators (e.g. gabapentin)

### Pressure sores
Are avoidable with good care; however, pressure damage may occur before admission but manifest only later (see ⮞ 'Pressure sores', pp. 504–5).

### Psychological problems
Low mood is extremely common post-stroke (at 4 months, 25% will be depressed, and over half of these remain depressed at a year). This is unrelated to the stroke type but is associated with a worse outcome (perhaps because of lower motivation in therapy). It should be actively sought (the screening question 'Do you think you are depressed?' is quick and effective; it may also be noticed by nurses, therapists, or family; tools such as the GDS can also be used but may be confounded by dysphasia). Treatment is with psychosocial support and antidepressants (e.g. citalopram). Anxiety is also very common and often responds to explanation and empowerment.

Post-stroke cognitive impairment is common (up to 80% prevalence). Delirium associated with acute stroke may improve, but cognitive deficits are often permanent (either fixed deficits or more global functioning).

## Non-dominant hemisphere syndromes

Usually MCA strokes of the right hemisphere where language is crudely preserved, but there are issues with fluency, semantics, and interpretation of language (a kind of acquired neglect dyslexia). Deficits in assimilating information to make sense of reality can cause complex issues with insight and empathy and disease denial.

## Thromboembolism

Very common post-stroke. Ensure well hydrated. Mobilize early. Intermittent pneumatic compression devices should be used in the acute phase. Low-dose low-molecular-weight heparin is used after the acute stage (when risk of haemorrhage into the brain diminishes). Have a low threshold for investigating a leg that becomes swollen or painful. Ensure careful VTE risk assessment is documented at each stage.

---

**HOW TO . . . Manage urinary incontinence after stroke**

This is very common, more so after severe stroke. It does, however, improve over time, and a flexible approach is required to ensure that a patient does not get catheterized and remains so.
- Initially, try to manage with pads and regular toileting
- If the skin starts to break down, or if the burden on carers is heavy, then a catheter can be inserted for a limited time span
- Once mobility improves, try removing the catheter—ensure this is seen by all as a positive and exciting step back towards independence, as it can cause considerable anxiety
- If this fails, check for, and treat, UTI and then try again
- If this fails, then replace the catheter and use bladder-stabilizing agents for about 2 weeks (e.g. tolterodine) before removing it again
- If all this fails, consider sheath catheter devices or bottles (with non-return valves for use in bed) in men; commodes next to the bed for women

▶ The need for a permanent catheter post-stroke should be reviewed regularly, as the condition is likely to improve (see ➲ 'Urinary incontinence: causes', pp. 534–5.

---

# Longer-term issues

### Return to the community

Best coordinated by the stroke MDT. Early supported discharge may be useful if the patient can transfer and there is a specialist community stroke team available. Later discharges are planned by the team, usually after careful assessment of needs (home alterations, care packages, etc.). The GP should be alerted to continue medical monitoring, in particular optimizing 2° prevention. Community teams (district nurses, community rehabilitation teams, home carers, etc.) should be aware of the patient's needs (continence, diabetic monitoring, ongoing therapy needs, etc.) and ideally be involved in the discharge planning. The patient and family should have adequate information and training, as well as a contact point in case of problems (stroke coordinators often take this role). Voluntary agencies (e.g. the Stroke Association) are helpful, and the patient should be informed about them.

### Driving regulations with cerebrovascular disease

- TIA/stroke with full neurological recovery—1 month off driving
- Recurrent TIAs—3 months off driving following last TIA
- Stroke with residual neurological deficit after 1 month—the patient must notify the DVLA, and the decision is made on a case-by-case basis, with evidence from medical reports
- Hemianopia, inattention, and impaired cognition are definite markers of lack of fitness to drive (can be decided by a GP or hospital physician). Subtle visual deficits need formal perimetry testing
- Dysphasia is harder—cognitive state is difficult to assess, and associated impairments (such as problems reading street signs or misinterpreting the environment) are not readily identified out of context
- Pure limb weakness can often be safely managed with car adaptation. If there are any doubts and the patient wishes to drive, then they should be seen in a driving assessment centre (the patient will have to pay)
- Stroke with seizure—this is treated as a provoked seizure. May be <1 year ban, depending on circumstances

See ℘ https://www.gov.uk/guidance/assessing-fitness-to-drive-a-guide-for-medical-professionals.

### Follow-up

Some follow-up should be offered to all stroke survivors. The intensity and duration of inpatient care can contrast sharply with home. The realities of living with disability begin to sink in, and many questions and anxieties arise. Even minor strokes or TIAs require a further point of contact, as they will have been committed to lifelong medication and will need monitoring of risk factors. In addition, stroke recovery continues (albeit at a slower pace) for years and management plans made at discharge may need to be adapted.

*The Stroke Association*
Helpline: 0303 303 3100. ℘ http://www.stroke.org.uk.

### Checklist for follow-up
(Usually 1–4 months after discharge)
*Secondary prevention*
Check drugs, BP, diabetic control, and cardiac rhythm.

*Continence*
- Are there continence problems?
- If a catheter is *in situ*, has mobility improved to a point at which trial removal can be done?
- If the patient was discharged on bladder-stabilizing drugs and has remained continent, can these be tailed off?

*Nutrition*
- Is nutrition adequate? (If not, refer to a dietician.)
- If a PEG tube is in place, is it still required?
- Does the patient warrant another assessment of swallowing (by SALT) to allow oral nutrition to begin?

*Communication and speech*
- Are there problems still?
- Is there a need for a SALT review?

*Mood*
- Is the patient depressed?
- Do they need referral to a psychologist or (rarely) a psychiatrist?
- If discharged on an antidepressant, can it be discontinued?

*Physical progress*
- Is there ongoing physical therapy?
- If not, is there continued improvement? If there has been deterioration, then refer back for assessment for further therapy (Royal College of Physicians' guidelines)

*Contractures*
- Are there any contractures developing? (If so, refer to PT.)

*Muscle spasms*
- Have these developed or lessened since discharge?
- Review need for antispasmodic medication—titrate down if no longer required

*Pain*
- Commonly in shoulder, or post-stroke pain
- Has this developed or lessened?
- Review need for medications

*Daily living*
- Are there any issues in managing day to day?
- Is all the necessary equipment in place? (And is it still needed, e.g. a commode can be returned when the patient is able to mobilize to the toilet alone?)
- Is there anything that they would like to be able to do that they cannot? (e.g. read a book, take a bath)
- Would a further review by a therapist be helpful?
- Do they wish to drive? (See ➋ 'Longer-term issues', p. 196)

*Support*
- Are they in contact with a community stroke coordinator (if available)?
- Are they aware of voluntary organizations?

# Transient ischaemic attack clinics

Rapid outpatient assessment of TIA and minor stroke, to establish diagnosis, commence 2° prevention, and lower risk of subsequent event.

## How fast?

This depends on how high a risk the patient is. Use the ABCD$^2$ score (see Table 8.3), and if the score is ≥4, the patient should be seen within 24h—in some services, these patients are admitted to hospital, but larger centres may provide 7-day/week outpatient services. Patients who have recurrent symptoms within a week or those in AF on anticoagulation should also be seen urgently. Those at lower risk should be seen within 7 days.

Currently, early antiplatelet agents, antihypertensives, and statin use have been shown to substantially reduce the chances of stroke at 1 week. Anticoagulation for patients with AF and early endarterectomy are also known to be beneficial for a subset of patients.

## Function

- *Confirm diagnosis*—very variable, but up to half of referrals to a TIA clinic are non-stroke. Main alternatives are migraine, epilepsy, cardiac dysrhythmias, orthostatic hypotension, or rarely brain tumour
- *Arrange investigations*—to aid diagnosis (e.g. CT brain) or investigate risk factors (e.g. FBC, ESR, HbA$_{1c}$, cholesterol, ECG, carotid Doppler, 24h tape, and echocardiogram)
- *Modify risk factors*—(see ➲ 'HOW TO . . . Protect your patient from another stroke', p. 193) set targets for BP and glucose control; advise about antiplatelet agents (there is significant regional variation in the therapy chosen, including aspirin with modified-release dipyridamole, or aspirin with clopidogrel for 1 month and then clopidogrel alone) and anticoagulation in AF; advise about statin use; refer for carotid endarterectomy urgently; advise about smoking cessation
- *Education*—of patients, relatives, and 1° care doctors. Discuss stroke disease and its modification, time frame for recovery, psychological aspects of stroke, and driving restrictions

## Structure

Varies enormously. Ideally would have:
- *Rapid referral protocol*
- *Stroke specialist nurse*—can take history, including standardized risk factor analysis, measure BP, provide education (leaflets, individual action plans), and coordinate investigations and follow-up. Role can be extended into the community—point of access for patients
- *Time for explanation*—many patients will feel overwhelmed by the amount of information they are being given. The specialist nurse can be very helpful in clarifying things, and information leaflets allow the information to be revisited at home. There are often several new tablets, or even suggesting surgery for a patient who feels well. Comprehension is vital for concordance

- *Rapid access to investigations*—particularly carotid Doppler and CT scanning. Many clinics run a 'one-stop' service where all assessments, investigations, and conclusions are completed at a single visit
- *Prompt communication to GP*—advice about risk reduction must be relayed promptly to the GP for maximum benefit. Ideally same day

**Table 8.3** The ABCD$^2$ score for TIA

|    |                   |                                     | Score |
|----|-------------------|-------------------------------------|-------|
| A  | Age               | ≥60                                 | 1     |
| B  | BP                | ≥140/90mmHg                         | 2     |
| C  | Clinical features | Unilateral weakness                 | 2     |
|    |                   | Speech disturbance without weakness | 1     |
| D1 | Duration          | ≥60min                              | 2     |
|    |                   | 10–59min                            | 1     |
|    |                   | <10min                              | 0     |
| D2 | Diabetes          | Diabetes                            | 1     |

ABCD$^2$ score—risk of stroke at 2 days: 0–3—1%; 4–5—4%; 6–7—8%.

# Further reading

Johnson SC, Rothwell PM, Nguyen-Huynh MN, *et al*. Validation and refinement of scores to predict very early stroke risk after transient ischemic attack. *Lancet* 2007; **369**: 238–92.

# Psychiatry

# Cognitive ageing

Cognitive, or thinking, ability is the product of:
- 'Fixed intelligence', the result of previous thinking, which often ↑ with age, i.e. 'wisdom'
- 'Fluid intelligence', i.e. real-time information processing, which declines modestly in older age

There are structural changes in the brain with age (see 'The ageing brain and nervous system', p. 150), but these correlate poorly with cognitive changes. Broadly, intellectual function is maintained until at least 80 years, but processing is slower. Non-critical impairments include forgetfulness, modestly reduced vocabulary, and slower learning of, e.g. languages. These changes are to be expected, their consequences can be managed, and they do not cause significant reduction in functional level.

Three factors support a diagnosis of normal ageing, rather than disease:
- The ability to maintain function in normal life through aids (e.g. *aides memoire*: lists or calendars) or adaptations (of one's environment or one's expectations)
- Very long time scale of decline: 10–30 years, compared with months or a few years in disease
- Relative decline, e.g. the academic who no longer holds his own at the graduates' reunion

# Impairments in cognitive function without dementia

## Age-associated memory impairment or benign senescent forgetfulness

Older people learn new information and recall information more slowly, but given time, their performance is unchanged. This is distinct from the impairment in dementia, in that in age-associated memory impairment (AAMI), overall function is unimpaired and usually only less important facts are forgotten. It is often more bothersome to the patient than a concern to relatives (compare dementia, when often the family are much more concerned than the patient).

AAMI can present early (age 40s–50s) when high achievers become frustrated by modest deterioration in speed of new learning. It may be exacerbated by performance anxiety, creating a vicious cycle, and is often helped by psychological strategies to assist memory.

## Minimal/mild cognitive impairment (MCI)

Impairments are more broad than memory alone and are felt to be pathological (e.g. $2°$ to cerebrovascular disease), but the full criteria for a diagnosis of dementia are not met, e.g. because there is not yet significant impact on day-to-day functioning.

Progression to dementia occurs in between 5% (community studies) and 10% (memory clinic studies) annually. Thus, with time, many patients do develop dementia, but many do not, and in some, there is no deterioration.

Diagnosis is important in order to:
- Reassure the patient (by distinguishing from dementia)
- Modify risk factors for progression
- Monitor deterioration such that intervention can begin promptly if progression occurs

# Dementia: overview

Dementia is:
- an acquired decline in memory and other cognitive function(s)
- in an alert (i.e. non-delirious) person
- sufficiently severe to affect daily life (home, social function)

All three elements must be present in order to make the diagnosis.

Prevalence ↑ dramatically with age: 1% of 60–65 year olds, >30% of over 85s. Over 50% of care home residents have dementia.

Age-specific incidence is falling (perhaps with improvements in risk factor management), although the national burden continues to ↑ with the ageing population.

Major dementia syndromes (and proportion of cases in older people) include:
- Mixed pathology—(especially Alzheimer's and vascular) is the most common type in post-mortem studies
- Dementia of Alzheimer type (60%)
- Vascular dementia (30%)
- Other neurodegenerative dementias (15%), e.g. dementia with Lewy bodies, Parkinson's disease with dementia, frontotemporal dementia
- Reversible dementias (<5%), e.g. drugs, metabolic, subdural, NPH

Diagnostically, there are many false-positive and false-negative cases. Mild to moderate dementia is easy to miss on a cursory, unstructured assessment. Patients labelled incorrectly as having dementia may be deaf, dysphasic, delirious, depressed, or under the influence of drugs.

## Triggers for considering a dementia diagnosis
- Delirium (much more common with underlying dementia)
- 'Unmasking' of poor cognition after spouse's death
- Social withdrawal
- Request for social services help
- Poor concordance with prescribed drug therapy
- Domestic crisis (e.g. fire, road traffic accident)
- Spouse/family disproportionately in control or speaking for patient

## UK National Dementia Strategy
The first national strategy was published by the UK government in 2009 with focus on accelerating the pace of improvement in dementia care, through local delivery of quality outcomes and local accountability for achieving them. This was updated in 2015 and challenges the UK to achieve global improvements in approaches to dementia across society, as well as health and social care, by 2020.

## HOW TO . . . Distinguish delirium from dementia

The most common issue in diagnosing the older patient with confusion ('brain failure') is whether the patient has delirium alone, dementia alone, or a delirium superimposed on a pre-existing dementia.

Achieve this by combining information from the history with a physical and mental state examination.

▶ The history is key. The duration of symptoms is the most important. Information from medical records, carers, and family will help determine whether dementia was present before the onset of delirium. 'When was his memory last as good as yours?' (See Table 9.1.)

Table 9.1 Features distinguishing delirium from dementia

| Feature | Delirium | Dementia |
|---------|----------|----------|
| Mode of onset | Acute or subacute | Chronic or subacute |
| Reversibility | Often reversible | Rarely reversible |
| Fluctuation | Diurnal or hour-to-hour fluctuation common | Generally little diurnal variation, although some deteriorate during the evening; 'sundowning'. Day-to-day fluctuation more common in Lewy body dementia |
| Poor attention | Yes (but variable hour to hour) | In severe dementia |
| Conscious level | Usually affected but may be subtle and variable | Normal |
| Hallucinations and misinterpretations | Common | Usually occurs late in the disease. Visual hallucinations earlier in the disease, especially when symptoms fluctuate, suggests Lewy body dementia |
| Fear, agitation, aggression | Common | Uncommon in early stages |
| Disorganized thought, unreal ideas | Common | Late. Often poverty of thought |
| Motor signs | Tremor, myoclonus, asterixis common | Late only |
| Speech | May be dysarthric, dysnomic | Normal |
| Dysgraphia | Often present | Usually late |
| Short- and long-term memory | Poor | Long-term memory often normal until late |

# Dementia: assessment

History is the most important component of assessment. Obtain information from both patient and family/friends. Note the onset, speed of progression, and symptoms. Take a careful drug history, including over-the-counter drugs and recreational drugs (especially alcohol). Also ask about a family history of early dementia and a personal psychiatric history of, e.g. depression.

Usually there is a progressive decline in cognitive function over several years, ending with complete dependency and death (usually due to dehydration, malnutrition, and/or sepsis).

Deterioration may be:
- Insidious and gradual (e.g. Alzheimer's)
- Stepwise (suggesting stroke/vascular aetiology)
- Abrupt (after a single critical stroke)
- Rapid over weeks/months, suggesting a drug, metabolic, or structural cause (e.g. tumour, subdural)

Abnormalities occur in:
- Retention of new information (e.g. appointments, events, working a new household appliance); short-term memory loss is often severe, with repetitive questioning
- Managing complex tasks (e.g. paying bills, cooking a meal for family)
- Language (word-finding difficulty with circumlocution, inability to hold a conversation)
- Behaviour (e.g. irritability, aggression, poor motivation, wandering)
- Orientation (e.g. getting lost in familiar places)
- Recognition (failure to recognize first acquaintances, then friends or distant family, then close family, e.g. spouse)
- Ability to self-care (grooming, bathing, dressing, continence/toileting)
- Reasoning: poor judgement, irrational or unaccustomed behaviours
- Ability to recognize familiar objects, people, and places (agnosia)
- Ability to carry out complex, coordinated movements (apraxia)

## Physical examination

- To determine possible causes of a dementia syndrome, including reversible factors
- Look for vascular disease (cardiovascular, peripheral vascular, and cerebrovascular), neuropathy, parkinsonism, thyroid disease, malignancy, dehydration, (alcoholic) liver disease
- In advanced dementia of any type, primitive reflexes (e.g. grasp, suckling, palmar-mental) and global hyperreflexia with extensor planters may occur

## Mental state

- *Exclude delirium.* Features include agitation, restlessness, poor attention, and fluctuating conscious level (see ➲ Appendix, 'CAM', p. 706)
- *Exclude depression.* Features include low affect, poor motivation, and a negative perspective. Perform a GDS (see ➲ Appendix, 'Geriatric Depression Scale', p. 701)

- *Measure cognitive function.* Serial testing may be helpful in borderline cases—is there evidence of progression? Many measurement tools are available, e.g. MMSE™, Montreal Cognitive Assessment (MoCA), Mini-Cog, number of animals named in 1min, clock-drawing test (see ❷ 'Measurement instruments', pp. 76–7, ❷ Appendix, 'The abbreviated mental test score', p. 704, and ❷ Appendix, 'Clock-drawing and the Mini-Cog™', p. 707)

Full *neuropsychological assessment* (detailed, prolonged assessment by a specialist psychologist) may be helpful in:
- Distinguishing between dementia and depression
- Distinguishing between different subtypes of dementia
- Distinguishing between AAMI and early dementia
- Distinguishing between focal impairments (e.g. aphasic or amnesic syndromes) and dementia
- Measuring progression and response to treatment

### Disclosure of dementia diagnosis
Each case should be considered individually, but in general, the diagnosis should be revealed. Disclosure:
- Is consistent with the patient's right to know (autonomy). Most older people say that they would want to know the diagnosis
- Facilitates medical, financial, and care planning, e.g. ADs, POA, living arrangements
- Allows for consent to treatment and facilitates participation in research
- Facilitates discussion between patient and carer

Arguments against disclosure include a possible depressive reaction, accentuated by a perceived lack of effective treatments. Such a reaction is minimized by sensitive multidisciplinary support that emphasizes the positive therapeutic solutions available.

## HOW TO . . . Investigate a patient with dementia

Cases of reversible dementia are uncommon, but their identification is important, as effective treatment may reverse the impairment and prevent progression. Therefore, screen for them.

### Blood tests

The following are generally considered useful: FBC, ESR, $B_{12}$, folate, U, C+E, calcium, LFTs, TSH, CRP, random glucose.

Request syphilis and human immunodeficiency virus (HIV) serology only if there are atypical features or special risks.

### ECG and CXR

Evidence of heart disease, occult malignancy.

### Neuroimaging

Every person with dementia should undergo brain imaging at some stage. Prompt imaging is indicated where there is:

- Early onset (<60 years)
- Sudden onset or brisk decline
- High risk of structural pathology (e.g. known cancer, falls with head injury)
- Focal CNS signs or symptoms

There are patients, usually in late-stage dementia, for whom the benefits of imaging are outweighed by the practical difficulties.

### Imaging modality

- *CT* is the usual imaging modality; dementia protocols allow volumetric assessment of medial temporal structures
- *MRI* gives superior images and provides additional diagnostic information for selected patients
- *SPECT/positron emission tomography (PET)* is used rarely, usually in specialist centres, to more reliably differentiate between Alzheimer's and vascular dementia

### Additional testing as clinically indicated

- *EEG* is used for suspected frontotemporal dementia or Creutzfeldt–Jakob disease (CJD), or where seizure activity is a possibility
- *Lumbar puncture* where CNS infection is considered

# Dementia: common diseases

## Alzheimer's disease (dementia of Alzheimer type)

- The most common cause of a dementia syndrome
- Diagnosis is made clinically, based on the typical history, mental state examination, and unremarkable physical examination
- *History*—insidious onset, with slow progression over years. Early, profound short-term memory loss progresses to include broad, often global, cognitive dysfunction, behavioural change, and functional impairment. Behavioural problems are common, usually occurring in moderate to severe dementia, but sometimes preceding overt cognitive impairment
- *Physical examination*—normal
- *Neuroimaging*—demonstrates no other causes of dementia (e.g. tumour or infarct) and may show disproportionate medial temporal lobe atrophy
- Treatment with acetylcholinesterase inhibitors may be indicated (see ➋ 'Dementia: acetylcholinesterase inhibitors', pp. 222–3)
- Early-onset Alzheimer's disease (<65 years) is uncommon, has a stronger genetic component, and is more rapidly progressive

## Vascular dementia

- The next most common cause
- Suggested by vascular risk factors, e.g. diabetes mellitus, hypertension, smoking, or other vascular pathology, with other supporting evidence on history, examination, or tests
- *History*—cognitive impairment may be patchy, compared with the more uniform impairments seen in Alzheimer's disease. Onset is often associated with stroke, or the deterioration is abrupt or stepwise; however, using 'multi-infarct dementia' as a synonym for vascular dementia is imprecise and its use should be discouraged. Frontal lobe, extrapyramidal, and pseudobulbar features and emotional lability are common. Urinary incontinence and falls without other explanation are often early features. Other features may be mostly cortical (mimicking Alzheimer's disease) or subcortical (e.g. apathy, depression)
- *Physical examination* often shows:
  - Focal neurology suggesting stroke or diffuse cerebrovascular disease (hyperreflexia, extensor plantars, abnormal gait, etc.)
  - Other evidence of vascular pathology, e.g. AF, peripheral vascular disease
- *Neuroimaging* shows either:
  - Multiple large-vessel infarcts, or
  - A single critical infarct (e.g. thalamus), or
  - White matter infarcts or periventricular white matter changes, or
  - Microvascular disease, too fine to be seen on neuroimaging, which may cause a significant proportion of vascular dementia, apparent only at post-mortem

## Differentiating between Alzheimer's and vascular dementia

The importance of differentiating between Alzheimer's and vascular dementia can be overemphasized. Their presentations overlap, and pathologies commonly coexist. Increasingly, it is believed that much of Alzheimer's disease pathology has a vascular component.

Pragmatically:

- In cases where vascular risk factors and/or signs exist, treat vascular risk factors aggressively, whether or not there is significant cerebrovascular pathology on brain imaging
- A trial of acetylcholinesterase inhibitors is now suggested for both conditions

# Dementia and parkinsonism

Dementia with Lewy bodies and Parkinson's disease with dementia may be considered as extremes of a continuum. In the latter, motor impairments precede cognitive impairments and are more severe. In dementia with Lewy bodies, cognitive and behavioural impairments precede motor phenomena and are more severe. There are frequently additional contributions from Alzheimer's or vascular pathology. There are believed to be common pathological processes in all these dementia syndromes.

## Dementia with Lewy bodies

- Progressive dementia, often with a faster course than other dementias
- Shorter-term fluctuations in cognitive function and alertness
- Prominent auditory or visual hallucinations, often with paranoia and delusions
- Parkinsonism is commonly present, but often not severe
- Typical antipsychotics (e.g. haloperidol) are very poorly tolerated, leading to worsening confusion or deterioration of parkinsonism. Atypical antipsychotics (e.g. risperidone, and especially quetiapine) may be better tolerated, but great caution is advised in their use
- Levodopa or dopamine agonists may worsen confusion
- Anticholinergics (e.g. rivastigmine) are effective, especially for hallucinations and behavioural disturbance

Note that several features are common to both dementia with Lewy bodies and delirium, e.g. fluctuations, effect of drugs, perceptual and psychotic phenomena. When comparing the two, the following is true of dementia with Lewy bodies:

- Onset is insidious and progression gradual
- No precipitating illness (e.g. infection) is found
- Hallucinations are complex and not the result of misperception of stimuli
- Delusions (commonly complex auditory or visual) are well formed and may be persistent
- Orthostatic hypotension and falls frequently occur
- Antipsychotics worsen status (not indicated as a diagnostic trial)

## Parkinson's disease with dementia

- People with Parkinson's disease are much more likely to develop dementia, especially older people, those in the later stages of the disease, and those who become confused on Parkinson's medication
- Typical motor features of Parkinson's disease are present and may be severe
- The presentation and neuropathology are variable and may resemble Alzheimer's disease, vascular dementia, or dementia with Lewy bodies
- By definition, if features of Parkinson's precede dementia by more than a year, then the diagnosis is of Parkinson's disease with dementia, not dementia with Lewy bodies. This applies even if the dementia syndrome is otherwise typical of dementia with Lewy bodies
- Multiple system atrophy, progressive supranuclear palsy, and corticobasal degeneration also present with both parkinsonism and dementia

**Minimal cognitive impairment in Parkinson's disease**
Many patients with Parkinson's disease have subtle impairments of cognition, too mild to justify a diagnosis of dementia. Slowed thinking and deficits in visuospatial, attention, and executive function are commonly seen.

# Normal pressure hydrocephalus

NPH classically presents with the triad:
- Gait disturbance (wide-based)
- Incontinence of urine
- Cognitive impairment (psychomotor slowing, apathy, appear depressed)

▶ Most patients with this triad have other (unrelated) causes or have diffuse cerebrovascular disease.

## Assessment

*Neuroimaging*
- Shows ventricles that are enlarged disproportionately, compared with the degree of cerebral atrophy
- Neuroimaging for unrelated reasons (e.g. TIA) may reveal ventricular enlargement that appears disproportionate to the degree of cerebral atrophy, suggesting possible NPH. In the absence of clinical features of NPH, the diagnosis cannot be supported and the patient may be reassured

*Investigation*
Lumbar puncture is being used less frequently in favour of external lumbar drainage (ELD) in specialist centres. This involves spinal catheter insertion for a period of up to 3 days, during which large volumes of cerebrospinal fluid (CSF) can be removed and the clinical impact assessed.

## Treatment

Ventriculoperitoneal shunting is effective for some, but many do not benefit. Gait is more likely to improve than is cognition.

It is a major procedure, and complications are common, e.g. infection and subdural haematoma. Decision to proceed requires:
- A confident diagnosis (may require specialist neurological review)
- Support of patient and carer for the procedure
- An assessment that the likelihood of benefit is high

Benefit is more likely in those who:
- Have a short history
- Have a known cause—usually trauma or subarachnoid haemorrhage
- Have normal brain substance on neuroimaging
- Have no significant comorbidities. Cerebrovascular disease is especially relevant
- Benefit from large-volume CSF removal

## Further reading

BMJ Best Practice. *Normal pressure hydrocephalus.* ℘ http://bestpractice.bmj.com/best-practice/monograph/712.html.

# Dementia: less common diseases

### Frontotemporal dementia

- Neurodegenerative disease, with insidious onset and slow (several years) progression
- Family history is positive in 50% of cases
- Onset is often early (age 35–70), and either behavioural or language difficulties dominate the clinical picture. Forgetfulness is mild. Insight is lost early. Difficulties at work may be the first sign
- Commonly used assessment tools (e.g. MMSE™) do not test frontal lobe function, so do not be put off the diagnosis by 'normal' cognitive screening tests
- Behavioural problems are the most common and include disinhibition, mental rigidity, inflexibility, impairment of executive function, ↓ personal care, and repetitive behaviours
- Language dysfunction may include word-finding difficulty, problems naming or understanding words, and lack of spontaneous conversation or circumlocution
- Later, impairments become broader, similar to severe Alzheimer's
- Primitive reflexes (e.g. grasp, palmar-mental) may be found
- Neuroimaging usually demonstrates frontal and/or temporal atrophy
- Frontotemporal dementia presents as a clinical spectrum. More specific conditions within that spectrum include:
  - *Frontal lobe degeneration*. Frontal greater than temporal degeneration
  - *Pick's disease*. Similar to frontal lobe degeneration, but uncommon. Classical 'Pick bodies' seen post-mortem
  - *MND* with dementia. Usually late in the progression of MND (see ➔ 'Motor neuron disease', pp. 168–9)
  - *Progressive non-fluent aphasia* and *semantic dementia*. Temporal degeneration

### Dementia and infection

- *Neurosyphilis* is becoming more common again. Serological tests for syphilis should be performed if a dementia syndrome has atypical features (e.g. seizures) or risk factors for sexually transmitted disease (STD) (including mental illness, history of other STD, drug/alcohol abuse). Beware false-positive serological tests in African Caribbeans with a history of yaws. If neurosyphilis seems possible, sample the CSF and seek microbiology advice with a view to penicillin treatment
- *HIV-associated dementia* generally affects younger people, reflecting the epidemiology of HIV infection. It occurs late in HIV, rarely, if at all, at presentation
- *CJD* is a prion-mediated, rapidly progressive cortical dementia. Myoclonus is found on physical examination. Psychosis occurs early

## Vasculitis

- Suggested by elevated CRP/ESR without other cause or characteristic CT/MRI (periventricular lesions)
- Heterogeneous presentation, including as delirium or dementia
- Examine the patient for evidence of systemic vasculitis
- Perform serology (e.g. ANA) and lumbar puncture with CSF tests to exclude infection/neoplasm
- Potentially treatable, so pursue this diagnosis vigorously if necessary. Specialist referral usually indicated

## Dementia and drugs/toxins

- Alcohol-associated dementia may occur after many years of heavy drinking, presenting with disproportionate short-term memory impairment (see ➲ 'Confusion and alcohol', p. 242)
- Psychoactive drugs may cause a dementia-like syndrome that is substantially reversible

# Dementia: general management

### General

- Modify *reversible aggravating factors*, commonly multiple but minor (e.g. constipation, low-grade sepsis, mild anaemia, drug side effects)
- Treat *depression*. SSRIs are much preferred to tricyclics. Repeat cognitive assessment 2–4 months after treatment to determine if cognitive impairment remains

### Social

- Encourage physical and mental activity, including social activities (e.g. social clubs, day centres; see ➋ 'Day hospitals', pp. 22–3)
- Create a safe, caring environment, usually in the patient's own home. A predictable routine is helpful. OT home assessment identifies hazards, provides visual safety cues, etc.
- Organize carers to assist with ADLs, prompt medication, etc.
- Support caregivers:
  - Enquire about caregiver burden and psychiatric symptoms
  - Caregiver support groups
  - Respite care—usually in care homes, for a few days to 2 weeks
  - Sitting services—usually for 2–3h once or twice weekly
  - Family support visitor—provides emotional and practical support
- Educate patients and families about the disease and how to cope with its manifestations. This includes appropriate modifications to the home environment and learning to communicate and interact with the patient with dementia. Counselling and support delay admission to care homes

### Practical

- Suggest simple interventions to improve coping (e.g. lists, calendars, alarms)
- Simplify medication, and provide dosette boxes or similar, to aid concordance. In the later stages, drugs such as antihypertensives may become pointless, if not harmful (i.e. risk > benefit)
- Support and educate patient and carers about legal and ethical issues including:
  - Driving (see ➋ 'HOW TO . . . Manage the driver who has dementia', p. 219)
  - Lasting power of attorney (LPA) (see ➋ 'Making financial decisions', pp. 658–9)
  - Wills (see ➋ 'Making a will', p. 678)
  - Discussion of end-of-life issues (clinically assisted nutrition, comfort versus life prolongation) may be appropriate

## HOW TO . . . Manage the driver who has dementia

Road traffic accident and injury risk ↑ with the severity of dementia. In most countries, it is mandatory for the driver to report important health factors to the licensing authority, which will then request further information from the patient's medical team. Patients and carers should be reminded of this responsibility at diagnosis.

Assessment of driving ability during a hospital outpatient or GP consultation is often difficult. In some cases, whether a patient is safe to drive will be obvious—either in the very earliest stages of cognitive impairment or in more severe dementia. In other cases, usually of mild (to moderate) cognitive impairment, the following evidence is useful:

• Reports of driving problems, incidents (e.g. near-misses), or accidents. Are relatives/friends concerned to get into the passenger seat? Have they tried but failed to limit or prohibit driving? Some evidence is of less value, e.g. getting lost is a poor indicator of safety
• Reports of how driving patterns have changed, and why. Are journeys now brief, infrequent, and confined to quiet local roads?
• Clinical evidence of major impairment in visuospatial function, attention, or judgement. However, a combination of modest impairments may be as important
• Presence of non-cognitive impairments (e.g. visual, joint function) or other conditions that affect driving safety (e.g. seizures, syncope)

Each case should be reassessed, either at regular intervals or at points prompted by critical incidents. The best assessment of driving ability is by a professional driving assessor, in the patient's own vehicle on the public roads or in a driving assessment centre (℘ http://www.rdac.co.uk). Such professionals, often OTs, can deliver the confident, robust opinion that is often required, as well as offering useful practical advice to the cognitively or physically impaired driver. In general:

• It is preferable that the patient, family, and doctor should agree that stopping voluntarily is advisable. Compulsory licence withdrawal by the authority generates great anger and distress
• The issue is best discussed early in the course of the disease, when the patient has best insight
• If driving is safe for the moment, encourage the patient and family to think ahead, to a time when driving cannot be continued—is local public transport sufficient, or will a spouse have to hone long-lost driving skills?

Rarely, a patient continues to drive when clearly unsafe and having been informed that they must stop. In most cases, further clear statements of this, backed up by the threat of medical reporting to the authorities, are sufficient to prompt cessation. If driving continues, the clinician is ethically justified in reporting this to the authorities and will usually have the strong support of the family.

## Further reading

Driver and Vehicle Licensing Agency (2016). *Assessing fitness to drive: a guide for medical professionals.* ℘ https://www.gov.uk/government/publications/assessing-fitness-to-drive-a-guide-for-medical-professionals.

# Dementia: risk management and abuse

Risk management is an essential part of care.

- Is there a risk of harm to the patient or to others?
- How great is the risk, over how long is the patient (or other person) exposed to it, and how severe are the consequences of the risk?

▶ There is no such thing as 'safe', only 'safer' and risk management demands careful balancing between autonomy/quality of life and safety.

Common risks include:

- *Falls*. Moving from own home to institutional care is rarely the answer. Supervision is far from continuous in any institution; the environment is less familiar, and the floors are often uncarpeted and unforgiving
- *Purposeful walking/wandering*. Usually more distressing to carers than presenting risk to the patient
- *Aggression by a patient towards carers or family*. Usually verbal, but sometimes physical or sexual. May lead to carers refusing to work with patient
- *Aggression towards a patient by carers or family*. Less easy to identify, as the patient may not complain, through fear or due to cognitive problems. Be concerned if there are unexplained 'falls' or unusual patterns of bruising (see ➋ 'Elder abuse', p. 674)
- *Self-neglect*. Often with denial. May manifest as poor diet, poor hygiene, etc.
- *Fire risk*. May be easily modifiable, through removal or modification of kitchen appliances, gas fires, etc. Cigarette smoking is more problematic
- *Driving* (see ➋ 'HOW TO . . . Manage the driver who has dementia', p. 219)
- *Financial abuse* (see ➋ 'Elder abuse', p. 674)
- Theft or fraud
- Modification of wills
- Misuse or transfer of a patient's money

Having determined the nature and magnitude of a risk, consider 'Can the risk be reduced?' and 'Should it be reduced?'

Consider whether the patient is competent to make their own decisions about risks or whether you are required to act in the patient's 'best interests'.

If risk reduction can be done without impacting on the patient's independence or enjoyment of life, then go ahead.

If reducing risk involves curtailing liberty or restricting enjoyable activity (walking, living alone), then consider:

- If competent, what is the patient's attitude to risk?
- If unable to express this, what was his/her premorbid attitude, and what would he/she now want?
- What is the view of carers?

Commonly, discussions around risk occur when a patient is perceived by some (carers, relatives, nursing or therapy staff) to have become unsafe to remain at home. This should prompt multidisciplinary assessment and discussion, including whether a move to institutional care would involve a change of risk patterns, rather than a reduction in overall risk.

# Dementia: prevention

## Lifestyle interventions

- *Physical activity*. Physical activity may protect against dementia and should be encouraged for other reasons
- *Cognitive activity*. Observational studies suggest that games, reading, etc. are protective, but these associations may not be causal, and there are no good randomized controlled trials
- *Diet*. Again, observational studies suggest benefits from a high fish oil diet, but there is no high-quality prospective evidence. Alcohol intake should be reduced
- *Social activity*. Likely to be protective

## Drugs

Multiple drugs have been proposed (HRT, NSAIDs, antioxidants, antihypertensives, statins), but there is no firm evidence that any should be given for this indication alone.

Usual practice is to encourage physical and mental and social activity ('use it or lose it'), to optimize BP, and to encourage low-dose aspirin in those with, or at high risk of, cerebrovascular disease.

# Dementia: acetylcholinesterase inhibitors

Work by blocking acetylcholinesterase which breaks down acetylcholine, an important neurotransmitter for memory.

## Effectiveness

Far from miracle drugs, with very variable response. In general:

- They offer symptomatic benefit through a one-off increment in cognition. The underlying disease continues to progress and some patients stopping the drug may revert to where they would have been without treatment
- Of the dementias, Alzheimer's disease, dementia with Lewy bodies, and Parkinson's disease with dementia have the greatest cholinergic deficit, and these are the dementia types known to benefit most from acetylcholinesterase inhibitor treatment
- About half of patients show no benefit; a significant minority show moderate improvements ('clock turned back a few months'), and for a small minority there is substantial improvement
- In some, there is a worsening in cognition, or onset of agitation that may be temporary or respond to a change in drug
- Early studies focused on effects on cognitive function, and these are overall modest. However, small improvements in cognition can translate into significantly improved day-to-day function, reducing carer burden
- Some evidence that acetylcholinesterase inhibitors can reduce the requirements for home care and can delay placement in nursing home
- Benefit has been demonstrated for mild to moderate dementia, not in severe dementia, although established treatment should not be automatically discontinued as disease advances

## Choosing a drug

The three acetylcholinesterase inhibitors currently available are:

- *Donepezil*
- *Galantamine*
- *Rivastigmine*

All should be initiated by a specialist and uptitrated. Effectiveness seems broadly similar. There is most evidence for donepezil in Alzheimer's disease and it has fewer adverse events than rivastigmine which is probably better for Lewy body dementia. Overall, the evidence for acetylcholinesterase inhibitors is strongest in Alzheimer's and Lewy body dementia, and weakest in vascular dementia.

## HOW TO . . . Treat with acetylcholinesterase inhibitors

Introducing and monitoring acetylcholinesterase inhibitors is a specialist area, usually undertaken by psychogeriatric teams or by geriatricians or neurologists working in the setting of a memory clinic. Increasingly, they are prescribed in 1° care as part of a locally agreed shared care protocol.

In general, acetylcholinesterase inhibitors should not be initiated in inpatient medical or rehabilitation settings, as the effects of environmental changes, physical illness, or drugs may dominate those of the acetylcholinesterase inhibitor, rendering assessment of effect impossible. It is preferable to initiate treatment when the patient is physically well and living in their own home.

Where given for behavioural disturbance or non-cognitive symptoms (e.g. hallucinations), acetylcholinesterase inhibitors may be initiated more urgently in an institutional setting.

*Before treatment*
- Consider the relative risks and benefits and discuss them with the patient and carer
- Explain that the drugs do not provide a cure and may reasonably be deferred until symptoms worsen
- Consider how concordance can be assured
- Perform an ECG, looking for conduction problems
- Check for relative contraindications, e.g. bradycardia or heart block

*Treatment trial*
- There are significant side effects, commonly gastrointestinal (nausea, dyspepsia, diarrhoea, anorexia). These occur especially during the dose titration phase at higher doses, are often short-lived
- An acetylcholinesterase inhibitor should be given for an initial treatment period of 2–3 months. If there is no effect at the maximum tolerated dose, the drug should be discontinued. There is probably little benefit from trying other acetylcholinesterase inhibitors if one has failed

*Assess impact using*
- Clinician's subjective global assessment, based on the views of the relative(s) or carer(s) and serial clinical observations
- The results of cognitive tests, e.g. MMSE™, clock-drawing test

*Continuing therapy*
- If benefit appears to have occurred, the drug should be continued at that dose. Benefit may be absolute or relative—a small decline would be expected during the 2- to 3-month evaluation period, so an absence of deterioration may be attributed to drug benefit
- Acetylcholinesterase inhibitors can be given indefinitely and there is some evidence that withdrawal in advanced disease reduces function
- As more patients are given an acetylcholinesterase inhibitor at an earlier stage of disease, monitoring falls more to 1° care

## Further reading

National Institute for Health and Care Excellence (2011). *Donepezil, galantamine, rivastigmine and memantine for the treatment of Alzheimer's disease.* Technology appraisal guidance TA217. ℔ http://guidance.nice.org.uk/TA217.

# Dementia: other drug treatments

## Memantine

- This is a blocker of *N*-methyl-D-aspartate (NMDA) receptors that may reduce glutamate-mediated destruction of cholinergic neurons
- It appears to have a beneficial effect in severe dementia of Alzheimer's or vascular aetiology and may be used in those with behavioural disturbance
- Recommended by NICE for moderate Alzheimer's where the patient cannot tolerate acetylcholinesterase inhibitors and in severe disease
- It is well tolerated. Uncommon side effects include hallucinations and worsening confusion
- Avoid in severe renal failure
- Memantine enhances the effect of levodopa and dopamine agonists

## Other drugs to prevent progression

No drugs have been proven to slow or halt progression, although dementia is seen as so catastrophic, the following are often used:

- *Vascular 2° prevention*, e.g. aspirin, lipid-lowering drugs, ACE inhibitors, and other antihypertensives. For patients with vascular dementia and mixed (Alzheimer's–vascular) dementia, aggressive risk factor modification and tailored drug treatment akin to that following stroke is logical but is without evidence. There is better evidence for 1° prevention, e.g. in those with hypertension
- *Vitamin E*. High doses are widely used by patients, but evidence is limited
- *Ginkgo biloba*. A supplement widely used by people with memory impairment or dementia to enhance memory and other cognitive functions, but not convincingly supported by trial evidence. Preparations are expensive, vary in strength, and have antiplatelet activity—caution with anticoagulants

### HOW TO . . . Manage patients with dementia in hospital

▶ Beware iatrogenic deterioration. Modest behavioural deterioration in a patient with moderate dementia at home may lead to hospital admission, with a loss of all familiar routine, physical environment, and caregivers, thus further behavioural decline, administration of sedatives, and further worsened confusion.

Over a quarter of UK hospital beds house patients with dementia. Patients with dementia stay in hospital longer than patients with similar problems but without cognitive impairment, and often leave hospital in a worse physical and mental state than when they arrived.

- Where appropriate, manage the patient at home, with a brief but thorough outpatient attendance if there is concern about physical precipitants. Community outreach may be available to help avoid unnecessary admissions
- If hospital admission is required, then, if possible, admit them directly to a dementia-friendly ward where staff are skilled in managing patients with cognitive impairment. This has been shown to improve outcomes, including length of stay
- Try to minimize disorientation by:
  - Avoiding admission and ward moves at night
  - Avoiding multiple changes of location/ward
  - Quiet room with window (so daylight seen)
  - Minimal distractions (e.g. turn off background radio/TV)
  - Visible clocks and calendars
  - Well-labelled facilities, e.g. toilets—images often better
  - Regular ward routine
  - Encouraging unrestricted family visitation
- Actively ascertain and treat symptoms such as pain or shortness of breath which patients may not spontaneously describe
- Good nursing management of hydration, nutrition, continence (avoid constipation), pressure areas, and falls prevention
- Where psychoactive medication is required, use it sparingly for short courses. Remember that sedation is a side effect and NOT the desired outcome (which is behaviour modification)
- Take time to communicate with the patient and their relatives
- Minimize the length of admission with proactive early discharge planning

### Further reading

Alzheimer's Society. ℛ http://alzheimers.org.uk.

# Dementia: managing behavioural problems

Behavioural problems include agitation, anxiety, phobias, irritability, purposeful walking (wandering), hoarding, aggression, socially inappropriate behaviour (e.g. sexual disinhibition, inappropriate urination, attention-seeking), hallucinations, and delusions.

These are common in dementia, including Alzheimer's, and may occur early in the disease. Often it is behavioural problems, rather than cognitive impairment, that lead to institutionalization; managing them successfully may enable a patient to remain in their own home.

## General

- Consider whether acute illness (e.g. sepsis), pain (e.g. urinary retention), or changes in drug treatment (e.g. anticholinergics) have contributed, especially if behaviour has deteriorated rapidly
- Consider whether agitation or aggression is a manifestation of depression (consider an SSRI) or of fear (which may respond if care is given in a non-challenging way by a familiar team)
- Medication may not be needed if symptoms are transient, do not cause the patient significant distress, and are not threatening care of the patient in the current environment

## Non-drug management

These are preferred and may be sufficient alone.

- Avoid precipitants
- Effective therapies include music, bathing, exercise, pets, art therapy, and aromatherapy
- The environment should be home-like, familiar, and interesting
- Activities may reduce boredom, wandering, and aggression
- Delusions and hallucinations may be helped by distraction and reassurance
- Anxiety may respond to relaxation or a discussion of worries
- Specialist teams (geriatricians or psychiatrists) may be able to offer helpful advice

## Drug treatment

The best drug is that which, for that patient with that problem, has worked well previously.

For *agitation, anxiety*, and *irritability*:

- Benzodiazepines, e.g. lorazepam, are often successful, but long-term treatment should be avoided due to side effects and dependence
- If depression is prominent, try an SSRI such as citalopram
- If this fails or side effects (usually oversedation) occur, introduce an atypical antipsychotic such as quetiapine—if considered necessary, use the lowest dose for the shortest period possible. Risperidone and olanzapine are now rarely recommended because of the ↑ risk of stroke, IHD, and death

- Haloperidol and phenothiazines are slow-acting and have many side effects so should be avoided in the absence of psychotic symptoms
- Memantine can be used with good effect in extreme agitation

For *problematic psychotic symptoms* (delusions, hallucinations, paranoia):
- Cholinesterase inhibitors may improve behaviour as well as cognition. They may be given 'first line', especially if symptoms are moderate and not acute in onset
- Atypical antipsychotics should be used at the lowest dose that is effective
- Trazodone, an antidepressant, may be useful, especially where sleep disturbance is a problem and aggression is only verbal
- In dementia with Lewy bodies, use antipsychotics with great caution, in low dose, under close supervision, and only when other non-pharmacological and pharmacological measures have been exhausted. Atypical antipsychotics are preferred

Review drug use regularly, being aware of potential side effects such as falls, immobility, or confusion. Behavioural problems are often periodic or provoked, so consider stopping treatment as soon as possible.

# Compulsory detention and treatment

Older people in need of medical assessment, treatment, or continuing care commonly lack the capacity to judge the risk and benefit of interventions. They may therefore refuse care when its benefit is clear to others.

In the UK, there are several legal procedures which may support a doctor in the compulsory treatment, admission, or detention of patients.

## Mental Capacity Act (2005)

The most commonly used legal support for actions when the patient lacks capacity to make a certain decision (see ➲ 'The Mental Capacity Act 2005', p. 656). Actions may include:
- Admission to hospital
- Treatment and detention on a ward or within a hospital
- Treatment in the home (e.g. in delirium 2° to infection, but refusing antibiotics)
- Detention in the home (e.g. wandering presents danger to the patient)

Actions should be:
- Justifiable, reasonable, and proportionate to the situation. Based on a consideration of the risks/benefits for that patient, and their likely wishes were they competent. Consider alternatives and always opt for the least restrictive (see ➲ 'Deprivation of Liberty Safeguards', p. 657)
- Carefully documented and reviewed regularly

## Section 5(2) of the Mental Health Act (1983)
- This permits the detention of an inpatient in a general or psychiatric hospital for up to 72h after submission of a report, while their mental health needs are assessed. Outpatients or DH patients do not fall within this section
- It should be considered if a patient is highly resistive to treatment or restraint, formalizing actions taken under common law
- It is sensible to seek the advice of a psychogeriatrician to confirm that it is appropriate, and during the 72h period to perform assessment and help guide further management
- Detention is authorized when the registered medical practitioner in charge of treatment or a fully registered deputy (not pre-registration junior) completes a report ('Form 12') and submits it to the duty hospital manager

## Section 2 of the Mental Health Act (1983)
- This permits the admission to hospital and detention of a patient for assessment and treatment
- The patient must have a mental disorder that warrants detention in the interests of the patient or for the protection of others
- Application is made by a relative or an approved social worker, and supported by two registered medical practitioners
- The assessment period is up to 28 days and is not renewable

## Deprivation of Liberty Safeguards

- This code of practice was published in 2007 and provides supplementary guidance to the Mental Capacity Act (2005). It lays down a framework for when and how Deprivation of Liberty (DoL) may be authorized (see ➋ 'Deprivation of Liberty Safeguards', p. 657)
- The impetus for these guidelines arose out of a well-publicized case dating back to 1997 in which an autistic patient who was incompetent was detained informally in Bournewood Hospital for assessment. The 'Bournewood Gap' was identified as a gap in the law by the European Court of Human Rights. Incompetent patients who were sectioned were subject to stringent rules (Mental Health Act), while 'informal patients' held under the common law of necessity did not have similar protective mechanisms and regulations and potentially could be held for indefinite amounts of time
- Deprivation of Liberty Safeguards (DoLS) are applicable in hospitals and care homes. There are detailed requirements about assessment, authorizing detention, renewing, and challenging decisions
- The underlying principle is that a patient should be detained in the least restrictive manner that is practical
- Despite the huge number of patients who potentially come under these legal safeguards in acute geriatric medicine wards, most remain under simple common law. DoLS teams provide assessment and support decision-making and documentation when the deprivation is particularly stringent, long-standing, or is challenged by family or friends

---

### HOW TO . . . Manage the older person refusing treatment

In practice, compulsion is possible only in hospital. Brief interventions against a patient's will are sometimes possible at home (e.g. restraint to prevent dangerous wandering; forced administration of antibiotics in a sepsis with delirium) but can rarely be sustained because of resource restraints and staff feeling legally and physically vulnerable.

Use guidance from the *Mental Capacity Act* to admit to acute medical wards in cases of:
- Dementia with acute physical illness
- Delirium with moderate behavioural disturbance

Use the *Mental Health Act* to admit to psychiatric wards in cases of:
- Dementia, with risk to self, but alternatives must be explored and considered
- Delirium with severe behavioural disturbance (to psychiatric or medical or geriatric ward)
- Psychotic state, severe with risk to self or others, e.g. severe depression with psychosis or risk of self-harm

Compulsory admission is not justified and/or not legal in cases of:
- Physical illness, refusing treatment without psychiatric illness
- Psychotic state or other psychiatric illness of moderate severity, without significant risk to self or others

These are guidelines. If in any doubt, seek emergency advice from the local psychogeriatric team.

# Psychosis

Psychotic symptoms, e.g. delusions and hallucinations, are common in older people, particularly in those who are acutely unwell, hospitalized, or in care homes. Symptoms range from benign and non-distressing to those that cause anxiety among patients and caregivers, and often indicate important, treatable disease.

## What is psychosis?

A state of severe impairment of assessment of reality. The results include:

- Distortions of perception, e.g. illusions (misperceptions—distortions of actual perceptions) and hallucinations (perceptions not the result of external stimulus)
- Distortions of thought content, i.e. delusions—beliefs held with great conviction despite contrary evidence. These are usually 2°, i.e. a response to abnormal occurrences such as hallucinations or low mood

## Causes of psychotic symptoms in older people

The most common causes are 'organic'. In order of frequency:

- Dementia
- Depression
- Delirium
- Drugs, e.g. levodopa
- Other neurological causes, e.g. cerebrovascular disease, brain tumour

Less common causes are 'functional' or 'non-organic', e.g.:

- Persistence into late life of chronic schizophrenia
- Delusional disorder of later life ('late-onset schizophrenia-like psychosis')
- Psychotic presentation of affective disorder (mania or depression)

## Treatment of patients with psychotic symptoms

- Can usually be managed on the general medical wards or at home, but early specialist psychogeriatric team support is advised
- Avoid reinforcing a patient's paranoid beliefs: do not avoid contact, do not seek rapid transfer from the ward, etc.
- Make a diagnosis and treat the underlying cause, e.g. stop drugs leading to delirium
- Attend to hearing and visual impairments
- Treat underlying mood disorder
- In dementia, especially Alzheimer's and dementia with Lewy bodies, consider acetylcholinesterase inhibitors
- If symptoms are distressing and persistent, consider the use of antipsychotics, e.g. haloperidol, risperidone, olanzapine; usually after specialist advice. Be cautious in patients who may have dementia with Lewy bodies
- On discharge, offer opportunities for social interaction and practical home support

# Delirium: diagnosis

Delirium is a syndrome of disturbance of consciousness accompanied by change in cognition not accounted for by pre-existing dementia. The term delirium (acute confusional state) refers to an acute brain syndrome, effectively acute brain failure, characterized by impairment of consciousness (however slight).

Beware sloppy language—the term confusion means only that: muddled thinking or an inability to think clearly. It is an important symptom of acute 'organic' brain disorders such as delirium but is not confined to them, i.e. low specificity. It may also be seen in depression, dementia, and less commonly in some 1° psychotic disorders. Use the term confusion when describing a presentation, but never as a diagnosis.

## Key features

- A *disturbance of consciousness* (↓ clarity of awareness of the environment). May be hypoactive, hyperactive, or mixed (see Box 9.1). ↓ ability to focus, shift, or sustain attention. Distractability. Lose thread of conversation. Leads to uncertainty about time of day. Impairment is often not obvious, especially if onset gradual; but, after recovery, memory for the period will be poor. This feature is not seen in early dementia or in 1° psychotic disorders
- *Change in cognition*. Often widespread, e.g. memory impairment (often recent memory), disorientation (time, place; person less common), language disturbance (e.g. dysgraphia, dysnomia), perceptual impairment (misinterpretations, e.g. slamming door = gunshot), illusions (usually visual, e.g. bedclothes animated), hallucinations. Thinking may be slow and muddled, but is often rich in content
- *Acute onset and fluctuates*. Usual onset over hours or a few days. Sometimes changes are subacute (weeks to a few months) and may be misdiagnosed as dementia. Severity varies during the day, e.g. 'sundowning' is a syndrome of worsening confusion in the later part of the day or at night

## Other features (not essential to make the diagnosis)

These include:
- Disturbance of the sleep–wake cycle. May be complete reversal
- Disturbed psychomotor behaviour. May be 'up' (restless, picking, wandering) or 'down' (slow, immobile)
- Emotional disturbance, e.g. fear, depression, anger, euphoria, lability. Fear and aggression may be a consequence of threatening hallucinations or delusions. The patient may call out, scream, or moan continually. In an institutional setting, this may be problematic, especially at night. At a lesser level, the patient may appear simply perplexed and bewildered
- Delusions (often persecutory) are common, but usually transient and poorly elaborated
- Poor insight is typical

## Box 9.1 Pitfalls in diagnosis

Making the diagnosis can be difficult, but early identification is vital as early treatment will improve prognosis. Delirium is a varied syndrome. As well as fluctuating day-to-day or hour-to-hour, it is variable in nature, manifesting distinctly in different patients, or in the same patient at different times. For example, two patterns (ends of a spectrum) have been described:

- Hyperactive or 'up': oversensitive to stimuli, psychomotor agitation, repeatedly getting out of bed, noisy, psychotic symptoms, aggression
- Hypoactive or 'down': psychomotor retardation, lethargy, quiet, paucity of speech, few psychotic symptoms. This variety is more commonly not recognized and has a worse prognosis
- A mixed picture can also occur

Delirium may be misdiagnosed when it is not present (e.g. in deaf, or blind or dysphasic patients). More commonly, the diagnosis is not made when it is present. Therefore, screening tests (typically the AMTS, and see ➜ Appendix, 'CAM', p. 706) are valuable and should be performed in all cases when delirium is possible—certainly at the time of admission, and during admission if changes in clinical condition occur.

Usually there is evidence of the medical condition that has led to delirium. Although this is not necessary to make the diagnosis, it is necessary to treat it effectively.

Ensure you document your assessment and diagnosis well.

# Delirium: causes

A particular case is often multifactorial, i.e. several factors (individually modest and alone insufficient) combine to push a patient across a threshold to frank delirium. Chronic factors (e.g. overt or incipient dementia) may maintain a person closer to that threshold, and impaired homeostasis of older age ↑ the systemic—and cerebral—effects of illness.

Delirium is therefore especially likely to occur in very elderly people, in the physically frail, or if there is pre-existing dementia, defective hearing or vision, or brain damage of any kind, e.g. idiopathic Parkinson's disease. In these cases, more minor acute illnesses may cause delirium.

## Factors that may contribute to delirium

▶ Usually, there is evidence from either the history or examination or simple tests, of the factor(s) that have contributed to delirium.

These factors include:

- *Infection*. Viral or bacterial. Not necessarily severe, especially in those with MCI, dementia, or other contributory factors. Common sources are chest, urine, skin (cellulitis). Remember other infections, e.g. CNS, endocarditis, biliary infection, diverticulitis, pancreatitis, abdominal perforation, and abdominal or pelvic collection
- *Drug intoxication*. Especially anticholinergics, anxiolytics/hypnotics, anticonvulsants, opiates (see Box 9.2)
- *Disorders of electrolyte/fluid balance*, e.g. dehydration, uraemia, hypo-/hypernatraemia, hypercalcaemia. Modest degrees of hyponatraemia (>130mmol/L) are unlikely to be the sole cause of delirium
- *Alcohol or drug withdrawal*
- *Organ failure*, e.g. cardiac, respiratory, liver
- *Endocrine*. High or low blood sugar, hypo- or hyperthyroid
- *Epileptic*. Post-ictal state following unrecognized seizures. Consider if there has been an unwitnessed 'collapse', with amnesia, and any ictal features (incontinence, tongue biting). If conscious level is low, consider ongoing ictal activity or even non-convulsive status
- *Intracranial pathology*, e.g. head injury, space-occupying lesion, ↑ intracranial pressure of whatever cause, infection, pre-existing cognitive impairment, or acute/chronic cerebrovascular disease
- *Pain*
- *Constipation/urinary retention*
- *Surgery, trauma, any anaesthesia*

These factors may be accentuated on admission to hospital by environmental disorientation, a lack of information, sensory over- or under-stimulation, impersonal setting, changes in staff or wards, poorly understood investigations and treatments, and being away from a familiar home and family/carers.

## Box 9.2 Drugs causing delirium

Drug-induced delirium is common. Incidence of delirium is closely associated with anticholinergic activity (anticholinergic burden scales exist; see ➔ Further reading below). Many more drugs are less frequently associated with delirious reactions:

- *Anticholinergics* (used for either urinary or gastrointestinal effects, e.g. oxybutynin, hyoscine)
- *Antipsychotic drugs* ('neuroleptics'), e.g. chlorpromazine, trifluoperazine
- *Antihistamines*, e.g. chlorphenamine
- *Hypnotics/anxiolytics*, e.g. benzodiazepines, 'Z-drugs' (zolpidem)
- *Antidepressant drugs*, especially tricyclics
- *Anticonvulsant drugs*, e.g. phenytoin, carbamazepine
- *Opiates and opiate-like drugs*, including codeine, dihydrocodeine, and tramadol
- *Corticosteroids*, including prednisolone
- *Lithium*
- *H2 receptor blockers*, e.g. ranitidine (rarely)
- *L-dopa* (co-beneldopa, co-careldopa), *dopamine agonists*. Caution in treating parkinsonism in patients with Lewy body dementia
- *Digoxin*

'Recreational' drugs that may cause delirium include alcohol, marijuana, LSD, amphetamines, cocaine, opiates, and inhalants.

A drug may be the 'final straw' that leads to overt delirium. For example, a dry, septic patient who has tolerated co-codamol when well may become delirious when it is again administered in hospital.

## Further reading

Aging Brain Care. *Aging brain care tools.* ℬ http://www.agingbraincare.org/index.php/tools/.

# Delirium: clinical assessment

### History and examination

- Most factors leading to a presentation with delirium can be identified by taking a history and examining the patient. Even confused, forgetful patients report ongoing symptoms (e.g. pain, dysuria) if asked
- Always obtain a collateral history, paying careful regard to recent minor/major symptoms (e.g. cough), as well as drug history, and an exploration of the nature and duration of memory/cognitive symptoms
- Always assess cognition objectively, e.g. using the AMTS or clock-drawing test. This may yield surprising results (better or worse than expected) and permits tracking of progress
- If a patient is non-compliant with examination, use distraction (e.g. chatting while examining) or complete the examination in sections. Sedation will only rarely be necessary
- Focus the examination on important areas—is there evidence of infection (examine all lung areas, abdomen) or of new focal neurology? Is the patient dehydrated or overloaded?
- Repeat vital signs regularly, especially temperature
- Check arterial oxygen saturation off oxygen—even modest hypoxaemia (sats ≤95%) may indicate important cardiopulmonary pathology

### Investigation

- One contributing factor may be obvious (e.g. UTI), but do not assume that this is the sole—or even the most important—factor, until others have been excluded
- All patients should have some baseline tests (see Box 9.3). These will vary according to the clinical picture, the availability of tests, and whether a clear cause is already apparent
- If the cause remains unclear despite a careful history, examination, and 'simple' tests, then repeat clinical assessment, consider less common causes, and consider more advanced tests such as CT/MRI brain, EEG, or CSF examination

## Box 9.3 Baseline investigations in delirium

- *FBC, ESR.* Evidence of infection, anaemia (unlikely on its own to cause delirium)
- *U, C+E.* Hypo-/hypernatraemia, dehydration, renal impairment
- *Glucose.* Hypo-/hyperglycaemia. The sugar may now be normal—but what was it an hour/day ago?
- *LFTs and amylase*
- *TFTs.* Hypo- or- hyperthyroidism are common and treatable. Both may contribute to a presentation of delirium
- *CRP.* A very useful test but may be normal early in the course of infection
- *Calcium and phosphate*
- *CXR.* Clinical examination is relatively insensitive to early/localized pathology, e.g. infection
- *ECG.* Silent ischaemia/infarction common in older people. Consider troponin
- *Urinalysis ± urine microscopy and culture.* Asymptomatic bacteriuria is common; a positive dipstick may not therefore explain a patient's delirium. Look for additional causes
- *Blood culture.* Always send before starting antibiotics. Occult bacteraemia is common
- *Blood gases.* Hypoxaemia or hypercapnia may contribute to delirium
- *Drug levels*, e.g. digoxin, lithium

# Delirium: treatment issues

▶ Initiate treatment early—delirium is a medical emergency.

## Where to treat?

In all cases, the patient should be thoroughly assessed by appropriately trained clinicians who have access to baseline investigations. If further investigations are required (e.g. CT), assessment at an acute hospital may be appropriate. Outside an acute hospital—in a domestic setting, care home, community or psychiatric hospital—the medical team must balance the benefits of advanced diagnostics, treatment, and monitoring with the possible detrimental effect of transfer. There is place for a 'treat at home' approach which may improve outcomes, provided that:

• The dominant cause is clear
• Effective treatment can be given
• Appropriate care and supervision can be assured

Keep the admission brief. With appropriate support and monitoring, discharge home or transfer to a less acute environment can often be achieved early before complete resolution.

## The underlying cause

▶ Making the diagnosis of delirium is half the job. The second part is eliciting and treating the cause(s).

• Use targeted antibiotics. Broad-spectrum antibiotics, with the associated risk of *Clostridium* colitis, should be reserved for patients with severe sepsis of unknown origin
• Always check the drug chart. Consider each drug in turn—at this time, does risk equal or exceed benefit? If so, stop the drug, at least temporarily
• Ensure adequate fluid and nutrition. The patient may not be dry or malnourished on admission (though they commonly are) but may soon become so
• If alcohol dependency or severe malnutrition is known or suspected, high-dose parenteral vitamin B supplements may be needed
• Occasionally, the cause of delirium is not apparent. In such cases:
  • Initiate general supportive measures (fluid, pressure care, nutrition, etc.)
  • Continually re-examine and consider more advanced tests

## Competency

Patients with delirium are not usually competent to direct treatment. The law allows assessment and treatment in their best interests. This may include:

• Holding within a ward or hospital if a patient attempts to leave
• Temporary restraint (e.g. while drugs are administered)
• Covert administration of essential drugs

Clear explanations should be given to staff and family of the need for such interventions, and their ethical and legal justification. Document clearly in the medical notes why the team considers that such measures are necessary. Reassess competence continually. Once the acute illness is over, a 'Deprivation of liberty assessment' may be needed (see ➲ 'Deprivation of Liberty Safeguards', p. 657).

# Delirium: non-drug management

Delirious patients feel ill, frightened, bemused, and disorientated. There are problems with attention, memory, and perception. Therefore, do what you can to make life easier for the patient:

- Provide a quiet environment free from worrying sounds; appropriate clothes; quality lighting, at an appropriate level for the time of day; a clock or outside view to aid orientation
- Optimize visual and auditory acuity by providing spectacles and hearing aids that work
- Reassure the patient repeatedly and calmly
- Explain who you are and what you wish to do, and confirm understanding
- Patients will sense a doctor's manner, particularly aggression or frustration. At all times, appear relaxed, unhurried, and pleasant
- Use non-verbal communication—sit down, smile, and appear friendly rather than professional
- Do not argue or correct delusions—the product will be aggravation and lesser compliance
- Educate visitors who are heightening emotion—ask them to modify their behaviour or even ask them to leave
- Explain to relatives and enlist their help in supervising, feeding, and bringing in items familiar to the patient

## Physical restraint

Restraint is terrifying and has adverse mental and physical sequelae. It is only rarely needed but is sometimes (inappropriately) used as a substitute for supervision and guidance by an experienced carer/nurse.

In cases of severe aggression, where parenteral drugs are required, brief immobilization of the patient using the minimum force necessary may, on balance, be in the patient's best interests.

## Recovery phase

▶ Patterns of recovery from delirium vary. Most patients recover completely in a few days; some take much longer, but some never return to baseline cognitive and/or physical function. Delirium can 'unmask' a previously unrecognized dementia. In those whose functional status declines significantly, remember that full recovery may take weeks or months—beware making irreversible decisions (e.g. home versus residential care)— before the final functional level is known.

Once a patient is admitted, multiple barriers to discharge often appear:

- Carers and family will fear that recent deterioration will persist and may resist discharge
- Care packages may be cancelled, taking weeks to restart
- Therapists may assess function as suboptimal in the unfamiliar hospital environment, judging that discharge is unsafe

Therefore, once the acute event has been diagnosed and treatment begun, encourage the team to begin promptly to plan for home. Delay in discharge leads to ↑ prescription of psychotropic drugs, institutionalization, and care home placement.

# Delirium: drug treatments

Drugs are needed only when the agitation that accompanies delirium is:
- Causing significant patient distress
- Threatening the safety of the patient or others
- Interfering with medical treatment (e.g. pulling out of iv lines, aggression preventing clinical examination)

Having decided that drug treatment is in the patient's interests, remember that:
- Drugs should complement, not replace, non-drug approaches
- The correct dose is the minimum effective dose
- The response (adverse and beneficial) and prescription must be reviewed regularly
- It is preferable to use only one drug, starting at low dose, and ↑ the dose incrementally at intervals of 30–60min
- Delirium can resolve quickly, so avoid regular prescription—each dose should be as needed (PRN).

The relative merits of differing drug classes and drugs are debated, but a reasonable consensus is presented in ➋ 'HOW TO . . . Prescribe sedating drugs in delirium', p. 241.

In cases where behaviour remains problematic, seek urgent advice from the local psychogeriatric team.

## HOW TO . . . Prescribe sedating drugs in delirium

*Short-acting benzodiazepines (e.g. lorazepam)*
- Have recently replaced antipsychotics as first-line treatments. Useful if sleep disturbance is prominent or for severe distress or agitation
- Short-acting benzodiazepines are preferred, e.g. lorazepam po, im, or sublingual, repeated as necessary/tolerated
- Dependence and tolerance are possible, so review regularly and discontinue as soon as possible. Avoid inclusion on 'to take out' (TTOs), if possible
- Long-acting benzodiazepines are especially useful for the treatment of delirium caused by alcohol or benzodiazepine withdrawal. Use chlordiazepoxide in reducing dose
- In extreme cases only (e.g. severe distress/agitation, with imminent danger to self/others), consider giving a small iv dose of a short-acting benzodiazepine (e.g. midazolam), carefully titrated to response. Monitor closely both clinically and with oximetry—the major risk is respiratory depression

*Typical antipsychotics (e.g. haloperidol)*
- Compared with low-potency antipsychotics, there are fewer side effects (e.g. sedation, hypotension, anticholinergic)
- Begin with a small dose, e.g. 0.5mg po, as tablet or liquid, prn. Repeat doses after 1–2h, and ↑ the dose size as needed and tolerated. Total daily oral dose is usually 0.5–4mg
- Response is idiosyncratic—some patients are very sensitive to low doses, others only to very large doses
- In older people, the half-life of haloperidol may be as long as 60h. Dosing can be cumulative. Failure to titrate the dose correctly may render the patient semi-conscious for days
- The oral liquid formulation of haloperidol is colourless and odourless, aiding covert administration (e.g. in a drink) if required
- In the very agitated, consider haloperidol 1–2mg im repeated after 1h (~2:1 oral to intramuscular dose equivalence)
- The incidence of extrapyramidal side effects is high. Avoid haloperidol in dementia with Lewy bodies and Parkinson's

*Atypical antipsychotics (e.g. olanzapine, risperidone)*
- Should be used second line following concerns of ↑ risk of stroke/cardiac events
- Risperidone liquid can be diluted in water, black coffee, or orange juice

*Combination treatment*
Benzodiazepines and antipsychotic medications are sometimes combined in the management of delirium symptoms, generally under specialist advice.

*Stopping treatment*
Once behaviour has improved, consider stepwise dose reduction, aiming to stop the drug as soon as possible without prompting relapse.

# Confusion and alcohol

It is an error to consider alcohol abuse as exclusively a disease of younger people. Even if the clinician remembers to ask about alcohol, they are often deceived by the patient who is embarrassed. ↓ alcohol metabolism means that older people should probably be recommended lower 'safe' drinking levels than younger adults. ↓ balance and cognitive reserve may mean that even very small doses of alcohol can have detrimental effects.

*Alcohol withdrawal*—occurs when habitual excess alcohol intake is stopped, e.g. when a patient is admitted to hospital. Agitation and confusion can occur along with physical signs such as diarrhoea, fever, and hypertension. Visual or tactile hallucinations or illusions can occur.

*Delirium tremens*—severe form of alcohol withdrawal with a high mortality. There are delusions, tremor, autonomic hyperactivity, and sometimes seizures.

*Wernicke's encephalopathy*—triad of confusion, ataxia, and ophthalmoplegia. May respond to prompt thiamine administration, but many go on to develop Korsakoff's syndrome.

*Korsakoff's syndrome*—irreversible brain damage caused by thiamine deficiency, most commonly seen in alcoholism. May follow an episode of Wernicke's encephalopathy or develop gradually. Amnesia and confabulation occur with lack of insight and apathy. Ataxia and tremor may also be found.

*Alcohol dementia syndrome*—a dementia almost indistinguishable from Alzheimer's, can occur without the typical features of Korsakoff–Wernicke syndrome.

## Managing alcohol withdrawal in hospital

- Make the diagnosis
- If necessary (not routinely—heavy drinkers get withdrawal symptoms in about half of cases), use a decreasing-dose schedule of benzodiazepine, e.g. chlordiazepoxide to control symptoms and behaviour. Clomethiazole should not be used in older patients.
- Always prescribe B vitamins—either parenterally or po (multivitamins plus thiamine)
- Offer support

# Squalor syndrome

Also referred to as senile self-neglect (inappropriately derogatory) or Diogenes syndrome.

## Clinical features

- Affected people, usually elderly, live in conditions of severe self-neglect, are socially withdrawn, and lack insight into the unusual nature of their behaviours and effects on others
- Financial problems are rare
- Homes are typically dirty, their upkeep neglected, and are often the repository for hoarded rubbish. This often causes distress and anxiety to neighbours, social and health professionals, much more so than to the patient themselves. Thus they come to the attention of many agencies—health, social, and public (e.g. environmental health)

The syndrome is not uncommon. Diagnosis is made when the clinical features listed exist, without major psychiatric illness (dementia, depression) to explain it. The best guess is that the syndrome is an unusual manifestation of long-standing personality disorder and that isolated frontal lobe dysfunction commonly plays a part.

## Risk factors

- Borderline personality ('eccentricity')
- Early dementia or depression
- Recent bereavement (commonly spouse)
- Lack of close family
- Social isolation
- Sensory impairment (often visual)

## Management

- This should include identification and treatment of contributing psychiatric illness and 2° physical illness, e.g. malnutrition
- Patients often decline ongoing social support. Psychiatric day care may maintain more mainstream behaviour for a time, but relapse is common. Institutional care is a long-term solution, if accepted
- Usually such people are competent to decide to maintain their unusual lifestyle and to decline offers of support
- Caring for them can be frustrating, but adverse consequences for the patient are often surprisingly few, and a watching brief is usually sufficient, with prompt intervention when decompensation occurs

# Depression: presentation

The most common psychiatric illness in older people. Probably 10–15% prevalence over 65 years, severe in 3%.

Risk factors for depression include:
- Disability and illness (especially if serious)
- Care home residents
- Bereavement. Reactive depression is more common in older people, who suffer more bereavement, illness, and other life events. The reaction may be understandable, but there is benefit from treatment (see ➲ 'Bereavement', p. 640)
- Social isolation
- Chronic pain
- Sensory impairment (e.g. hearing or sight)

Comorbidity may mask or precipitate depression and may be:
- Physical (Parkinson's, stroke, cancer, or post-acute illness)
- Psychiatric (dementia)

Depression is underdiagnosed in older people, for the following reasons:
- Perception that depression carries a social stigma, so not volunteering symptoms
- Presentation with symptoms suggesting physical, rather than psychiatric, disease (e.g. weight loss, rather than sadness)
- Perception that low mood is a normal part of ageing (e.g. 'Of course she is depressed—she is in a nursing home with chronic disability and pain')

▶ Have a low threshold for opportunistic screening.

## HOW TO . . . Distinguish dementia from a depressive pseudodementia

*Pseudodementia* is a depression that presents with poor memory and concentration and impaired functional capacity, e.g. for ADLs. Also known as dementia of depression.

It is usually distinguishable from dementia, because:
- The history is often short and the onset relatively abrupt
- Patients often complain about poor memory and are despairing
- Assessment of cognition often results in 'don't know' responses
- Memories are often accessible with 'hints' or cues from the assessor—they remain 'stored'
- There is often a past history of depression, or an identifiable precipitant

The prognosis is variable. In some, mood and cognition respond to antidepressants. However, many go on to develop dementia, usually of Alzheimer type.

### Coexistence of depression and dementia
- Both depression and dementia are relatively common and may coexist coincidentally
- Over 20% of people with an early dementia may be depressed, suggesting a depressive reaction to the onset of dementia—especially common and understandable if insight is preserved
- This is quite different from pseudodementia (where there is no actual dementia)

### General guidance
- Treat depression whatever the cause—whether a 'true' pseudodementia or a combination of dementia and depression
- Avoid mislabelling a depressed patient as also having dementia—the management and prognoses are very different
- Always screen for depression when assessing patients with cognitive disorders, including short-term memory loss alone

# Depression: clinical features

### Sadness

Commonly denied, and not necessary in order to make a diagnosis of depression. Tearfulness is uncommon, especially in men. Also ask about biological symptoms, anhedonia (inability to enjoy—ask 'What do you enjoy or look forward to?'), and depressive thoughts (guilt, worthlessness, low self-esteem, self-blame, suicidal thoughts, hopelessness, and helplessness).

### Anorexia and weight loss

Common to both depression and serious physical illness. In the patient who presents in this way, without evidence of a physical cause after clinical examination and basic tests, it is a matter of judgement whether and when an antidepressant trial should begin, and whether more invasive tests should be delayed pending the results of that therapeutic trial (see ➔ 'HOW TO . . . Manage weight loss in older patients', p. 355).

### Sleep disturbance

Typically early morning wakening, but a full sleep history is useful, as early wakening may be appropriate, e.g. if sleeping during the day. Some older people do sleep much less than when younger—the key is whether they wake refreshed or wake anxious and fearful, keen to return to sleep but unable to do so (see ➔ 'Sleep and insomnia', pp. 174–5).

### Disturbance of behaviour

May include attention-seeking, aggression, irritability, cries for help (e.g. intentional falls), self-neglect, malnutrition, and social withdrawal.

### Cognitive impairment

Poor attention and concentration may result in impairments in several cognitive domains, typically memory. If severe, this may manifest as a 'depressive pseudodementia'.

### Suicidal ideation and self-harm

Should always be taken seriously, as completed suicide is relatively common in older people, especially those with physical illness. Self-harm (e.g. drug overdose) may be medically trivial, but psychiatrically very serious, and should mandate psychiatric referral. Parasuicide—a 'cry for help' or 'manipulative' self-harm event—is very rare; most older people who self-harm are at least moderately depressed.

### Physical slowness

Exclude physical causes, including parkinsonism, cerebrovascular disease, and hypothyroidism. May manifest as ↑ dependence or 'failure to cope'. May be severe, with very reduced mobility or total immobility—the depressed, bed-bound, motionless, anorexic patient must be treated as an emergency.

## Somatization

This expression of psychological problems as physical symptoms is common, as is hypochondriasis (disproportionate concern over health). In the patient presenting with somatization or hypochondriasis, the risks are of failing to investigate and treat when a true physical illness is present, or conversely of failing to appreciate that antidepressant treatment is actually what is needed.

---

### HOW TO . . . Assess depression

*Depression rating scales*

For example, GDS (see ⬤ Appendix, 'Geriatric Depression Scale', p. 701), which is known to be valid in community and hospital settings and maintains specificity in mild to moderate dementia.

Two or three simple questions can be effective screening tools. Simply asking 'Do you feel low?' has reasonable sensitivity and specificity for depression.

*Psychiatric history and examination*

*Physical history and examination*

Targeting evidence of physical illness contributing to, or mimicking, depression, and contraindications to drug treatments.

*Cognitive assessment screen*

For example, MoCA, clock-drawing test. Is there coexisting cognitive impairment? If so, does it improve with treatment for depression, i.e. pseudodementia? (See ⬤ 'HOW TO . . . Distinguish dementia from a depressive pseudodementia', p. 245.)

*Blood tests*

- FBC (anaemia leading to lethargy; high mean corpuscular volume (MCV) in alcohol excess)
- ESR (malignancy, vasculitis)
- $B_{12}$ and folate (low levels may contribute to depression or result from anorexia)
- U, C+E (uraemia, dehydration)
- Calcium (hypercalcaemia leading to depression and fatigue)
- Thyroid function (hypothyroidism, and occasionally hyperthyroidism, may present as depression)
- Liver function (malignancy, alcohol excess)

# Depression: non-drug management

Depression is undertreated as well as under-diagnosed. Treatment should be started promptly.

### Supportive treatment

- Includes counselling and relief of loneliness
- Treat physical symptoms and pain
- Address rational anxieties, e.g. financial, housing, physical dependency
- Consider stopping contributory drugs (β-blockers, benzodiazepines, levodopa, opiates, steroids)

### Psychotherapy

As effective as antidepressants for mild to moderate depression and is without physical side effects. For severe depression, should be combined with drug treatment. Cognitive behavioural therapy has the most evidence. Is resource-intensive and often has limited availability and/or long waiting lists.

### Electroconvulsive therapy

Electroconvulsive therapy (ECT) offers a safe, rapid, and reasonably certain response in cases where:

- Rapid response is necessary
- Patients with depression have been intolerant to, or have not responded to, drug treatment
- When depression is very severe and manifests as psychosis, severe physical retardation, depressive stupor, or food/fluid refusal

Relative contraindications include coronary, cerebrovascular, and pulmonary disease.

### Specialist referral

Consider psychogeriatric assessment if:

- Treatment is unsuccessful after 6–8 weeks
- Depression is severe, e.g. with delusions
- The diagnosis is unclear, e.g. when depression and significant cognitive impairment coexist
- A patient is refusing treatment or otherwise threatening self-harm
- There are questions of competency
- ECT is being considered

# Depression: drug treatments

Drug treatment is generally effective, well tolerated, and non-addictive, although patients often believe otherwise.

▶ There is significant stigma associated with taking antidepressants, which is more prevalent in older age populations, and this may need to be explored and addressed.

## General

- In reactive depression, consider saying 'This won't stop you feeling sad, that's understandable, but it will help you to cope better with those feelings'
- Inform the patient that response takes time but is usual
- No antidepressant class has been shown to be more effective, so choice depends on side effects, speed of onset, response to previous treatment, drug interactions, and associated conditions, e.g. anxiety or pain

## Selective serotonin reuptake inhibitors

For example: citalopram or sertraline.
- Now generally the first class of antidepressant prescribed
- Compared with tricyclic antidepressants such as amitriptyline, they are less sedating, have fewer anticholinergic and cardiotoxic side effects, have fewer drug interactions, and are much safer in overdose
- Symptomatic response commonly starts after 2 weeks but may take up to 8 weeks
- Common side effects include gastrointestinal symptoms (nausea and diarrhoea), postural hypotension, anxiety, and restlessness, and hyponatraemia. Hyponatraemia is usually moderate (sodium >125mmol/L) and asymptomatic, and especially common in combination with diuretics
- Rarely causes serotonin syndrome (see ● 'Neuroleptic malignant syndrome', p. 167)
- Start at low doses to minimize side effects and build up, as needed, to give a useful response
- If there is no response to an adequate dose of one SSRI, there is little point trying another. Instead, switch class

## Serotonin antagonist

For example: mirtazapine.
- An atypical antidepressant which tends to cause weight gain (so may be particularly useful in malnourished)
- It has fewer anticholinergic side effects but is more sedating than tricyclics (so consider when a degree of sedation is desirable)
- Also less commonly complicated by hyponatraemia than SSRIs

### Serotonin and noradrenaline reuptake inhibitors (SNRIs)

For example: venlafaxine or duloxetine.
- For severe depression or when poor response to SSRIs after 6 weeks
- Also useful for anxiety and obsessive–compulsive disorder
- May cause less orthostatic hypotension than the SSRIs, but other side effects similar

### Tricyclic antidepressants

For example: amitriptyline, nortriptyline.
- Much less prescribed than previously
- They still have a role, e.g.:
  - If anticholinergic effects are desirable (urge incontinence)
  - When there is neuropathic or other pain that may respond to its co-analgesic effect
  - In depression resistant to other drugs
- The 2° amines (e.g. nortriptyline) are preferred, causing less orthostatic hypotension than tertiary amines (e.g. amitriptyline, imipramine). Anticholinergic side effects are less troublesome if doses start low and are ↑ weekly

### Monoamine oxidase inhibitors

For example: moclobemide.
- Occasionally used, under expert guidance, but dietary and drug interactions are problematic
- Treatment should be continued for up to a year. If depression has been severe and/or recurrent, consider continuing indefinitely

### Stopping drugs

Withdrawal reactions (anxiety, mania, delirium, insomnia, gastrointestinal side effects, headache, giddiness) may occur if drugs are stopped abruptly after 8 weeks or more. Therefore, reduce the dose gradually, over 4 weeks. In those on long-term treatment, reduce over several months.

### Switching drugs

'Cross-tapering' is generally advised, i.e. the incremental reduction of the 'old' drug, and incremental ↑ of the 'new' drug usually over 2–3 weeks. Rarely, a washout period between drugs is required (e.g. before MAOIs).

# Suicide and attempted suicide

Older people, especially men, have a higher risk of completed (rather than attempted) suicide than all other groups. Following an attempted suicide, further attempts—and successful suicide—are common.

Risk factors include being ♂, single (i.e. unmarried, divorced/separated, or widowed), being socially isolated, having financial problems, having made previous attempts, and recent bereavement. Unlike younger people, the substantial majority of older people who attempt suicide are psychiatrically unwell at the time of the attempt; most are depressed. Many seek contact with medical services prior to the attempt, although they may not express depressive or suicidal thoughts at that visit.

Suicidal behaviours may be overt or covert.

*Overt* behaviours include:
- Intentional drug overdoses (opiates, antidepressants, paracetamol, benzodiazepines; more common in women)
- Self-injury (hanging, shooting, jumping, drowning; more common in men)

*Covert suicide* is relatively more common in older people and includes
- Social withdrawal
- Severe self-neglect
- Refusal of food, fluid, or medication

This may manifest in subtle ways that encourage extensive investigation to exclude physical illness, while the psychiatric problem goes unrecognized and untreated.

Suicidal ideation is more common in institutional settings (acute and rehabilitation hospital wards, and care homes) and in people with acute or chronic physical illness. Risk factors here include depression, chronic pain, sleep disturbance, functional impairment, drug abuse, and psychotropic drug prescription. At their mildest, suicidal ideas manifest as common and relatively benign doubts about whether life is worth living. At their most worrying, they are carefully considered, well formulated, and strongly held beliefs that death is preferable to life, and how that could be achieved.

Assessment of the 'severity' of an attempt requires an effort to determine perceived risk from the patient's perspective at the time of the attempt. This may not parallel the medical seriousness. Consider:
- Degree of planning versus impulsivity
- Likelihood of interruption during attempt
- Reaction to interruption to attempt (disappointment or relief?)
- Suicide note and its contents
- Planning for future (e.g. making of will, contents of suicide note)
- Personal view of suicide as a reasonable 'life choice'

*Specialist referral*. Always in cases of attempted suicide, suicidal ideation, or 'covert suicide'. Probably not in cases of non-persistent or poorly formulated views that life is not worth living.

# Cardiovascular

# The ageing cardiovascular system

Advanced age is the most potent risk factor for cardiovascular disease. This vulnerability stems from the following.

## Cumulative exposure to risk factors (extrinsic ageing)

- This was looked at in more detail in the WHO MONICA project (see ➔ 'Further reading', p. 255), which looked at coronary risk factors in 38 populations across 21 countries for a decade
- This showed that not all risk factors ↑ with age—♂ smoking ↓ (although not ♀), and cholesterol showed a small downwards trend. Body mass index (BMI) ↑ for both sexes
- Thus, it is not inevitable and can be modified by behaviour, e.g. athletes who continue to exercise into older age may show fewer signs of cardiovascular ageing than an unfit younger person

## Disease acquisition

- Often occult
- Affected by risk factor accumulation

## Intrinsic ageing

The relative contributions of these factors to the clinical picture are unclear. Table 10.1 addresses the three important questions:
- What are the common changes with age?
- How does that impact on function?
- What are the clinical implications?

**Table 10.1** An overview of age-related changes and their effects

| Age-related change | Impact on function | Clinical implications |
|---|---|---|
| Proximal arteries become thicker, dilated, elongated, and less elastic | Systolic pressure peak ↑, causing hypertension↑ peripheral vascular resistance (variable) | Intimal thickening probably predisposes to atheroma<br>Systolic hypertension common in older patients<br>CXR may show enlarged aortic knuckle 'unfolding' of the aorta |
| Fibrosis and fat infiltration of the sinoatrial (SA) node and conducting system | Slower conduction from the SA node and through the conducting system | First-degree heart block and bundle branch block common<br>Left axis deviation more frequent<br>More vulnerable to clinically significant bradyarrhythmias |
| Maximum heart rate falls by 10% at rest and 25% during stress | ↓ capacity for cardiac output—largely compensated for at rest but limits response to stress | Less able to mount a tachycardia, so less reliable sign of acute illness |
| LV wall thickens as myocyte size ↑ | ↑ cardiac filling pressures and allows compensation for drop in heart rate | A degree of cardiac enlargement seen on CXR is normal. Worse with hypertension, so always check BP and treat as needed |
| Left atrial size ↑ due to alterations in cardiac filling | | Predisposes to AF |
| Myocardial contractility impaired at high demand | Contractility preserved at low stimulation, but with stress cannot ↑. Means that (along with heart rate factors) cardiac output cannot be ↑ | ↓ cardiac reserve to stress—may become haemodynamically compromised in response to acute illness earlier than younger patients |
| ↑ circulating catecholamines with downregulated receptors (especially β-adrenergic) | Impairs ability to mount a stress response | As above in this table—↓ cardiac reserve to stress<br>More prone to heart failure |
| Impaired oxygen consumption on exercise | Varies considerably between individual older patients—unchanged in those used to exercise, up to 60% reduction in unfit | Contributes to reduced cardiovascular reserve to stress |

## Further reading

World Health Organization. *The WHO MONICA Project.* ℘ http://www.thl.fi/publications/monica/manual/index.htm.

# Chest pain

A common complaint in all settings. May be 1° symptom (presenting to GPs and general medical take) or mentioned only in response to direct questioning. Also occurs during inpatient stays for other reasons.

There are very many causes, the majority of which become more common with age. Many are benign, but some are serious and even life-threatening, so a thorough and sensible approach is needed.

Common conditions not to be missed include: cardiac pain; pleuritic pain due to pulmonary infarction or infection; peptic pain (including bleeding ulcers); and pain from dissecting aortic aneurysm and pneumothorax (especially in COPD).

Other possibilities include: muscular pain (e.g. after unaccustomed exertion); costochondritis (local tenderness at sternal joint); pain from injury (e.g. after a fall); referred pain from the back and neck (e.g. osteoarthritis); and referred pain from the abdomen.

Differentiating these depends on accurate history taking and careful examination, both of which can be more of a challenge in older patients. Presentation may be atypical, and the patient may have many other problems, so teasing out which the important symptoms are can be difficult (experience improves the ability to 'feel' your way around the history). ▶ It may be the last symptom mentioned in a long list; however, mention of chest pain should always trigger a careful assessment.

## History

- Is this a new symptom? (may suffer from chronic angina)
- If not, is it any different from the usual pain? (intensity, pattern)
- What is the nature of the pain? (pleuritic, heavy, tight. This is often hard to do, and hand gestures can help—a clenched fist for a heavy pain, a stabbing action for a sharp pleuritic pain)
- Where is it located? (including radiation)
- How acute is the onset and what is the duration?
- Are there any associated symptoms?

Patients with cognitive impairment can be particularly difficult to assess, but allowing free conversation may reveal symptoms, followed by closed questions that may prompt appropriate answers. Family members may have noted signs or symptoms and are an invaluable aid to assessment, e.g. clutching the chest after walking.

Remember that cardiac symptoms may differ for each patient and they will describe the pain in their own terms. Many older adults with ischaemia will deny 'pain' and instead describe 'discomfort'. Some will just experience weakness, dyspnoea, or nausea.

## Examination

- How does the patient look? A sweaty, clammy patient needs urgent and exhaustive assessment, whereas a patient drinking tea and chatting is less likely to have a devastating condition
- What are the basic observations?

- Signs of shock alert to a serious condition—IHD, pulmonary infarction, dissection, sepsis, blood loss—but remember these may be late signs and are less useful in older patients. The patient may usually be hypertensive, so a BP of 120/80 may be very low for them; they may be on a β-blocker, so unable to mount a tachycardia, etc.
- Temperature may be raised in sepsis
- Low oxygen saturation always needs explaining (unless chronic) and may indicate an intrapulmonary problem
- Is the jugular venous pressure (JVP) elevated? (heart failure)
- Look at the chest wall for shingles, bruising, and localized tenderness
- Different BPs in the arms may indicate dissection (but may also occur with atheroma)
- Listen to the heart—are there any new murmurs (dissection or infarction) or a rub (pericarditis)?
- Listen to the lungs—is there consolidation (sepsis) or a rub (consolidation or infarction)?
- Look at the legs—is there any clinical DVT?

### Investigations

Some tests can be less useful in older patients and should be individually tailored to the patient. Sending off every single test on all patients with chest pain will only lead to confusion.

- ECG—should be done on the majority of patients with chest pain. Remember the baseline ECG may well be abnormal in an elderly person, and comparison with old traces is extremely useful. If your patient has a very abnormal ECG (e.g. left bundle branch block (LBBB)), it is useful to give them a copy to carry with them
- CXR—looking for lung abnormalities and widening of the mediastinum. Remember that the aorta often 'unfolds', so a careful look at the contours of the aortic arch and/or comparison with old films is needed to assess possible dissection. Remember that a patient can look fairly well in the early stages of aortic dissection
- Blood tests—basic haematology, biochemistry, and inflammatory markers are often useful. Remember that in acute blood loss, the Hb level may not drop immediately and that an elderly septic patient may take a day or two to develop an elevated white cell count and CRP
- Troponin—useful in a patient with suspected cardiac chest pain (for risk stratification). It is NOT a useful test if you do not think this is cardiac pain—there are many false positives that will only cause confusion
- D-dimer—only useful if negative in cases of suspected thromboembolism. There are a huge number of causes of a positive D-dimer (including old age itself); a positive result does not imply the diagnosis of PE
- Further tests (e.g. CT thorax for suspected dissection, exercise testing for angina, lung perfusion scans for thromboembolism, etc.) depend on clinical factors

▶ Always attempt to explain a chest pain—both for the patient and future clinicians. A 'diagnosis' of non-cardiac chest pain is rarely helpful.

# Stable angina

Coronary artery disease is clinically evident in 20% of those >80 years. Management is often sub-optimal. It is unacceptable to leave a patient with symptoms, however frail, until all available options have been looked at, and it has been proven (by trying it) that a certain treatment cannot be tolerated. A stepwise, slow introduction of tablets allows insight into adverse effects and may require multiple clinic visits. Symptom diaries can assist with this process.

## Stable angina

*Risk factor reduction*
- Cholesterol and BP less likely to be lowered in older patients, but the risk reduction is equal to, if not greater than, for younger subjects
- Diabetic control is less likely to be tight, in part due to justifiable concerns about the dangers of hypoglycaemia
- Lifestyle advice (exercise, smoking, and diet) should be given

*Aggravating conditions*
More common in older people. Correcting such conditions, where possible, often more effective than increasing antianginal meds.
  Can be divided into:
- ↓ myocardial *supply*, e.g. anaemia, blood loss, hypoxia, fever, hypotension
- ↑ myocardial *demand*, e.g. tachycardia, fever, valvular heart disease, heart failure, hypertension, hyperthyroidism

*Medication*
- Under-utilized, particularly aspirin (concerns about bleeding) and β-blockade, but there is evidence that they are both equally useful in reducing risk
- A trial and error approach to treatment is needed—add one or two treatments at a time to minimize the risk of side effects (most commonly orthostatic hypotension), and stop if there are problems, trying something else instead
- Start on low doses, and titrate upwards (e.g. bisoprolol 2.5mg)
- Long-acting agents (e.g. diltiazem modified-release) reduce compliance problems
- Nicorandil (10–20mg bd) is often better tolerated than other antianginals in this age group
- Choice of medication should be pragmatic—if a patient has a bradycardia, for example, a negatively chronotropic drug is usually inappropriate (consider using amlodipine 5–10mg). If a patient has heart failure, a cardioselective β-blocker (e.g. carvedilol, metoprolol, bisoprolol) is a better choice than a fluid-retaining calcium channel blocker
- GTN can cause considerable problems with hypotension, and instruction on correct use is essential. Tablets can be spat out once the pain starts to settle, so (in theory) the dose can be titrated to symptoms. In practice, the spray is often easier to use. It should be used sitting down, if possible, and prophylactically before significant exertion

*Revascularization*

Should be considered (ideally after risk stratification by stress testing), as for younger patients, if symptoms persist despite maximal medical therapy (see ➔ 'Revascularization procedures', p. 262).

*Palliation*

Consider if diffuse disease, not amenable to revascularization with ongoing symptoms (e.g. home oxygen therapy, opiates to allow sleep), particularly if angina occurs in the context of heart failure syndrome.

---

**HOW TO . . . Rationalize antianginals in older patients**

*When?*
- With advancing age and frailty, mobility may reduce and so angina symptoms may become less frequent, or even stop
- It is not uncommon to find an octogenarian on four antianginals, who has not had angina for many years
- Use a low pulse or BP reading as a trigger to review the medication
- Do not hesitate to rationalize this—there are many pitfalls from polypharmacy, and requirements will change with time

*How?*
- If cognitive impairment, confirm with carers that they are genuinely asymptomatic from angina
- Review observations—if bradycardic, stop β-blockade first; if hypotensive, start with the symptomatic medications first (e.g. nitrates) before those with disease-modifying properties
- Select one drug to modify, then reduce in a stepwise fashion (e.g. reducing dose and/or frequency)
- Patients and family may be resistant to medication changes after years of healthcare professionals emphasizing the importance of their tablets. Some are frightened of a recurrence of disabling symptoms, so explain to the patient, carers, and GP what you are doing
- Clarify the contingency plan: 'This is a trial, and if it does not suit you, you may get angina pains again. If that happens, please just start taking your old doses again'
- Ensure there is backup if there are concerns (e.g. telephone number)

*Review*
- Set a date for review of impact
- Assess whether there have been any symptoms, and reassess the pulse and BP
- If all is well, continue with careful reduction in medication

*Goal*
- Aim to use as few medications as possible, while maintaining control of symptoms
- If the BP allows, continue those with disease-modifying properties (β-blockade, ACE inhibitors), but in frail older people, it is more important to avoid orthostatic hypotension and falls
- Once the medication has been titrated down to an optimum level (balancing pulse, BP, symptoms, and disease modification), communicate the final list to others, especially the GP

# Acute coronary syndromes

Coronary heart disease (CHD) incidence rises with ↑ age. An acute coronary syndrome describes a scenario in which the myocardial cells are not receiving enough blood and oxygen to meet their demands. This can be due to an acute coronary event (type 1 ischaemia) or ↑ demand which outstrips supply (type 2 ischaemia).

## 'Troponinitis'

With ↑ sensitivity of tests for myocardial damage (e.g. troponin) and ↑ (often inappropriate) screening, older people are being increasingly diagnosed as ACS coinciding with other illness, rather than as 1° pathology. In these cases, ↑ demand, rather than coronary artery disease, is driving the process and treatment should primarily aim at optimizing management of the other conditions (e.g. sepsis, dehydration, etc.) (see ➲ 'Aggravating conditions', p. 258).

▶▶ In these cases, the ACS treatment bundle (e.g. anticoagulant, antiplatelet, β-blockade, etc.) is often contraindicated and risks detracting clinicians from the underlying pathology.

ACS has a range of syndromes from unstable angina to non-ST elevation MI (NSTEMI) to ST elevation MI (STEMI). Management in general is as for younger patients, but there are some points relating to older patients in particular.

## Atypical presentation

- More likely to present with atypical or vague symptoms (e.g. intense dyspnoea, syncope, weakness, abdominal pain)
- Symptoms may be obscured by comorbidity
- ECG changes may not be present in up to a quarter of acute MI, with the full diagnostic triad (chest pain, ECG changes, and biochemical changes) present in under a third of those >85 years
- ECG may be difficult to interpret because of pre-existing abnormalities (LBBB, pacing)
- Vital signs or symptoms may be obscured by medication (β-blockade, pain medication)

## Different pathology

- More pre-existing coronary artery disease with more multivessel disease
- NSTEMI more likely than an STEMI
- More likely to develop heart failure, AV block, AF, and cardiogenic shock after a coronary event

## Later presentation

- ↑ prevalence of angina, so less alarmed by chest pains
- May modify lifestyle to avoid symptoms (if climbing a hill gives them chest pain, they may just stop doing it)
- ↑ occurrence of 'silent ischaemia' (especially in people with diabetes)
- ↑ social/attitudinal factors ('I didn't want to bother the doctor')
- A third of patients >65 with MI will present later than 6h after symptom onset

**Increased comorbidity**
- Making diagnosis difficult (e.g. a patient with COPD who has exertional breathlessness) and therapy less well tolerated (e.g. β-blockers with peripheral vascular disease)
- Also as comorbidities add up, so frailty ↑ and medications are generally less well tolerated

Older patients with ACS have a higher inpatient mortality so should be prioritized for specialist monitoring where there are limited resources; however, it is known that they are:
- Less likely to receive aggressive acute therapy (e.g. less angiography and angioplasty, and coronary artery bypass grafting (CABG), and maximal medical treatment)
- Less likely to have full 2° prevention measures implemented

Management of the older cardiac patient is therefore more difficult and more likely to result in death than in younger patients. Sometimes there are good reasons for withholding therapy (e.g. patients presenting later are less often eligible for thrombolysis, side effects may restrict 2° prevention), but often the justification is less robust. Lack of evidence in older people does not mean that there is no benefit—rather that it has not been proven.

Common sense dictates when to use an aggressive approach, considering the patient as a whole, including:
- Patient preference where possible
- Comorbidities (alter risk profile)
- Current medication
- Frailty and likely life expectancy
- Apparent biological age, rather than chronological age

There are many well-defined treatment algorithms, and older patients should be included at every step unless there are good reasons not to. If you plan to exclude a patient from treatment, you should clearly document your rationale. There is some evidence that the excess IHD mortality for older people is diminishing (see below), probably due to improved risk stratification and the application of more evidence-based interventions to this group.

## Revascularization procedures

Includes percutaneous coronary angiography and intervention (PCI) and CABG.

### When?

- Used when stable symptoms persist despite maximal medical therapy, when unstable symptoms fail to settle, or for acute MI (1° PCI)
- Risk-stratify with exercise testing and troponin measurements. Older patients may be unable to exercise, but consider bicycle exercise, stress echocardiography, or an isotope myocardial perfusion scan to look for evidence of reversible ischaemia

### What are the risks?

- PCI—higher risk of death, renal failure, and infarction in the elderly. Age is an independent predictor of ↑ complication, but so too are diabetes, heart failure, and chronic renal impairment, all of which are more common in older patients
- CABG—↑ early mortality and stroke in older patients

### What are the benefits?

- PCI—may be the only way to control intrusive symptoms in stable angina, with better quality of life but no change in mortality. 1° management of STEMI, rarely for NSTEMI that is not responding to other treatments. Variable evidence from studies—all agree ↑ early complications, but longer-term benefits in older patients are reported as equivalent or even better
- CABG—probably better with triple vessel disease, poor exercise tolerance, poor LV function, and diabetes. Generally well tolerated in the elderly, with similar long-term improvements in symptoms and quality of life to younger patients. New minimally invasive techniques that do not require bypass are likely to reduce the early complications without impairing outcome

### Overall recommendations

Consider all patients who fail medical treatment for revascularization procedures, regardless of age. The early complication rate is higher in older patients, but the eventual benefit is equal to, if not better than, for younger patients.

Approach a cardiologist with a record of treating older patients. Crucial to include the patient in the decision, with a frank and individualized discussion about risks and benefits.

## Further reading

Gale CP, Cattle BA, Woolston A, *et al*. Resolving inequalities in care? Reduced mortality in the elderly after acute coronary syndromes. The Myocardial Ischaemia National Audit Project 2003–2010. *Eur Heart J* 2012; **33**: 630–9.

Thygesen K, Alpert JS, White HD. Universal definition of myocardial infarction. *Eur Heart J* 2007; **28**: 2525–38.

# Myocardial infarction

This includes both NSTEMI and STEMI. Around two-thirds of all MIs occur in patients >65 and a third in patients >75. Overall, the incidence of MI has ↓, but this is not the case for older patients. Despite this, evidence regarding optimal management is lacking, as older patients tend to be underrepresented in clinical trials.

Consult NICE guidelines (which do not suggest differences in approach for most areas for older people). While evidence is lacking in older patients, it is more reasonable to extrapolate from a younger population than to deny treatment. This approach must, of course, be tempered with common sense and individually tailored decision-making. Table 10.2 summarizes some evidence specifically relating to older people.

## Prior to discharge

*Medication*
- May include aspirin ± clopidogrel, statin, β-blockade, ACE inhibitor, and GTN spray
- Use medications, unless they are contraindicated or the risk > benefit
- Be alert for common side effects (more likely with advancing age), e.g. orthostatic hypotension, gastrointestinal bleeding

*Education*
- Diet, nutrition, cholesterol control
- Smoking cessation
- Activity restrictions and graded reintroduction
- Recurrent symptoms and what to do
- Routine follow-up after stents

## Cardiac rehabilitation

- Used after ACS and multiple presentations of congestive heart failure
- Involves structured exercise programme
- Proven to improve exercise tolerance and ↓ readmission
- Underused for older cardiac patients—less referral and sometimes there are upper age limits in place
- Benefit seen in older patients is equivalent to that in younger patients, although they start from a less fit baseline
- Older people adhere well to programmes and seem to suffer no complications
- Some adaptations are needed (more time to warm up and cool down, longer breaks, avoidance of high-impact activity, lower intensity for a longer time)
- Benefits include improved fitness, ↑ bone mineral density, improved mood and fewer falls, as well as improved cardiovascular fitness

**Table 10.2** MI treatment evidence for older people

| Therapy | Evidence |
| --- | --- |
| Aspirin | Equivalent risk reduction in elderly population |
| 1° PCI | This is usually the strategy of choice where presentation is early. It reduces death and recurrent MI, compared with a conservative strategy. Procedural risks are greater with frail patients, and the role for PCI in those >80 with multiple comorbidities has not been well studied. Resource limitations may impact |
| Thrombolysis | Not indicated for unstable angina or NSTEMI |
| | Has a role in STEMI, regardless of age |
| | Must be administered <12h after onset (ideally <3h) and is used where PCI is not available or feasible |
| | ↑ risk of complications, e.g. cerebral bleeding (but can predict those at higher risk if hypertensive, low body weight, previous stroke, or on warfarin) |
| | Contradictory evidence regarding mortality—early large RCTs suggest ↑ absolute risk reduction of mortality in elderly patients but had selected probably fitter patients and do not include the very old. Observational trials of actual practice suggest equivalent benefit in older patients, or possibly even a survival disadvantage. Probable equivalent proportional mortality reduction, so absolute reduction greatest in the elderly who have the highest mortality |
| | Overall, the consensus is that thrombolysis can be used in older patients, with rare exceptions for the very frail or where individual risk seems to outweigh benefit |
| Low-molecular-weight heparin | Full dose is effective in NSTEMI, and possibly more effective in older patients |
| Glycoprotein IIb/IIIa inhibitors | Rarely used (e.g. for NSTEMI while awaiting reperfusion) Older people have ↑ risk of bleeding but have equal benefit overall |

Carro A, Kaski JC. Myocardial infarction in the elderly. *Aging Dis* 2011; 2: 116–37.

# Hypertension

Hypertension is an important risk factor for vascular disease. Historically under-diagnosed and undertreated, especially in older patients, although improved in the UK when GPs had national guidelines/targets and financial incentives to treat.

The incidence of hypertension overall rises with age, reaching a prevalence of 60–80% beyond 65. After this age, systolic BP (SBP) rises linearly, while diastolic BP (DBP) falls, leading to widening of the pulse pressure and relative frequency of isolated systolic hypertension (see Table 10.3). Isolated systolic hypertension reflects reduced arterial compliance, which is disease-related and not part of 'normal' ageing per se. It is treated in the same way as normal hypertension.

Hypertension is an independent risk factor for stroke, IHD, peripheral vascular disease, congestive heart failure, renal failure, and dementia in all age groups, but in older patients, it is SBP and widened pulse pressure that are the strongest predictors of adverse cardiovascular outcome.

## Assessment

- *Ask about* symptoms (including hypotensive), comorbidity, and smoking
- *Measure* with a well-maintained, calibrated device, with an appropriate-sized cuff:
  - Check supine and standing BP (orthostatic hypotension can cause symptoms when treatment initiated)
  - Take at least two measurements in a single consultation and use the lowest reading
  - Ambulatory or home BP measurement is now considered essential for confirming a new diagnosis in almost all cases. Ambulatory or home BP thresholds and goals are 5–10mmHg below clinic readings. Most cognitively intact older patients tolerate this well, and having a BP cuff at home can be useful to monitor for adverse effects during treatment
- *Examine* for evidence of target organ damage (stroke, dementia, carotid bruits, cardiac enlargement, IHD, peripheral vascular disease, renal disease, retinal changes)
- *Investigations* to look at target organs (urinalysis, blood urea, and electrolytes, ECG) and for risk factor analysis (glucose, lipids)
- *Consider* 2° *hypertension*—rare in older patients, but consider if drug-resistant, severe hypertension, or with suggestive examination or laboratory findings. Consider medications (NSAIDs, steroids, SSRIs), Cushing's syndrome, sleep apnoea, 1° aldosteronism, phaeochromocytoma, or renal artery stenosis

## Treatment thresholds

- NICE suggests treating <80 years who have stage 1 hypertension (BP >140/90 in clinic (or 135/85 at home) if they also have other risk factors, e.g. diabetes mellitus, proteinuria, CKD, stroke, etc.
- For patients aged >80, only treat if stage 2 hypertension (BP >160/100 in clinic or 150/95 at home)
- Lower thresholds (>140mmHg) for diagnosis and treatment exist for very high-risk patients, e.g. CKD and diabetes

## Treatment goals

- Target ranges are similar to treatment thresholds, i.e. 140/90 under age 80 and 160/100 for over age 80
- In older patients, the most common limit to treatment is symptomatic postural hypotension; consider using alternative agents which may cause less orthostatic drop (e.g. ARBs, calcium channel blockers)
- There are even fewer data for very elderly (>90) people, and a pragmatic approach based on apparent biological age is appropriate

# Hypertension: treatment

Similar approach to that used in younger patients, but it is important to bear the following in mind:
- Side effects are more common and more debilitating in older patients (due to more sluggish baroreceptors and reduced cerebral autoregulation)
- There is a greater risk of drug interactions, as older patients are more often victims of polypharmacy
- Comorbidity is common and should direct the choice of antihypertensive agents (see ➲ 'HOW TO . . . Use antihypertensives in a patient with comorbid conditions', p. 269)
- Hypertension should be seen as a risk factor, and the decision to treat should be weighed along with other risk factors. In a very frail older person with a limited life expectancy, the side effects might far outweigh any future benefits from risk factor modification. This, however, should be an active decision reached, if possible, with the patient, and not a simple omission
- Begin with lower doses and titrate up slowly ('start low and go slow') to minimize adverse reactions. It is better to be on something at a low dose than nothing at all

## Non-pharmacological measures

Lifestyle modifications are as important and effective in reducing BP in older patients as in the young. Salt restriction, weight reduction, and regular exercise are particularly effective. Moderate or absent alcohol intake is advised. Smoking cessation and ↓ saturated fat intake help with overall risk reduction.

## Choice of medication

Many large trials have compared the different classes of antihypertensive, but with little consistency in results. Overall, it seems that it is lowering the BP per se that is the important factor, and this benefit continues up until at least 84 years (possibly beyond—evidence pending). In older patients, with much comorbidity, there may be compelling reasons for using, or not using, certain agents (see ➲ 'HOW TO . . . Use antihypertensives in a patient with comorbid conditions', p. 269).

The 2011 UK guidelines suggest, in the absence of reasons to modify therapeutics, drugs should be introduced for all adults over age 55 in the following order:
1. Calcium channel blocker
2. Add ACE inhibitors or ARBs
3. Add thiazide diuretic
4. In resistant hypertension, consider adding an α-blocker, spironolactone, or a β-blocker

## HOW TO . . . Use antihypertensives in a patient with comorbid conditions

*Calcium channel blockers*
- Use rate-limiting options (e.g. diltiazem) to slow the heart rate in AF or reduce angina with normal LV function
- May make heart failure worse or cause constipation
- Dihydropyridine calcium channel blockers (e.g. amlodipine, felodipine) are excellent in isolated systolic hypertension

*ACE inhibitors*
For example: ramipril 2.5–10mg.
- Use for 2° prevention after vascular event (stroke, TIA, heart attack), and in diabetes, heart failure, and chronic renal impairment
- Avoid in renal artery stenosis
- Monitor potassium and renal function

*ARBs*
For example: losartan 50mg.
- Use when ACE-intolerant (usually cough) where an ACE is indicated
- May cause fewer orthostatic symptoms than ACE inhibitors
- Monitor potassium and renal function

*Thiazide diuretics*
For example: bendroflumethiazide 2.5mg.
- Useful first-line therapy in most older patients—may help with ankle swelling and heart failure symptoms
- Avoid if severe gout, urinary incontinence, or profound dyslipidaemia
- May worsen urinary incontinence
- Need to monitor for hyponatraemia

*Beta-blockers*
For example: atenolol 25mg.
- Useful with angina, AF, and stable heart failure (cardioselective better)
- Avoid with peripheral vascular disease, asthma, and heart block

*Alpha-blockers*
For example: doxazosin 1mg.
- Excellent for resistant hypertension in older patients
- Use if prostatic hypertrophy
- Commonly cause orthostatic symptoms
- May exacerbate stress incontinence

## Further reading

Beckett NS, Peters R, Fletcher AE, *et al.*; HYVET Study Group. Treatment of hypertension in patients 80 years of age or older. *N Engl J Med* 2008; **358**: 1887–98.

National Institute for Health and Care Excellence (2011). *Hypertension in adults: diagnosis and management.* Clinical guideline CG127. ℘ https://www.nice.org.uk/guidance/cg127.

# Arrhythmia: presentation

Arrhythmias are very common in older people but are not so common as a presenting complaint. A patient with recurrent presyncope preceded by palpitations presents very little diagnostic challenge. What is much more common is for an arrhythmia to be the explanation for a rather more vague presentation such as:

- Recurrent falls
- Patient covered in bruises who has been explaining them away as clumsiness
- General fatigue
- Dizzy spells
- Light-headedness
- 'Collapse query cause'
- Blackouts
- Worsening/new angina or heart failure

## History

It is important to ask about palpitations with any of these problems, (indeed it should form part of the systems review in all older people), but be aware of the following points:

- *Clarify carefully* what you mean—many people do not understand what we mean by 'palpitations' and may be describing an ectopic heartbeat followed by a compensatory pause, or even just an awareness of the normal heartbeat, e.g. when lying in bed at night. Getting the patient to tap out what they feel can be very revealing
- Do not exclude the possibility of an arrhythmia just because the patient does not complain of palpitations—especially with confused patients
- Where there are palpitations/light-headedness, *establish an order* wherever possible. Postural hypotension (see ➋ 'Orthostatic (postural) hypotension', pp. 116–17) is very common in older patients and can produce a similar set of symptoms (falling BP causing light-headedness, then a compensatory tachycardia)—in theory, the palpitations should come first in an arrhythmia
- Are there any *constant features*? For example, dizziness occurring:
  - On standing is more likely to be postural hypotension
  - On exertion may have an ischaemic component
  - On turning the head may be due to vestibular problems or carotid sinus hypersensitivity (see ➋ 'Carotid sinus syndrome', p. 120)
  - In any situation or at any time is much more likely to be due to an arrhythmia
- A history of *SIGNIFICANT injury* (especially facial bruising) with a blackout ↑ the chances of finding an arrhythmia, particularly a bradycardia requiring pacing
- Always take a *full drug history*—antiarrhythmics can be pro-arrhythmogenic, drugs that cause bradyarrhythmias (commonly β-blockers, digoxin, or rate-limiting calcium channel blockers such as diltiazem), and antidepressants (especially the tricyclics) that can predispose to arrhythmias. Medications containing ephedrine, thyroxine, caffeine, and β-agonists can cause tachyarrhythmias

## Examination

- Should always include lying and standing BP; assessment of the baseline pulse character, rate, and rhythm; full cardiovascular examination to look for evidence of structural cardiac disease (e.g. cardiomyopathy, heart failure, valvular lesions), all of which may predispose to arrhythmias
- General problems require a full general examination—it is rarely appropriate to examine a single system only in an elderly patient. A rectal examination, for example, may reveal a rectal tumour causing anaemia, and hence palpitations
- It may also be appropriate to examine the vestibular system (see ⊃ 'HOW TO . . . Examine the vestibular system', p. 563) and CNS

## Investigations

- Blood tests—including FBC (anaemia), U, C+E (low potassium predisposes to arrhythmias), thyroid function, and digoxin levels where relevant
- ECG—look for baseline rhythm and any evidence of conducting system disease (e.g. a bundle branch block or any heart block). Measure the P-R and the Q-T interval. Also look for LV hypertrophy (arrhythmias more likely) or ischaemia. A totally normal ECG diminishes the possibility of a clinically significant arrhythmia
- CXR—look at the cardiac size
- Holter monitoring—a prolonged ECG recording. Usually a 24h period initially. Remember this is a very small snapshot and of limited value, especially if symptoms are infrequent. Can be useful if the symptoms are experienced while the monitor is on and the ECG trace shows normal sinus rhythm. If the suspicion of arrhythmias is high, then repeat the test or arrange for trans-telephonic event recording or even an implantable loop recorder where the symptoms are severe enough (e.g. sudden syncope)

# Arrhythmias: management

Management of arrhythmias in older patients does not differ significantly from management in other age groups, but consider the following.

## Precipitants

- Always check for common precipitants in older patients:
  - Electrolyte abnormalities (especially hypo- or hyperkalaemia and hypocalcaemia)
  - Anaemia
  - MI
  - Antiarrhythmic toxicity (especially digoxin)
  - Sepsis
  - Hypothermia
  - Any other acute illness
- If the precipitant cannot be reversed quickly (e.g. sepsis), then the arrhythmia is likely to be recurrent. Consider cardiac monitoring if cardiovascular compromise or if arrhythmia recurrence is likely

## Effect of arrhythmia

- Tachycardia may be less well tolerated than in younger patients, causing significant hypotension, angina, or heart failure
- Hypotension itself may be less well tolerated than in younger patients (risk of cerebral injury), and so prompt action is required
- Where there is heart failure because of an arrhythmia, fluids cannot be used for resuscitation, and so definitive action is required sooner rather than later. Begin by using standard treatment for acute heart failure (oxygen, iv diuretics, and opiates, etc.), while organizing cardioversion (usually electrical for speed) or rate limitation (appropriate for AF)

## Diagnosis

- There is more likely to be an underlying cardiac pathology—always check for ischaemia and structural heart disease, even for apparently benign arrhythmias (e.g. SVT)
- Bundle branch block is common, and so there may be confusion between supraventricular and ventricular arrhythmias. There are numerous subtle ways of distinguishing between these, but in an emergency:
  - If the patient is compromised, electrical cardioversion will treat both effectively
  - If the patient is unwell, but stable, an amiodarone infusion will treat both effectively and has the advantage of causing little myocardial depression

## Treatment

- Elderly patients are much more likely to be on an antiarrhythmic drug already.

▶ Check the medication carefully before administering any therapy. See Box 10.1 for common pitfalls.

- *Electrical cardioversion* is well tolerated by most older patients, usually effective and less likely to cause side effects than many medications. It should be considered early where there is significant compromise. Anaesthetic support is required, which can take some time to arrange, so prompt referral is recommended. It is less useful in acute sepsis where the arrhythmia is likely to recur, and it is hard to establish whether compromise is caused by the sepsis or the arrhythmia
- *Implantable cardiovertor–defibrillators* are lifesaving for malignant ventricular arrhythmias (VT and ventricular fibrillation (VF)). Regardless of patient age, they should be considered for survivors of sudden cardiac arrest, ventricular arrhythmias associated with EFs of <35%, and recurrent or refractory ventricular tachycardias with syncope. However, they are very expensive, can cause debility and pain, and do not allow a natural death (they must be turned off during palliative care). There is therefore reluctance to use them in older, frail patients in whom non-arrhythmic deaths are common.

## Box 10.1 Common pitfalls with antiarrhythmic medication

*Adenosine*
- Its action is prolonged by dipyridamole (commonly prescribed with aspirin in stroke), so avoid using together
- Exacerbates asthma and is antagonized by theophylline, so avoid in asthmatic people

*Amiodarone*
- Risk of ventricular arrhythmias when used with disopyramide, procainamide, and quinidine, so avoid concomitant use
- ↑ plasma half-life of flecainide, so reduce dose

*Atropine*
- Can precipitate glaucoma, so avoid in patients with this condition

*Flecainide*
- Contraindicated when there is IHD, heart failure, and haemodynamic compromise
- Probably best avoided in most older patients who may well have occult cardiac disease

*Verapamil*
- Do not use iv in a patient already on a β-blocker (high risk of asystole and hypotension)

*General guidance*
Most antiarrhythmic medication used concomitantly ↑ the risk of myocardial depression and arrhythmias. This effect is more pronounced in older patients. Caution when using >1, and consider using sequentially, rather than additively, if one alone is ineffective.

# Atrial fibrillation

Common arrhythmia, becoming more common with age (risk doubles with each additional decade of age, rising to 7% in >85 year olds). Often associated with other disease (e.g. hypertension, coronary artery disease, mitral valve disease, thyrotoxicosis) but also occurs in 1–2% of otherwise healthy elderly people. Unlike other arrhythmias, it is often chronic.

Disorganized atrial activity with variable conduction to the ventricles leads to an irregularly irregular pulse rate and volume. Up to a third of older patients with AF will have AV nodal disease that limits the rate to <100bpm, often making it asymptomatic. It is therefore often noted incidentally during routine examination—but should never be ignored.

## Assessment

Should include examination for hypertension and valve disease, blood tests for thyroid disease, and an ECG to confirm the diagnosis. Paroxysmal AF may cause intermittent symptoms and should be looked for with Holter monitoring.

## Complications

AF causes an ↑ in morbidity and mortality, even if there is no underlying cardiac disease.

- Pulse >120 often causes palpitations, light-headedness, or syncope
- Rapid rate may also cause dyspnoea, angina, or heart failure
- General malaise may also result from a chronically sub-optimal cardiac output
- AF is often associated with periods of AV conduction delay ('pauses') and if >3s, these may cause syncope
- The main complication is stroke from cardiac emboli

## Atrial flutter

- Rapid, regular atrial activity (usually 300/min)
- Characteristic sawtooth appearance on ECG (revealed by carotid sinus massage if rate high)
- Rate depends on degree of AV block (150bpm if 2:1 block, 75bpm if 4:1 block, etc.)

▶ Always think of atrial flutter when the pulse rate is 150bpm.

- Commonly associated with COPD or IHD
- Similar embolic risk to AF, and as the patient will often flip in and out of flutter and fibrillation, they should be managed in the same way
- Treat with rate control and stroke prophylaxis. This rhythm is usually amenable to cardioversion, but if there are significant comorbidities, structural heart disease, or ablation therapy, then sinus rhythm is unlikely to be sustained

# Atrial fibrillation: rate/rhythm control

## Acute atrial fibrillation

- Aim to return to sinus *RHYTHM*, i.e. cardioversion
- Treat underlying condition, e.g. sepsis, ischaemia, heart failure
- If compromised, consider electrical cardioversion
- Otherwise, control rate (usually with cardioselective β-blocker, e.g. bisoprolol, or rate-limiting calcium channel blocker, e.g. diltiazem; add digoxin if resistant) and wait to see if resolves once precipitant has been dealt with
- Chemical cardioversion is an option—give amiodarone (initially 200mg po tds for a week, then 200mg bd for a week, then 200mg od thereafter). May be able to drop dose further to 100mg a day, or even every other day). Long-term amiodarone for permanent AF rate control is no longer recommended
- Remember anticoagulation (stroke prophylaxis) during the episode

## Persistent/permanent atrial fibrillation

- Persistent is lasting >7 days; it is classed as permanent when attempts at cardioversion have failed
- Guidelines suggest *RATE* control with cardioselective β-blockade (e.g. bisoprolol) or calcium channel blockers (e.g. diltiazem)
- In practice, many frail, largely sedentary old patients will tolerate digoxin better, and this remains the first choice of many geriatricians (see ➲ 'HOW TO . . . Use digoxin', p. 281)

▶ Remember that amiodarone interacts with warfarin, and regular monitoring of INR will be needed if the two are used together—as is often the case. Also can cause thyroid abnormalities, and this should be monitored with TFTs.

- Dronedarone is a newer agent that is simpler to use than amiodarone but cannot be used in severe heart failure, and safety in permanent AF is unclear
- Electrical cardioversion for chronic AF should only be attempted after a period of anticoagulation (minimum 3 weeks). It is more likely to succeed (and less likely to recur) where there are fewer of the following present:
  - Structural heart disease (hypertrophy, atrial enlargement, valvular heart disease, etc.)
  - Comorbidity (especially hypertension, heart failure)
  - ↑ age

Recent evidence suggests that an older patient with several of the factors listed is better off being treated with rate control and anticoagulation only, without attempting cardioversion.

- Atrial catheter ablation is used in selected, usually younger, patients, but consider referral if a patient remains symptomatic and has failed trials of medical treatment or to destroy/isolate abnormal electrical impulses

### Paroxysmal atrial fibrillation

- Equal embolic risk, so consider anticoagulation as for chronic AF
- Remember that digoxin does not prevent paroxysms of AF
- Amiodarone, dronedarone, or cardioselective β-blockers (e.g. bisoprolol) are useful to prevent paroxysms of AF
- Ablation therapy may be useful in those with normal-sized atria and few comorbidities, although the recurrence rate is probably higher than in younger patients

# Atrial fibrillation: stroke prevention

This is a complex and often emotive issue. Many older people will have very strong views about stroke ('I'd rather die than ever have a stroke') or warfarin (many know it as 'rat poison' or have known someone who had a bleed while on warfarin). As we are dealing with population risks and benefits, it is impossible to accurately predict for a single individual what will happen to them if they do, or do not, take preventative therapy. Conveying this concept is difficult, but because the decision is complex, involvement of the patient becomes key. This takes time and patience. A decision aid with visual aids, such as that available from NICE clinical guideline CG180, can help.

It is important to have a simple way of explaining the facts as they are known, perhaps writing them down for clarity, then allowing time for them to sink in before coming to a final decision. There is no enormous urgency—the stroke risks quoted are per annum, and it is worth giving the patient time to think things over, if required.

Address each of the following questions.

### What is the risk of stroke in this patient with atrial fibrillation?

Overall, the risk is about five times greater than a person with similar health and age who does not have AF. Paroxysmal AF carries the same embolic risk.

Risk may be more accurately quantified by using $CHA_2DS_2VASc$ scoring system (see Table 10.3).

Without anticoagulation, annual stroke rate is ~1% for a score of 1, 2% for a score of 2, 3% for a score of 3, 5% for a score of 4, 7% for a score of 5, and 11% for a score of 7.

▶ In clinical practice, most older patients with AF will have a risk of stroke that warrants consideration of anticoagulation.

### What is the risk of anticoagulant therapy?

- Warfarin, when taken correctly and monitored carefully, has around 1% per year risk of major bleeding in 1° prevention of stroke, and 2.5% risk in 2° prevention
- Direct, non-vitamin K thrombin inhibitors (NOACs/DOACs), e.g. dabigatran, require no INR monitoring and no dietary changes, and have lower bleeding risks (probably about half the rate of warfarin)
- Falls alone are not a contraindication to anticoagulation
- Risk can be more accurately assessed using HAS-BLED criteria (see Table 10.4).

Annual major bleed risk on anticoagulant is 1% for score of 1, ~2% for score of 2, ~4% for score of 3, and ~9% for score of 4.

**Table 10.3** CHA$_2$DS$_2$VASc scoring system

| | |
|---|---|
| Cardiac failure | 1 |
| Hypertension | 1 |
| Age over 75 | 2 |
| Age 65–74 | 1 |
| Stroke, TIA, or thromboembolism | 2 |
| Vascular disease | 1 |
| Sex ♀ | 1 |
| Total (maximum 8) | |

**Table 10.4** HAS-BLED criteria

| | |
|---|---|
| Hypertension—systolic >160mmHg | 1 |
| Abnormal liver function | 1 |
| Abnormal renal function | 1 |
| Stroke | 1 |
| Bleeding tendency | 1 |
| Labile INR | 1 |
| Elderly (age >65) | 1 |
| Drugs, e.g. aspirin, NSAIDs | 1 |
| Alcohol abuse | 1 |
| Total (maximum 9) | |

### How effective is therapy at reducing risk?

- Anticoagulation reduces stroke risk in AF by around 60–70%
- Aspirin at any dose is no longer used in AF as monotherapy but is sometimes co-prescribed with anticoagulants if there is a separate reason (e.g. coronary artery disease).

### What are the recommendations?

- NICE recommends anticoagulant treatment for anyone with a CHA$_2$DS$_2$VASc of ≥2 (and as age >74 scores 2, that means almost everyone, all older patients), unless there is a very high bleeding risk.

### Other options

There is limited trial evidence that occlusion of the left atrial appendage using a percutaneous device is equivalent to warfarin in the prevention of stroke. Pace and ablate therapies can also be used to control AF. This may be an option for high-risk patients in whom anticoagulation is not feasible.

**HOW TO . . . Discuss warfarin for AF**

Your patient is an 86-year-old woman with hypertension, IHD, and mild heart failure. She currently takes aspirin, bisoprolol, bendroflumethiazide, furosemide, and ramipril. She has newly diagnosed AF, which is rate-controlled because of the bisoprolol.

You wish to discuss starting warfarin with her. The conversation may go as follows:

*Doctor:* 'You have a condition called atrial fibrillation—where the heart beat is irregular. It is not causing you any problems at the moment; it is common, and it is not a dangerous heart condition. However, there is a risk that this irregular beat could send a clot to the brain and cause a stroke and I would like to consider a treatment to reduce the risk of this happening.'

*Patient:* 'A stroke? I'm going to have a stroke?'

*Doctor:* 'If we took 100 people in your situation, then in a year about 10 of them would have a stroke—but 90 would not.'

*Patient:* 'I would hate to have a stroke. What can you do?'

*Doctor:* 'We can thin your blood with a drug called warfarin.'

*Patient:* 'I've heard of that—isn't it very dangerous?'

*Doctor:* 'You would need to have regular blood tests to make sure the dosage was right. If those 100 people all took warfarin, then one of them would have a serious problem with bleeding.'

*Patient:* 'But it will stop me from having a stroke?'

*Doctor:* 'Going back to those 100 people—if they all take the warfarin, then only three or four will have a stroke instead of the original 10. The risk is reduced by about two-thirds.'

*Patient:* 'Which three or four people?'

*Doctor:* 'There is no way of predicting who will benefit from treatment and who will have a problem. What we do know is that overall, the risk is lower with warfarin, and so we do recommend treatment for someone like you.'

*Patient:* 'Do I have to?'

*Doctor:* 'No, of course not. It is your decision. I will give you an information leaflet—why don't you go away and think it over—we will talk again.'

## HOW TO . . . Use digoxin

*Indications*
- Rate control of AF in sedentary patients intolerant to β-blockers
- Mild positive inotrope sometimes used in heart failure

*Not useful for*
- Paroxysmal AF prevention
- Exercise-induced fast AF

*Loading with digoxin*
- 1mg in divided doses over 24h

This dose is always required, regardless of renal function—modify *maintenance* doses only in renal impairment.
  Example:
- Day 1—8 a.m. digoxin 500 micrograms po, 8 p.m. digoxin 500 micrograms po
- Day 2—8 a.m. digoxin at maintenance dose

*Deciding a maintenance dose*
- Main determinant is renal function—digoxin is excreted this way, so use a low dose with renal impairment
- Consider also body mass, e.g. start with 62.5 micrograms for a small older woman—the dose can always be ↑ if there is inadequate rate control
- Dosage is determined clinically, but serum levels can be used to assess toxicity or adherence

*Digoxin toxicity*
- Hypokalaemia predisposes to this, so always monitor potassium and supplement if needed. Target [K⁺] >4.0mmol/L
- Symptoms include confusion, nausea, vomiting, arrhythmias (especially nodal bradycardia and ventricular ectopics), and yellow or green visual haloes
- ECG may show ST depression and inverted T wave in V5 and V6 (reversed tick pattern) or any arrhythmia
- Treat by stopping medication, rehydrating, and correcting hypokalaemia
- Life-threatening poisoning can be treated with digoxin-specific antibody fragments

## Further reading

Heidbuchel H, Verhamme P, Alings M, *et al*. Updated European Heart Rhythm Association Practical Guide on the use of non-vitamin K antagonist anticoagulants in patients with non-valvular atrial fibrillation. *Europace* 2015; **17**: 1467–507. ℘ http://europace.oxfordjournals.org/content/europace/early/2015/08/29/europace.euv309.full.pdf.

National Institute for Health and Care Excellence (2014). *Atrial fibrillation: management*. Clinical guideline CG180. ℘ https://www.nice.org.uk/guidance/cg180/resources.

National Institute for Health and Care Excellence (2014). *Atrial fibrillation: medicines to help reduce your risk of a stroke – what are the options?* Patient decision aid. ℘ https://www.nice.org.uk/guidance/cg180/resources/patient-decision-aid-243734797.

# Bradycardia and conduction disorders

As the heart ages, the function of the cardiac pacemaker (the SA node) and the conducting system (bundle of His and Purkinje fibres) tends to decline, due to:

- Declining numbers of cells in the SA node
- ↑ prevalence of disease (atheroma, amyloid, and hypertension)
- Degeneration with fibrosis and fat infiltration

This is not inevitable, but around 50% of older patients will have some ECG evidence of conduction delay (prolonged PR and QT interval, left axis deviation, etc.) and be prone to symptomatic bradycardia and conduction disorders.

## Causes

- *Medication*—digoxin, amiodarone, β-blockers (including some eye drops), calcium channel blockers, donepezil, tricyclic antidepressants
- *Sick sinus syndrome*—isolated sinus node dysfunction, very common in older patients, with uncertain cause (theories include vascular insufficiency or amyloid infiltration, but often no cause is found)
- *IHD*
- *Structural heart disease*, e.g. hypertrophic cardiomyopathy
- *Systemic disease*—hypothyroidism, liver failure, hypothermia, hypoxia, hypercapnia, cerebral disease (e.g. stroke, raised intracranial pressure, haemorrhage)

## Presentation

- Often picked up incidentally on an ECG
- When symptomatic, bradycardia causes low output syndromes ranging from fatigue, dizziness, dyspnoea, and presyncope, syncope, and falls, angina to heart failure and shock
- May be intermittent (with paroxysmal bradyarrhythmias), chronic (with stable arrhythmias), or occur acutely (usually post-MI)

## Management

This depends on the clinical presentation, not on the rhythm; a patient with complete heart block can be moribund or asymptomatic, and treatment will obviously be dramatically different in these scenarios. Seek advice from the local cardiology service if in doubt.

*Is the patient acutely compromised?*

- If so, then urgent treatment is required in order to minimize cerebral injury. For shock, lie the patient down, and elevate the legs. Use iv fluids and/or try to ↑ the heart rate using atropine (0.6mg iv, repeated up to a total dose of 3mg), an isoprenaline infusion, or temporary pacing (external pads are quick and often well tolerated; if the situation persists, insert a temporary pacing wire)

- Always look for underlying causes, e.g. sepsis, stroke, hypothermia, hypothyroidism; treating an underlying cause may be equal or greater priority than the bradycardia. Reversible bradyarrhythmia commonly occurs after acute inferior MI, in which case support the patient during the acute episode as needed (non-invasively if feasible). Acutely, hypothermia can also cause bradycardia which reverses when patient is normothermic again
- Tailor your treatment to each individual—if the cause of the bradycardia is a catastrophic intracerebral event, then putting the patient through a temporary wire is not appropriate

*A stable patient with intermittent symptoms*

- Symptoms can be insidious, and sometimes patients do not recognize their symptoms until after the bradycardia is corrected. Ask specifically about tiredness, exercise tolerance, worsening symptoms of heart failure or angina, as well as syncope and presyncope symptoms
- Check medication. Digoxin (especially with toxicity), amiodarone, β-blockers, and calcium channel blockers can all cause or exacerbate bradycardia. Referral for a pacemaker should not occur unless patients remain bradycardic off any culprit drugs for at least a week
- Check and correct thyroid function
- Very few patients need admission and urgent permanent or temporary pacemaker insertion, but consider admission for frequent syncope or severe persistent symptoms. Most cardiology services have a 'fast track' outpatient service to avoid admission for symptomatic patients who cannot wait for a routine list
- Patients or their relatives can sometimes reject the idea of a pacemaker because they believe it is a 'big' operation or it will stop them dying. A pacemaker is a relatively low-risk intervention which can dramatically improve quality of life, even in frail patients or those with cognitive impairment, so ensure they fully understand the proposed procedure before rejecting it

*Asymptomatic patients*

- Older patients can be truly asymptomatic and can tolerate pulses of 50bpm for many years. Action is not required unless there is a high risk of future asystole. Asystole is a major risk with complete heart block and also with second-degree heart block type II where there is also bundle branch block—even if asymptomatic, a pacemaker should be offered for these two conditions

## Permanent pacemakers

### Indications

- Over 85% are used for patients >64 years old
- 50% are for sick sinus syndrome and AV block
- Occasionally used for vasodepressor carotid sinus hypersensitivity
- Occasionally used for recurrent syncope where no cause is found
- Used with AV node ablation with refractory AF
- Resynchronization therapy for heart failure

### Pacemakers

- Dual-chamber pacemakers are preferred, as they produce a better cardiac output and less AF than single-chamber ones
- Permanent pacing should be programmed to minimize paced beats, allowing the intrinsic rhythm to get through as much as possible
- In LV dysfunction, pacing may need to include multisite pacing, as right ventricular pacing can worsen dyssynchrony and exacerbate LV failure
- Cardiac resynchronization therapy (biventricular pacing) may reduce heart failure symptoms in patients with reduced LV function, if they have wide QRS complexes

### Insertion

- Relatively simple procedure, done while awake using local anaesthetic, which is usually well tolerated by even very frail patients; however, technical problems can occur with insertion if the patient cannot lie still and flat
- Rare complications during insertion include arrhythmias (commonly AF) and rarely perforation of the right ventricle
- Later problems include sepsis and failure of pacemaker output
- Regular follow-up is required to check the pacemaker function and battery reserve

## Further reading

National Institute for Health and Care Excellence (2005). *Dual-chamber pacemakers for symptomatic bradycardia due to sick sinus syndrome and/or atrioventricular block*. Technology appraisal guidance TA88. ℳ http://www.nice.org.uk/ta88.

# Common arrhythmias and conduction abnormalities

(See Table 10.5.)

Table 10.5 Common arrhythmias and conduction abnormalities

| Condition | Clinical features | Treatment |
|---|---|---|
| Sinus bradycardia | Intrinsic SA nodal disease<br>Pulse rate <60<br>Common incidental finding<br>Drugs are common cause<br>Acute onset associated with inferior MI and raised intracranial pressure<br>Consider hypothyroidism | Treat only if symptomatic (rarely causes problem)<br>Check thyroid function |
| Supraventricular ectopics | Narrow complex QRS without a P wave, followed by a compensatory pause<br>Patient may be aware of this and describe an 'early beat' with a gap afterwards | Benign<br>Reassure the patient<br>No action required |
| SA block | Intermittent inability of SA node to depolarize the atrium<br>ECG shows pauses that are multiples of the PR interval | Usually asymptomatic<br>Treat only if symptoms |
| Slow AF | Combination of AF and SA nodal disease very common<br>Symptomatic pauses frequent | Anticoagulation for stroke prevention<br>High index of suspicion for pauses if suggestive symptoms—check with Holter monitor and treat with pacemaker |
| Sick sinus syndrome | SA node dysfunction (degenerative or due to IHD) causing a bradycardia—includes sinus bradycardia and slow AF<br>Often associated with other conduction problems | Treat symptoms |
| Tachy-brady syndrome | Combination of slow underlying rate (sinus bradycardia or slow AF) with tendency for runs of SVT that often terminate with a long pause<br>Symptoms due to both slow and fast pulse | Usually requires pacemaker for bradycardia and rate-limiting drugs to control tachyarrhythmias |

**Table 10.5** (*Contd.*)

| Condition | Clinical features | Treatment |
|---|---|---|
| First-degree heart block | PR >0.2s | Benign if isolated, but always check for coexisting second- or third-degree block<br><br>No action required |
| Second-degree heart block, Mobitz type I (Wenckebach) | PR interval ↑ progressively until a QRS is dropped | Often occurs transiently post-MI<br><br>Usually appropriate to monitor until resolves |
| Second-degree heart block, Mobitz type II | Fixed PR interval, but conduction to the ventricles does not occur on every beat. Usually in a fixed pattern (conducting every second, third or fourth beat)<br><br>Often associated with bundle branch block | Often symptomatic<br><br>High risk of progression to complete heart block<br><br>Usually requires elective pacing |
| Complete heart block (third-degree) | Complete dissociation of atrial and ventricular activity. P waves visible, but not conducted. QRS originates at ventricular pacemaker (escape rhythm). If this is in the AV node, then the rate is around 60 and the QRS morphology narrow. If it is more distal, then the rate tends to be around 40 with wide QRS complexes | Usually symptomatic, although if rate >50, may only be on exertion<br><br>If chronic, limit activity until permanent pacing arranged<br><br>If acute (e.g. post-MI), likely to resolve<br><br>When associated with hypotension, angina, or heart failure at rest, may need urgent pacing |
| Bundle branch block | Widened QRS due to delayed conduction<br><br>Not related to rate, usually asymptomatic<br><br>RBBB is a common finding in healthy elderly and is usually benign, but if acute, consider acute PE<br><br>LBBB is associated with hypertension and IHD | Acutely, LBBB may indicate acute infarct<br><br>If found incidentally, tell the patient (aids future emergency treatment and consider giving a copy of the ECG to the patient |
| Trifascicular block | Prolonged PR, RBBB, and left anterior or posterior fascicular block (causing left axis deviation) | High risk of intermittent complete heart block. Pacemaker is considered |

# Heart failure: assessment

Heart failure is very common, occurring in 1 in 10 of the >65s and accounting for 5% of admissions to medical wards and 1–2% of all healthcare costs. Overall prevalence is 3–20 cases per 1000 population, but this doubles with each decade after 45 years. Becoming more common as the population ages and survival from coronary events improves.

## Pathology

- Poor LV function (systolic or diastolic) ↓ cardiac output, resulting in ↑ pulmonary pressures and oedema
- Sympathetic nervous system activated (↑ pulse, myocardial contractility, peripheral vasoconstriction, and catecholamines)
- Renin–angiotensin system activated (↑ salt and water retention)
- Vasopressin and natriuretic peptides ↑

## Causes

Usually due to CHD (especially in Caucasians—CHD risk factors are markers for heart failure) and hypertension (especially African Caribbeans). Other causes include valve disease, arrhythmias, pericardial disease, pulmonary hypertension (e.g. with COPD or multiple PEs), high output states (look especially for anaemia, thyroid disease, and Paget's disease), and cardiomyopathy (check alcohol history).

## Diagnosis

Heart failure is a complex clinical diagnosis, with no universally agreed diagnostic criteria. Often difficult to diagnose accurately, particularly in older patients with ↑ comorbidity and symptoms. Many older people are put on a diuretic for presumed heart failure, but diuretic use as a marker of heart failure is 73% sensitive but only 41% specific. This predisposes to postural symptoms and adds to polypharmacy.

## Symptoms

Ask 'are these symptoms cardiac' and 'what is the underlying disease causing them?' Exertional dyspnoea is 100% sensitive for heart failure (i.e. every case has it), but only 17% specific (i.e. many other causes of exertional dyspnoea exist—the main one being respiratory). Fatigue and ankle swelling are also very common in heart failure but occur in many other diseases too. Orthopnoea and paroxysmal nocturnal dyspnoea are much more specific but, occurring late in the disease, are not sensitive.

## Signs

Again, early signs are sensitive, but not specific (e.g. tachycardia, pulmonary crepitations, peripheral oedema). Later signs are more specific, but not sensitive (e.g. elevated JVP—98% specific, 17% sensitive; gallop rhythm—99% specific and 24% sensitive).

▶ Overall, clinical features tend to be sensitive OR specific, but not both. The multiple pathology of older patients poses a particular challenge in diagnosis. Clinical suspicion should then be supported by investigation before embarking on a trial of treatment.

**HOW TO . . . Investigate a patient with suspected heart failure**

Use investigations to support a clinical diagnosis and establish the cause.
- *ECG*—abnormal in over 90% of cases (Q waves, T wave/ST segment changes, LV hypertrophy, bundle branch block, AF). Consider Holter monitor if paroxysmal symptoms
- *CXR*—look for cardiac enlargement (although this is absent with acute onset, e.g. post-MI or PE), upper lobe blood diversion, fluid in the horizontal fissure, Kerley B lines, bat wing pulmonary oedema, pleural effusions (usually bilateral; right > left if unilateral), and any other cause for breathlessness

▶ Combination of a normal CXR and ECG makes heart failure very unlikely indeed.
- *Blood tests*—B-type natriuretic peptide (BNP) (see Box 10.2), FBC (? anaemic), biochemistry (? renal function, sodium low in severe heart failure), glucose and lipids (CHD risk factors), liver function (? congestion), thyroid function
- *Echocardiography*—echo should be done for all with suspected heart failure (NICE guidelines) to help confirm diagnosis, establish cause, and grade disease severity. Looks for LV function (systolic and diastolic; see ➋ 'Heart failure with preserved left ventricular function', pp. 298–9), estimates EF, and looks for evidence of valve disease, cardiomyopathy, regional wall abnormalities from IHD, pericardial disease, intracardiac shunts, LV aneurysms, or cardiac thrombus. Open access echo (i.e. direct GP referral) has improved the number of patients who have an echo, but the results are only as good as the echo technician and there can be problems with interpreting results (e.g. diastolic problems). Patients may need a repeat echo after several years, especially if symptoms progress or change
- *Pulmonary function tests*—may help distinguish cardiac from respiratory breathlessness (peak expiratory flow rate (PEFR) and forced expiratory volume in 1 s ($FEV_1$) reduced in heart failure, but less than in COPD). Remember many patients have both

## Box 10.2 B-type natriuretic peptide

Three types of natriuretic peptide known, with effects on the heart, kidneys, and nervous system. B-type is found mainly in the heart and ↑ with volume and pressure overload of the heart, acting as a biochemical marker for heart failure. BNP rises slightly with age but remains below 100pg/mL (which is the most common threshold used for diagnosis).

▶ Overall, a 'negative' (i.e. very low) result in a breathless patient makes heart failure very unlikely, and other causes should be sought.

BNP is a highly sensitive test (negative predictive value of 96%). Causes of false positives include pulmonary hypertension, e.g. PE, sepsis, acute kidney injury.

BNP concentration correlates with the severity of heart disease—very high levels carry a poor prognosis. It is equally useful in systolic and diastolic heart failure.

*Where and how is it used?*

• *1° care screening.* BNP should be used in all patients before referring for heart failure services. Patients with a normal BNP should not be referred to cardiology, as they are extremely unlikely to have heart failure causing their symptoms, and other diagnoses should be considered

• *Acute first presentation of heart failure.* A single BNP measurement can be helpful, alongside clinical features and other tests (e.g. echo). Remember that acutely unwell patients (e.g. sepsis and kidney injury) can have false-positive elevations, and in these patients, an interval measurement when stable is indicated, especially if only a minor elevation is detected acutely

• *Chronic heart failure.* A single measurement is all that is required to aid diagnosis (usually by the GP as above) and does not usually need repeating

• *Future uses.* Research shows BNP is a powerful predictive tool for future morbidity and mortality in lots of different populations (including asymptomatic patients). BNP may therefore have a role in population screening and targeting interventions for the highest-risk groups. It can be used by cardiologists to monitor response to treatment

# Acute heart failure

### Treatment

- Immediate treatment with oxygen, iv loop diuretic, and nitrates given iv or sublingually (if adequate BP), opiate, and antiemetic
- Address the cause (e.g. acute MI, arrhythmia)
- Stop any exacerbating medications (NSAIDs, β-blockers)
- Consider thromboprophylaxis (e.g. low-molecular-weight heparin)
- Consider ventilatory support (non-invasive positive pressure ventilation, which can be done in a non-ITU setting, can produce dramatic resolution of symptoms)
- After improvement is seen, begin to plan ongoing treatment—write up regular loop diuretic and usually an ACE on the drug chart, and make plans for further assessment
- Monitor electrolytes, BP, and weight

### Prognosis

Patients with acute heart failure look extremely unwell yet can often make apparently 'miraculous' recoveries as the precipitant is dealt with. Remember that it is the premorbid state and the nature of the acute injury, never age alone, that should determine how aggressively to manage the acute condition.

### Rapid atrial fibrillation and heart failure

- A common combination in older patients
- It is rarely clear which came first
- Treat both simultaneously
- Digoxin may slow AF in this situation without depressing the myocardium (may occur with β-blocker or amiodarone). Load 1mg of digoxin over 24h in divided doses, e.g. 500 micrograms iv or po, repeated at 12h, followed by the maintenance dose
- Always look for a precipitant—sepsis, MI, PE, etc.

# Chronic heart failure

A specialist multidisciplinary approach is preferable, as management is best done by those with an interest and with facilities for ongoing follow-up. Settings can vary, e.g. DHs (particularly suited to the frailer patient), heart failure clinics, and by heart failure specialist nurses or GPSIs.

Education and involvement of the patient are key to successful monitoring (e.g. daily weighing) and management (improves adherence and satisfaction).

## Subtypes
- LV failure
- Right ventricular failure/cor pulmonale
- LV failure with preserved LV function, previously known as diastolic heart failure (see ➔ 'Heart failure with preserved left ventricular function', pp. 298–9)

There is a strong evidence base for management of LV failure subtype with life prolonging therapies.

## Diagnosis

Use a combination of clinical features, ECG, CXR, BNP, and echo. Always review a historical diagnosis of heart failure, particularly if the appropriate investigations were not completed.

## Lifestyle interventions

Address cardiovascular risk actors, stop smoking, stop/reduce alcohol intake, and ↑ aerobic exercise (ideally as part of a rehabilitation programme). Offer annual influenza vaccination annually and pneumococcal vaccine once.

## Treating underlying cause/comorbidities
- AF should be slowed and anticoagulation started (cardioversion unlikely to succeed once LV dysfunction)
- Hypertension should be treated until disease progression drops cardiac output and hence BP
- Valvular disease should be assessed for surgical correction where appropriate (especially aortic valve disease—discuss with the patient early after onset of heart failure)
- Optimize management of anaemia (iv iron or erythropoietin), thyroid disease, and diabetes

## Medication

There is a large evidence base for many drugs (see Box 10.3). It may be tempting to limit the number of drugs in older patients, justified by concerns about side effects, but if the diagnosis is secure, then all classes should be attempted. It is probably better to prescribe a low dose of an ACE with a β-blocker, rather than a maximum dose of an ACE when the BP may be insufficient to introduce the β-blocker.

## Monitoring
Should include:
- Clinical assessment of symptoms and functional capacity (how far they can walk without stopping, etc.)
- BP, including postural measurements

## Box 10.3 Medication for chronic heart failure

- *Loop diuretics*—(e.g. furosemide) used to control symptoms. Begin with 40mg (20mg in the very elderly) and titrate upwards (guided by symptoms and examination findings). Monitor renal function and electrolytes
- *ACE inhibitors*—should be started early in all with a diagnosis of systolic heart failure, unless valvular cause or renal artery stenosis suspected. Again begin low (e.g. ramipril 1.25mg) and titrate upwards, monitoring renal function and postural symptoms
- *β-blockers*—should be started in all stable patients with LV systolic dysfunction after diuretics, regardless of whether there are continuing symptoms (improves prognosis). Use a β-blocker licensed for heart failure, e.g. carvedilol 3.125mg, bisoprolol 2.5mg, and titrate upwards
- *Spironolactone*—use for continuing symptoms despite loop and ACE. Watch potassium levels, especially in combination with ACE
- *Digoxin*—use in AF and where there are continuing symptoms despite maximal other therapy in sinus rhythm
- *Thiazide diuretics*—can be added to loop diuretics in end-stage heart failure, e.g. bendroflumethiazide 2.5mg or metolazone 5mg (monitor electrolytes closely; may be used on alternate days if causes excess diuresis)
- *Warfarin*—use in AF or where echo has shown intracardiac thrombus
- *ARBs*—(e.g. candesartan) useful where ACE-intolerant; this class has benefits in heart failure, but its equivalence to ACE inhibition is debated
- *Aspirin/statins*—used for risk factor modification where the cause is IHD
- *Ivabradine*—useful in some patients in sinus rhythm who have a tachycardia but cannot tolerate a β-blocker

- Fluid status (weigh regularly. Estimate the dry weight, record it, and use this to titrate future management. Examine for JVP, oedema, and lung crepitations)
- Cardiac rhythm (clinically and by ECG)
- Cognitive state (commonly impaired in heart failure due to vascular disease and low BP)
- Nutritional state (malnutrition common in heart failure. Ask about appetite, assess muscle bulk, check albumin—consider build-up drinks or dietician input)
- Medication review (are they on all appropriate drugs at maximum tolerated doses?)
- Side effects (especially ask about postural symptoms, check U, C+E)
- Psychological and social review, done by an MDT (how are they and carers coping with problems of chronic disease? Do they need any social support?)
- Routine monitoring with tests such as BNP, CXR, and echo are expensive and largely unhelpful

## Further reading

National Institute for Health and Care Excellence (2010). *Chronic heart failure in adults: management.* Clinical guideline CG108. ℘ http://www.nice.org.uk/cg108.

# Dilemmas in heart failure

## Terminal care

- Chronic heart failure is a grim diagnosis with a poor outlook (only 25% will survive 3 years—worse than many cancers)
- Consider broaching this with all patients in clinic (ideally in a stable phase of the illness) to allow future plans to be made and resuscitation issues discussed. Monitoring of any cognitive impairment allows the timing of this conversation to be carefully judged
- As the disease progresses, ensure appropriate palliative care measures are taken with careful review of symptoms and patient/family anxieties
- Consider hospice care if available
- Opiates (e.g. morphine sulfate solution 2.5–10mg) can be given to help relieve the distress of dyspnoea and allow sleep
- Continuous oxygen therapy may ease discomfort
- Intermittent iv boluses of furosemide in DH or sc at home can keep people out of hospital

## Mixed cardiac and pulmonary disease

It is very common to see older patients presenting with mixed pathology, e.g. a 92-year-old ex-smoking ♀ may well have breathlessness due to a combination of:

- Significant emphysema
- LV impairment
- Kyphoscoliosis with restrictive ventilatory problems
- Chronic anaemia
- Rhythm disturbance with poorly controlled AF
- Physical deconditioning

In this sort of case, the signs can be confusing or contradictory, and trying to balance management is very challenging. Recognition of all the contributing factors is important—small changes across all factors may be a much more successful strategy than intense focus on a single element. A geriatrician may be better placed to do this than involvement of a multiple organ specialist.

## HOW TO . . . Manage the heart failure see-saw

One of the most common dilemmas is balancing drugs in a patient with both heart failure and chronic renal failure. When the see-saw is unchecked, this can lead to multiple unnecessary admissions to hospital and, more importantly, reduced quality of life for the patient.

*Aggressive diuretic use* will improve the heart failure but lead to thirst, malaise, hyponatraemia, uraemia, postural hypotension, and ultimately anuria.

*Hydrating* to improve renal function will lead to worsening pulmonary and peripheral oedema.

Each patient will need a carefully planned balance, accepting moderate elevations in urea and/or a bit of oedema, which enables the patient to exist in the greatest comfort. This balance will take time and skill to achieve.

The following will help:

- Make all changes slowly and wait for impact—large-dose changes ↑ oscillation between wet and dry states
- If a patient is still losing/gaining weight on a treatment regimen, they are likely to continue to do so. Keep the patient under continuing close review until stability is reached
- Get to know the ideal weight, and use this to guide therapy
- Involve patients and carers wherever possible
- Get to know the patient—continuity of care is very helpful, and community heart failure nurses may play a key role in this. The patient must know how to access a review and advice quickly when they detect a swing in their symptoms
- Communicate between different health care settings. Many mistakes are made when a carefully constructed medication balance is not continued when a patient moves from hospital to home, or vice versa

# Heart failure with preserved left ventricular function

- Previously known as 'diastolic heart failure'
- Clinical syndrome of heart failure with normal LVEF seen on echocardiography (>50%) where there is no major valvular disease
- The use of BNP in combination with echo has helped identify these patients (BNP equally sensitive in heart failure with preserved left ventricular function (HFPLVF))
- NICE guidelines suggest diagnosis should be done by a specialist
- Accounts for around a third of clinically diagnosed heart failure and is more common in older patients, especially women, hypertensive patients, and those with LVH
- *Not* a benign condition—ambulatory patients do better than those with systolic heart failure, but the mortality is equivalent in older patients or hospitalized. Fourfold ↑ in mortality when compared with controls without heart failure

▶ Important to recognize and treat, and not to discontinue heart failure treatment on basis of normal LV function alone.

## Pathology

Thick-walled LV with a small cavity. Slow to relax and slow filling in diastole, causing ↑ diastolic pressures (hence pulmonary pressures and so dyspnoea) and a low cardiac output (hence fatigue).

## Diagnosis

- *Clinical suspicion* (history as for systolic heart failure) and *examination* findings (elevated JVP, pulmonary oedema, hypertension, murmur in the aortic area, fourth heart sound) are key
- *CXR* may show pulmonary congestion, and the *ECG* may have evidence of hypertension
- *Echocardiography* shows preserved LV function and, in skilled hands, may show evidence of abnormal diastolic relaxation (Doppler studies show a reduced ratio of early (E) to late or atrial (A) ventricular filling velocities—E:A <0.5 is suggestive of diastolic dysfunction). However, these changes are very common in older patients (E:A often <1). Thus, treatment is based on symptoms, not echo
- *BNP* (see Box 10.2) useful particularly in cases where there are multiple possible aetiologies of dyspnea, as a negative result makes heart failure unlikely, helping to limit polypharmacy

## Management

- *Prevention*—by BP control at population level
- *Relieve precipitants*—treat arrhythmias, anaemia, thyroid disease, ischaemia, and malnutrition
- *Acute symptoms*—control BP with oral agents as priority. Use loop diuretics, as for LV failure
- *Chronic disease management*—much less evidence than for systolic heart failure. Control of BP is key. Diastolic relaxation agents (e.g. β-blockade) not proven, but rate control with these, especially where there is dual indication, e.g. AF or IHD. Diuretics improve symptoms, but ensure you do not dehydrate patients as these patients are vulnerable to reductions in preload. Improve exercise tolerance with physical activity

# Valvular heart disease

The majority of valvular heart lesions in the UK are degenerative (e.g. senile calcification is the main cause of aortic stenosis), so valve defects are very common in older patients. The following must be remembered:

- Listen to the heart of all elderly people—many valve lesions are detected incidentally
- Think of valvular disease when a patient presents with dyspnoea, heart failure, angina, palpitations, syncope, or dizziness. Examine them carefully (see Table 10.6)
- When a murmur is heard, an echo should be requested in order to document the valve lesion and formulate a management plan
- Following a review of evidence by NICE in 2008, antibiotic prophylaxis is no longer recommended for invasive dental procedures

▶ Remember endocarditis if a murmur is heard in the context of an unexplained fever.

## Surgical treatment

- Once the valve lesion is known, decide whether *valve replacement* is indicated yet (see Table 10.5). In many lesions (e.g. mitral valve disease and aortic regurgitation), the progression of symptoms alerts to the need for pre-emptive surgery. In aortic stenosis, however, a prompt response to the development of early symptoms is required, and so the approach is different
- Consider whether or not the patient is a surgical 'candidate'. Remember that many lesions are amenable to *percutaneous interventions* which are feasible in much frailer patients
- Bioprosthetic (pig) valves can be used in older patients, which have a shorter lifespan than metal valves but obviate the need for anticoagulation
- If surgery is not yet indicated, then ensure there is some sort of call-back/surveillance system in place—whether repeat echocardiography or clinic review, or simply ensuring that the patient knows what symptoms should trigger medical review

## Talking to patients about potential surgery

- Always ask the patient what they think—often there will be strong views that come as a surprise to the physician. Many older people are terrified at the prospect, others are keen to proceed, and others will not want to decide—'whatever you think, doctor'
- Make it clear that obtaining a surgical opinion is not committing the patient to surgery, indeed the surgeon may feel that the risks outweigh the benefits, but that it is an important first step
- Having a frank and useful discussion about risks and benefits is often difficult but should always be attempted before referral is made
- Ensure you have enough time and take it slowly, giving plenty of opportunity for questions. They may wish to go away and think about it, perhaps returning with a family member—encourage this and do not force a decision

Table 10.6 Common valve lesions

| Valve lesion | Symptoms | Complications | Treatment | Who to consider for surgery? |
|---|---|---|---|---|
| Mitral stenosis | Dyspnoea<br>Fatigue<br>Palpitations<br>Chest pain<br>Haemoptysis | AF<br>Systemic emboli<br>Pulmonary hypertension<br>Pulmonary oedema<br>Pressure effects from large LA<br>Endocarditis | Rate control of AF (digoxin and/or β-blocker)<br>Anticoagulation for AF<br>Diuretics if heart failure | Symptoms despite medical management<br>If pliable valve, may be candidate for balloon valvuloplasty |
| Mitral regurgitation | Dyspnoea<br>Fatigue<br>Palpitations | Pulmonary oedema<br>AF<br>Endocarditis | Rate control of AF<br>Anticoagulation if AF<br>Diuretics if HF | Deteriorating symptoms—aim to replace valve before extensive LV damage<br>Condition progresses slowly, so not if asymptomatic |
| Aortic sclerosis | None | None | None | Not applicable |
| Aortic regurgitation | Dyspnoea<br>Palpitations<br>Heart failure | Pulmonary oedema<br>Endocarditis | Diuretics if heart failure | Worsening symptoms, worsening cardiomegaly, ECG deterioration<br>Aim to replace valve before extensive LV damage |

# Peripheral oedema

Swollen ankles are extremely common in older patients. As with all geriatric medicine, a careful assessment, diagnosis, and appropriate treatment should be carried out.

▶ Swollen ankles do not always indicate heart failure—starting a diuretic must not be an immediate reaction, as this treats only one of several causes and may cause harm.

## Causes

- Often, mild ankle swelling occurs in an otherwise fit person—this tends to be worse on prolonged standing and in the heat (sometimes referred to as 'dependent oedema'). It is likely that there is some minor venous disease causing the oedema, but it is essentially benign
- *Peripheral venous disease*—chronic oedema due to damage to deep veins causing venous hypertension, ↑ capillary pressure, and fibrinogen leakage ➲. Usually bilateral, but one side is often worse than the other (see ➲ 'Chronic venous insufficiency', p. 592)
- *Heart failure*—usually bilateral. Look for associated signs, e.g. raised JVP, cardiac enlargement, pulmonary crepitations, etc.
- *Superficial thrombophlebitis*—acute oedema with a red, hot, very tender venous cord with surrounding oedema
- *DVT*—acute-onset, painful swollen calf with pitting oedema of the ankle. Review thrombotic risk factors

▶ Always consider DVT with new-onset unilateral swelling.

- *Drug side effect*—commonly calcium channel blockers (especially amlodipine) and NSAIDs
- *Low serum albumin*—nephrotic syndrome, gastrointestinal loss, malnutrition, chronic disease, acute sepsis, etc.
- *Lymphatic obstruction*—consider obstructing pelvic tumours. If oedema is severe, perform rectal and groin examination
- *Traumatic*—after forcefully dorsiflexing the foot (usually when walking), leading to rupture of the plantar tendon or injury to the gastrocnemius. This oedema tends to be unilateral, tender, above the ankle, and with associated bruising to the calf. Treat with rest and NSAIDs
- *Other*, e.g. hypothyroidism, osteoarthritis of the knee, ruptured Baker's cyst, post-stroke paralysis

## Assessment

- *History*—how acute was the onset? Is it unilateral or bilateral? Is it painful, red, and hot? What are the associated physical symptoms—importantly dyspnoea (may indicate PE or heart failure)?
- *Examination*—look for physical signs. Always listen to the heart and lungs, and look for sacral oedema when ankle swelling is found. Consider rectal/groin examination
- *Investigations*—be guided by your clinical suspicion. Consider ECG (unlikely to be normal in heart failure), urea and electrolytes, albumin, FBC, TFTs

▶ D-dimer in elderly patients with swollen ankles is rarely helpful. While a negative result effectively rules out DVT, many elderly patients will have an elevated D-dimer—only use the test if you would proceed to ultrasound scanning in the event of a positive result.

## Treatment

All patients with ankle swelling should have a careful assessment for disease, with treatment dependent on cause:

- Stop drugs if they are responsible (consider alternatives)
- If heart failure, then full assessment and treatment are required
- For chronic venous disease, use leg elevation and compression bandaging or stockings (see ➋ 'Chronic venous insufficiency', p. 592)
- With severe lymphoedema, massage and pneumatic boots can be useful. Consider referral to specialist lymphoedema clinics
- If low albumin, treat the cause and ↑ dietary intake

If no disease is found, then management is pragmatic. Patients may find the ankle swelling unsightly, have difficulty fitting on their shoes, or even complain of an aching pain. Support hosiery may help. Many patients may be happy to tolerate the minor inconvenience once they have been assured that there is no serious pathology.

It may then be appropriate to start a low dose of thiazide or loop diuretic, but this will necessitate occasional monitoring of electrolytes and clinical review to ensure the benefits of treatment still outweigh the risks.

## Ankle swelling and nocturnal polyuria

- During the day, a large amount of fluid can collect in the interstitial space in the ankles
- At night, when the legs are elevated, this fluid is partly returned to the circulating volume and can cause a diuresis—hence nocturnal polyuria
- Paradoxically, treating such a patient with diuretics to limit the swelling may ultimately help with the polyuria

# Preventing venous thromboembolism in an older person

VTE, which incorporates DVT and PE, is a major cause of morbidity and mortality in hospitalized patients on both medical and surgical wards. The UK Department of Health has recently introduced national initiatives to reduce rates.

## Recognition

- Older patients present atypically, so diagnosis is often delayed
- They less frequently complain of pain and ↓ ability to walk, and their legs more commonly have asymmetrical swelling due to other conditions, e.g. chronic venous insufficiency, arterial or joint disease, etc.

## Prophylaxis

- Most hospitals now use a standardized risk assessment score/tool for all patients
- Age >60 is known to be a risk factor for VTE, as is reduced mobility, compared to normal, so almost all older patients will qualify for prophylactic treatment unless risks of treatment (bleeding risk) outweigh benefits
- Contraindications are sometimes absolute (e.g. immediately after stroke, haematemesis) but more commonly are relative (e.g. extensive bruising after a fall), and the geriatrician must weigh risks and benefits on a case-by-case basis
- Aspirin is no longer considered effective VTE prophylaxis, but patients on aspirin for other reasons are at higher risk of some bleeding complications (especially gastrointestinal) when low-molecular-weight heparin is given

## Review

- Reassessment is required every few days or when there is a material change in the patient condition
- Patients who move into rehabilitation settings often regain mobility, and it is unclear from the evidence when prophylactic low-molecular-weight heparin is no longer required. Options include stopping at:
  - Premorbid mobility level
  - Steady state
  - Discharge

Heparin injections should usually be stopped for patients receiving palliative care.

## Options for thromboprophylaxis
(See Table 10.7.)

**Table 10.7** Thromboprophylaxis options for older patients

| Prophylactic treatment | Risks/disadvantages in older patients | Notes |
|---|---|---|
| General measures, e.g. promote mobilization, avoid dehydration | | Earlier mobilization may ↑ falls risk and ↑ nursing time |
| Graduated anti-embolism stockings | Contraindicated in arterial disease, neuropathies, skin fragility/breaks, and heart failure<br><br>Not always well tolerated<br><br>Older patients need help to put on and maintain correct position, so ↑ nursing time | Incorrectly applied stockings (wrinkles) can worsen venous return<br><br>Proven to be of no help in patients with stroke |
| Low-molecular-weight heparin | Bleeding risks more common in older patients, include risk of falls, low platelets, and anticoagulant treatment | A reduced dose should be used in patients with low eGFR or weight |
| DOACs | | Low dose used for prevention after elective hip or knee surgery |
| Inferior vena cava (IVC) filter | | Only in very high-risk (e.g. PE despite warfarin) patients who need additional or alternative prophylaxis to full anticoagulation |

## Further reading
National Institute for Health and Care Excellence (2010). *Venous thromboembolism: reducing the risk for patients in hospital.* Clinical guideline CG92. ℰ http://www.nice.org.uk/cg92.

# Peripheral vascular disease

Peripheral vascular disease is common in older patients—causing symptoms in 10% of those over 70 years.

## Symptoms

- Only a third of older patients will have the classic symptoms of intermittent claudication, and often ↓ activity levels will mask developing disease. It may be difficult to distinguish the pain from that of osteoarthritis
- Claudication pain may progress to ischaemic rest pain (night-time pain, often relieved by hanging the foot over the bed), then to ulceration (due to trauma with poor healing—small, punctate, painful ulcers at pressure points, e.g. toes, lateral malleolus, metatarsal heads), and possibly gangrene
- Around 80% of patients with claudication remain stable or improve; only 20% deteriorate, and 6% require amputation (ongoing smokers and diabetics are most at risk)

## Examination

- Loss of pulses (best discriminator is an abnormality of the posterior tibial pulse)
- Possibly bruits
- Coolness to touch
- Slow capillary refill (over 2s)
- Shiny, hairless skin with atrophic nails and poor wound healing

## Peripheral vascular disease as a marker of other vascular disease

- 5-year mortality in peripheral vascular disease is 30%, mostly due to cardiovascular disease
- It is easy to detect peripheral vascular disease non-invasively by measuring the ankle–brachial pressure index (ABPI) (see ➲ 'HOW TO . . . Measure ABPI', p. 307)
- The impact of broad vascular risk management on subsequent vascular disease burden has yet to be quantified but is likely to be substantial

▶ If a patient complains of leg pains, screen for peripheral vascular disease and if detected, initiate full vascular 2° prevention.

## Management

Although very common, many elderly people will modify their lifestyle to reduce symptoms. It is important to actively seek out symptoms.

Adopt the following treatment approach:

- Modify risk factors (especially smoking)
- Advise ↑ exercise (NOT ↓). This is best done in a supervised exercise programme
- Commence antiplatelet agent—commonly aspirin; clopidogrel may have slightly more efficacy

- Consider other drugs—naftidrofuryl oxalate is the only vasodilator drug supported by NICE. The herbal remedy *Ginkgo biloba* probably has no impact but does no harm
- Do not necessarily stop β-blockers (traditionally thought to worsen claudication). The evidence for this is weak and β-blockers have a major role in modifying cardiac risk
- Refer for revascularization when appropriate. Percutaneous revascularization is relatively low-risk and should be considered for lifestyle-limiting claudication that does not respond to medical therapy, where there is a focal stenosis, a non-healing arterial ulcer or when there is limb-threatening ischaemia. Elective surgery is usually reserved for low-risk patients (under 70 years with no diabetes and no distal disease) who are fit enough to tolerate the procedure. Age has a significant impact on surgical risk—relative risk of mortality ↑ by 1.62 with each decade

## HOW TO . . . Measure ABPI

*When?*
- To confirm peripheral vascular disease as a cause of claudication
- To diagnose vascular disease before implementing 2° prevention
- To diagnose the aetiology of (venous) ulcers
- To ensure compression bandaging is safe

*Equipment*
- BP cuff with sphygmomanometer
- Hand-held Doppler probe

*Method*
- Inflate the cuff around the upper arm as usual, and use the Doppler probe over the brachial artery to measure the SBP
- Repeat in the other arm, and use the highest value
- Next inflate the cuff around the ankle, and use the probe to measure the systolic pressure in the dorsalis pedis and posterior tibial arteries
- Take the highest of the four ankle readings, and divide by the higher of the two arm readings to give the ABPI

*Interpretation*
- >1.3—non-compressible, calcified vessels; reading has limited value
- 1.0–1.3—normal range
- <0.9–angiographic peripheral vascular disease very likely
- 0.4–0.9—likely to be associated with claudication
- <0.4—advanced ischaemia

# Gangrene in peripheral vascular disease

The onset of gangrene is relatively common in people with severe peripheral vascular disease and causes considerable distress. It often poses management difficulties, as many frail older patients are judged inappropriate for open surgery.

## Slowly progressive disease with dry gangrene

- Cyanotic anaesthetic tissue with necrosis
- Distal, with clear demarcation
- Often a low-grade inflammatory response (elevated white cell count and CRP)
- The patient may feel unwell and anorexic
- Non-urgent surgical review is appropriate, but the approach is often to allow auto-amputation—a lengthy, and sometimes distressing, process, for the patient and family. This may be managed as an outpatient
- Surgical amputation may be considered, but as there is often inadequate local circulation to allow healing, this may need to be extensive or combined with bypass (the latter carrying a significant operative risk). Sometimes amputation vastly improves the quality of life for a bed-bound patient with gangrene. Discussion about possible amputation should be approached with tact and sensitivity—patients are often very against loss of a limb, even when they have not walked for years. Ensure that the patient and family are aware of the rationale for treatment and that there is regular review of analgesia requirements

## Wet gangrene

- Moist, swollen, and blistered skin—usually in people with diabetes

▶ This is a life-threatening condition, and urgent surgical review is required in all but the most terminal of patients

- The usual approach to management is to start iv antibiotics prior to debridement and amputation

## Acute ischaemia

▶ This is a limb-threatening condition and demands urgent action
- Usually due to embolization
- *Distal emboli* cause so-called 'blue toe syndrome'. The main object of treatment is to prevent recurrence, as little can be done to salvage occluded small vessels. This may include angiography to establish the source, and/or anticoagulation depending on the fitness of the patient
- *Proximal emboli* cause diffuse acute ischaemia. Revascularization of the limb is nearly always attempted (unless there is already irreversible ischaemic changes), and the approach can be tailored to the frailty of the patient—ranging from thrombolysis and percutaneous thromboembolectomy (possible under local anaesthesia) to emergency bypass procedures

# Vascular secondary prevention

(See Table 10.8.)

Atheromatous vascular disease (cardiac, peripheral vascular, and cerebral) accounts for a huge amount of morbidity, mortality, and expenditure.

2° prevention measures evolve continually, as individual clinical trials reach completion. Although some interventions are primarily applied to a specific pathology, most impact on all vascular systems. The cumulative effect of therapies is not yet known, but the consensus is that they will substantially reduce the burden of future vascular events.

Traditionally, older patients have been under-provided with 2° prevention measures, for a number of reasons:

• There is often polypharmacy, and reluctance among patients and health-care professionals to add to this
• It was thought that 2° prevention benefits were seen only with long-term (perhaps 5–10 years) treatment. Unless life expectancy was greater than this, therapy was not begun
• It may be 'shutting the door after the horse has bolted'—the damage has already been done

But consider several contrary points:

• Recent evidence suggests that some therapies (statins and ACE inhibitors) act quickly, possibly due to endovascular stabilization
• Although older patients are underrepresented in clinical trials, where older patients have been included (e.g. the Heart Protection Study), the benefits have been equal, if not greater than in younger patients
• Do not assume that a disabled person will not benefit from prevention of further events. In a bed-bound stroke patient who has to be spoon-fed, a further stroke that removes swallowing ability altogether may deprive that person of their only pleasure in life
• As with much of geriatric medicine, frank discussion with the patient is advised. Many patients will have strong views and fall into one of two groups—the fatalists, who prefer not to take medication 'just in case', and the 'belt-and-braces' patients who welcome all possible measures
• Drug doses are determined by clinical trial evidence—often a high dose in generally robust patients. Adopt a pragmatic approach in frail patients with lower doses, as these may be effective with fewer side effects
• Reduce doses of renally cleared medication with low glomerular filtration rate (GFR)

We do not advocate the blind prescription of all 2° prevention to all of older patients—such an approach would be clinically inappropriate for some and unlikely to be cost-effective. What we do suggest is that each patient is considered on a case-by-case basis and, where possible, included in the discussion to reach an individually tailored action plan.

## Further reading

The Heart Protection Study Collaborative Group. MRC/BHF Heart Protection Study of cholesterol lowering with simvastatin in 20,536 high-risk individuals: a randomised placebo-controlled trial. *Lancet* 2002; **360**: 7–22.

Table 10.8 The main secondary prevention agents

| Agent | Dose | Action | Outcome | Special points |
|-------|------|--------|---------|----------------|
| Aspirin | 75–300mg od | Antiplatelet activity | Prevention of all vascular events | Use lower doses<br>Beware gastric irritation<br>Consider co-prescription of proton pump inhibitor/H2 antagonist<br>Enteric-coated formulations unlikely to be very useful |
| Clopidogrel | 75mg od | Antiplatelet activity | Mainly as an alternative to aspirin where not tolerated, or as an addition in cardiac and some stroke disease | Reportedly, lower gastric side effects.<br>Slightly higher efficacy than aspirin as monotherapy |
| Dipyridamole MR | 200mg bd | Antiplatelet activity | Addition to aspirin in cerebrovascular disease<br>NOT for cardiac disease (can exacerbate angina) | Start slowly as commonly causes headache<br>Low bleeding risk |
| Antihypertensives | Various agents | Blood pressure reduction | Prevention of all vascular events | The lower the BP, the greater the benefit, but take care to avoid hypotensive side effects |
| ACE inhibitors | e.g. ramipril 10mg od | Blood pressure reduction and possible endovascular effect | Prevention of all vascular events | Dose stated is often not tolerated in older patients—aim as high as tolerated, but start with 1.25mg |
| Statins | e.g. atorvastatin 40mg od | Cholesterol lowering and possible endovascular effect | Prevention of all vascular events | Should be prescribed for vast majority<br>Lower doses may be better tolerated<br>\watch for myalgia and raised LFTs |

Note: consider also smoking cessation, increasing physical activity, and for stroke–endarterectomy and AF prophylaxis.

# Chest medicine

# The ageing lung

Most of the functional impairment of the lungs that is seen in older people is due to disease, often smoking-related. Intrinsic ageing leads only to mild functional deterioration. The respiratory system has a capacity well in excess of that required for normal activity, so intrinsic ageing:

- Does not lead to symptoms in the non-smoker without respiratory disease, although reduced physical activity can lead to a reduction in physical fitness
- In those with respiratory disease (e.g. emphysema) will cause progressively worsening symptoms with age, even if the disease itself remains stable
- In acute disease, e.g. pneumonia, may cause earlier decompensation or a more severe presentation

### Specific respiratory changes

Seen in healthy older people are similar to those seen in mild chronic obstructive pulmonary disease and include:

- ↓ elastic recoil causing small airways to collapse at low lung volumes and ↑ residual volume
- ↑ chest wall stiffness, due to:
  - Degenerative change in intercostal, intervertebral, and costovertebral joints
  - Osteoporosis and kyphoscoliosis
  - Weaker respiratory muscles that may have lower endurance
- Reduced gas exchange and ↑ ventilation–perfusion (V/Q) mismatch, due to collapse of peripheral airways while perfusion remains intact
- Impaired chemoreceptor function, leading to lessened ventilatory response to ↓ $P_aO_2$ or ↑ $P_aCO_2$
- Impaired microbial defence mechanisms. Less effective mucociliary clearance and less sensitive cough reflex

### Observed consequences of these changes

These include:

- ↑ susceptibility to infection (underventilation of, and inability to clear sputum from, dependent lung zones)
- Lower maximum minute ventilation (weaker musculature acting against a stiffer chest)
- An approximately linear fall in $P_aO_2$ with age (~0.3%/year). Since alveolar oxygen tension remains stable, the alveolar–arterial (A–a) oxygen gradient rises
- Reduced exercise capacity. However, oxygen consumption and cardiac output decline in proportion to lung function, so the lungs are rarely the limiting factor in exercise performance

## Breathlessness in older people is often multifactorial

- Chronic breathlessness in an individual may be the result of, e.g. ↓ fitness, obesity, an inefficient gait (osteoarthritis or stroke), kyphosis, previous lung damage (e.g. apical fibrosis due to tuberculosis (TB)), and intrinsic ageing. In this example, note that only one of the factors is specific to the lung
- In the acutely breathless patient, pathologies commonly coexist, e.g. infection, fast AF, and heart failure. The classic treatment triad of digoxin, furosemide, and amoxicillin is not a sign of diagnostic indecision but is often entirely appropriate treatment

# Respiratory infections

Cough with or without sputum, shortness of breath, fever, or chest pain are a very common presentation in older patients. It is very important to try to distinguish which part of the airway is primarily affected because this implies completely different pathogens, prognoses, and treatment strategies. Try to avoid aggregating all such patients together using the imprecise term 'chest infection'.

## Upper respiratory tract infections

These are caused by viruses, e.g. rhinovirus, respiratory syncytial virus, influenza, and parainfluenza. Symptoms include nasal discharge and congestion, fever, and sore throat. These may extend to the lower tract and then include cough, wheeze, sputum production, or worsening of existing cardiopulmonary disease.

With ↑ age:
- Upper respiratory tract infection becomes less frequent, but more severe
- The risk of complications ↑. These include:
  - Lower tract infection such as bronchitis or pneumonia, which may be bacterial or viral
  - Bronchospasm
  - Extrapulmonary manifestations such as falls, immobility, and delirium
- Post-infection weakness, fatigue, and anorexia are more severe and prolonged, maybe lasting several weeks
- Frequency of hospital admission and death ↑ substantially

## Acute bronchitis

Occurs with inflammation of the bronchial tree, with little or no involvement of lung parenchyma (which is pneumonia). Is more common in those with chronic airways disease (see ⭕ 'Asthma and COPD: assessment', pp. 340–1).

Compared with pneumonia, bronchitis:
- Has fewer systemic features and a better prognosis
- Has no chest symptoms and signs, e.g. pleuritic pain or crepitations, but may have prominent cough and wheeze
- CXR not routinely indicated
- Can be managed less aggressively, with more reliance on supportive treatment and bronchodilators than antibiotics. Often viral in origin; if an antibacterial is thought appropriate, give amoxicillin to cover *Streptococcus pneumoniae* (erythromycin or clarithromycin if penicillin-sensitive)

# Influenza

This is the most serious viral respiratory tract infection in older patients and is often a severe, systemic illness with pulmonary bacterial superinfection (*Staphylococcus aureus, Haemophilus influenzae, S. pneumoniae*). It occurs most commonly in December–February. Antigenic shifts result in periodic pandemics.

*Presentation* is similar in young and old, i.e. rapid onset of fever (rigors, chills), myalgia, headache, and fatigue, with variable degrees of prostration. Compared with less threatening viruses such as rhinovirus:

- Nausea, vomiting, diarrhoea, high fever, rigors, and ocular symptoms (e.g. photophobia) are more common
- Rhinorrhoea is less common

Less common serious complications include myocarditis and meningoencephalitis. Mild meningism is common and, if combined with other sinister features (e.g. altered conscious level), is an indication for CSF sampling.

*Diagnosis* is usually based on combining clinical assessment with epidemiological data, particularly current influenza incidence. Some other viruses can cause an identical clinical syndrome, and serological test results are not immediately available. Thus, an initial assessment cannot produce an absolutely confident microbiological diagnosis. The syndrome may therefore most precisely be labelled 'influenza-like illness'.

Positive virological diagnosis in the context of ↑ community incidence or a care home outbreak is helpful by prompting vigorous attempts to reduce transmission of infection.

## Reducing viral transmission

All >65yr olds in the UK are offered yearly influenza immunization. Mass outbreaks of respiratory viral infection are common in care homes and hospitals. They can occur at any time of the year but are most common from autumn to spring. Viruses are spread by aerosol or hand-to-hand contact (sometimes indirect, via fomites such as cutlery or drinking vessels).

*During an outbreak*
- Reduce transfers of healthy patients into, or symptomatic patients out of, the affected area
- Reduce staff movement across work areas (especially applicable to short-term staff who may work in many clinical areas in a short time)
- Care for symptomatic patients in single rooms, or in ward bays with similarly infected patients
- Exclude visitors with respiratory or viral symptoms from the ward
- Ensure that care staff have been immunized against influenza
- Ensure that scrupulous hand-washing procedures are followed
- Consider using face masks for staff caring for symptomatic patients

## HOW TO . . . Treat influenza-like illness in older people

The following guidance is generic and should be tailored to the patient, their illness, and their care environment. If the highest-quality care cannot be provided, then a prompt step-up of care should be arranged. This may include hospital admission.

- Do not underestimate the disease. Mortality and morbidity ↑ exponentially with age and frailty
- Give excellent supportive and symptomatic care. Its effectiveness should not be underestimated
  - Fluids. Reduced intake and ↑ losses (fever) lead to volume depletion and end-organ dysfunction. Encourage frequent oral fluid, and suspend any diuretic treatment. Consider early initiation of s/c or iv fluids if a vicious spiral of dehydration and poor intake seems likely to ensue
  - Nutrition. Encourage high-calorie, high-protein drinks or solids. If the illness is especially severe, prolonged, or complicated, or if the patient is especially frail or malnourished, consider a period of NG feeding. Involve a dietician early
  - Paracetamol. If fever, discomfort, or pain occur
  - Maintain mobility. Bed rest may sentence the patient to death or dependency. Carers may need clear, firm advice about this
- Identify and treat complications promptly
  - Carers may need information about important warning signs and the need to seek prompt medical advice
  - Perform regular observations of BP, pulse, and temperature where possible
  - Common serious complications include delirium, 2° bacterial infection, bronchospasm, pressure sores, and circulatory collapse
- Antiviral agents (the neuraminidase inhibitors zanamivir and oseltamivir) may reduce both the severity and duration of influenza
  - They are indicated in patients with severe symptoms if they are pregnant, >65 years, or with certain comorbidities (especially if hospitalized)
  - Zanamivir is inhaled; oseltamivir is taken po

## Further reading

National Institute for Health and Care Excellence (2009). *Amantadine, oseltamivir and zanamivir for the treatment of influenza*. Technology appraisal guidance TA168. http://www.nice.org.uk/ta168.

# Pneumonia

### Pneumonia

- This is a syndrome of acute respiratory infection with shadowing on CXR
- May be lobar, bronchial, or mixed pattern
- Symptoms may be mild and are often non-organ-specific, e.g. fever, malaise
- Common presenting scenarios include cough (often unproductive), delirium, reduced conscious level, lethargy, anorexia, falls, immobility, and dizziness. Rarely patients can present with shock, coma, and adult respiratory distress syndrome (ARDS)
- Chest pain, dyspnoea, and high fever are less common than in younger people. Signs may be minimal:
  - The patient may be well or unwell. Assess severity using the CURB criteria (see ➲ 'Characteristics of severe pneumonia: the CURB-65 score', p. 322)
  - Fever is often absent, but vasodilatation is common
  - Tachypnoea is a sensitive sign, as is at least moderate hypoxaemia (≤95% on air) on oximetry
- Tests often guide management:
  - Chest radiograph may reveal only minimal infective infiltrate. Also look for malignancy, effusion, or heart failure
  - Blood cultures should be sent, but sputum culture is rarely useful, unless TB is suspected
  - White cell count may be raised, normal, or even depressed
  - CRP is often normal early in the illness
  - U, C+E guide fluid management. Kidney impairment is a sign of poor prognosis
  - Arterial blood gas (ABG) sampling is not usually necessary, unless oxygen saturations are <90%; oximetry is much better tolerated and usually sufficient to guide oxygen therapy
- Organisms vary depending on the clinical setting in which pneumonia occurs (see Table 11.1)
  - Often no causative organism is identified
  - *Pneumococcus* is common in all settings, including hospital
  - Viral pneumonia, especially influenza, is under-recognized and is the second most common cause of community-acquired pneumonia
  - *Legionella* and *Mycoplasma* pneumonias are uncommon. *Mycoplasma* is much more frequent during epidemics, occurring every 3 years or so
  - Unusual organisms are more common in frail patients, in higher-dependency environments, and in those who have recently received courses of antibiotics. Organisms include Gram negatives (which colonize the oropharynx) and anaerobes (a result of aspiration of gut contents). MRSA pneumonia can occur in hospital or community. Health care-associated pneumonias can occur after discharge

**Table 11.1** Pneumonia pathogens in various care settings (in approximate order of frequency)

| Community-acquired | Care home-acquired | Hospital-acquired |
|---|---|---|
| S. pneumoniae (>30% of cases) | S. pneumoniae (>30% of cases) | Gram-negative aerobic bacilli, e.g. Klebsiella, Pseudomonas aeruginosa |
| Viral, e.g. influenza, parainfluenza, respiratory syncytial virus | Viral, e.g. influenza, parainfluenza, respiratory syncytial virus | Anaerobes, e.g. Bacteroides, especially in those at risk of aspiration, e.g. immobility, swallowing difficulty, prolonged recumbency, or impaired conscious level |
| H. influenzae | Gram-negative aerobic bacilli, e.g. Klebsiella, P. aeruginosa | S. aureus (including MRSA) |
| Gram-negative aerobic bacilli, e.g. Klebsiella, P. aeruginosa | H. influenzae | S. pneumoniae and H. influenzae. NB. These may be the most common pathogens—in non-acute settings, e.g. rehabilitation wards—in the well, less frail patient |
| Legionella pneumophila. Mycoplasma pneumoniae if epidemic | Anaerobes, e.g. Bacteroides, Clostridium. Especially in those at risk of aspiration, e.g. immobility, swallowing difficulty, prolonged recumbency, or impaired conscious level | Viral, e.g. influenza, parainfluenza, respiratory syncytial virus |
| Other, e.g. TB | Other, e.g. TB | |
| Following influenza, think of 2° bacterial infection, especially with S. pneumoniae (most common), H. influenzae, or S. aureus | Following influenza, think of 2° bacterial infection, especially with S. pneumoniae (most common), H. influenzae, or S. aureus | |

# Pneumonia: treatment

Multifactorial treatment should be started promptly. Ideally, antimicrobials should be administered within 1h, alongside the following:

- Assess and optimize fluid volume status; give po, sc, or iv fluid as appropriate. Concurrent heart failure is common, but volume depletion more so
- If there is subjective dyspnoea or moderate/severe hypoxaemia, then supplement *oxygen*, titrating the inspired oxygen concentration upwards to achieve arterial oxygen saturations of 94–98% (see ➲ 'Oxygen therapy', pp. 346–7). For lesser degrees of hypoxaemia, it is not necessary to subject patients to claustrophobic, uncomfortable oxygen masks—simply monitoring saturations may be sufficient
  - Exercise caution in COPD and other conditions that predispose to carbon dioxide ($CO_2$) retention. Target saturations of 88–92%. Observe the patient closely, both clinically and with serial ABG sampling
  - Avoid the use of nasal specs acutely; if ventilatory drive is poor, inspired oxygen concentrations are very uncontrolled
- Encourage *mobility*. If immobile, sit upright in bed, and sit out in a chair
- Request *physiotherapy* if there is a poor cough or lobar/lung collapse
- Use saline *nebulizers* to loosen secretions which are difficult to expectorate, and bronchodilator nebulizers when wheeze suggests associated bronchoconstriction
- Minimize the risk of *thromboembolism*, unless contraindicated, through prophylactic heparin and early mobilization
- Assess pressure sore risk and act accordingly (see ➲ 'Pressure sores', pp. 504–5)
- If dyspnoea, anxiety, or pain is very distressing, consider *opiates*. Side effects include respiratory depression, sedation, and delirium, so begin with small doses and assess effect

## Characteristics of severe pneumonia: the CURB-65 score

Five key criteria (acronym 'CURB-65') determine prognosis and can help guide location of treatment:

- *C*onfusion (AMTS ≤8)
- *U*rea (serum urea >7mmol/L)
- *R*espiratory rate (≥30/min)
- *B*lood pressure (<90 systolic and/or ≤60mmHg diastolic)
- *65* years of age or more

The score has a six-point scale (0–5 adverse prognostic features):

- 0 or 1: low risk of death (0–3%)
- 2: intermediate risk of death (13%)
- 3, 4, or 5: severe pneumonia, with high risk of death (score 3: mortality 17%; score 4: mortality 41%; score 5: mortality 57%)

A five-point scale using only four criteria (CRB-65; urea excluded) can be applied outside hospital and also discriminates effectively between good and poor prognoses (e.g. mortality score 1: 5%; score 3: 33%).

- Anticipate possible deterioration, and judge in advance the appropriate levels of intervention. Would renal dialysis, ventilation, and/or cardiopulmonary resuscitation be effective and appropriate? (See ➲ 'Diagnosing dying and estimating when treatment is without hope', p. 666.)
- Keep the family informed. Where possible, enlist their help, e.g. in encouraging eating and drinking

## Antimicrobials

Refer to local guidelines, reflecting pathogen sensitivities and drug costs.

*Community or care home settings*

- Amoxicillin po is usually effective (vs *S. pneumoniae* and *H. influenzae*). Erythromycin or clarithromycin if penicillin-allergic
- Add clarithromycin (or erythromycin which has more gastric side effects) if there are features of atypical pneumonia, there is a *Mycoplasma* epidemic, or the patient may have had influenza
- Co-amoxiclav po has added activity against some Gram-negatives and *S. aureus*, and may be more effective in the frail patient or where aspiration is likely
- Ciprofloxacin alone should be used rarely—it has Gram-negative activity but is less effective against *S. pneumoniae*, an important pathogen in most settings. If an antimicrobial is sought that will cover both chest and urinary sepsis, a better choice may be co-amoxiclav or trimethoprim
- iv antibiotics are only necessary if the patient is very unwell (CURB-65 score of 3 or above). Examples include co-administration of co-amoxiclav and clarithromycin. If you suspect MRSA pneumonia, add vancomycin. Convert to oral therapy and change broad- to narrower-spectrum drugs when the patient's condition improves and/or culture results are known, to minimize complications, e.g. CDAD (see ➲ '*Clostridium difficile*-associated diarrhoea', pp. 614–15). Often, only 48h or less of broad-spectrum iv therapy is needed

*Hospital-acquired infection*

This presents a difficult dilemma. Hospitalized patients, especially those who are more frail and have spent longer in hospital, are prone to Gram-negative and anaerobic pulmonary infections. However, they are also susceptible to the adverse effects (especially diarrhoea) of broad-spectrum antimicrobials.

A hierarchical approach is sensible, considering likely pathogens and illness severity, guided by local protocols:

- In the less frail patient who remains well, begin amoxicillin alone, co-amoxiclav, or a combination of amoxicillin and a quinolone (all po). Broaden the spectrum only if the patient deteriorates or culture results suggest that the likely pathogen is insensitive
- If a patient is at high risk of Gram-negative infection (frail, dependency, prolonged stay, invasive procedures, aspiration risk), begin with iv piperacillin/tazobactam (or equivalent). Narrow the antimicrobial spectrum when the patient's condition improves and/or a pathogen is identified
- If the patient has received multiple courses of treatment, seek microbiology advice
- In all cases, take blood cultures, and monitor the patient carefully

## HOW TO . . . Manage the patient with pneumonia who fails to respond to treatment

*Is the diagnosis correct?*
- Consider other chest pathology such as heart failure, PE, pleural effusion, empyema, cancer, or cryptogenic organizing pneumonia. Extrathoracic pathology mimicking pneumonia includes acidosis (tachypnoea) and biliary or pancreatic pathology
- Review the history, examination, and investigations
- Consider admission to hospital and further tests

*Is there a complication?*
- For example, effusion, empyema, heart failure, silent MI, or PE

*Is the antibiotic being taken regularly and in adequate dose?*
- Is adherence a problem? Could a friend or relative help prompt tablet-taking, or would a Multiple Dosing System help?
- Syrups may be swallowed more easily than tablets
- If swallowing remains ineffective, or drug absorption in doubt (e.g. vomiting), then consider iv/im therapy

*Is the organism resistant?*
- Take more blood cultures
- Consider a change in antimicrobial, taking into account likely pathogens and their known sensitivities
- Consider atypical infection; send urine for *Legionella* antigen test, especially if the patient is immunocompromised or if a patient appears disproportionately unwell. Remember MRSA pneumonia, especially in those known to be previously colonized

*Could other elements of care be more effective?*
- For example, fluid balance, oxygenation, nutrition, posture, and chest PT. Would this be more effectively delivered on ITU/high dependency unit (HDU)?

*Is this an end-of-life situation?*
- Is treatment to extend life now inappropriate, the failure to respond a sign that the diagnosis is of 'dying' (see ➔ 'Diagnosing dying and estimating when treatment is without hope', p. 666)? If the patient cannot tell you their wishes, determine their likely views by discussing with family and friends, a decision informed by your judgement of where in their life trajectory your patient sits
- In determining prognosis, consider comorbidity—is this an abrupt, potentially reversible illness in an otherwise fit person, or a further lurch downhill for a patient with multiorgan failure? Not for nothing is pneumonia referred to as 'the old man's friend', sometimes bringing to a brisk and welcome end a period of irrevocable decline and suffering

## Further reading

British Thoracic Society. Guidelines. ℘ https://www.brit-thoracic.org.uk/standards-of-care/guide-lines/.

# Vaccinating against pneumonia and influenza

## Vaccine delivery
- Both vaccines should be offered simultaneously in October or early November to all aged >65 years, especially:
  - Care home residents
  - The immunosuppressed
  - Those with comorbidity, e.g. heart failure, COPD, diabetes
- Pneumococcal vaccination is given once, whereas influenza vaccination should occur annually
- Reliable delivery of these vaccinations depends upon effective information management systems in GP, and substantial efforts by patients, carers, district nurses, and 1° care nurses
- A common reason to have missed immunization is to have been a long-term inpatient (e.g. undergoing rehabilitation) during the autumn immunization period. Hospitals should ensure that these inpatients are immunized
- Vaccinating health-care workers, especially those working in long-term care settings, reduces the spread of infection, and therefore death due to influenza, among patients

## Pneumococcal vaccine
- Pneumococcal polysaccharide vaccine (PPV) is effective against 65% of serotypes
- Immunity remains for at least 5 years, perhaps for life
- Bacteraemia is reduced by at least 50%. The effect on incidence of pneumonia itself is less clear

## Influenza vaccine
- The trivalent vaccine is prepared from currently prevalent serotypes
- Immunity develops in <2 weeks, and it is therefore useful during epidemics
- Immunity remains for up to 8 months
- The risk of pneumonia, hospitalization, or death due to influenza is reduced by over half

## Post-exposure antiviral prophylaxis
- Pharmacological prophylaxis of influenza is currently recommended when an unimmunized, high-risk group adult (e.g. care home resident) has had close contact with a person with influenza-like illness during a period when flu is prevalent[1]
- Treatment with neuraminidase inhibitors must be initiated promptly (within 24h)
- Consider why immunization was not performed. Is it too late to administer this year (this contact may not have 'flu, but the next one might)? If not, then optimize the chances of immunization next year

---

[1] National Institute for Health and Care Excellence (2008). *Oseltamivir, amantadine (review) and zanamivir for the prophylaxis of influenza.* Technology appraisal guidance TA158. ℘ https://www.nice.org.uk/guidance/ta158.

# Pulmonary fibrosis

This common problem is much underdiagnosed in older people due to a combination of under-investigation and overlap of clinical signs with common pathologies such as heart failure.

Consider when breathlessness coexists with profuse fine chest crepitations, with or without clubbing, or is slow to recover from apparently minor respiratory infection. On CXR, there may be bilateral pulmonary shadowing indistinguishable from pulmonary oedema, but with little supporting evidence (e.g. normal heart size, absent Kerley B lines).

## Causes

- Idiopathic. The most common type in older people, known as usual interstitial pneumonia
- Connective tissue disease, e.g. rheumatoid arthritis (most common), systemic lupus erythematosus (SLE), sarcoidosis. Lung involvement is sometimes the first manifestation of the multisystem disease
- Drugs, e.g. amiodarone, nitrofurantoin rarely
- Occupational exposure, e.g. asbestos, silica
- If localized, consider TB, bronchiectasis, and radiotherapy

## Tests

- The diagnosis is usually confirmed by high-resolution CT scanning, which can also help distinguish subgroups likely to respond to immunosuppressive treatment
- Respiratory function tests may be useful (a restrictive picture with ↓ transfer factor is usual) but typically adds little in the frail older person
- Consider referral to a respiratory physician to confirm diagnosis and guidance on management

## Prognosis

This is very variable—about a third are clinically stable, a third improve, and a third deteriorate at rates that vary greatly between individuals. Some can live with pulmonary fibrosis for years without significant functional impairment.

## Treatment

- Treat or remove any underlying cause, e.g. drugs
- A minority respond slowly (over weeks) to immunosuppression (e.g. prednisolone and azathioprine or pirfenidone). Ensure bone protection with calcium, vitamin D, and bisphosphonates
- Home oxygen therapy is often useful
- Give opiates for distressing dyspnoea
- In those in whom dyspnoea progresses, consider end-of-life issues, including treatment limitation, and a change of focus from life-extending measures to a purely palliative approach

# Rib fractures

Common in older people.
- Often a result of falls or even minimal bony stress such as coughing in a person with osteoporosis
- Consider the possible contribution of alcohol, which causes both falls and osteoporosis

## Diagnosis

Rib fractures should be diagnosed clinically.
- Point tenderness and crepitus are often found
- Pressure over the sternum may provoke the pain in a lateral rib
- CXR, even with multiple projections, may miss the fracture but is useful in excluding early complications such as pneumo- or haemothorax
- Radioisotope bone scans are very sensitive but not specific (hot spots are often found without clinical fracture), so they are rarely indicated

## Management

Rib fractures heal without specific treatment. The major problem is pain, which commonly leads to voluntary splinting of the injured area. There is hypoventilation and a failure to clear secretions, and 2° pulmonary infection can occur.
- The patient should be encouraged to breathe deeply and to cough. Supporting the injured area when coughing, using a small pillow, minimizes pain. Strapping of the affected area is no longer done, as it ↑ complication rates
- Regular analgesia should include paracetamol, plus a weak opiate in most cases. A short course of NSAIDs with gastric protection may be helpful
- Anticipate and treat complications (usually infection) promptly
- In cases of severe pain (e.g. multiple fractures), consider strong opiates or intercostal/paravertebral blocks. Involve the local pain team
- Surgical repair is an option, e.g. for flail chest, multiple fractures

The patient is often reassured with a diagnosis and explanation that the injury itself is not severe and will heal without immobilization, and that coughing will prevent complications, not cause further damage.

# Pleural effusions

A frequent (clinical or radiological) finding, sometimes incidental. Common causes are heart failure, post-pneumonia, PE, and malignancy (especially lung 1°, mesothelioma, leukaemia, lymphoma, and metastatic adenocarcinoma (ovary, stomach)).

The differential diagnosis is wide, but narrowed when the results of CXR and pleural fluid aspiration are known (see Table 11.2).

**Table 11.2** Differentiating cause by fluid type

| Transudate | Exudate |
|---|---|
| Heart failure | Malignancy |
| Hepatic cirrhosis | Infection, including TB |
| Hypoproteinaemia, e.g. malabsorption, sepsis | Gastrointestinal causes, e.g. pancreatitis |
| Nephrotic syndrome | Multisystem disorders, e.g. rheumatoid |
| (Exudative causes if low serum protein) | (Heart failure after diuresis) |

Pleural aspiration (diagnostic and therapeutic) is now mainly done under ultrasound guidance by a clinician with appropriate competencies.

*Light's criteria* is used to differentiate fluid type.

Exudate is likely if one of the following is present:

- Effusion protein:serum protein ratio >0.5
- Effusion lactate dehydrogenase (LDH):serum LDH ratio >0.6
- Effusion LDH level > two-thirds the upper limit of the laboratory's reference range of serum LDH
- Empyema, malignancy, and TB produce exudates with low pH (<7.2), low glucose (<3.3mmol/L), but high LDH
- Transudates are usually not due to focal lung pathology and so usually affect both lungs. Unilateral effusions due to transudates occasionally do occur, more commonly on the right side
- Effusions due to heart failure are typically bilateral, with cardiomegaly; they can be unilateral, but usually a tiny contralateral effusion is seen, manifesting as blunting of the costophrenic angle; if the angle remains sharp, other causes are more likely
- A massive unilateral effusion is usually due to malignancy
- A uniformly bloodstained effusion is usually due to infection, embolism, malignancy, or trauma

## Chronic effusions

- If bilateral transudates, should be treated as for heart failure
- If the diagnosis is not clear after CXR and aspiration, consider CT chest and/or chest physician referral
- For large, recurrent effusions, consider chest physician referral for continuous outpatient external fluid drainage via a semi-permanent intrapleural catheter or pleurodesis

- Frail patients may not tolerate, or desire, the more invasive tests. In this case, consider:
  - Repeated aspiration, combining diagnostic with therapeutic taps and sending larger volumes of fluid for cytology and acid-fast bacilli culture
  - 'Watching and waiting', with regular clinical review
  - A trial of diuretics, especially if the effusion is a transudate

## Further reading

Light RW, Macgregor MI, Luchsinger PC, Ball WC Jr. Pleural effusions: the diagnostic separation of transudates and exudates. *Ann Intern Med* 1972; **77**: 507–13.

# Pulmonary embolism

PE is common yet, as 'the great pretender' (of other pathology), is under-diagnosed and underreported on death certificates. It commonly coexists with, and is confused with, other lung disease, e.g. pneumonia, heart failure, and COPD—and is a common cause of deterioration in such patients.

## Presentation

The classic symptom triad of pain, dyspnoea, and haemoptysis is seen less commonly in older people.

Common presentations include:

- Brief paroxysm(s) of breathlessness, or tachypnoea
- Collapse, cardiac arrest, syncope, presyncope, or hypotension
- Pulmonary hypertension and right heart failure, presenting as chronic unexplained breathlessness
- Puzzling signs, e.g. fever, wheeze, resistant heart failure, arrhythmia, confusion, or functional decline

## Investigations

Determining the likelihood of PE rests on combining clinical judgement (the product of history, examination, and immediately available tests such as CXR) with appropriate imaging such as V/Q scan or CT pulmonary angiography (CTPA). The common clinical features of PE—tachypnoea, tachycardia, and modest degrees of hypoxaemia—are common in ill older people, so clinical judgement alone is rarely enough.

Moreover, a confident diagnosis is essential because in older people:

- The risk of anticoagulation is higher
- The risk of a missed diagnosis is higher (less physiological reserve)

Possible PE in older people should be investigated in the usual way, with the choice of tests guided by local facilities and expertise. The following issues are especially relevant:

- In a patient without known lung disease, the combination of breathlessness and a CXR showing clear lung fields strongly suggests PE. Further test(s) (V/Q or CTPA) are indicated. Ensure adequate hydration prior, to minimize the risk of contrast nephropathy
- CXR abnormalities may be minor (atelectasis, raised hemidiaphragm, small effusions) or major (usually reflecting comorbid conditions, rather than PE itself). Classical wedge shadows or unilateral oligaemia are rare
- PE in the absence of lower limb DVT is common (10–20% of cases), so do not be put off by an absence of clinical signs of the leg or a negative Doppler ultrasound
- D-dimer can be a useful screening test to rule out PE, but because many older people have coexisting conditions, e.g. infection, false positives are very common (i.e. sensitivity high, specificity low)
- ABGs have some value in diagnosis, but the common abnormalities (low $PaO_2$, low $PaCO_2$, and ↑ A–a oxygen gradient) are neither sensitive nor specific
  - In healthy older people, an ↑ A–a gradient is common
  - In older people following PE, a normal A–a gradient is seen in >10%

- Echocardiogram may be normal following PE. However, in a patient with a high clinical probability, typical features of PE on echocardiogram may provide sufficient diagnostic confidence to permit anticoagulation without further imaging
- In the patient with unexplained right heart failure, consider PE—obtain an ECG and echocardiogram (ask for PA pressures) and request imaging that details the lung parenchyma (high-resolution CT: pulmonary fibrosis?) and the vasculature (CTPA: PE?)
- In the patient who does not respond to treatment for chest infection, heart failure, or acute exacerbation of COPD, consider whether PE may be responsible

## Treatment

### Anticoagulation

Standard treatment is low-molecular-weight heparin (e.g. dalteparin, enoxaparin), followed by warfarin, with a goal for INR of 2–3. DOACs (e.g. apixaban, dabigatran) are also recommended and achieve full anticoagulation after the first dose. Once the possibility of PE is raised, it is essential to treat with treatment-dose low-molecular-weight heparin pending investigation results, unless there are particular treatment risks.

To minimize bleeding risk:
- Anticoagulate with caution. Check baseline clotting
- Beware the older patient with mild anaemia/low MCV—do they have occult blood loss?
- In the very frail, sick, unstable patient in whom oral anticoagulation would present significant risk, consider a period of anticoagulation with low-molecular-weight heparin. Start an oral agent when clinical stability returns

### Thrombolysis

Consider thrombolysing, balancing risks and benefits, where there is life-threatening PE manifesting as acute right heart strain and systemic hypotension. Both risk and benefit ↑ with age, so age itself is not a contraindication.

### Inferior vena cava filter

An IVC filter can be inserted under local anaesthesia by an interventional radiologist. Follow-up should be arranged to consider timing for removal.

Indications include:
- Strong contraindication to anticoagulation, e.g.:
  - Active bleeding
  - A high risk of bleeding, e.g. newly diagnosed peptic ulcer or very recent haemorrhagic stroke
- Massive thromboembolism with contraindication to thrombolyis
- Ongoing thromboembolism despite anticoagulation
- Embolism from a septic focus

# Aspiration pneumonia/pneumonitis

The involuntary entry of extrinsic material into the pulmonary airways. This is a common problem, ranging from subclinical micro-aspiration of oro-pharyngeal mucus to major inhalation of gastric contents.

## Risk factors
- Swallowing problems
- Gastro-oesophageal disorders leading to reflux
- Impaired conscious level, including seizures
- Sedative drugs
- Previous aspiration or non-aspiration pneumonia
- Clinically assisted nutrition—either NG or gastrostomy

## Diagnosis
Commonly, the occurrence of pneumonia in a patient with risk factor(s) suggests the diagnosis.

CXR may show consolidation in dependent lung zones, e.g. right lower lobe, although any zone may be affected.

## Treatment
- The role of antibiotics is debated. Much of the radiographic response may be chemical pneumonitis, i.e. inflammatory reaction to caustic gastric contents, rather than infective pneumonia
- The choice of antibiotics is also contentious. Many cases respond well to amoxicillin or co-amoxiclav, but consider broad-spectrum iv antibiotics to cover Gram-negatives and anaerobes in:
  - The unwell and frail
  - High-dependency settings
  - Where aspiration has been major
- If possible, treat the underlying cause. If risk factors persist (e.g. impaired swallow or continual seizures), consider a 'nil by mouth' order until they are addressed
- Where the swallow may be impaired, perform a formal swallowing assessment (see ➔ 'HOW TO . . . Manage swallow after stroke', p. 187) and manage according to the results
- In palliative care;
  - Consider anticholinergics to dry secretions
  - In advanced dementia, it is often appropriate to accept the risk of aspiration. Insertion of a gastrostomy (commonly a PEG) risks medicalizing the final months while achieving nothing—aspiration is common in patients with a PEG
  - It is often cruel and futile to deny a dying patient food that he or she may enjoy, even if the risk of aspiration and a life-shortening pneumonia exists. 'Nil by mouth' orders are usually inappropriate in end-of-life situations. Instead consider using thickened fluids, pureed diet, supervised feeding, and avoiding eating in a recumbent position, with straws or feeder cups

# Chronic cough

A common problem, with causes ranging from the trivial to the sinister. Even where the underlying cause is benign, chronic cough can be both distressing and disabling.

## Causes

- Asthma. Cough is a common presenting symptom in older people
- Silent pulmonary aspiration
- GORD
- Post-nasal drip can be due to sinusitis or chronic rhinitis. Frequently allergic in origin, but in older people, symptoms are often not seasonal
- Drugs, e.g. ACE inhibitors (may take weeks or months to develop), β-blockers (leading to bronchospasm)
- Persistent benign cough following upper respiratory tract infection. May persist for 2–3 months
- Chronic pulmonary pathology, e.g. COPD, TB, bronchiectasis
- Heart failure, with high pulmonary pressures
- Thoracic malignancy, either 1° or 2°

## Investigation

Consider both tests and trials of treatment. Their pace and extent depend on the differential diagnosis following careful history and examination. Consider the following tests:

- CXR (mandatory)
- Sinus imaging
- Spirometry, with assessment of response to bronchodilators
- Monitoring of PEFR, looking for morning drops suggesting asthma
- Sputum microscopy and culture are unlikely to be helpful

Next, consider a trial of treatment for the most likely cause, e.g.:

- Bronchodilators (and inhaled steroids) for possible asthma
- A PPI for possible GORD
- Assess the effect of treatment of possible chronic rhinitis with:
  - Nasal corticosteroids. Probably the treatment of choice, e.g. beclometasone, budesonide
  - Decongestants. Should be used in short courses only (since rebound phenomenon)
  - Antihistamines. Most useful for obvious allergic rhinitis. Can be topical spray or tablet. Should be used with caution; select those with fewer anticholinergics properties, e.g. cetirizine or loratadine

In all cases, trials of treatment need to be prolonged (≥8 weeks).

## Treatment

This is of the underlying cause. Where this cannot be treated effectively (e.g. advanced malignancy), specific treatments aimed at reducing cough may be of benefit. These include opiates such as codeine or morphine. Simple cough linctus may be useful for irritating dry cough following an upper respiratory tract infection.

# Lung cancers

The most common cause of cancer deaths, and largely a disease of older people.

- Symptoms may be non-specific (e.g. fatigue, weight loss), or else pulmonary in origin but attributed to existing non-malignant pathology (e.g. dyspnoea in a patient with COPD)
- Have a high index of suspicion and a low threshold for further investigation. Have an even higher degree of suspicion in older smokers presenting with pneumonia

*Sinister features* in those presenting with pneumonia include:

- Haemoptysis, especially if significant, e.g. with persistent blood clots
- Regional or generalized symptoms of cancer (e.g. hoarse voice, weight loss)
- Cough and consolidation without obvious infective symptoms (e.g. fever)
- Symptoms that continue to be troublesome despite antibiotics

If sinister features are present, it is unacceptable to wait (up to 6 weeks) before repeating a CXR to confirm resolution. Refer promptly for urgent specialist assessment, and consider CT scanning, bronchoscopy, or lung biopsy.

## Treatment

- Treatment has improved and is now more effective, both in extending life and in palliating symptoms. Therefore, 'benign neglect', i.e. simply observing an older person with probable lung cancer, is now only rarely acceptable. It may be appropriate, for example, in cases of extreme frailty or severe cognitive impairment
- Older people with probable lung cancer remain under-investigated and undertreated:
  - Tests such as bronchoscopy and a histopathological diagnosis are less commonly obtained. This makes palliative treatment and prognostication difficult
  - Treatment such as surgery or chemotherapy are less commonly considered or administered. To an extent, this reflects appropriate decision-making based on functional status
- Treatment decisions should be made by expert MDTs that consider the patient's functional status, comorbidities, and cancer characteristics

▶ Refer all patients with suspected or confirmed lung cancer for a specialist opinion.

## Non-small cell carcinoma (squamous cell, adeno-, and large cell carcinoma)

- Surgery may lead to cure if:
  - There is adequate pulmonary function (arbitrarily, $FEV_1$ ≥1.5L)
  - There is no distant spread (but >50% of cancers have spread at presentation)
  - The patient is relatively well with good functional status and no serious comorbidity

- Surgical procedures are high-risk, but the condition is always fatal without treatment, so the patient's view is critical
- Radiotherapy. When surgery is not feasible, either because of the nature of disease or the fitness of the patient, then radiotherapy may be used either palliatively (to control symptoms), neoadjuvantly (to reduce tumour volume and sometimes to convert a non-operable tumour into an operable one), or occasionally curatively
- Molecular characterization of tumour tissue enables tailored treatment. Chemotherapy, molecularly targeted therapy, and/or immunotherapy can be useful

## Small cell carcinoma

- Relatively more common in older people: >20% of cases
- Most cases are advanced at presentation
- Most patients are treated with combination chemo- and radiotherapy. Frail patients are unlikely to tolerate aggressive treatment and it risks reducing the quality of the brief life that remains. Therefore, regimens are tailored to the patient, determined by structured assessment of performance status. In general, frail patients undergo fewer, but similar, therapy cycles, compared to the more robust
- Prophylactic cranial irradiation ↓ the incidence of brain metastases and prolongs survival in patients with limited disease
- Very advanced disease is managed supportively or with chemotherapy alone
- Surgery is seldom useful because tumours are rarely localized at presentation

## Palliative interventions

- Radiotherapy for superior mediastinal obstruction, bronchial obstruction, chest pain, haemoptysis, or painful bony metastases. This is generally well tolerated, although ~10% develop radiation pneumonitis weeks after treatment, and it is on average more severe in older people
- Opiates for cough
- Aspiration of pleural effusion for breathlessness
- Endobronchial therapy (e.g. stenting, diathermy)

# Tuberculosis: presentation

In older people:
- Incidence of TB is much higher, especially in the very old and certain immigrant populations
- Outcomes, including mortality, are much less good
- TB is most commonly due to reactivation of previous disease, the 1° infection having been asymptomatic or unrecognized. In the early twentieth century, 1° infection of young adults was common. By the mid-late twentieth century, 1° infection in younger people had diminished. When this cohort reaches old age, TB reactivation will be much less common
- Reactivation (post-1° disease) occurs due to ↓ immunity, itself due to intrinsic ageing, disease (e.g. diabetes mellitus, renal failure), malnutrition (e.g. chronic alcohol excess), or drugs (e.g. steroids)
- A few patients develop new infection from open cases. Care home residents are most vulnerable, infection passing from fellow residents or from care home staff
- Consider HIV infection when TB diagnosed

## Presentation

### Pulmonary disease
- Sometimes similar to that in younger people, i.e. cough, sputum, fatigue, weight loss, and anorexia
- Night sweats, fevers, and pulmonary symptoms may be less common
- May present as pneumonia that fails to resolve or as an incidental finding suggested on CXR

### Extrapulmonary disease
Most (>75%) presentations are pulmonary, but extrapulmonary cases are relatively more common in older people, e.g.:
- *Miliary*. Diffuse, overwhelming infection with fever, weight loss, and hepatosplenomegaly. Pancytopenia can occur
- *Urogenital and renal*. May affect any part of the renal tract. Sterile pyuria, haematuria, abdominal or back pain, genital sinuses, or pelvic masses may occur, or disease may be asymptomatic
- *Meningeal*. Consider this in the very frail, malnourished, or immunosuppressed patient with non-specific cerebral signs (e.g. confusion, dementia-like syndrome, headache, or reduced conscious level). Meningism may be absent, and the CSF virtually acellular
- *Skeletal*. Bone infection most commonly affects the spine (usually thoracic or lumbar), presenting as pain and tenderness. TB arthritis usually affects large weight-bearing joints
- *Other*, e.g. lymph nodes, intestine

### Sequelae of previous treatment
Lung collapse therapy was used widely in the treatment of pulmonary TB in the 1930–50s. Procedures included therapeutic pneumothorax, thoraco-plasty, and plombage (expanding the extrapleural space with artificial materials). Sequelae include empyema, sinus formation, bronchopleural fistulae, and ventilatory failure. TB pyogenic or fungal organisms may be isolated. Early specialist input is essential.

# Tuberculosis: investigation

## Chest X-ray

Changes are more variable than in younger people and may mimic other benign or malignant disease (e.g. bacterial pneumonia, cancer).

- Usually upper zone infiltrates with cavities, but more common features in older people include mid-/lower zone infiltrates, and miliary (diffuse nodular) and bilateral changes
- Healed old disease is usually seen, i.e. calcified hilar nodes, a peripheral 1° complex, pleural thickening, and diffuse apical fibrosis and calcification
- Pleural effusions are common
- Rare changes include mass lesions or isolated lymphadenopathy
- The CXR may be normal, e.g. occasionally in miliary or endobronchial disease. If clinical suspicion persists, repeat at an interval

## Sputum for microscopy and culture

The standard method of confirming TB:

- Conventionally, three early morning sputum specimens are obtained and stained by acid fast staining (e.g. Ziehl–Neelsen). The quality and persistence of the microscopist is important, as the scanty organisms can be easily missed on cursory examination
- If a patient cannot expectorate, obtain 'induced sputum' through PT or nebulized normal saline (rarely nebulized hypertonic saline). If this fails, or clinical suspicion is high despite negative smear and culture, consider bronchoscopy with washings

## Other tests

- Raised *ESR* and *CRP* are usual
- *FBC*. Mild (normocytic) anaemia and reduced white cell count are more common in older people. Lymphocytosis or pancytopenia can occur
- Obtain three *early morning urine* specimens in case of possible genitourinary infection
- *Tissue sampling*. Where possible, sample tissue, e.g. lymph node, pleura, bone marrow. Send samples to both microbiology (microscopy and culture) and histology. Typical histological features of caseous necrosis with granuloma formation (with or without acid-fast bacilli) support strongly the diagnosis of TB
- *Polymerase chain reaction (PCR) testing* on smear-positive sputum can identify the type of *Mycobacterium* and help guide appropriate antimicrobial therapy
- *Tuberculin skin testing* (Mantoux test) is used to diagnose latent TB and is done in high-risk individuals where treatment would be considered. Tuberculin purified protein derivative (PPD) is injected in a standardized manner, and the reaction assessed quantitatively. Previous bacille Calmette–Guérin (BCG) vaccination can cause a reaction, but this usually reduces over about a decade. Age can reduce the immunological response to tuberculin, and the test and its interpretation are best done by specialist clinicians
- *Interferon γ release assay* is a newer type of blood test for TB that is becoming more widely available and is used to help diagnose latent TB

# Tuberculosis: treatment

Given the complexities of treatment, specialist referral is mandatory. This is a notifiable disease, and public health local authorities will investigate contacts, especially in the care home setting. Respiratory isolation precautions are necessary for patients with pulmonary TB treated in hospital.

Pulmonary disease is treated for a total of 6 months:
- Usually 6 months of rifampicin and isoniazid, with pyrazinamide and ethambutol for the first 2 months only
- Longer-treatment periods may be needed for extrapulmonary disease

In older people:
- Drug resistance is rare, as most infections are recurrences of 1° disease, contracted decades ago
- Failures of treatment are usually due to poor adherence. Combination drug preparations may improve this
- Side effects are more common, including ocular toxicity from ethambutol (reduce dose in renal impairment) and hepatitis from isoniazid. Close monitoring is important
- Atypical mycobacteria, e.g. *Mycobacterium avium intracellulare* or *kansasii*, can occur in those with structural lung disease such as bronchiectasis. This requires even broader and more prolonged courses of antibiotics, but isolation is not required as it does not spread from person to person

# Asthma and COPD: assessment

### Presentation

Asthma and COPD (see Table 11.3) in older people:

- Are both diseases characterized by airflow obstruction
- Commonly coexist, e.g. in the childhood asthmatic who has smoked
- May be both mimicked by other common diseases, e.g. cancer, PE, heart failure
- May present late—older people are less aware of hypoxaemia, breathlessness, or bronchoconstriction, or may interpret it as 'normal' ageing
- Are under-diagnosed and undertreated, especially in older people

*Asthma*

- May present in old age as true 'late-onset asthma'. There are also ↑ numbers of people who have grown old with their asthma
- In older people, cough may dominate, symptoms fluctuate less, triggers (e.g. cold, smoke, allergens) are less frequent, and the association with hay fever or eczema is less strong
- Nocturnal cough or dyspnoea, including paroxysmal nocturnal dyspnoea, may be caused by asthma
- NSAIDs and β-blockers (oral or ocular) may worsen bronchoconstriction

*COPD*

- Is much more common in older age, the consequence of intrinsic ageing and progressive disease
- Is caused by environmental exposure, usually to tobacco smoke, in genetically susceptible people. Significant disease can develop in those who have not smoked for years, as acquired lung damage depends more on 'total pack years' smoked, rather than duration alone
- Symptoms are usually more chronic and slowly progressive, without significant variability
- If bronchitis is significant, there is a productive cough
- Fatigue and sleep disturbance are common. Daytime somnolence suggests ventilatory failure
- There may be associated anaemia of chronic disease, osteoporosis, malnutrition, and depression

### Investigations

- *Pulse oximetry* will determine the presence and degree of hypoxaemia. In moderately or severely hypoxaemic patients (oxygen saturation <92%), consider *ABGs* to determine whether long-term oxygen therapy (LTOT) may be of benefit (see ➲ 'Oxygen therapy', pp. 346–7) and, in the acutely unwell, to guide oxygen administration
- *CXR, ECG,* and *FBC* will help to exclude other pathology, e.g. anaemia, dysrhythmia
- *α-1 antitrypsin* should be considered in atypical cases

**Table 11.3** Distinguishing asthma from COPD

| Asthma | COPD |
| --- | --- |
| Modest degree of fixed airways obstruction (this is uncommon in younger people) | Greater degree of airways obstruction |
| Significant or full reversibility | No, or only minimal, reversibility |
| ≥20% variability in PEFR | <20% variability in PEFR |
| | Greater age |
| | Significant smoking history |

- *PEFR*, measured regularly (bd–qds) for up to 2 weeks, helps determine whether variable airways obstruction (asthma) exists. Variability of ≥20% is significant. Older people may find using PEFR meters and charting the results difficult. Ask them to demonstrate the technique, reading the device, and charting in clinic
- *Spirometry*. Obtain at least $FEV_1$ and forced vital capacity (FVC). An $FEV_1$:FVC ratio of <0.7 suggests obstruction
  - Older people often have difficulty performing pulmonary function tests; an experienced technician in a respiratory laboratory will help provide accurate results
  - Assessments for *bronchodilator responsiveness* using inhaled bronchodilators are now considered less helpful, as they are poorly predictive of the response to treatment and do not distinguish reliably between asthma and COPD. However, airflow obstruction that completely and repeatedly resolves after bronchodilator administration does exclude COPD
  - Assessments for *steroid responsiveness* can be helpful in distinguishing between asthma and COPD (response is greater in asthma than COPD, although there is overlap). Perform spirometry before and after steroids (either 2 weeks of prednisolone 30mg od or 6 weeks of inhaled beclometasone 400 micrograms bd)
  - Some patients show improvement in FVC or functional status (walking distance or speed) despite no significant change in $FEV_1$

# Asthma and COPD: drug treatment

In general, treatment principles are similar to those in younger people and are described in detail in British Thoracic Society guidelines. However, some differences and some similarities benefit from emphasis.

### Bronchodilators

- Older people perceive symptoms less reliably, so where there is evidence of variable airways obstruction, give bronchodilators regularly, rather than as required
- These include short-acting β2-agonists (SABA), short-acting muscarinic antagonists (SAMA), long-acting β2-agonists (LABA), and long-acting muscarinic antagonists (LAMA)
- Protocols exist for up-titration of these, starting with short-acting agents, then adding in the long-acting agents in a stepwise fashion
- In older age, response to antimuscarinics, e.g. ipratropium, tiotropium, may be better than to β-agonists, e.g. salbutamol
- High-dose β-agonists, e.g. from nebulizers, may cause tremor, tachycardia, or rate-related angina. Nebulizers may not be required—try higher inhaled doses via a spacer or long-acting agents
- Antimuscarinic bronchodilators uncommonly cause side effects such as dry mouth or blurred vision, more often with higher (nebulized) doses and with long-acting preparations. Acute glaucoma is a rare, but important, complication—reduce ocular exposure by nebulizing via a mouthpiece, rather than a face mask

### Corticosteroids

- Inhaled corticosteroids have a role in the protocols
- Long-term oral steroids are rarely beneficial
- In those receiving regular courses of oral steroids for acute exacerbations, give osteoporosis prophylactic treatment. Inhaled steroids alone probably do not cause osteoporosis

### Theophylline

- Toxicity is common in older people. Plasma levels are ↑ by febrile illness, heart failure, and drugs, e.g. erythromycin/ciprofloxacin. Serious side effects, e.g. convulsions, may be the first sign of toxicity
- Check levels when titrating the dose. Most of the therapeutic effect is seen at the lower end of the therapeutic range, so target this first
- Before introducing oral theophylline, optimize inhaled bronchodilator and steroid therapy, including the use of long-acting and higher-dose preparations, if necessary

## HOW TO . . . Improve drug delivery in asthma or COPD

- The traditional metered-dose inhaler alone is rarely adequate, due to difficulties in coordinating device activation and the onset of inhalation
- Adding a large-volume spacer device reduces the need to coordinate activation with inhalation, improving drug delivery and reducing side effects (e.g. oral thrush). Spacers are generally better tolerated by older patients who do not tend to attach the same social stigma as youngsters
- Breath-activated devices provide an alternative to the metered-dose inhaler, although lung volumes may not be adequate to activate the device. They vary widely in design, and patients vary greatly in the ability to use them
- Assess and advise on the technique regularly, involving both hospital and community teams (doctor, nurse, and pharmacist), as well as the family and other carers
- Nebulizers are rarely required. A metered-dose inhaler via a large-volume spacer device is usually just as effective. Patients in whom nebulized drugs are being considered should be referred for specialist assessment
- Where adherence is an issue, e.g. in a person with dementia living alone:
  - Give long-acting preparations where possible
  - Give combined preparations
  - Once-daily inhaled steroid is better than none
  - Supervise the taking of medication as often as possible, but accept that for pulmonary drugs, taking medications irregularly is probably better than taking them not at all
- Rarely, inhaled drugs are administered too frequently by cognitively impaired people. This very rarely causes side effects, but relatives may need reassurance that this is the case
- Occasionally, oral β-agonists are useful in patients in whom all inhaled preparations have been unsuccessful

## Other

- Influenza and pneumococcal vaccine should be given
- Exercise extreme caution in the use of *respiratory depressants*, e.g. benzodiazepines or opiates. In general:
  - In acutely unwell patients with $CO_2$ retention, stop them, reintroducing only if withdrawal effects occur
  - In stable patients with or without $CO_2$ retention, withdraw or reduce them where possible
  - In severe end-stage COPD, if dyspnoea or cough are distressing and cannot be otherwise relieved, consider giving opiates. Give small doses initially, but ↑ as needed to relieve distress, even if respiratory function deteriorates. Explain the rationale to staff, relatives, and the patient, if appropriate

## Further reading

British Thoracic Society. Guidelines. ℘ https://www.brit-thoracic.org.uk/standards-of-care/guidelines/.

# Asthma and COPD: non-drug treatment

- *Smoking cessation* should be advised, except in the very advanced or terminal phase where it may lack benefit and be unkind. Consider referring for support and/or nicotine replacement therapy
- *Exercise* is beneficial, sometimes available as part of a pulmonary rehabilitation scheme. Elements should include aerobic and strength-based exercises, as well as specific breathing exercises
- *Pulmonary rehabilitation* is as effective as inhaler therapy and should be a key part of treatment. It is a complex intervention tailored to the individual, with exercise, behavioural, and educational components. Individual action plans can be followed by older people, facilitating self-management and early intervention
- *Weight reduction* is beneficial in the obese. However, weight commonly falls in advanced disease as the work of breathing exceeds calorific intake, and *nutritional supplements* may be needed
- *Comorbidities*, including depression, are common and should be treated aggressively
- *Social and practical interventions*. A comprehensive multidisciplinary assessment may be warranted. Provide appropriate mobility aids, e.g. electric wheelchairs, stairlifts, and alarm systems, e.g. pendant alarms. Treat social isolation

## Assisted ventilation

- Consider this in cases of respiratory acidosis, delirium, exhaustion, or deteriorating respiratory function despite full treatment. Hypercapnia, rather than hypoxaemia, is usually the key contributor to delirium; sedation is likely to worsen ventilation and precipitate coma
- For some patients with acute-on-chronic deterioration, ventilation will be futile and inappropriate. Make such a decision after considering:
  - The nature of the chronic illness and recent deterioration
  - The presence of reversible factors
  - The patient's current physiological status
  - The views of the patient or others who represent them
  - If in doubt, request guidance from the ITU team
- Non-invasive ventilation (NIV), e.g. nasal intermittent positive pressure ventilation, provides an acceptable alternative to invasive ventilation (usually endotracheal intubation). NIV is often well tolerated, can be delivered on specialist or high-dependency wards, and provides a modest level of ventilatory support that can be weaned promptly as the patient recovers

## Palliative interventions

- Reassure—many patients are frequently terrified. Assure them that their symptoms of suffocation can, and will be, treated. Consider advance care planning
- Positioning—sit up, day and night
- Involve the palliative care team. Their advice and support are often valuable and can continue into the community if discharge occurs

# Oxygen therapy

- Oxygen is a drug—it has clear indications and common and important side effects. Precision and care in prescribing maximizes benefit and reduces harm
- Controlled oxygen therapy targeted to pulse oximetry (94–98% for most, 88–92% for those at risk of type 2 respiratory failure)
- In older people, dyspnoea may be more frequently accepted, leading to underprescribing
- However, indiscriminate prescribing, particularly the use of high-concentration oxygen, risks respiratory depression and $CO_2$ narcosis. This is common in older people with COPD

### High-concentration oxygen therapy

- Previously used in emergency situations (15L/min via a non-rebreathe bag); this is rarely required to achieve the target saturations of 94–98%.
- Hyperoxaemia can be harmful (it can cause vasoconstriction and depressed respiratory drive)

### Oxygen delivery systems

Supply patients with an administration device applicable to their circumstances which should be prescribed on the drug chart.

*Constant performance oxygen delivery systems* (e.g. Venturi mask) provide a stable concentration of inspired oxygen ($FiO_2$) (24%, 28%, 35%, etc.) for a range of ventilation rates. These must always be used for hypoventilating patients with elevated $P_aCO_2$.

*Variable performance oxygen delivery systems*—the $FiO_2$ varies. The system delivers oxygen at a given rate which mixes with room air at rates dependent on ventilation. Systems include:

- Nasal cannulae. Often better tolerated by patients and allow them to eat and talk. With oxygen flows of 1–2L/min, $FiO_2$ is usually low (<28%) but can approach 30% if the patient hypoventilates
- Simple face mask, e.g. Hudson. Provides variable $FiO_2$ up to 40%
- Non-rebreathing mask with a reservoir bag. Provides variable $FiO_2$ of up to 60%

### Long-term oxygen therapy

This improves prognosis in severe COPD and in moderate COPD with features of cor pulmonale. To reduce pulmonary hypertension, arterial $pO_2$ should be raised to above 8kPa for at least 15h each day. $FiO_2$ of 24–28% usually achieves this. Respiratory depression is very rarely a problem in patients with stable respiratory failure who receive low oxygen concentrations.

Specific criteria must be met before prescribing LTOT. Measure ABGs twice, on air, at least 3 weeks apart and at least 4 weeks after an acute exacerbation.

Criteria include:

- $P_aO_2$ 7.3–8.0kPa in COPD with complications such as peripheral oedema, evidence of pulmonary hypertension, or polycythaemia
- $P_aO_2$ <7.3kPa in COPD without the complications already listed

## Intermittent oxygen therapy (IOT)

This is useful for a variety of cardiorespiratory conditions, e.g. COPD, advanced heart failure, lung cancer. It relieves distress and improves exercise tolerance and mobility. Low concentrations (24–28%) can achieve significant symptomatic benefit. Prognosis is unaltered.

## Oxygen gas supply

*Oxygen concentrators* are costly to purchase, but running costs are low. They are cost-effective when needing low-flow oxygen for prolonged periods (≥8h per day). Oxygen is piped to convenient position(s) in the home and usually administered via nasal cannulae. Urgent installations can usually be arranged within 24h.

*Oxygen bottles* are useful for:
- Patients on LTOT via an oxygen concentrator who wish to leave their home for short periods
- Patients needing oxygen as required, who do not meet the LTOT criteria
- Patients who are likely to have a short-term need for continuous oxygen, e.g. for end-of-life palliation, for whom installation of an oxygen concentrator may not be worthwhile

A small oxygen cylinder (300L, lasting 2h) is available which is convenient for wheelchair excursions or travel in a car.

▶ Smokers should stop smoking before beginning oxygen therapy. The risk of burns and household fires is substantially ↑.

# Asbestos-related disease

The period between asbestos exposure and overt (or covert) disease is usually long, often over 20 years. Almost all new cases are in older people because asbestos exposure is so carefully regulated now. The exposure may not be clearly recollected by the patient, but always consider in high-risk occupations, including building, dock work, and heavy engineering. Confirming the diagnosis is important because compensation may be due if disease can confidently be shown to have arisen as a consequence of asbestos exposure. If the diagnosis could not be confirmed during life, then post-mortem confirmation may lead to compensation payments to relatives.

### Pleural plaques

Discrete areas of thickening of the pleura that often calcify. Benign. A marker of asbestos exposure, but of no further clinical significance. Compensation for this is not universally available.

### Asbestosis

Progressive fibrosis, clinically and radiographically similar to idiopathic pulmonary fibrosis. Usually due to prolonged and substantial occupational exposure.

### Mesothelioma

A malignant, incurable tumour of the pleura, presenting as cough, chest pain, effusion, or dyspnoea. Very poor prognosis; few survive over 2 years. Treatment is nearly always palliative; the tumour is not resectable and is relatively insensitive to chemotherapy or radiotherapy. Asbestos exposure may have been only transient.

### Bronchial carcinoma

There appears to be a synergistic effect between asbestos and tobacco.

# Gastroenterology

# The ageing gastrointestinal system

### Teeth
- Change colour—yellow and less translucent
- Become worn (enamel does not regenerate)
- ↓ vascularity and sensitivity of dentine and pulp
- Caries, periodontitis, and tooth loss are common, but not inevitable in older patients. Being 'long in the tooth' refers to gum retraction seen with periodontal disease which ↑ with poor oral hygiene and xerostomia, both common in older people

### Mouth
- Mucosa—thinner and more friable, rarely a functional problem
- Salivary glands do not produce less saliva, but causes of xerostomia (see ➔ 'Xerostomia', p. 353) are more frequent with ↑ age
- Bone resorption occurs in the mandible alongside osteoporosis. This is accelerated with periodontitis and progresses fast once teeth are lost, leading to a change in facial appearance
- Orofacial muscle tone can diminish with consequent dribbling

### Taste
Olfactory function, and hence taste discrimination, ↓ gradually with normal ageing, but an acute change or complete absence of taste should prompt investigations for a cranial tumour.

### Oesophagus
- Slight changes in innervation produce clinically insignificant changes in swallow and peristalsis
- The misnamed presbyoesophagus (see ➔ 'Oesophageal motility disorders', p. 361) is a disorder of oesophageal motility, not a universal age change
- Hiatus hernias and reflux are very common—probably related to anatomical and postural changes

### Stomach
- ↑ incidence of atrophic gastritis (with reduced acid production), but in the absence of disease, most older patients maintain normal pH levels
- Reduction in gastric emptying is common
- ↑ mucosal susceptibility to damage
- ↑ *Helicobacter pylori* carriage, but this is less likely to cause ulceration

### Small intestine
- Function well preserved, except for calcium absorption which is ↓
- ↑ incidence of bacterial overgrowth with malnutrition and diarrhoea

**Large intestine**
- ↓ rectal sensation contributes to high incidence of constipation

**Pancreas**
- Structural changes including atrophy, but function is well preserved

**Liver**
- Hepatic weight and volume ↓ by around 25% and there is brown (lipofuscin) pigment build-up, but liver function (and therefore LFTs) is not affected
- Some older patients have a slightly low bilirubin and albumin level, but results still remain within the normal range

**Gall bladder**
- Incidence of gallstones ↑ (40% ♀ >80), probably related to reduced rate of synthesis and excretion of bile
- Most gallstones are asymptomatic

# The elderly mouth

## Mouth examination

Use gloves. Be systematic. Important and often not done—serious pathology may be missed. Check:

- *Parotid glands* (enlarged in parotitis, alcoholism, chronic lymphoid leukaemia)
- *Temporomandibular joint* (arthritis causes crepitus, subluxation, pain). Dislocation can cause pain and inability to close the mouth
- *Soft tissues*: tongue and floor of the mouth most common site for oral cancer in smokers/alcoholics. Angular stomatitis
- *Salivation*: (see ➲ 'Xerostomia', p. 353)
- *Teeth*: how many missing, how many restorations, pain/sensitivities. Caries is ↑ by poor brushing and low fluoride exposure, diet of soft sweet foods, xerostomia, poor fitting dentures, and infrequent dentist visits
- *Dentures*: cleanliness, integrity, and fit

## General management

- Nursing help with dental/mouthcare is vital for anyone unable to help themselves
- Referral to a dentist. Dental check-ups should continue every 6 months, regardless of age/disability. This is very difficult to arrange for inpatients, but maxillofacial surgeons (who are also trained as dentists) will sometimes help out in severe/urgent cases
- Consider chlorhexidine mouthwash for patients with poor oral self-care, e.g. stroke, dementia
- Severe periodontal disease may require antibiotics (topical or systemic) and surgical debridement to arrest progress
- Poor oral and dental health contributes to poor appetite and malnutrition—consider nutritional support (see ➲ 'Nutrition', pp. 354–5)

## Facial pain

Consider trigeminal neuralgia, TA, parotitis, temporomandibular joint arthritis, dental caries/abscess, aphthous mouth ulcers, or the idiopathic benign 'burning mouth syndrome'.

## Sore tongue

Can be a side effect of drugs, glossitis ($B_{12}$, iron, or folate deficiency), candida/thrush, especially after antibiotics or in diabetes. A black tongue may be due to *Aspergillus* colonization and is treated with nystatin lozenges/mouth rinse.

## Parotitis

Acute bacterial parotitis is not uncommon in frail older patients who are not eating. Low salivary flow (dehydration and not eating) and poor oral hygiene predispose to parotid gland infection with mouth flora (staphylococci and anaerobes). Treat with aggressive rehydration, iv flucloxacillin, and chlorhexidine mouth rinses. Response to treatment is usually dramatic—if not, consider abscess formation or MRSA.

### Xerostomia

Perception of dry mouth is closely related to salivary flow. Saliva is needed for:

- *Taste*: dissolves food to present to taste buds
- *Swallow*: helps form food bolus
- *Protection* of teeth and mucosa: contains antibacterials, buffers, and mucin. Rapid tooth decay is a risk of xerostomia

Xerostomia is not a normal ageing change and should always be investigated. Causes include:

- Drugs with anticholinergic side effects (e.g. tricyclic antidepressants, levodopa)
- Sjögren's syndrome (an autoimmune destruction of salivary glands) can be 1° or associated with other autoimmune conditions
- Irradiation, salivary stones, tumours, sialadenitis (viral or bacterial infections)

Treatment depends on cause—stop or ↓ causative drugs, stimulate saliva with grapefruit juice/sugar-free sweets or mints, and promote frequent careful mouthcare. Artificial saliva can provide symptomatic relief for some patients.

### Oral candidiasis

May manifest as oral thrush (with removable white plaques on an erythematous base), angular stomatitis (sore cracks in the corner of the mouth), or rarely atrophic forms (e.g. under dentures, may not have creamy plaque). Consider and reverse risk factors such as antibiotics, steroids, hyperglycaemia, and immunosuppression, where possible. Use nystatin 1mL qds, rinsed around the mouth for several minutes. In cases with painful swallowing/dysphagia (i.e. might have oesophageal involvement) and those that cannot comply with rinses, use oral fluconazole 50–100mg od for 7–14 days. Dentures should be kept out where possible and soaked in chlorhexidine during treatment.

### Mouth ulcers

Simple aphthous ulcers and ulcers due to poorly fitting dentures should be treated with topical anti-inflammatories (salicylate gel or triamcinolone), hydrocortisone lozenges, or steroids. Ulcers can occur as part of a systemic disease such as inflammatory bowel disease. Any oral lesion persisting >3 weeks merits referral and/or biopsy to exclude cancer, but most mouth cancers are painless.

### Oral manifestation of systemic diseases/drugs

A very long list of manifestations, including common and general (e.g. oral candidiasis in immunosuppression), as well as rare and specific (e.g. oral lichen planus). Remember that many drugs also affect the mouth, e.g. xerostomia (see ➲ 'Xerostomia', p. 353), tardive dyskinesia with antipsychotics, and gum hypertrophy with phenytoin.

### Systemic manifestation of dental diseases

Poor oral hygiene with dental or periodontal disease can cause septicaemia or infective endocarditis. Poor teeth can contribute to poor nutrition.

# Nutrition

With normal ageing, there are:
- Reduced calorie requirements due to reduced activity and lower resting metabolic rate (↓ muscle mass)
- Reductions in appetite (anorexia of ageing)
- Lower reserves of macro- and micronutrients (vitamins and minerals)

In the presence of disease, older patients quickly become malnourished, which is a powerful predictor of outcome (↑ functional dependency, morbidity, mortality, and use of health-care resources).

Malnutrition is extremely common in the older, frail or institutionalized population, and studies have shown that once in hospital, most patients' nutritional status actually declines further. Protein–energy undernutrition affects:
- 15% of community-dwelling older patients
- 5–12% of housebound patients with multiple chronic problems
- 35–65% of patients acutely admitted to hospital
- 25–60% of institutionalized older persons

## Nutritional assessment
- BMI (weight in kg/(height in m)$^2$) is often impractical, as height cannot be accurately measured in immobile patients or those with abnormal posture (although approximations can be made, e.g. using ulnar length)
- Simple weight is still useful, especially if the patient knows their usual weight—rapid weight loss (>4kg in 6 months) is always worrying, even in obese patients. Mid-arm circumference can be used to approximate
- Nutrition screening tools are often employed by nursing staff to target interventions. The MUST score (see ⦿ Appendix, 'Malnutrition universal screening tool (MUST)', p. 709) is widely used in UK hospitals and is sensitive for detection of protein–energy undernutrition in hospitalized patients
- More complex tools (e.g. Mini Nutritional Assessment) are helpful, but time-consuming, and are rarely used outside research
- Biochemical measures (e.g. hypoalbuminaemia, anaemia, hypocholesterolaemia) develop at a late stage and are confounded by acute illness

## Nutritional support
- Identification is key to allow targeted intervention (improves outcome)
- The cause is usually multifactorial and a holistic approach is needed, e.g. medical (immobile, unwell, reflux, constipation, etc.), social (poverty, isolation), psychological (depression, dementia), and age-related (altered hunger recognition)
- Involve a dietician early (especially if anorexia is prominent)
- Record food intake carefully—this highlights deficiencies in intake and helps identify where interventions might help
- Make mealtimes a priority (protected mealtimes) and provide assistance with feeding (care assistants or family)

- Schemes such as using a red tray can highlight those in need of assistance
- Establish food preferences and offer tempting, high-calorie foods (e.g. substitute full-fat milk and yogurt if they are on the lower-fat variety)
- Prescribe dietary supplements according to patient preference (e.g. milky or fruit drinks, soups, puddings, or high-calorie shots)
- Appetite stimulants, e.g. prednisolone, can ↑ weight, but side effects usually outweigh benefits
- Consider the role of enteral feeding

---

### HOW TO . . . Manage weight loss in older patients

Peak body mass is reached at age 40–50, and weight loss can occur after this due to ↓ lean mass, although the proportion of fat is relatively ↑, so overall weight is often remarkably stable.

As a rule of thumb, unintentional weight loss of >2.3kg (5lb)/5% of body weight in a month or 4.5kg (10lb)/10% body weight in 6 months is worrying.

Always try to get recorded weight (rather than relying on patient/carer memory)—a search of old outpatient clinic and 1° care records can help. Record weight regularly while you investigate to look for ongoing trends.

Dramatic weight loss should always prompt a search for remediable pathology. The cause is often multifactorial. It is important to consider:
- Dementia
- Depression
- Malignancy
- Chronic infection/disease, e.g. COPD, heart failure, TB
- Inflammatory conditions, e.g. GCA
- Malabsorption (see ➔ 'Diarrhoea in older patients', p. 374)
- Mesenteric ischaemia (recurrent postprandial abdominal pain)
- Drug causes, e.g. digoxin, theophyllines, cholinesterase inhibitors
- Metabolic disorders, e.g. hyperthyroidism, uraemia
- Swallowing problems
- Persistent nausea or abdominal pain/reflux
- Social causes, e.g. inability to cook, poverty, social isolation, alcoholism

A careful history (including dietary history and mental state with collateral history where possible), examination, and routine screening tests (see ➔ 'Investigations', pp. 64–5) will usually give clues of significant underlying pathology. If preliminary investigations are negative, a 'watch and re-weigh and wait' plan is reasonable—be reassured if weight is actually stable or rising; re-examine and re-screen if further loss occurs.

Obviously if a remediable cause is found and treated, then weight loss may be halted or reversed. Where no such cause is found, or where it is not reversible, interventions are still possible.

# Enteral feeding

Consider enteral feeding early if there is dysphagia (e.g. stroke, MND, Parkinson's disease) or failure of oral feeding (e.g. severe anorexia syndromes, intensive care unit) with an intact gastrointestinal tract.

There are three common methods:

- *Fine-bore NGTs*: simple, quick, and inexpensive. The preferred method for short-term feeding. Some patients (usually confused/drowsy) repeatedly pull out NGTs. Interference with the tube ↑ the risk of aspiration. Persistence, supervision, and careful taping can sometimes help, but often a PEG or RIG is required (also described here). There is ↑ experience using NGTs which are held in place via a nasal loop (Bridle™). Trained practitioners can insert these by the bedside, and removal by the patient is very rare
- *PEG*: the risks of insertion include perforation, bleeding, and infection for a patient who is usually already frail. The patient has to be fit to undergo sedation. Problems obtaining consent from a competent patient and 'agreement' from the next of kin for an incompetent one are not uncommon. Once established, this method is discreet and better tolerated than NGTs and is the method of choice for medium/long-term enteral feeding
- *RIG*: useful if gastroscopy technically difficult (e.g. pharyngeal pouch) and sometimes if small bowel feeding preferred over gastric feeding. Similar complication rate to PEG

## Complications for all methods include

- *Aspiration pneumonia*: there is a common misconception that enteral feeding eliminates aspiration in dysphagic patients. This is not true—reflux of food into the oesophagus is common and this, along with salivary secretions and covert oral intake, may still be aspirated. Always check the position of the tube if the patient becomes unwell, feverish, or breathless. If aspiration is ongoing despite correct tube position, slow the feed, feed the patient sitting upright (i.e. not at night), and add pro-motility drugs, e.g. metoclopramide or erythromycin (pre-meals). A nasojejunal tube or jejunal extension to a PEG tube can also reduce aspiration rates (see ➲ 'Aspiration pneumonia/pneumonitis', p. 332)
- *Re-feeding syndrome*: occurs when the patient has been malnourished for a long time. When feeding commences, insulin levels cause minerals (especially phosphorus) to move rapidly into the intracellular space and fluid retention occurs causing hypophosphataemia, hypomagnesaemia, and hypokalaemia. This, in turn, can cause life-threatening heart failure, respiratory failure, arrhythmias, seizures, and coma. Avoid by 'starting low and going slow' when introducing feed. It is important to check and correct any abnormal biochemistry before feeding starts and then monitor frequently (check urea and electrolytes, calcium, magnesium, phosphate, and glucose daily for a few days, then weekly). Supplementation of minerals may be done iv or by adding extra to NG feed
- *Fluid overload and heart failure*: ↓ volume and add diuretics
- *Diarrhoea*: exclude infection (especially *Clostridium difficile*). Try slowing the feed rate or changing the feed to one containing more or less fibre

## Parenteral feeding

Should be considered when the gut is not functioning. It requires large venous access and should only be undertaken when supervised by an experienced nutrition team. It is usually a temporary measure, e.g. post-gastrointestinal surgery. Complications such as fluid overload, electrolyte disturbance, and iv catheter sepsis are common in older patients.

---

### HOW TO . . . Insert a fine-bore NG feeding tube

This task is often performed by nursing staff who may be very experienced. Doctors are often asked to help when insertion is proving difficult.

1. Get the patient's consent—if they refuse, come back later. They may well have just had several uncomfortable failed attempts. It is rarely appropriate to perform against the wishes of the patient
2. Have the patient sitting upright with the chin tucked forward (patients often hyperextend their neck which makes it harder). Draw the curtains (this can be an unpleasant procedure to have done or to watch)
3. Leave the guide wire in the tube and lubricate with lots of jelly
4. Feed the tube down one nostril about 20cm (until it hits the back of the throat). In stroke, start with the inattentive side, as it may be better tolerated
5. If there is a proximal obstruction, try the other nostril
6. If possible, ask the patient to swallow and advance the wire
7. Check the back of the throat carefully—you should be able to see a single wire going vertically down. Start again if there is a loop
8. Secure the tube yourself immediately with tape to both the nose and cheek

Once you believe the tube is in place, you need to check it is in the stomach by one or both of the following methods BEFORE you use the tube.

- Aspiration of gastric contents that are clearly acidic (pH <5)
- CXR is used if there is no aspirate or the pH is equivocal. If you leave the guide wire in, the tube shows more easily. The tip of the tube should be clearly below the diaphragm

The method of blowing air down the tube and listening for bubbles has now been discredited, as a bubbling sound can be generated due to saliva and pulmonary secretions.

# The ethics of clinically assisted feeding

Feeding is a highly emotive issue. It is seen by many (especially relatives) as a basic need, and hence failing to provide adequate nutrition is seen as a form of neglect or even euthanasia. In contrast, others feel that artificial enteral feeding is a cruel and futile treatment performed on incompetent patients that only postpones a 'natural' death that involves anorexia or dysphagia.

The use of the term 'clinically assisted nutrition and hydration' has been suggested by the General Medical Council (UK) to replace the term 'artificial nutrition and hydration' underlining the fact that this is a form of treatment.

There are numerous high-profile legal cases regarding feeding (usually withdrawal of), and controversial cases that cannot be resolved locally should always be referred to the courts via the local legal team.

▶ The key to steering a course through this minefield is communication.

## Initiating treatment

- Establish if the patient is competent—even dysphasic patients may understand a little with non-verbal cues, etc.
- If the patient has capacity (see ➲ 'Capacity', pp. 654–5), ensure they understand the chosen method (and its risks) and projected duration of feeding. Patients with dysphagia must realize that they will be expected to dramatically ↓, or stop, oral feeding
- For patients who lack capacity, ensure you have communicated with all interested carers, family, and the GP. There is sometimes disagreement between interested parties, and these are best detected and 'thrashed out' early. A case conference is often helpful
- Establish that everyone accepts the indications for feeding and the aims of treatment, and set a date for review, e.g.:
  - 2 weeks of NG feeding in a patient with dysphagia following a stroke, which is hoped will resolve
  - PEG insertion in a patient with MND and malnutrition with recurrent aspiration pneumonia, to be reviewed if the patient requests or if enters the terminal phase of the disease
- Do not be afraid of a therapeutic trial (e.g. if you do not know whether the patient's lethargy/drowsiness/depression is related to malnutrition). Always ensure everyone understands and agrees on review dates and criteria for reassessment. Patients/relatives can be reassured that PEG tubes can be removed if improvement occurs
- Record discussions and plan carefully in the medical records
- If there is still dispute, get a second opinion. As a last resort, legal advice may be needed

## Withdrawing treatment

▶ Withholding treatment is not morally different to withdrawing it.

There are, however, technical and emotional differences, which is why many more ethical problems arise when withdrawing and why some doctors are resistant to trials of treatment.

Artificial feeding can be withdrawn because:
- It is no longer required (rarely controversial)
- A therapeutic trial has failed (see ➲ 'Initiating treatment', pp. 358–9; this is sometimes controversial)
- Although feeding is successful, the patient's quality of life is felt to be unacceptable (nearly always controversial)
- A patient with a long-term feed is dying from another condition (sometimes controversial)

When considering withdrawal of long-term feeding for stable conditions (e.g. persistent vegetative state), decisions should be referred to the courts.

### Accepting aspiration risk

There is also a group of patients who have dysphagia, weight loss, and recurrent aspiration due to progressive neurological conditions such as dementia, who merit special consideration.

It is not always appropriate to aggressively manage such patients, who are frequently incompetent and derive pleasure from eating normally. It may be appropriate to allow the patient to eat, accepting that there is a risk of aspiration. 'Feeding at risk' protocols are becoming more common to document the process and improve interface communication.

Adopting such a palliative policy is impossible, unless everyone, including the whole MDT and relatives, understand and sympathize with the aims of management.

## Further reading

General Medical Council. Guidance. ℅ http://www.gmc-uk.org.
Royal College of Physicians of London (2010). *Oral Feeding Difficulties and Dilemmas*. London: Royal College of Physicians of London.

# Oesophageal disease

### Gastro-oesophageal reflux disease

- The symptoms (retrosternal burning, acid regurgitation, belching, atypical chest pain) correlate poorly with the pathology (normal mucosa to severe oesophagitis)
- Sinister features which might suggest malignancy include sudden or recent onset, dysphagia, vomiting, weight loss, and anaemia. They should guide management:
  - In the absence of sinister features, a 4-week trial of treatment is given
  - If there are sinister features, then a gastroscopy should be arranged
- Oesophageal pH monitoring is rarely necessary

*Treatment*

Check if the patient is taking prescribed or over-the-counter NSAIDs, steroids, or bisphosphonates, and stop or minimize the dose. PPIs have revolutionized treatment, making antacids and H2 blockers, such as raniti-dine, almost redundant. They are very effective (for symptoms and healing) and generally safe. They are used for prophylaxis with aspirin in high-risk/symptomatic patients—often at lower dose, as well as treatment, and some are licensed for intermittent symptomatic use. Some are available over the counter. Rarely elderly patients can have side effects of diarrhoea or confu-sion (see ➲ 'Proton pump inhibitors', p. 144).

### Barrett's/columnar-lined oesophagus

Gastric mucosa replaces the oesophageal squamous cell mucosa. It is asso-ciated with an ↑ risk of malignancy and should have endoscopic surveillance based on Prague Criteria, regardless of symptoms.

### Hiatus hernia

- Very common in older patients, occurring to a degree in almost all
- Laxity of structures at the gastro-oesophageal junction allows the oesophago-gastric junction or portions of the stomach to move up (permanently or intermittently) into the thorax
- May be asymptomatic but often presents with GORD symptoms and occasionally with dysphagia
- Very large intrathoracic hernias can impair respiratory function and strangulate/perforate
- Diagnosis on CXR (stomach or fluid level behind the heart), at endoscopy, or on contrast radiology

*Treatment*

To reduce reflux, suggest: lose weight; avoid alcohol and caffeine; eat small meals often; avoid eating before bed; and sleep propped up on pil-lows or elevate the head of the bed on blocks. PPIs will nearly always relieve symptoms; consider investigations if they do not. Prokinetic agents, e.g. metoclopramide, sometimes help. Younger patients with intractable problems can be assessed for surgery—laparoscopic surgery now available.

## Achalasia

- An idiopathic neurological degeneration causing impaired peristalsis and a lack of lower oesophageal sphincter relaxation, causing a functional obstruction
- Dysphagia for solids and/or liquids is the most frequent presenting complaint
- Onset is insidious and slowly progressive
- CXR may reveal a dilated oesophagus
- Endoscopy is usually performed to exclude malignancy but may be normal
- Barium swallow has characteristic abnormalities (dilated oesophagus terminating in a beak-like narrowing)
- Manometry is the gold standard for diagnosis
- Treatment is aimed at facilitating lower oesophageal sphincter relaxation and can include drugs (calcium channel blockers or nitrates), botulinum toxin injection, endoscopic dilation of the sphincter, or surgical myotomy

## Oesophageal motility disorders

- Group of disorders where oesophageal motility is significantly different from normal (excluding achalasia, which is a distinct pathological entity)
- Incorporates those patients previously described as having presbyoesophagus (motility abnormalities ascribed to age, probably incorrectly)
- Presenting features include heartburn, chest pain, and dysphagia
- Syndromes include diffuse oesophageal spasm, nutcracker oesophagus, and hypertensive lower oesophageal sphincter
- Motility disorders can also arise 2° to other diseases (e.g. diabetes, systemic sclerosis, chronic GORD)
- Diagnosis may be made with barium swallow, but manometry is the gold standard
- Treatment is difficult and depends on the condition/dominant symptoms. Try prokinetics or PPIs. Calcium channel blockers or tricyclic antidepressants can relieve chest discomfort. Botulinum toxin and endoscopic dilation are also occasionally used

## Oesophageal candidiasis

- Can present with dysphagia or pain
- Consider in frail or immunosuppressed patients, especially if oral candidiasis is present
- Characteristic appearance on endoscopy (biopsy confirms) or barium swallow
- Treat with fluconazole for 2 weeks

# Dysphagia

Dysphagia (difficulty in swallowing) is a common symptom in older patients.

## History

- Ask what type of food is difficult (solids or liquids) and the level at which food sticks (mouth/throat, retrosternal, or epigastric)
- Distinguish dysphagia from early satiety and regurgitation (when successfully swallowed food returns after seconds/minutes), which usually occurs with gastric outlet obstruction or pharyngeal pouch
- If the swallow 'tires' through a meal, consider myasthenia
- Cough, wheeze, or recurrent aspiration pneumonia can be a presentation of swallowing problems which cause aspiration

## Signs

Look for weight loss, oral thrush (may be associated with oesophageal candida), supraclavicular lymphadenopathy, and a gastric splash (implies gastric outlet obstruction). Watch the patient swallow some water and food—the diagnosis might be clear.

## Causes

These can be divided into two:

- *Structural lesions* (worse with solids)
  - Oesophageal or gastric cancer
  - Benign strictures—scarring following, e.g. oesophagitis, scleroderma, polymyositis, radiotherapy
  - Pharyngeal pouch
  - Oesophageal candida or severe oesophagitis
  - Hiatus hernia can produce obstruction symptoms
  - External obstruction, e.g. bronchial tumour, aortic aneurysm, or cervical osteophyte
  - Foreign bodies
- *Functional problems* (often worse with fluids)
  - Pharynx/throat—the most common neurological cause is stroke but can occur in advanced dementia and MND. Rarer neurological conditions include myasthenia gravis, inclusion body myositis, multiple sclerosis, and parkinsonian syndromes
  - Oesophagus—dysmotility problems are relatively common in older patients and include achalasia and diffuse oesophageal spasm

## Investigations

Gastroscopy is now the 1° investigation and is well tolerated, even in frail patients. Use a barium swallow first if there is felt to be a high risk of perforation with an endoscope (e.g. suspect pouch), but gastroscopy allows biopsy and therapy, e.g. dilation. Videofluoroscopy provides functional imaging and is useful diagnostically, but the correlation between observed aspiration and clinically significant problems is poor.

## Treatment

- An empirical trial of PPI can be used in patients who are deemed unfit for investigation
- If oral thrush is present (suggesting oesophageal infection), try fluconazole for a week
- Oesophageal dilation ± stenting can be very successful for benign or malignant strictures
- For functional problems, always involve a speech therapist. Changing the consistency of food and fluids, and positioning the patient correctly can minimize problems
- Oesophageal dysmotility—try prokinetic/calcium channel blocker
- Gastroparesis causes early satiety and vomiting. It can be very hard to treat—try a prokinetic. Electrical gastric 'pacing' or surgery may provide relief (rarely used)
- Nutritional support—elderly patients with dysphagia are usually malnourished to start with and are then put nil by mouth for investigations. Refer to the dietician, and consider dietary supplements and early enteral feeding by NGT or PEG (see ➋ 'Enteral feeding', p. 356)

*Aspiration pneumonitis* (see ➋ 'Aspiration pneumonia/pneumonitis', p. 332) is largely a chemical, rather than infective, insult that may be complicated by infection. It is treated by:

- Preventing/minimizing aspiration (nil by mouth, NG feeding)
- Oxygen therapy
- Chest PT
- Antibiotics are often given to prevent/treat superinfection

# Peptic ulcer disease

This disease is becoming much rarer with the advent of effective medical treatment. It remains predominantly a disease of the elderly population. NSAID use is the most common cause, followed by *H. pylori*.

*H. pylori* is a spiral Gram-negative bacterium which colonizes the gastric mucosa causing gastritis. Carriage rates ↑ with age. Infection is usually asymptomatic but is the most common cause of dyspepsia in older patients. *H. pylori* is strongly associated with duodenal ulcers and may have a link with NSAID-associated ulceration.

## Presentation

Acute bleeding, pain (epigastric, retrosternal, or back), indigestion, 'heartburn', dysphagia, anorexia, weight loss, perforation (peritonitis), iron deficiency anaemia, or an incidental finding (e.g. on endoscopy). Older patients may present non-specifically ('off food' or vague abdominal pains).

### Investigations

- Upper GI endoscopy is very safe and well tolerated in older patients. It can often be performed using local anaesthesia in the throat only
- *H. pylori* can be detected with gastric biopsy and histology or with a test for urease activity (Clo test®). Serological tests remain positive, but titres gradually decline after eradication. Breath tests can detect *H. pylori* colonization but obviously do not demonstrate pathology

### Treatment

Dietary restriction is unnecessary (worth specifically mentioning because older patients can remember harsh or bizarre anti-ulcer diets). Stop any NSAIDs. Stop aspirin if possible, and plan for safe reintroduction depending on risk/benefit of the individual patient. Where there is *H. pylori* and ulceration/gastritis, treat with one of the many 'triple therapy' antibiotic PPI regimens. In the absence of *H. pylori*, just a PPI will suffice. Arrange a repeat scope at 6 weeks to check healing of all gastric ulcers and malignant-looking duodenal ulcers.

*For bleeding*

- Effective resuscitation is lifesaving
- Early interventional endoscopy with adrenaline injection (or other modalities, e.g. heater probes or clips) into the bleeding point is suitable for almost all patients—do not delay because of age/comorbidity
- iv PPI reduces the risk of re-bleeding
- Continued bleeding/re-bleeding despite endoscopic treatment is an indication for surgical intervention or radiological embolization
- Scores using clinical, laboratory, and endoscopic features can stratify risk of re-bleeding (e.g. Rockall score)

*For perforation*

(See ➔ 'The "acute surgical abdomen" ', p. 378.)

Remember 'silent' perforation (without signs of peritonitis) is more common in the elderly population (especially if on steroids or diabetic). Mortality is high due to delayed diagnosis, reluctance to perform surgery, and post-operative complications.

## HOW TO . . . Investigate and manage persistent unexplained nausea and vomiting

This group of patients can be very challenging, but you should actively manage them from an early stage because they are often very uncomfortable and bed-bound. There is frequently reversible disease and they are at high risk of dehydration/malnutrition and complications of immobility.

Nausea and vomiting can be the major presenting feature of illnesses as diverse as pneumonia, MI, intracerebral haemorrhage, Addison's disease, UTI, and constipation.

- Start with a careful history (especially drug history)
- Thorough examination (including rectal examination and neurological assessment)
- Regular observations of vital signs (looking for intermittent pyrexia, arrhythmia, etc.)
- Screening blood tests (including calcium, thyroid function, CRP, iron studies, liver function, coeliac screen), urinalysis, CXR, and ECG

*Drugs*

Look very carefully at the drug history—almost any drug can cause nausea and vomiting, but digoxin (even with therapeutic serum levels), opiates, tramadol, antiparkinsonian drugs, antidepressants, NSAIDs, and PPIs are some of the common candidates. New drugs are the most likely, but remember poor compliance with drugs at home which are prescribed in hospital, e.g. co-codamol used occasionally at home may be written as 2 qds in hospital. If there is polypharmacy, try stopping the drugs one at a time, remembering that some can take days to 'wash out'.

*Central causes*

Raised intracerebral pressure can occasionally present this way. A CT scan is needed if there is drowsiness, focal neurology, or a past history of intraventricular blood (exclude hydrocephalus). If there is vertigo or tinnitus, consider labyrinthitis or posterior circulation stroke (see Table 21.1).

*Gut causes*

- *Constipation* is a very common cause of nausea
- *Obstruction* should be excluded with an abdominal X-ray (AXR). Consider repeating this if symptoms persist and you remain suspicious. Plain radiology will remain normal in high obstruction, and an oesophagogastroduodenoscopy (OGD) or small bowel follow-through may help
- *Severe gastritis/peptic ulceration* can present with nausea and vomiting without pain/bleeding
- *Gastroparesis* is most common in people with diabetes and is very hard to treat—try prokinetics

# The liver and gall bladder

## Cirrhosis

Chronic liver disease can present for the first time in older people. The presentation is often non-specific. The prognosis is worse than for a younger person with the same degree of liver damage. Common causes include alcohol, hepatitis C, autoimmune hepatitis, and non-alcoholic fatty liver. A proportion are cryptogenic (thought to be 'burnt-out' autoimmune hepatitis or non-alcoholic fatty liver disease).

- *Hepatitis C* may have been transmitted from blood products received before 1991 when screening was introduced. Alcohol consumption is known to ↑ the percentage of those infected with hepatitis C who develop cirrhosis
- *Alcohol excess* can present with falls, confusion, and heart failure at any age, but older patients are less likely to volunteer (or be asked) their alcohol history. ▶ Always enquire about alcohol

*Investigations*

If you suspect cirrhosis, should include: α-1 antitrypsin, autoimmune profile (ANA, smooth muscle antibody (SMA), liver–kidney microsome antibodies (LKM), antimitochondrial antibody, and immunoglobulins), ferritin and iron studies, caeruloplasmin, hepatitis B and C serology, and ultrasound including Doppler of the portal and hepatic vein.

## Non-alcoholic fatty liver disease

Is not always a benign condition (half will be progressive and 15% develop cirrhosis; outlook worse with advancing age). Obesity, hyperlipidaemia, and type 2 diabetes are risk factors, so this condition is more common in older patients. If an ultrasound scan reveals fatty liver, advise about weight reduction and alcohol cessation.

## Gallstones

- Very common (1:3 elderly ♀) and mostly asymptomatic, although troublesome symptoms often misdiagnosed as GORD or diverticulitis in older age groups
- Management largely as for younger patients, but the risks with endoscopic retrograde cholangiopancreatography (ERCP)/surgical intervention are higher, so conservative/less invasive approaches often adopted
- Acute cholecystitis in older patients may present atypically (e.g. without pain) and is not always associated with gallstones. It has a 10% mortality and should be aggressively treated with iv antibiotics and supportive care. Failure to improve should prompt early surgical review

## HOW TO . . . Approach an older patient with abnormal liver function tests

This is not an uncommon finding, and investigation is as for younger patients. However, the following should be considered:

- Drug injury to the liver is common and may occur up to 6 months after exposure (e.g. statins, co-proxamol, penicillins, some over-the-counter medications)
- Liver metastases may present this way (more common in older patients)
- Deranged LFTs may occur as part of a systemic illness, e.g. sepsis (consider gall bladder/biliary infection if the LFTs are very abnormal), cardiac failure (with hepatic congestion), inflammatory conditions (PMR), ischaemic liver damage (after prolonged hypotension), Addison's disease, and thyroid disease
- The picture is often mixed, with both cholestatic and hepatocellular components

A careful history should be taken, looking for duration of the problem and whether (if old) it has been previously investigated. If new, ask about possible drug or toxin exposure, associated symptoms (e.g. heart failure, sepsis, 1° malignancy), and alcohol use (do not make lifestyle assumptions—alcohol excess is under-recognized in older people).
Clarify that that abnormality is from the liver:

- An isolated elevated ALP is often from a bone source (commonly Paget's disease), but do not assume this—liver metastases can present this way
- Isoenzymes can be measured, but clinical judgement is usually sufficient to guide investigation
- Muscle disorders can cause transaminase elevation

Persistent elevation should always prompt investigations:

- Bloods including electrolytes, clotting, TFTs, autoimmune screen (serum electrophoresis, ANA, antimitochondrial antibodies, SMA, and LMK), viral serology (hepatitis B and C), iron studies (haemochromatosis), caeruloplasmin (Wilson's disease), coeliac disease screen, and α-1 antitrypsin
- Liver ultrasound—a good screening test that will usually identify liver metastases, as well as highlighting any biliary duct dilation prompting referral for ERCP

If the liver damage is progressive, or the diagnosis elusive, then refer to a hepatologist for consideration of liver biopsy.

# Constipation

The term constipation is used in different ways, indicating one or more of the following:

- The time between bowel evacuations is longer than normal
- The stool is harder than normal
- The total faecal mass present within the abdomen is ↑

The most precise definition may be delayed alimentary tract transit time, but this is hard to measure and is delayed in age, in the institutionalized, and in those eating a Western diet.

There are said to be three types of constipation:

- Hard faeces present in the rectum (often in massive amounts)
- The whole distal large bowel loaded with soft, putty-like faeces that cannot be evacuated
- High (proximal) impaction which may be due to obstructing pathology (e.g. diverticular disease, carcinoma)

## Diagnosis

The diagnosis is largely clinical (based on history and examination alone).

▶ Ask specifically, as some patients are embarrassed to trouble doctors with bowel symptoms.

Constipation may rarely be the 1° cause of delirium but commonly contributes to the presentation of frail older patients with other pathology such as sepsis or renal failure.

Rectal examination may be diagnostic, and sometimes the rectum will barely admit the examining finger. If the rectum is empty, consider high impaction. In a thin patient, high impaction is unlikely if the loaded colon cannot be felt during abdominal examination. In more obese subjects, a plain AXR will be necessary to confirm high impaction but is insensitive in the very obese.

▶ Do not exclude constipation as the cause of faecal incontinence until there has been an adequate therapeutic trial for high faecal impaction.

## Causes

- *Reduced motility of the bowel*: drugs (e.g. opiates, iron, anticholinergics, antidepressants, antipsychotics, calcium channel blockers, calcium preparations), immobility, constitutional illness, electrolyte disturbances, dehydration, hypothyroidism, lack of dietary fibre, hypercalcaemia
- *Failure to evacuate the bowels fully*: any painful condition of the rectum or anus, difficulty in access to the toilet, lack of privacy, altered daily routine
- *Neuromuscular*: Parkinson's disease, diabetic neuropathy pseudo-obstruction
- *Mechanical obstruction of the bowel*: carcinoma of the colon, diverticular disease

## Prevention and treatment

Precipitating causes, such as dehydration, hypothyroidism, hypercalcaemia, and drugs, should be identified and reversed.

*Non-pharmacological measures*, including regular exercise, improving access to the toilet, adequate dietary fibre, and adequate hydration, are effective.

*Laxatives* should be used in combination with non-pharmacological measures. Unless there are reversible factors, always prescribe regular laxatives. Waiting for constipation to occur, then using 'PRN' doses is far less effective. You will need to titrate the laxative dose with time and changing patient circumstances.

There is little good evidence to guide the choice of laxative, and prescription varies with geography and personal choice. Here are some guiding principles:

- Stimulant laxatives, such as senna or bisacodyl, or stimulant suppositories may be appropriate for those with bulky, soft faecal overloading
- Avoid stimulant laxatives in patients with hard rocks of faeces, as this may produce abdominal pain. Use a stool softening (osmotic) laxative instead such as lactulose or a macrogol
- Long-term use of stimulant laxatives has been said to cause 'bowel tolerance'/neuronal damage, leading to a dilated, atonic colon that required even more laxatives. There is very little evidence to support this, and stimulant laxatives are now considered safe, in moderate doses, for long-term use
- Sometimes stimulant and osmotic laxatives are used in combination, typically in severe constipation (e.g. opiate-induced) that has been unresponsive to a single drug
- Stool-bulking agents, such as methylcellulose or ispaghula, are useful in prophylaxis but are less effective in treating established constipation; both fibre and other bulking agents will ↑ stool volume and may ↑ problems
- Newer agents with novel mechanisms of action are available as third-line agents (e.g. prucalopride and lubiprostone)
- Costs of laxatives vary enormously, and there is no correlation between cost and patient acceptability. Try cheaper preparations first (fibre, senna)

Faecal retention severe enough to cause incontinence nearly always needs a determined effort to clear the colon (see ➔ 'HOW TO . . . Treat "overflow" faecal incontinence', p. 547).

# Diverticular disease

Narrow-necked pockets of colonic mucosa which occur adjacent to blood vessel penetrations of the muscle bands, like 'blowouts' on a tyre. Occur anywhere in the large bowel, but most commonly in the sigmoid.

- *Rare* in <40 years, ↑ frequency with age and almost universal in >85 years
- *Cause:* thought to be raised intraluminal pressure due to low-fibre Western diet
- *Investigation:* colonoscopy/flexible sigmoidoscopy and barium enema are usually diagnostic and rule out other pathology. CT colonography (abdominal CT with oral contrast) is increasingly used as a better tolerated test in older patients

▶ The majority of cases are asymptomatic the majority of the time. On other occasions, innocent diverticulae are blamed for symptoms that arise from other pathology, e.g. constipation, irritable bowel disease, or gastro-enteritis. The previous diagnosis of diverticular disease should not stop the careful evaluation of new bowel symptoms to exclude important diagnoses such as colitis or cancer.

Pain may occur and, especially if associated with constipation, can be improved by a high-fibre diet with or without extra stool-bulking drugs (e.g. ispaghula).

## Complications

### Diverticulitis

Should be thought of as 'left-sided appendicitis'. Infection occurs within a pocket and may be due to a faecolith blocking the neck, so avoiding con-stipation is key to prevention. Abdominal pain and tenderness, diarrhoea, and vomiting occur with fever and raised inflammatory markers. Treat with antibiotics (include anaerobic cover)—mild cases oral antibiotics at home, severe cases may need admission for iv rehydration, antibiotics, and liaison with surgical services.

### Haemorrhage

Selective angiography can be used to demonstrate bleeding point.

### Diverticular abscess

Ultrasound or CT for diagnosis. Surgical or interventional radiographically guided drainage is required.

### Perforation/peritonitis

See ➋ 'The "acute surgical abdomen" ', p. 378.

### Fistula

Most commonly to the bladder, causing urinary infection and bubbles in the urine (pneumaturia). Cystoscopy or CT scan for diagnosis. Surgery is required, but simple defunctioning colostomy is often sufficient.

## HOW TO . . . Image the older colon

This requires careful consideration of the risk and discomfort of a test, balanced against the quality of the information obtained. Discussing the pros and cons of each investigation with the patients and/or relatives will often help. It is useful to clarify that a patient is fit for bowel preparation on the request form, if relevant.

- *Flexible sigmoidoscopy* is safe and generally well tolerated, requiring only an enema in preparation, allowing direct visualization and biopsy of rectal and lower colonic pathology. Sedation is usually not needed
- *Colonoscopy* allows direct imaging and biopsy of more of the colon, and is the preferred method for general population investigation but carries an ↑ risk of bowel perforation in the over 75s. Full bowel clearance and sedation are required
- *CT colonography* involves using a CT scanner to produce two- and three-dimensional images of the colon, which are interpreted by a radiologist. This requires full bowel clearance and air insufflation during the procedure, both of which can be difficult to tolerate. It is less invasive than colonoscopy but is equivalent for detection of lesions of a reasonable size. The technique is improving all the time and is the investigation of choice for patients >75 who are able to tolerate full bowel clearance
- *Minimal preparation CT colon* involves ingestion of a contrast agent 48–72h before the scan, which then tags the faecal matter and removes the need for bowel clearance. It is therefore a better investigation for frailer patients, although it misses smaller lesions
- *Plain CT abdomen* has reasonable sensitivity for large colonic lesions, may reveal other pathologies, and requires no bowel preparation. It is therefore useful in emergency assessment or where the pathology is not clearly colonic
- *Barium enema* requires bowel clearance and is less sensitive than CT colonography, so is becoming less frequently used

# Inflammatory bowel disease

Ulcerative colitis and Crohn's disease are chronic, relapsing conditions caused by inflammation of the bowel wall. Inflammatory bowel disease is idiopathic and has an ↑ incidence in the population as a whole. Initial presentation is usually in adolescence, but there is a second peak of incidence in older patients. Diarrhoea and urgency in this age group can be particularly disabling and may result in incontinence and social isolation.

## Features

- Diarrhoea (often with blood), malaise, weight loss, and abdominal pain. Delayed presentation may result from embarrassment or fear of cancer. Delayed diagnosis more common in older people because symptoms are ascribed to one of the common differential diagnoses such as diverticular disease, CDAD, colonic carcinoma, and ischaemic colitis
- Associated conditions include arthritis, iritis, sclerosing cholangitis, ankylosing spondylitis, and skin disorders (pyoderma gangrenosum, erythema nodosum)
- Complications include thromboembolism, malabsorption and malnutrition, perforation, stenosis with obstruction, fistula formation, and colonic and biliary malignancy

## Investigations

- Exclude infection with stool culture and examination for ova, cysts, and parasites and *Clostridium* toxin (if in hospital or recent antibiotics)
- ESR and CRP are usually elevated but may be normal in localized disease
- A normochromic normocytic anaemia is common, but if there is excessive bleeding, iron deficiency can develop
- Plain X-rays are usually normal, but contrast studies are often diagnostic
- Sigmoidoscopy/colonoscopy and biopsy have high diagnostic yield

## Treatment

Confirmed cases are best managed by gastroenterology teams. Treatment in older patients is not greatly different and is aimed at obtaining and then maintaining remission. Some principles for treating older patients include:

- Exacerbations of distal colitis are usually treated with topical mesalazine and steroids given as enemas—this may be impractical in older patients, unless a carer can help, and oral steroids can be a better option
- Budesonide is a steroid with high topical potency (poor absorption and rapid first-pass metabolism), so equivalent doses cause fewer side effects
- Side effects, drug interactions, and polypharmacy may be more problematic, e.g. always consider bisphosphonates with oral steroids therapy
- Look for, and treat, proximal constipation which can impair the efficacy of treatment of a distal colitis
- Oral 5-aminosalicylic acid preparations (e.g. slow-release mesalazine) are often successful (for exacerbations and maintenance) and well tolerated

- The risk of malignancy is higher the longer the patient has active disease, so theoretically many older patients should be under surveillance by a gastroenterologist. Unfortunately the risk of colonic perforation during colonoscopic screening is higher in the elderly population, so many screening programmes stop at age 75
- For failure of medical management, elective colectomy is well tolerated and may give the best quality of life. In contrast, emergency surgery in older patients has high mortality

# Diarrhoea in older patients

## Acute

Short-lived bouts of diarrhoea are commonly due to viral gastroenteritis. Supportive management (rehydration, light diet) is usually sufficient for this self-limiting condition. It can spread rapidly in institutions (especially if due to norovirus—responsible for much of the so-called 'winter vomiting'), and appropriate infection control measures should be put in place. In frail, hospitalized patients, especially with recent antibiotic exposure, consider CDAD earlier rather than later.

If diarrhoea persists, always send samples for culture, ova, cysts, and parasites, and *C. difficile* toxin (see ⊃ '*Clostridium difficile*-associated diarrhoea', pp. 614–15).

## Chronic

There is a group of elderly people who have chronic or recurring episodes of diarrhoea that merit active investigation—untreated, they suffer high morbidity (especially if diarrhoea induces faecal incontinence) and many causes are treatable. See ⊃ 'HOW TO . . . Investigate and manage chronic diarrhoea', p. 375 for a suggested plan of investigation.

## Malabsorption

Patients do not always have diarrhoea. Look for low BMI and falling weight despite reasonable oral calorie intake. Biochemical markers of malnutrition, e.g. hypoalbuminaemia, may be present. Anaemia is caused by malabsorption of iron, $B_{12}$, or folate and is therefore microcytic, macrocytic, or normocytic.

The common causes of malabsorption in older patients often coexist and include:

- *Coeliac disease/gluten-sensitive enteropathy*:
  - Peak incidence at age 50 but can manifest for the first time in old age with weight loss, bone pain (osteoporosis), fatigue (anaemia), and mouth ulcers
  - Duodenal biopsy should be performed in all who present with iron deficiency undergoing endoscopy
  - Anti-endomysial or tissue transglutaminase antibodies have very high specificity (100%) and reasonable sensitivity (around 85%). False negatives can occur with low immunoglobulin A (IgA), so always check serum immunoglobulins at the same time
- *Pancreatic insufficiency* can occur without a history of pancreatitis, alcoholism, or gallstones. Request a faecal elastase—a low level supports pancreatic insufficiency
- *Bile salt malabsorption*. Ileal resection or disease allows bile salts to reach the colon which causes diarrhoea
- *Bacterial overgrowth* is particularly common in any person with an anatomical abnormality of the gut (e.g. post-gastrectomy, small bowel diverticula) but can also occur with normal gut architecture

## HOW TO . . . **Investigate and manage chronic diarrhoea**

Diagnoses to consider in the elderly population include:
- Colonic tumour
- Diverticular disease
- Chronic infections
- Constipation with overflow diarrhoea
- Drugs—many drugs can cause diarrhoea; review the list and stop any that may be implicated. Common culprits include laxatives, antibiotics, bisphosphonates, NSAIDs, and PPIs
- Inflammatory bowel disease or microscopic colitis
- Malabsorption

*History*

Ask about foreign travel, antibiotic exposure, full drug history, previous gut surgery/pancreatitis, and family history of inflammatory bowel disease. Ask the patient or carer to make a record of stool frequency/texture.

*Examination*

Abdominal and digital rectal examination. If rectum is loaded, be highly suspicious of overflow diarrhoea.

*Investigations*
- Stool: culture, *C. difficile* toxin, ova, cysts, and parasites
- Blood tests: FBC (anaemia), haematinics (Iron, $B_{12}$, folate deficiency), tissue transglutaminase antibodies (and IgA levels), CRP, and ESR
- Radiology: plain AXR is rarely diagnostic (except unexpected, left-sided faecal loading)
- Sigmoidoscopy: biopsy in several places, even if the mucosa looks normal to exclude microscopic colitis (see ➔ 'Other colonic conditions', pp. 376–7)
- More extensive colonic imaging may be needed (see ➔ 'HOW TO . . . Image the older colon', p. 371)
- Faecal calprotectin is useful to rule out inflammatory bowel disease

*Treatment*

Obviously depends on the cause, but in patients in whom diagnosis is not clear and are not fit for, or refuse, more complex investigations, there is a place for trial of empirical treatment. One such strategy is at least 2-week trials of:
- Metronidazole (for overgrowth/diverticular disease)
- Pancreatin, e.g. Creon® (pancreatic disease)
- Bile acid sequestrants, e.g. colestyramine (bile salt malabsorption)
- Steroids (for colitis)

Pick the most likely, or try each in turn for a few weeks.

# Other colonic conditions

### Irritable bowel syndrome

A chronic, non-inflammatory condition characterized by abdominal pain, altered bowel habit (diarrhoea or constipation), and abdominal bloating, but with no identifiable structural or biochemical disorder.

* New onset is rare in older age, and this diagnosis should not be made '*de novo*' in older patients without very careful exclusion of structural disease (particularly colonic tumours and diverticulitis)
* Lifelong sufferers may continue with symptoms in later life, but if the symptoms change, the patient should also undergo investigations
* Pain or diarrhoea that wakes a patient at night, blood in stool, weight loss, or fever are NEVER features of irritable bowel syndrome
* Some drugs used to treat irritable bowel syndrome (e.g. tricyclic antidepressants) are less well tolerated in older patients. Mebeverine might be better tolerated for spasm
* Dietary advice should be given (low fibre for bloating or wind, high fibre for diarrhoea or constipation, exclude exacerbating foods)
* Stool-bulking drugs can be useful for constipation
* Loperamide or codeine can be used for disabling diarrhoea

### Angiodysplasia

Tiny capillary malformations (like spider naevi) that can occur anywhere in the gut are important only because they bleed.

* Slow blood loss leads to unexplained recurrent iron deficiency anaemia; brisk loss may produce life-threatening haemorrhage
* Unless they are inherited in a syndrome (e.g. hereditary haemorrhagic telangiectasia), they are acquired and therefore have ↑ prevalence with age (most cases aged over 70)
* Asymptomatic angiodysplasia in older patients is common. Diagnosis is often by exclusion of other causes of iron deficiency anaemia. Many patients are reinvestigated for recurrent anaemia, and the absence of sinister features over a period of time with no demonstrated pathology on standard tests may suggest angiodysplasia is the cause
* Sometimes colonoscopy can visualize lesions (which can then be treated by diathermy), but CT does not reveal this pathology
* Selective mesenteric angiography can demonstrate lesions that are actively and rapidly bleeding
* Tranexamic acid, oestrogens, and thalidomide are sometimes successful in controlling chronic blood loss

## Microscopic colitis

Also known as collagenous or lymphocytic colitis. An idiopathic condition causing chronic or episodic watery, non-bloody diarrhoea, but with no gross structural changes seen on colonoscopy.

- Biopsy changes are diagnostic with collagenous thickening of the subepithelial layer and infiltration with lymphocytes
- Peak incidence in 50s
- There is no ↑ risk of cancer
- Keep treatment as simple as possible—start with diet and anti-diarrhoeal drugs (e.g. loperamide), then try steroids (e.g. budesonide)

## Intestinal ischaemia

There is a variety of presentations. Pain out of proportion to the abdominal examination findings is common in these syndromes and should always make you consider them. An elevated lactate ± acidosis should alert you to the possibility of dead bowel.

- *Intestinal angina* results from chronic arterial obstruction of the coeliac axis or superior mesenteric artery. Epigastric pain occurs after eating. Diagnosis is tricky, as the pain is similar to peptic ulcer pain, but angiography is diagnostic. Treat with antiplatelet agents. Angioplasty or stenting may be useful
- *Small bowel ischaemia* results from mesenteric artery occlusion, often by an embolus (more common in AF). There is acute colic with rectal bleeding, followed by circulatory collapse. Laparotomy is required, but outcome is poor
- *Ischaemic colitis* is an under-diagnosed cause of acute diarrhoea ± blood in dehydrated, hypotensive elderly patients with vascular disease. Often self-limiting if volume depletion corrected and the bowel is rested. May result in colonic stricture
- *Colonic gangrene* occurs after profound hypotension typically in older ITU patients with heart failure and sepsis. Laparotomy and colectomy are required, but fatality is high

# The 'acute surgical abdomen'

▶ Peritonitis/perforation often presents in a non-specific way. Patients often present to medicine, rather than surgery. The diagnosis is easily missed, so always have a high index of suspicion and examine the abdomen carefully and repeatedly in sick elderly patients without a diagnosis.

Common causes in older patients include:

- Complications of diverticular disease
- First presentation of a tumour (gut, pancreatic)
- Ischaemic bowel (emboli in patients with AF)
- Strangulated hernias (always remember groin examination)
- Ruptured abdominal aortic aneurysm
- Duodenal ulcer perforation (becoming less common)
- Biliary stones/sepsis (stones) and pancreatitis
- Appendicitis

## Signs

Peritonitis/perforation may not have guarding or rigidity, particularly in the very old, those on steroids, or people with diabetes. Lack of bowel sounds can be helpful. Signs may develop with time, so repeated assessments are mandatory.

## Investigations

Erect CXR can reveal air under the diaphragm (this is sometimes the only indication of a 'silent' perforation). Ultrasound or CT imaging will often reveal the cause.

## Management

Always involve the surgical team, even where the patient is unsuitable for operation, as they can advise on conservative management and occasionally an 'interval' procedure is appropriate (e.g. gallstone surgery once cholecystitis has settled).

▶ Ensure that surgical decisions are made on the basis of frailty assessment and comorbidity, not just age alone. Aim to achieve a senior medical, surgical, and anaesthetic consensus about treatment, and then discuss with the patient (or their advocate).

Medical management involves:

- Broad-spectrum iv antibiotics
- Resting the bowel (nil by mouth, NGT if vomiting)
- Careful monitoring of fluid balance—heart failure from fluid overload or renal failure from dehydration are often the mechanisms of death. A urinary catheter and central venous pressure monitoring are sometimes necessary
- Prophylactic low-molecular-weight heparin

It is surprising how often patients survive with conservative measures, so continue to monitor the patient and adjust treatment carefully. Once the signs/symptoms recede, try to get the patient eating, on oral antibiotics, and mobilizing as soon as possible to avoid the complications of malnutrition, pressure sores, VTE, and *C. difficile* colitis which may be more lethal than the initial peritonitis.

# Obstructed bowel in older patients

As with peritonitis, this often presents in a non-specific or non-dramatic way. Common causes in older patients include:
- Constipation
- Colonic tumours
- Sigmoid volvulus
- Strangulated hernias (remember to examine the groins)
- Adhesions (look for old abdominal scars)
- Complications of diverticular disease (abscess, localized perforation, stricture)

## Signs

Consider excluding obstruction (with plain X-ray) in any patient with persistent vomiting and/or abdominal bloating (ask the patient if their tummy is a normal size for them). Pain/colic, absence of defecation, tinkling bowel sounds, and gastric splash are helpful when present (but are often absent). Always examine the groins in both sexes for obstructed herniae.

## Investigations

Plain AXR shows dilated bowel—standing AXRs have fluid levels but are often impractical in older patients and rarely add diagnostic information to a supine film. CT imaging may localize a cause. Contrast radiology and gastroscopy are sometimes useful.

## Management

Always involve the surgical team who can advise on diagnosis and conservative management, e.g. insertion of a flatus tube for sigmoid volvulus.
General management usually involves:
- Resting the bowel (nil by mouth and wide-bore NGT)
- Careful monitoring of fluid balance—heart failure from fluid overload or renal failure from dehydration are often the mechanisms of death
- Therapeutic oral Gastrografin® (hyperosmolar 'lubricating' agent and can relieve small bowel obstruction due to adhesions)
- Consider broad-spectrum antibiotics if there is fever or features of coexistent perforation
- Prophylactic low-molecular-weight heparin

Where conservative management fails and an operation is necessary, less invasive/palliative procedures are often more appropriate (e.g. defunctioning colostomy, rather than anterior resection).

*Pseudo-obstruction* presents with vomiting and dilated bowel on X-ray but is due to an atonic bowel, so bowel sounds are absent or ↓, rather than ↑. Frail, older, immobile, debilitated patients are more at risk. Can occur with electrolyte abnormality (especially low potassium), post-surgery, with drugs (e.g. opiates, anticholinergics), in neurological disease (e.g. Parkinson's or Alzheimer's), or any severe illness (e.g. septicaemia). Supportive care with hydration and bowel rest is needed, along with correction of the underlying abnormality. Often resolves with this approach, but decompression or surgery is occasionally needed.

# Obesity in older people

In developed countries, there is a general ↑ in body weight and BMI until about 60 years of age, after which both tend to decline. The body composition also changes, with an ↑ proportion of intra-abdominal fat.

Weight gain in older people usually relates to a reduction in activity and falling basal metabolic rate, rather than an alteration in calorie intake (which actually tends to get lower with age).

The ideal body mass for an older person has not been established, although it is probably higher than that for a younger person.

## Impact of obesity

The relationship between mortality and obesity in older people has not been established. The following should be considered:

- Weight loss has been reported to ↑ mortality—but all the studies have methodological problems, and weight loss is a marker of underlying disease which may be occult
- Those with chronic disabilities and diseases will reduce activity more than fit older people, and so may gain weight more easily
- In care home residents, only *severe* obesity (BMI >40) is clearly associated with an ↑ in mortality. Care homes may need special equipment (e.g. wider frames, wheelchairs) to allow for their care
- Obesity will ↑ morbidity from conditions such as arthritis and diabetes and ↑ cardiovascular risk
- Obese older people are more likely to have mobility problems, and their quadriceps strength-to-weight ratio is key to standing ability
- Obesity does not exclude frailty

## Treatment

The goal of treating obesity in older people is to reduce weight without losing lean mass or contributing to frailty—excessive weight loss in older people is associated with an ↑ in mortality.

In the very old, there is little to be gained from altering a lifelong dietary and exercise habit where there are few complications from obesity, but younger patients (60s and 70s) with diabetes or vascular disease may benefit greatly from healthier eating habits.

- ↑ physical activity is the mainstay of treatment. This may ↑ energy expenditure and promote weight loss, improve muscle strength and stamina, reduce intra-abdominal fat, and promote a feeling of well-being
- Calorie restriction should be undertaken with caution and include at least 800kcal/day with good fluid intake
- Dietary supplements can be used in patients who have a high BMI during acute illness but should not be continued indefinitely
- Drugs to enhance weight loss are rarely useful (risk > benefit), although inhibitors of fat absorption (e.g. orlistat) may be useful in people with diabetes
- Gastric surgery is higher risk in older obese people and not frequently undertaken

# Renal medicine

# The ageing kidney

Kidney function tends to decline with age, but unless there is additional disease, function is usually sufficient to remove waste and to regulate volume and electrolyte balance; it is only when stressed that lack of renal reserve becomes apparent. The relative contribution of cumulative exposure to risk factors (extrinsic ageing), disease acquisition (often occult), and intrinsic ageing is unknown, but not all the changes described are universal in an older population.

## Falling renal reserve

The GFR falls steadily after the age of 40 in most healthy older people, possibly due to the following age-related changes:
- Rise in BP within the normal range
- Numbers of glomeruli fall (~50% fewer at age 70 than at age 30)
- ↑ in sclerotic glomeruli

Renal blood flow ↓ by around 10% per decade (cortex more than medulla, leading to patchy cortical defects on renal scans).

Lower GFR and renal blood flow are the major causes of reduced renal reserve, with the following clinical implications:
- Renally excreted substances are likely to be retained longer (especially drugs), making prescription amendments necessary (see ➲ 'Pharmacology in older patients', pp. 124–5)
- Reduced threshold for damage with ischaemia or nephrotoxins

The normal range for plasma urea and creatinine does not change with age. However, as production of urea and creatinine ↓ with falling body muscle mass, renal function is often substantially diminished in an older person, even with apparently normal blood chemistry.

▶ GFR is a better estimate of renal function than plasma urea and creatinine (see ➲ 'HOW TO . . . Estimate the glomerular filtration rate', p. 391)

## Blunted fluid and electrolyte homeostasis

The following changes occur with age:
- A blunted response to sodium loading and depletion, so equilibrium is achieved more slowly
- Reduced ability to dilute and concentrate urine (falls 5% every decade)
- Lower renin and aldosterone levels (30–50% less than in young people)
- Loss of the sensation of thirst, even when plasma tonicity is high (reasons unclear—may relate to altered baroreceptor function, dry mouth, or altered mental capacity)
- Reduced response to vasopressin
- In addition, many commonly prescribed drugs interfere with renal function (diuretics, NSAIDs, ACE inhibitors, lithium, sedatives, etc.)

Hyponatraemia is therefore common (low sodium intake combined with renal sodium wasting), but in times of acute illness (↑ fluid demand and ↓ intake), the slower adaptive mechanisms make hypernatraemic dehydration more common.

Hypokalaemia is common because of poor intake and frequent diuretic use, but lower GFR and hypoaldosteronism lead to vulnerability to hyperkalaemia, especially when exacerbating drugs (NSAIDs, spironolactone, ACE inhibitors) are used.

## Structural changes

- Renal mass falls by 20–30% between 30 and 90 years, making kidneys appear smaller on ultrasound scanning, without necessarily implying disease
- Distal nephrons develop diverticulae (three per tubule by age 90) that may become retention cysts (benign finding in older people)

## Other changes

- Renal 1-hydroxylase activity ↓ with age, leading to ↓ vitamin D production. Combined with low phosphate intake, this can mildly elevate parathyroid hormone (PTH) levels
- There is loss of the circadian rhythm, owing to altered sodium handling and patterns of aldosterone secretion, so that over the age of 60, the proportion of water, sodium, and potassium excretion occurring at night ↑, causing nocturia

# Acute kidney injury

This is more common in older people, but with a similar prognosis if occurring *de novo* and treated correctly. Due to recognition of high mortality and
possible undertreatment of acute kidney injury (AKI), there is a national UK
initiative to flag and improve management for these patients.

▶ Do not deny treatment based on age alone—even anuric patients can
make a full recovery.

## Causes

Eighty per cent of cases of AKI are caused by pre-renal failure and ATN.

### Pre-renal causes

Due to poor renal perfusion. May be caused by:
• Dehydration (commonly associated with sepsis)
• Volume loss (e.g. bleeding, over-diuresis)
• Volume redistribution (e.g. with low serum albumin)
• Poor cardiac output (e.g. post-MI)
• Aggravated by many drugs (e.g. diuretics, ACE inhibitors, NSAIDs)

Older patients are prone to sepsis, have less capacity to maintain circulating
volume in the face of stress, and are more likely to be on aggravating medications, making this a very common problem (e.g. urinary sepsis in a patient
taking diuretics and NSAIDs can often cause pre-renal renal impairment and
responds well to antibiotics, fluids, and drug cessation).

▶ All unwell older patients should have renal function checked routinely
and repeatedly. Consider stopping diuretics and ACE inhibitors during an
acute illness.

### Renal causes

Due to direct damage to the kidney. Commonly ATN, which may be:
• Ischaemic (occurs when pre-renal failure is not corrected quickly,
  e.g. with sepsis, surgical procedures, prolonged hypotension, etc.)
• Nephrotoxic (usually medication such as aminoglycoside antibiotics,
  e.g. gentamicin)
• Due to pigment deposition (e.g. myoglobin in rhabdomyolysis;
  see ➋ 'Rhabdomyolysis', p. 507)

Not all renal failure is ATN. Other (rarer) causes include:
• Glomerulonephritis—diffuse inflammatory change to glomeruli with
  resulting haematuria and red cell casts
• Acute interstitial nephritis—consider drug-induced nephritis. May have
  flank pain, rash, fever, eosinophilia, and urine WBCs/casts, but consider
  if new drug recently, even in absence of these features

These less common causes are important because they are often responsive to specific treatment (usually steroids). The patient should be assessed
by a renal physician promptly and often needs a biopsy.

*Post-renal causes*
- Obstruction of the renal tract at some point, e.g. prostatic enlargement, renal stones, urethral strictures, pelvic tumours
- Ultrasound scan shows a dilated collecting system
- These conditions are all more common in older people and are very responsive to treatment if found early, often with full recovery of renal function

# Acute kidney injury: management

### Is this acute kidney injury?

Older people are more likely to have underlying CKD, and this confers a worse prognosis. Check old notes; ask the patient, family, and GP about history, and look back at blood test results. The more severe and persistent the episode of AKI, the greater the permanent deterioration in renal function.

Generally, management does not differ significantly from younger patients.

### Investigations

(See Table 13.1.)

- Treat the cause

Older people respond as well to most treatments.

### Monitor meticulously

- Pulse and BP, cardiac monitor, input (iv and po), and output (urine, faecal matter, vomit, drains, sweat)
- May be best done on HDU
- Aim for euvolaemia (assessed clinically, may need to correct deficit), then maintain by matching input to output on an hourly basis initially
- Management of fluid balance is likely to be harder in older people because of comorbidity (especially heart failure)

▶ The presence of peripheral oedema does not necessarily indicate fluid overload. Circulating volume is best assessed by BP, pulse, JVP, and skin turgor (see ➋ 'Challenges to volume status assessment in elderly patients', p. 403).

- May need central venous catheter and urinary catheter initially, but remove as soon as possible because of infection risk
- Document daily weight and total fluid balance summary
- Be prepared for polyuria in the recovery phase, and ensure that the patient does not become fluid-depleted

### Treat complications

Importantly hyperkalaemia, acidosis, and pulmonary oedema.

Refer early for further renal support (filtration or dialysis); a patient can remain oliguric for some time while renal recovery is occurring, but it is sensible to make the relevant teams aware of a potential patient. The indications for renal replacement therapy are as follows:

- Refractory pulmonary oedema (older people are particularly prone to this after over-enthusiastic initial fluid replacement)
- Persistent hyperkalaemia (potassium >7mmol/L) that cannot be controlled by insulin/glucose infusions and iv calcium
- Worsening acidosis (pH <7.2)
- Uraemic pericarditis
- Uraemic encephalopathy

## HOW TO . . . Perform a fluid challenge in AKI/anuria

Many older patients are clearly dehydrated with mildly impaired renal function tests, and these patients can be simply rehydrated orally or parenterally.

If the patient presents with established AKI or is found to be anuric despite simple rehydration, then a fluid challenge should be contemplated.

This is an important clinical skill to develop and requires advanced clinical acumen and an investment of time. The key is an accurate assessment of fluid status, with the aim of rendering the patient euvolaemic.

A urinary catheter is usually required, and a central venous pressure monitoring device is helpful if facilities exist.

- Start by assessing and clearly documenting baseline fluid status, as this will inform your management and will be helpful when the patient is reassessed
- If the patient is already fluid-overloaded, then a single bolus of iv loop diuretic and early contact with the renal specialist team is needed
- If the patient appears to be hypovolaemic, give 500mL of normal saline (sodium bicarbonate may be considered if they are profoundly acidotic) over 30–60min, and review
- If the patient appears to be euvolaemic, then the fluid challenge should be more cautious. Give a 100mL bolus iv, and review after about 15min
- For the review, repeat and document the fluid status and urine output. Repeat this cycle of fluid prescription, and do a careful review as the clinical progression becomes clear

**Table 13.1** Acute kidney injury—investigations

| Investigation | Rationale | Special points in older people |
|---|---|---|
| Urea and creatinine | Elevated in renal failure | Older people with very little muscle mass will have lower baseline levels, so a urea of 10 in a small elderly woman will represent significant renal impairment |
| | | Urea:creatinine ratio can be useful—elevated in pre-renal and post-renal failure, acting as a marker of dehydration or obstruction |
| Electrolytes | Potassium rises dangerously in AKI | More prone to cardiac complications of electrolyte disturbance—monitor carefully |
| Arterial blood gases | Monitor pH which falls in AKI | pH can also be checked on a venous sample |
| Inflammatory markers (ESR, CRP, white cell count) | Check for infection | Common precipitant of AKI in older people (may be occult) |
| Urine dipstick | Check for leucocytes and nitrites (infection), blood, and protein (active renal lesion likely) | High rate of positive urine dipstick in older people—does not always imply infection |
| Urine microscopy | Looking for casts (red cell casts in glomerulonephritis, white cell casts in infection, etc.) and blood cells | Always send for culture, even when the dipstick is negative |
| Blood and urine cultures | Identify microbes | Ensure these are sent on all patients (who may have occult infection) prior to starting antibiotics |

| Creatinine kinase | Elevated in rhabdomyolysis | Always check after falls (especially after a long period on the floor before being found). Even if there is not full blown rhabdomyolysis, an elevated CK level indicates the need for hydration and monitoring of renal function |
|---|---|---|
| Urinary sodium | Helps distinguish between pre-renal failure (urinary Na <20 mmol/L as kidney still functioning to preserve sodium) and ATN (urinary Na >40 mmol/L as kidney not functioning, so losing Na) | Particularly useful in older people where clinical assessment of fluid balance may be harder because of peripheral oedema etc. Not helpful if the patient has taken diuretics (increase sodium excretion) |
| CXR | Looking for evidence of cardiac disease, source of infection, pulmonary oedema or pulmonary infiltrates (vasculitis) | More prone to pulmonary oedema—extra caution with fluid replacement if there is cardiomegaly, even where there is no history of cardiac failure |
| ECG | Looking for evidence of cardiac disease and monitoring for hyperkalaemia | Again alerts to occult cardiac disease if ECG is abnormal |
| Renal ultrasound | Assess renal size and look for evidence of hydronephrosis | Very useful in older people to help establish if renal failure is truly acute (small kidneys with chronic failure). Also checks for treatable obstructive causes—common in this age group |
| Other tests | All should have FBC and LFTs Usually also send autoantibodies (ANA, antineutrophilic cytoplasmic antibodies (ANCA)), immunoglobulins, complement and electrophoresis of blood and urine | |

# Chronic kidney disease

CKD is a substantial irreversible, long-standing, and usually progressive loss in renal function. CKD is more common in older people (incidence in the over 75s is ten times higher than in the under 40s). Half of all renal replacement therapy is now started for patients >65 years, and this underestimates the burden of renal impairment, as the majority will die with, and not of, kidney disease, many never encountering a renal physician.

Much renal impairment is discovered incidentally by finding elevated creatinine and low eGFR levels. There are adaptive mechanisms that maintain reasonable health with failing renal function until severe damage has occurred (GFR of 10–15mL/min).

## Causes

Common causes include hypertension, diabetes, obstruction (usually due to prostatic enlargement), glomerulonephritis, and renovascular disease. A significant proportion presenting late remains idiopathic.

## Management

When abnormal renal function is discovered, firstly consider the circumstances—is the patient acutely unwell? Are they being over-diuresed? Correct all of remediable factors, and recheck renal function in a stable clinical state. If it remains deranged, then:

- Estimate the GFR (see ➔ 'HOW TO . . . Estimate the glomerular filtration rate', p. 391). Consider checking the GFR, even when creatinine is within normal range for an older patient with a low body weight
- Identify and treat any modifiable factors (e.g. diabetes, hypertension, and obstructive uropathy)
- Delay disease progression by controlling diabetes and hypertension and by using an ACE inhibitor (or an ARB)
- Lipid-lowering diets and correcting anaemia should be considered
- Avoid exacerbating factors such as volume depletion, iv contrast, urinary obstruction, and nephrotoxic drugs
- Review drug treatment; some are better stopped (e.g. metformin), and others need the dose adjusting (e.g. digoxin)
- Identify and treat complications as they arise (see ➔ 'Chronic kidney disease: complications', pp. 392–3)
- Try to establish the rate of decline, using previous creatinine measurements. Deterioration tends to be steady, and so it is often possible to estimate when interventions are likely to be needed
- Prepare for the end-stage. A person with limited life expectancy and moderate impairment is likely to die of other causes before complex renal issues become a problem. Most other patients benefit from early renal specialist review (i.e. when impairment is moderate to severe) to clarify diagnosis, optimize management, and discuss renal replacement therapy. Late referral for dialysis is associated with a poor outcome

## HOW TO . . . Estimate the glomerular filtration rate

Although elevated urea and creatinine levels often alert the clinician to renal impairment, they give a poor estimate of extent, as the levels are determined by many factors, as well as the GFR, e.g. creatinine is directly related to muscle mass, which tends to fall with age, meaning that:

- A small rise in urea and creatinine in an elderly person is significant and should be taken seriously
- A creatinine within the normal range may represent renal failure in a small old patient

GFR is a better measure of renal function but requires a 24h urine collection which can be tricky in older people. Creatinine clearance approximates the GFR and can be estimated using various equations.

The Cockcroft–Gault formula is the best known:

$$\text{Creatinine clearance} = [(140 - \text{age in years}) \times \text{weight in kg}] /$$
$$\text{plasma creatinine (micromole/L)} \times 0.82$$

This figure needs to be reduced slightly for women.

It can be seen that a patient of 80, weighing 50kg with a creatinine of 140 will have an eGFR of 26 (i.e. severe failure). Another patient of 30, weighing 70kg with a creatinine of 140, however, will have an eGFR of 67 (i.e. mild failure).

The eGFR should be used in calculating dose adjustments for certain drugs, e.g. gentamicin, low-molecular-weight heparin.

Using this derived figure, renal impairment has been classified by the Kidney Disease Outcomes Quality Initiative (KDOQI) and this acts as a guide for management (see Table 13.2).

**Table 13.2** Kidney Disease Outcomes Quality Initiative

| GFR (mL/min) | Average creatinine for patient of 30 years weighing 70kg | Average creatinine for patient of 80 years weighing 50kg | Degree of renal failure |
|---|---|---|---|
| 60–89 | 125 | 50 | Mild failure |
| 30–59 | 220 | 85 | Moderate failure |
| 15–29 | 420 | 165 | Severe failure |
| <15 | >1500 | >700 | End-stage renal failure |

## Further reading

National Kidney Foundation. *The National Kidney Foundation Kidney Disease Outcomes Quality Initiative.* ℘ http://www.kidney.org/professionals/guidelines.

# Chronic kidney disease: complications

## Hypertension
- Can occur at any point in the disease and is a cause and a consequence of CKD
- Monitor BP regularly in all patients. Targets differ, depending on the degree of proteinuria—as low as 120–129/80 with higher levels of proteinuria
- Treat with an ACE inhibitor, especially if diabetic or microalbuminuric (preserves renal function)

## Hyperlipidaemia
- May contribute to renal damage
- Treat to target with a statin

## Atherosclerosis
- Accelerated atheroma occurs with renal impairment
- Ensure that all vascular risk factors are addressed

## Salt and water retention
- Onset with moderate impairment
- Consider loop diuretics for oedema (e.g. high doses of furosemide may be required, but start low and ↑ as needed)
- Restrict dietary salt and sometimes potassium intake
- Fluid restriction may be necessary with more severe renal impairment

## Secondary hyperparathyroidism
- Onset usually with moderate impairment
- Low calcium, high phosphate, low vitamin D, and appropriately high PTH
- Ensure calcium, phosphate, and PTH are checked
- Consider dietary phosphate restriction (milk, cheese, eggs, etc.), phosphate binders (e.g. calcium carbonate), calcium supplements, and vitamin D analogues (e.g. alfacalcidol) if there is a problem
- Risk of renal bone disease (renal osteodystrophy)

## Anaemia
- Onset usually with moderate impairment
- Check for alternative causes of anaemia (iron deficiency, chronic disease, etc.)
- Hb often responds to oral or parenteral iron
- If this fails, consider an erythropoiesis-stimulating agent to keep Hb 100–120g/L (usually initiated by the renal team)

## Nervous system
- Onset with severe impairment
- Includes peripheral neuropathy, autonomic neuropathy, and encephalopathy

## Acidosis and hyperkalaemia

- Onset with moderate or severe impairment
- Treated with oral bicarbonate and diet
- May indicate need for renal replacement therapy or plans for terminal care

# Renal replacement therapy: dialysis

This includes haemodialysis (usually done at a dialysis centre and accounting for around 80% of dialysis in the older age group) and peritoneal dialysis (mainly managed at home).

## Survival

Older patients have a shorter survival on dialysis than younger patients, probably because of an ↑ in complications (see ➲ 'Complications', p. 394), yet still can expect a 20–40% 5-year survival (mean life expectancy 3–5 years).

Those aged over 80 on dialysis have a median survival of 26 months, irrespective of the age at onset of treatment.

## Effectiveness

- Some older patients may mistakenly be under-dialysed (low muscle mass leads to lower urea and creatinine levels that do not reflect the need for dialysis). In addition, dialysis sessions are more commonly stopped early because of hypotension
- This adversely affects outcome. Using other means to calculate dialysis frequency and optimizing health with nutritional support, erythropoiesis-stimulating agents (to keep Hb >100g/L), and appropriate buffer selection can vastly improve effectiveness in older people

## Complications

*In older people*
- Nausea, vomiting, and hypotension during dialysis are more common (due to autonomic dysfunction and ↓ cardiac reserve)
- Malnutrition occurs in up to 20%
- There is ↑ risk of infection (ageing immune system and malnutrition), depression, and gastrointestinal bleeds (from uraemic gastritis, diverticulosis, and angiodysplasia)

## Quality of life

Many older patients on dialysis enjoy a high quality of life. They resent the intrusion of visits to a dialysis centre less than younger patients and can find it offers positive social interaction. Many of this highly selected cohort (frailer elderly patients with renal impairment are not appropriate for this service) retain their independence, with over 90% maintaining good community social contacts and over 80% regularly going outdoors. Around 40% rate their health positively. However, for some, it becomes tiring and burdensome, especially if relying on hospital transport for attendance.

## Who should be offered dialysis?

Dialysis is expensive, and the number of older people with end-stage renal failure is large. Many older patients with end-stage renal failure elect to have dialysis if offered, but offering it to all is not sensible or feasible.

It should not be offered to simply delay dying, rather used if the renal failure is the main threat to continued survival. Severe dementia, advanced malignancy (except possibly multiple myeloma), or advanced liver disease generally makes dialysis inadvisable. Caution should be exercised before offering dialysis to patients with severe heart or lung disease, or frail patients with multiple comorbidities.

## What next?

Many patients need to swap dialysis modalities for some reason. Forty per cent would like to proceed to transplant if an organ was available. The rate of voluntary withdrawal (overall about 5%) ↑ with age and is usually because of general dissatisfaction with life or the development of significant comorbidity (often cancer). Guidelines suggest that patients approaching the end of their life should have input into an individual palliative care plan, often in conjunction with palliative care services.

# Renal replacement therapy: transplantation

This is the gold standard of renal replacement therapy for end-stage renal failure, as it improves survival and quality of life when compared with dialysis, as well as releasing the patient from the burden of regular dialysis sessions. It is also cost-effective, being cheaper than dialysis after the first year.

Transplant recipients are getting older. However, as the majority of end-stage failures occur in the older population, this still represents an imbalance. Donated cadaver kidneys are in short supply and tend to be given to those who will get the most use out of them, namely younger patients with a longer natural life expectancy.

The most common cause of graft failure in older people is death of the host with a functioning graft. This is due to a number of factors:

- The most common cause of death after transplantation is cardiovascular disease
- Older people have altered immune responses—this makes it less likely that they will reject a donated kidney and allows for modified immunosuppressive medication. However, it also ↑ the risk of serious infection
- Older people have ↑ side effects to immunosuppressive medication, particularly steroids
- Other common conditions make the transplant procedure more complicated, e.g. peripheral vascular disease (technical surgical problems), diverticular disease (predisposes to post-transplant perforation), and cholelithiasis (predisposes to biliary sepsis)

There are limited outcome data for older patients, but:

- Patients >60 have a 70% 5-year survival post-transplantation, compared with >90% for younger patients, although graft survival is equivalent
- Transplant carries a greater chance of survival than dialysis, in older as in younger patients (around 10 years, compared with 6 years on dialysis for those aged 60–74)

Each individual must be considered separately, taking into account the biological, and not chronological, age. Careful screening for comorbidity will reveal those most likely to benefit, regardless of age. The use of older donors for older recipients could partially redress the imbalance, as the grafts themselves will have a limited lifespan and so be most appropriate for an age-matched recipient. Live organ donation is a rapidly expanding area which may improve kidney availability.

# Nephrotic syndrome

↑ glomerular permeability to protein causes proteinuria (>3g/day), hypoal-buminaemia, generalized oedema, and hyperlipidaemia. There is an ↑ susceptibility to infection, thrombosis, and renal failure.

More common in older people, but often missed as oedema may be attributed to cardiac failure and a low serum albumin to poor nutrition.

▶ Always dipstick the urine for protein in an oedematous patient.

## Causes

Membranous and minimal change nephropathy, glomerulonephritis, and amyloid are common pathologies. Look for associated conditions, including malignancy (e.g. carcinoma, lymphoma), infection (e.g. hepatitis B), systemic disease (e.g. SLE, rheumatoid arthritis, chronic infection), and diabetes. NSAID use may be the only cause.

## Presentation

Frothy urine, anorexia, malaise, muscle wasting, oedema (mobile, depending on gravity—moves from the sacrum and eyelids at night to the legs during the day), and effusions (pleural, pericardial, ascites). BP varies. Patients are prone to intravascular depletion with ↑ total body water, especially when over-diuresed due to assumed cardiac failure.

## Investigations

- Routine blood screen (FBC, U, C+E, glucose, LFTs)
- Urinalysis (high protein:creatinine ratio)
- 24h urinary protein
- ANA, antineutrophil cytoplasmic antibody (ANCA), complement
- Urine and serum electrophoresis, immunoglobulins
- Hepatitis serology
- Renal ultrasound
- Refer to the renal team for possible biopsy

## Treatment

- Usually requires admission and involvement of the renal physician
- Monitor proteinuria, urea and electrolytes, fluid balance, and BP
- Fluid and salt restriction
- Diuretics (e.g. furosemide)
- Prophylactic heparin s/c
- Monitor closely for infection
- Specific treatment with steroids/immunosuppressants after histology known (specialist advice)
- Control of hypertension in diabetic patients

# Glomerulonephritis

- A diffuse inflammatory process involving the glomeruli
- Presents with renal failure, hypertension, oedema, haematuria, red cell casts, and proteinuria
- Older people often present non-specifically (e.g. with nausea, malaise, arthralgia, and pulmonary infiltrates due to vasculitis)

▶ Often misdiagnosed initially, causing delay in treatment. In unwell older people, always dipstick the urine. Think of glomerulonephritis if there is haematuria (see ➲ 'Near-patient urine tests', pp. 618–19).

## Causes

- Post-infectious (usually streptococcal/staphylococcal, 2–6 weeks post-exposure)
- Systemic disease (vasculitis, lupus, Wegener's granulomatosis, Churg–Strauss, Goodpasture's syndrome, Henoch–Schönlein purpura, etc.)
- 1° renal (e.g. IgA nephropathy)
- Unknown aetiology is not uncommon

## Investigations

- As for nephrotic syndrome
- Usually best supervised by a renal physician
- Biopsy required for definitive diagnosis
- Specific investigations for individual causes, e.g. anti-glomerular basement antibodies for Goodpasture's syndrome

## Treatment

- Supportive
- 20% require dialysis
- Steroids can be used for all but post-infectious, so refer early to a renal team to confirm the diagnosis (usually by renal biopsy)

## Outcome

- Worse in older people. More die, and more progress to CKD

# Renal artery stenosis

More common with ↑ age. Usually due to atheroma (as opposed to intimal hyperplasia pathology in younger patients), so patients often have known vascular disease in other areas.

## Diagnosis

Think of renal artery stenosis when:

- Renal function deteriorates after starting an ACE inhibitor. Stopping the drug promptly should reverse the changes
- BP is hard to control
- There is unexplained hypokalaemia (due to low aldosterone levels)
- A renal bruit is heard on clinical examination
- There is a unilateral small kidney seen on imaging
- Flash pulmonary oedema

MRI or CT angiography can be useful in diagnosis as long as renal function allows (contrast contraindicated if eGFR <30ml/min/1.73m$^2$). Digital subtraction angiography is the gold standard and usually precedes stenting.

## Management

As there are often no symptoms, conservative management with BP control and optimizing vascular 2° prevention, but avoiding ACE inhibitors, is often appropriate. If, however, renal function declines or BP cannot be controlled, then percutaneous angioplasty or stent insertion is well tolerated, even in very old people.

# Homeostasis

# Volume depletion and dehydration

An important, common, easily missed clinical condition, especially in older people. Highly prevalent among acutely unwell older people admitted to hospital due to a combination of ↑ fluid loss (fever, gastrointestinal loss) and ↓ intake (nausea, anorexia, weakness).

## Causes

Often multifactorial and include:
- Blood loss
- Diuretics
- Gastrointestinal losses (e.g. diarrhoea, NG drainage)
- Sequestration of fluid (e.g. ileus, burns, peritonitis)
- Poor oral intake
- Fever

## Symptoms and signs

- Thirst is uncommon in older people
- Malaise, apathy, weakness
- Orthostatic symptoms (light-headedness or syncope) and/or postural hypotension. Use passive leg raising for recumbent patients (raise legs by 45° and recheck BP. Improvement suggests volume depletion)
- Nausea, anorexia, vomiting, and oliguria in severe uraemia
- Tachycardia, supine hypotension (late signs, also in *fluid overload*)
- ↓ skin turgor, sunken facies, absence of dependent oedema

The symptoms and signs of clinically important dehydration may be subtle and confusing. It is therefore under-recognized. Continual clinical assessment, assisted by basic tests (urinalysis; U, C+E), is essential. Invasive monitoring or other tests are rarely needed.

Older patients commonly become dehydrated because:
- They are 'run dry' on the wards, as medical (and nursing) staff fear precipitating acute pulmonary oedema through excessive iv fluid administration
- iv infusions often run more slowly than prescribed or cannot run for periods if iv access is lost
- Moderate leg oedema is very poorly specific for heart failure—do not treat this sign alone, in the absence of supporting evidence, with diuretic

▶ Poor urine output on the surgical (or medical) wards is more often a sign of dehydration than of heart failure. Improving urine volume with diuretics is the wrong treatment.

▶ There is no sensitive biochemical marker of dehydration—urea and creatinine are commonly in the normal range and may be abnormal when normally hydrated (e.g. in CKD).

## Challenges to volume status assessment in elderly patients

This can be difficult and requires care.

There is no gold standard in routine clinical examination, although a capillary wedge pressure will give a reliable estimate in ITU/HDU settings.

Most symptoms and signs can occur in both fluid overload and dehydration—use multiple indicators to make an overall decision about volume status.

Use serial assessments, and if the response to treatment is not as anticipated, review your judgement.

### Symptoms
- Thirst is often absent in dehydration
- Confusion can occur in dehydration and fluid overload
- Breathlessness may occur in fluid overload, but also in, e.g. chest sepsis with dehydration

### Signs
- Tachycardia may occur in dehydration (may be absent if there is β- blockade) but also occurs in cardiac failure
- Hypotension similarly occurs both in dehydration and cardiac failure. A postural drop is more likely to indicate dehydration but may also be induced by medication or autonomic dysfunction
- Look at the skin turgor—choose a site away from peripheral oedema, e.g. the forehead. Pinch the skin gently and see how quickly it returns to normal. A sluggish response indicates dehydration
- Check for peripheral oedema—remember that in a bed-bound patient, this may collect in the sacral region. It is possible to have peripheral oedema with intravascular depletion (e.g. in hypoalbuminaemia), so this is not a reliable indicator of fluid state
- Check the JVP, which is elevated in cardiac failure and also in tricuspid regurgitation

### Investigations
- Urine specific gravity may be high in dehydration, and also in heart failure, and is less helpful when diuretics have been used
- Elevated U, C+E often indicate dehydration—check for the patient's baseline, if possible. CKD will also elevate urea and creatinine but is likely to be chronic. Remember that frail older people will have a lower creatinine (perhaps even in the normal range) because of low muscle bulk, but this may still represent a marked abnormality for them
- Elevated Hb may occur in dehydration and in chronic hypoxia

# Dehydration: management

- Treat the underlying cause(s)
- Suspend diuretic and ACE inhibitors
- Continually reassess clinically, assisted by urinalysis/U, C+E. Measure and document intake, output, BP, and weight
- If mild: oral rehydration may suffice. A 'homemade' oral rehydration mixture can be made by adding a level teaspoon of salt and eight level teaspoons of sugar to a litre of water with a touch of fruit juice. Older people may need time, encouragement, and physical assistance with drinking. Enlist relatives and friends to help
- More severe dehydration, or mild dehydration not responding to conservative measures, will require other measures—usually parenteral treatment, either s/c (see ➲ 'HOW TO . . . Administer subcutaneous fluid', p. 405) or iv
- The speed of parenteral fluid administration should be tailored to the individual patient, based on volume of fluid deficit, degree of physiological compromise, and perceived risks of fluid overload. For example, a hypotensive patient who is clinically volume-depleted with evidence of end-organ failure should be fluid-resuscitated briskly, even if there is a history of heart failure. In the absence of end-organ dysfunction, rehydration may proceed more cautiously, but continual reassessment is essential to confirm that the clinical situation remains benign and that progress (input > output) is being made

## HOW TO . . . Administer subcutaneous fluid

This method was widely used in the 1950s but fell into disrepute following reports of adverse effects associated with very hypo-/hypertonic fluid. Fluids that are close to isotonic delivered by competent staff are a safe and effective substitute for iv therapy.

- A simple, widely accessible method for parenteral fluid/electrolytes
- Fluid is administered via a standard giving set and fine (21–23G) butterfly needle into s/c tissue, then draining centrally via lymphatics and veins
- s/c fluid administration should be considered when insertion or maintenance of iv access presents problems, e.g. difficult venous access, persistent extravasation, or lack of staff skills
- iv access is preferred if rapid fluid administration is needed (e.g. gastrointestinal bleed) or if precise control of fluid volume is essential

### Sites of administration

Preferred sites: abdomen, chest (avoid the breast), thigh, and scapula. In agitated patients who can tear out iv (or s/c) lines, sites close to the scapulae may foil their attempts.

### Fluid type

Any crystalloid solution that is approximately isotonic can be used, including normal (0.9%) saline, 5% glucose, and any isotonic combination of glucose–saline. Potassium chloride can be added to the infusion, in concentrations of 20–40mmol/L. If local irritation occurs, change site and/or reduce the concentration of added potassium.

### Infusion rate

Typical flow (and absorption) rate: 1mL/min or 1.5L/day. Infusion pumps may be used. If flow or absorption is slow (leading to lumpy, oedematous areas):

- Change site
- Use two separate infusion sites at the same time
- Using these techniques, up to 2L of fluid daily may be given. For smaller volumes, consider an overnight 'top-up' of 500–1000mL, or two daily boluses of 500mL each (run in over 2–3h), leaving the patient free of infusion lines during daily rehabilitation/activity. Some patients need only 1L/alternate nights to maintain hydration

### Monitoring

Patients should be monitored clinically (hydration state, input/output, weight) and biochemically as they would if they were receiving iv fluid.

▶ Be responsive and creative in your prescriptions of fluid and electrolytes. One size does not fit all.

### Potential complications

Rare and usually mild. They include local infection and local adverse reactions to hypertonic fluid (e.g. with added potassium).

### Contraindications

- Exercise caution in thrombocytopenia or coagulopathy
- s/c infusion is not appropriate in patients who need rapid volume repletion

# Hyponatraemia: assessment

A common problem. May be safely monitored, rather than treated, if modest in severity ([Na] >125mmol/L), stable, and without side effects, and if there is an identifiable (often drug) cause.

## Clinical features

- Subtle or absent in mild cases
- [Na] = 115–125mmol/L: lethargy, confusion, altered personality
- At [Na] <115mmol/L: delirium, coma, seizures, and death

## Causes

Iatrogenic causes are the most common. Acute onset, certain drugs, or recent iv fluids make iatrogenesis especially likely.

Important causes include:

- Drugs. Many are implicated (see Box 14.1)
- Excess water administration—either NG (rarely po) or iv (5% glucose)
- Failure of heart, liver, thyroid, kidneys
- Stress response, e.g. after trauma or surgery, exacerbated by iv colloid or 5% glucose
- Hypoadrenalism: steroid withdrawal or Addison's disease
- Syndrome of inappropriate antidiuretic hormone secretion (SIADH)

In older people, multiple causes are common, e.g. heart failure, diuretics, and acute diarrhoea.

## Approach

Take a careful drug history, including those stopped in the past few weeks. Examine to determine evidence of the cause and volume status (JVP, postural BP, pulmonary oedema, ankle/sacral oedema, peripheral perfusion).

## Investigations

Clinical history and examination, urine, and blood biochemistry are usually all that are needed. Ensure that the sample was not delayed in transit or taken from a drip arm. If genuine hyponatraemia, take:

- Blood for creatinine, osmolarity, TFTs, LFTs, glucose, random cortisol
- Spot urine sample for sodium and osmolarity

Consider a short adrenocorticotropic hormone (ACTH) test to exclude hypoadrenalism, particularly if the patient is volume-depleted and hyperkalaemic (see ➲ 'HOW TO . . . Perform a short ACTH stimulation test (short Synacthen® test)', p. 411).

# Hyponatraemia: treatment

(See Box 14.1 and Fig. 14.1.)
- Combine normalization of sodium with correction of fluid volume and treating underlying cause(s)
- The rate of correction of hyponatraemia should not be too rapid. Usually, correction to the lower limit of the normal range (~130mmol/L) should be achieved in a few days. Maximum correction in any 24h period should be <10mmol/L. Full correction can reasonably take weeks
- Acute, severe hyponatraemia with moderate/severe symptoms such as seizures, should be considered for treatment with hypertonic saline to reduce the risk of complications
- Rapid correction risks central pontine myelinolysis (leading to quadriparesis and cranial nerve abnormalities) and is indicated only when hyponatraemia is severe and the patient critically unwell

▶ By definition, hyponatraemia is a low blood sodium concentration. Therefore, a low level may be a result of low sodium, high water, or both. Dehydration and hyponatraemia may coexist if sodium depletion exceeds water depletion. This is common—do not worsen the dehydration by fluid-restricting these patients.

### Box 14.1 Drugs and hyponatraemia
- Most commonly diuretics (especially in high dose or combination), SSRIs, carbamazepine, NSAIDs
- Other drugs include opiates, other antidepressants (MAOIs, tricyclic antidepressants), other anticonvulsants (e.g. valproate), oral hypoglycaemics (sulfonylureas, e.g. glipizide), PPIs, ACE inhibitors, and barbiturates
- Combinations of drugs (e.g. diuretic and SSRI) are especially likely to cause hyponatraemia
- If hyponatraemia is problematic and the treatment is needed, consider other drugs that are less likely to cause a low sodium (e.g. mirtazapine for depression)

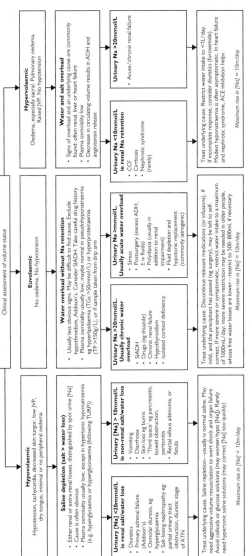

Clinical assessment of volume status

**Hypovolaemic**
Hypotension, tachycardia, decreased skin turgor, low JVP, dry tongue, minimal or no peripheral oedema

**Saline depletion (salt > water loss)**
- Either renal or extra-renal losses, distinguished by spot urine [Na]
- Cause is often obvious
- Plasma osmolality usually low, except in hypertonic hyponatraemia (e.g. hyperglycaemia or hyperglycinaemia (following TURP))

**Urinary [Na] <20mmol/L ie renal salt/water loss**
- Diuretics
- Primary adrenal failure (Addison's)
- Osmolar diuresis, eg: hyperglycaemia
- Salt-losing nephropathy eg: partial urinary tract obstruction, diuretic stage of ATN

**Urinary [Na] > 10mmol/L ie non-renal salt/water loss**
- Vomiting
- Diarrhoea
- Skin loss eg burns
- 'Third space' eg pancreatitis, bowel obstruction, peritonitis
- Rectal villous adenoma, or fistula

Treat underlying cause. Saline repletion—usually with normal saline. May need aggressive volume resuscitation to avert shock and organ failure. Avoid colloids or glucose solutions (may worsen hypo [Na]). Rarely need hypertonic saline solutions (may correct [Na] too quickly)

*Maximum rise in [Na] = 10m/day*

**Euvolaemic**
No oedema. No hypotension

**Water overload without Na retention**
- Usually less obvious signs. May be difficult to find cause. Exclude hypothyroidism, Addison's. Consider SIADH. Take careful drug history
- Plasma osmolality usually low; maybe normal in pseudohyponatraemia eg hyperlipidaemia (TGs >50mmol/L) or hyperproteinaemia (TP >150g/L), or if sample taken from drip arm

**Urinary Na >20mmol/L Usually chronic water overload**
- SIADH
- Drugs (eg thiazide)
- Chronic renal failure
- Hypothyroidism
- Isolated cortisol deficiency

**Urinary Na >mmol/L Usually acute water overload**
- Stress
- Postsurgery (excess ADH, ± iv fluids)
- Polydipsia (usually in addition to renal impairment)
- Fluid depletion and hypotonic replacement (commonly iatrogenic)

Treat underlying cause. Discontinue relevant medications (or infusions). If mild, and the precipitant has passed (eg surgery), may be left to self-correct. If more severe or symptomatic, restrict water intake to a maximum of 1000mL/day; more severe restriction may be needed in older people, whose free water losses are lower—restrict to 500-800mL if necessary

*Maximum rise in [Na] = 10m/day*

**Hypervolaemic**
Oedema, especially sacral. Pulmonary oedema. Raised JVP. No hypotension

**Water and salt overload**
- Signs of overload and an underlying cause are commonly found: often renal, liver or heart failure
- Plasma osmolality low
- Decrease in circulating volume results in ADH and angiotensin release

**Urinary Na <10mmol/L ie renal Na retention**
- CCF
- Cirrhosis
- Nephrotic syndrome (rarely)

**Urinary Na >20mmol/L**
- Acute/chronic renal failure

Treat underlying cause. Restrict water intake to <1L/day. If incomplete response, consider diuretics (furosemide). Modest hyponatraemia is often asymptomatic. In heart failure and nephrotic syndrome, ACE inhibition helps

*Maximum rise in [Na] = 10m/day*

Fig. 14.1 Hyponatraemia: aetiology and treatment. TG, triglyceride; TP, turgor pressure; TURP, transurethral resection of the prostrate.

# Syndrome of inappropriate antidiuretic hormone secretion

### Definition
Less than maximally dilute (i.e. inappropriately concentrated) urine in the presence of subclinical excess body water.

▶ SIADH is massively over-diagnosed, especially in older people, leading to inappropriate fluid restriction. Consider it a diagnosis of exclusion—drugs or organ impairment cause a similar clinical syndrome.

### Diagnosis
Essential features include:
- Hypotonic hyponatraemia ([Na] <125mmol/L and plasma osmolarity <260mOsm/L)
- Normal volume status, i.e. euvolaemia—there is slight water overload, but not clinically identifiable
- Normal renal, thyroid, hepatic, cardiac, and adrenal function
- Inappropriately concentrated, salty urine: osmolarity >200mOsm/L and [Na] >20mmol/L)
- No diuretics, or ADH-modulating drugs (opiates, anticonvulsants, antidepressants, NSAIDs, barbiturates, and oral hypoglycaemics). Drug effects may take days or weeks to diminish

### Causes
Common causes include:
- Surgical stress
- Neoplasms (especially bronchogenic, pancreatic)
- CNS disease (especially trauma, subdural haematoma, stroke, meningoencephalitis)
- Lung disease (TB, pneumonia, bronchiectasis)
- Some drugs cause low sodium by an SIADH-like effect, but this is not the true syndrome

### Treatment
- Treat the underlying cause
- If mild, and the precipitant has passed (e.g. surgery), may be left to self-correct
- If more severe and/or symptomatic, restrict water intake to a maximum of 1000mL/day; more severe restriction may be needed in older people whose free water losses are lower—restrict to 500–800mL, if necessary
- Drug treatments are generally reserved for refractory cases or where fluid restriction is not tolerated. Demeclocycline acts by blocking the renal tubular effect of ADH and is first line. Vasopressin receptor antagonists can also be used (e.g. tolvaptan)

## HOW TO . . . Perform a short ACTH stimulation test (short Synacthen® test)

The diagnosis of adrenocortical insufficiency is made when the adrenal cortex is found not to synthesize cortisol despite adequate stimulation. Within 30min of ACTH stimulation, the normal adrenal releases several times its basal cortisol output.

*Performing the test*
- The test can be done at any time of the day
- Steroid treatment (e.g. prednisolone) may invalidate results; these should be stopped at least 24h before the test. Oestrogens should also be suspended
- Take blood for baseline cortisol. Label the tube with patient identifiers and the time taken
- Give 250 micrograms of Synacthen® (synthetic ACTH, 1-24 amino acid sequence). Give iv if iv access is present; otherwise im
- Thirty minutes after injection, take more blood for cortisol. Label the tube with patient identifiers and the time taken

*Interpreting the test*
A normal response meets three criteria:
- Baseline cortisol level >150nmol/L
- 30min cortisol >500nmol/L
- 30min cortisol greater than baseline cortisol by 200nmol/L or more

The absolute 30min cortisol carries more significance than the baseline–30min increment, especially in patients who are stressed (ill) and at maximal adrenal output.

A normal Synacthen® test excludes Addison's disease. If the test is not normal:
- Consider further tests, such as the prolonged ACTH stimulation test, usually after specialist advice, e.g.:
  - ACTH level (elevated in 1°, and low in 2°, hypoadrenalism)
  - The prolonged ACTH stimulation test
- If the patient is very unwell, give hydrocortisone 100mg iv, pending confirmation of hypoadrenalism

# Hypernatraemia

## Causes
- Usually due to true 'dehydration', i.e. water loss > sodium loss
- Not enough water in, or too much water out, or a combination, e.g. poor oral intake, diarrhoea, vomiting, diuretics, uncontrolled diabetes mellitus
- Rarely due to salt excess—iatrogenic (iv or po), psychogenic, or malicious (poisoning)
- Very rarely due to diabetes insipidus (urine osmolarity low) or mineralocorticoid excess (Conn's syndrome)

Commonly seen in older people with sepsis: ↑ losses (sweating), reduced oral intake, and reduced renal concentrating (water-conserving) mechanism.

## Clinical features
- Hypotension (supine and/or orthostatic)
- Sunken features
- Urine scanty and concentrated
- Lethargy, confusion, coma, and fits

## Tests
Urea and creatinine are often high but may be in the high normal range; the patient is still water-depleted. Potassium is low in Conn's. Hb and albumin are often high (haemoconcentration), correcting with treatment.

## Treatment
- Encourage oral fluid
- Usually iv fluid is required; rarely s/c fluid will be sufficient
- Fluid infusion rates should not be too cautious, e.g. 3L/24h is reasonable, guided by clinical and biochemical response. Too rapid infusions risk cerebral oedema, especially in the more chronically hypernatraemic patient
- Ensure the patient becomes clinically euvolaemic, as well as normo-natraemic—most dehydrated patients have a normal [Na] and will correct into the normal range before the patient is fully hydrated
- Many patients are sodium-deplete, as well as water-deplete; therefore, consider alternating normal saline with 5% glucose infusions

▶ Even mild hypernatraemia is usually clinically important and needs attention.

# Hypothermia: diagnosis

A common medical emergency in older people, occurring both in and out of hospital.

### Definition

- Core temperature <35°C, but <35.5°C is probably abnormal
- Mild: 32–35°C; moderate: 30–32°C; severe: <30°C
- Fatality is high and correlates with severity of associated illness

### Causes

Often multifactorial.

- Illness (drugs, fall, sepsis)
- Defective homeostasis (failure of autonomic nervous system-induced shivering and vasoconstriction; ↓ muscle mass)
- Cold exposure (clothing, defective temperature discrimination, climate, poverty)

In established hypothermia, thermoregulation is further impaired and is effectively poikilothermic (temperature varies with the environment).

▶ Hypothermia is a common presentation of sepsis in hospital in older people, and probably an indicator of poor prognosis. Do not ignore the temperature chart.

### Diagnosis

Rectal temperature is the gold standard, but well-taken oral or tympanic temperature will suffice.

Ensure the thermometer range includes low temperatures (mercury-in-glass thermometer range usually 34–42°C, thereby underestimating severity in all but the mildest cases).

### Presentation

Often insidious and non-specific. The patient will frequently not complain of feeling cold. Multiple systems affected.

- *Skin*: may be cold to touch (paradoxically warm if defective vasoconstriction). Shivering is unusual (this occurs early in the cooling process). There may be ↑ muscle tone, skin oedema, erythema, or bullae
- *Nervous system*: signs can mimic stroke with falls, unsteadiness, weakness, slow speech, and ataxia. Reflexes may be depressed or exaggerated, with an abnormal plantar response and dilated, sluggish pupils. Conscious level ranges from confused/sleepy to coma. Seizures and focal signs can occur
- *Cardiovascular system*:
  - Initially vasoconstriction, hypertension, and tachycardia
  - Then myocardial suppression, hypotension, sinus bradycardia
  - Eventually extreme bradycardia, bradypnoea, and hypotension. May lead to false diagnosis of death; however, the protective effect of cold on vital organs means survival may be possible
  - Dysrhythmias include AF (early), VF, and asystole (late)
- *Renal*: there is early diuresis, with later oliguria and ATN

- *Respiratory*: respiratory depression and cough suppression occur with 2° atelectasis and pneumonia. Pulmonary oedema and ARDS occur late
- *Gastrointestinal*: hypomotility may lead to ileus, gastric dilation, and vomiting. Hepatic metabolism is reduced (including of drugs). There is a risk of pancreatitis with hypo- or hyperglycaemia
- *Other*: disseminated intravascular coagulation (DIC), pressure injuries, and rhabdomyolysis

## Investigations
- FBC, ESR
- U, C+E
- Glucose
- Amylase
- CRP
- LFTs
- TFTs
- Blood culture
- Drug/toxin screen
- CK and urinalysis (may show rhabdomyolysis)
- ABGs (looking for metabolic and respiratory acidosis and lactate. Do not correct for temperature)
- ECG (abnormalities include prolonged PR interval, J waves (peak between QRS and T in leads V4–6) at <30°C, and dysrhythmia)
- Serum cortisol (consider if there are features of hypoadrenalism or hypothermia is unexplained or recurrent)

▶ It is important to repeat key investigations during rewarming, e.g. U, C+E, ECG, and ABGs.

# Hypothermia: management

## Monitoring
Regular BP, pulse, temperature, respiratory rate, oxygen saturation, and glucose; continuous ECG; consider urinary catheter. Consider ITU.

## Treatment principles
- Mild hypothermia should be managed with gentle warming and close monitoring
- The features of severe hypothermia may mimic those of death. Begin resuscitation while gathering information that permits a decision as to whether further intervention is likely to be futile or else not in the patient's interests. Stop resuscitation according to clinical judgement; generally do not declare dead until re-warmed or re-warming fails
- Re-warming: rate should approximate that of onset (0.5–1°C/h if not critically unwell). Caution, as re-warming may lead to hypotension. A combination of the following modalities is usually sufficient:
  - Passive external: surround with dry clothes and blankets/space blankets
  - Active external: hot air blanket ('Bair Hugger™'), hot water bottle, bath
  - Active internal: heated oxygen, fluid, and food
- System support: maintain airway, ventilate as necessary. Good iv access. Warm iv fluid: may need large volumes as warming causes vasodilatation. Treat organ dysfunction as appropriate. Cardiac pacing only if bradycardia is disproportionate to reduced metabolic rate
- If severe, or multiple organ failure, consider ITU. Handle carefully—rough handling and procedures (including intubation) may precipitate VF

Sudden, severe hypothermia ± cardiac arrest (e.g. due to water immersion) is uncommon in older people. If it occurs, manage in the usual way with rapid, invasive re-warming, supported by ITU.

## Drug treatment
Consider:
- Empirical antibiotics (most have evidence of infection on careful serial assessment)
- Adrenal insufficiency (treatment: hydrocortisone 100mg qds)
- Hypothyroidism (treatment: liothyronine 50 micrograms, then 25 micrograms tds iv, always with hydrocortisone)
- Thiamine deficiency (malnourished or alcoholic) (treatment: B vitamins oral or iv) (as Pabrinex®)

Drug metabolism is reduced, and accumulation can occur. Efficacy at the site of action is also reduced. Exercise caution with s/c and im drugs (including insulin) that may accumulate and be mobilized rapidly as perfusion improves.

## Prevention
Before discharge, establish why this episode occurred—is recurrence likely? (Consider housing, cognition, hypoglycaemia, sepsis, etc.) Consider how further episodes may be prevented or terminated early.

## HOW TO ... Monitor temperature

No method is absolutely precise.
- Traditional mercury-in-glass thermometers are now rarely used in hospital, having been replaced due to risks to patients, staff, and the public
- Digital electronic and infrared thermometers can provide reliable results when used correctly and in accordance with the manufacturer's instructions
- Thermochromic (forehead) thermometers are imprecise, although they may be useful for screening or with uncooperative patients

*Digital electronic thermometers*

These may permit oral, axillary, or rectal measurement. They typically require a small period of equilibration and patient compliance.

*Infrared ('tympanic') thermometers*

These measure the temperature of tissue within, and close to, the eardrum, returning a value rapidly. Ensure that the earlobe is gently pulled posteriorly and superiorly, straightening the external ear canal, before inserting the probe fairly firmly.

Ear wax has only a slight effect, reducing measured temperature by <0.5°C.

Note that tympanic thermometers may offer a choice of displaying temperature as either 'true tympanic' or the derived value 'oral equivalent'. Ensure that you are familiar with the thermometer in use in your hospital and what output they give—tympanic or 'oral equivalent'.

*Measurement in practice*

- Precise temperature measurement is fundamental to detecting and monitoring disease
- Fever may be due to infection, malignancy, inflammation, connective tissue disease, or drugs
- A reduced or absent fever response to sepsis is seen in some elderly patients. Do not dismiss modest fever (<37.5°C) as insignificant or rule out infection because the patient is afebrile
- Hypothermia occurs inside and outside hospital and may be missed, unless thermometers with an appropriate range (30–40°C) are used
- Temperature varies continuously—lowest in peripheral skin, highest in the central vessels and brain. No site is truly representative of the 'core' temperature. Typically, when compared with oral temperature, axillary temperatures are 1.0°C lower, and rectal and tympanic temperatures 0.5–1.0°C higher (but see notes on tympanic thermometry, also in this box)
- Where clinical suspicion is high, make measurements yourself, complementing monitoring by nursing staff. Body temperature changes continuously, and a fever may manifest only after the patient has re-warmed following a cooling ambulance journey
- The hand on the forehead to assess core temperature (and on the palm of the hand to determine peripheral vasodilation) is of value in screening for sepsis and can be incorporated into daily rounds without time penalty

# Heat-related illness

An important cause of morbidity and mortality in older people, but the risk is much less appreciated than that of hypothermia. The contribution of heat stress to death is rarely mentioned on death certificates, but epidemiological studies indicate significant excess morbidity and mortality during extended periods of unaccustomed hot weather (e.g. France 2003: 15 000 excess deaths). There is an ↑ incidence of acute cerebrovascular, respiratory, and especially cardiovascular disease.

## Risk factors

- Consider older people as being relatively poikilothermic, i.e. lacking close control of body temperature in some circumstances
- Homeostasis is weakened due to raised sweating threshold, reduced sweat volume, altered vasomotor control, and behavioural factors (lessened sensation of temperature extremes)
- Climate: high temperature, high radiant heat (sitting in sunshine, indoors or out), high humidity
- Drugs, e.g. diuretics, anticholinergics, psychotropics
- Comorbidity: frailty, cerebrovascular and cardiovascular disease

## A spectrum of illness

The presentation is usually different in older people, typically occurring not after extreme exertion, but during heatwaves in temperate zones.

- *Prickly heat ('miliaria')*: itchy, erythematous, papular rash. Treatment: cool, wash, antihistamines
- *Heat oedema*: peripheral oedema, usually self-limiting
- *Heat syncope*: ↑ syncope risk due to fluid depletion and vasodilation
- *Heat exhaustion*: is a potentially catastrophic illness. Dehydration and heat stress leads to non-specific presentation with collapse, immobility, weakness, vomiting, dizziness, headache, fever, and tachycardia. However, treatment should result in rapid improvement
- *Heat stroke* occurs when untreated heat exhaustion progresses to its end-stage (hyperthermic thermoregulatory failure). Core temperature is generally >40°C; mental state is altered (confusion → coma); circulatory and other organ failure is common, and sweating is often absent. CNS changes may be persistent and severe. Prognosis reflects pre-existing comorbidity, severity, and complications, and is often poor

## Management

- *Individual response*. Emergency inpatient treatment required. Identify and reverse precipitants. Cool rapidly until temperature 38–39°C— fan, tepid sponging, remove clothing. Close monitoring (temperature, BP, pulse saturation, urine output); consider invasive central venous pressure monitoring. Cool iv fluids according to assessment of fluid/electrolyte status
- *Community response*. Local environment modification—fans, air conditioning, shade windows, open windows at night, seek cooler areas, avoid exercise, maintain or ↑ cool fluid intake, light/loose clothing. Education of patient and carers. Governments should have public health measures in place to reduce the impact of heat waves

# Endocrinology

# The ageing endocrine system

### Ageing and thyroid function

Normal thyroid function is preserved in healthy older people. Median TSH levels drift upwards very slowly with age but remain within normal limits in the absence of disease. Lower T3 and TSH levels seen in institutionalized older people and in very advanced old age (>95 years) are probably due to illness.

### Sick euthyroid syndrome

- TFTs are often abnormal in euthyroid patients who are ill with non-thyroid systemic disease; this reverses spontaneously when the underlying illness improves

▶ Do not automatically initiate thyroid treatment changes.

- Changes depend on illness severity and when TFTs are checked (during acute illness or recovery)
- TSH secretion ↓ early in the illness. Falls in T4 and (especially) T3 may follow, the result of reduced TSH, lower thyroid hormone binding, and reduced peripheral T4 → T3 conversion
- Changes are more likely due to true hypothyroidism if:
  - Free T4 levels are low
  - Changes are severe
- 2° hypothyroidism (due to hypothalamo-pituitary failure) causes a similar pattern of TFTs but is very much less common, and other features of pituitary failure are present (e.g. hypogonadism)
- In the convalescent phase following illness, TSH may be elevated as low thyroid hormone levels drive TSH production. For a time, TSH may be high and T4/T3 low, mimicking 1° hypothyroidism. TFTs repeated a few weeks later are usually normal

### Ageing and glucose metabolism

In older people:
- Glucose-induced insulin release is delayed and reduced in size
- Insulin-induced suppression of hepatic glucose production is delayed
- Insulin-mediated peripheral (muscle and fat) glucose uptake is reduced

In addition to reductions in physical activity and lean muscle mass, the factors listed here lead to higher frequency of impaired glucose tolerance (IGT) with age. IGT is associated with macrovascular disease, but not with specific diabetic complications. A minority of people with IGT progress to diabetes.

### Other hormone systems

There are complex changes in the hypothalamo-pituitary-adrenal axis, but little impact on function of the adrenal gland.

All sex hormones ↓ with age. The impact of this is well recognized in ♀ (menopause) and, to a lesser degree, in men.

Changes in growth hormone and other growth factors may have a role in altering muscle, fat, protein synthesis, and lean body mass, contributing to sarcopenia and frailty.

# Diabetes mellitus

Diabetes is much more common with age—about 40% of new diagnoses are in people over 65. Prevalence in people aged 70–79 is 24% in the UK, up to 50% in some ethnic groups and obese patients. It is estimated that 5 million people in the UK will have diabetes by 2025 (a mixture of population ageing and ↑ obesity).

## Comparing type 1 and type 2 diabetes

- Both type 1 (insulin-dependent; IDDM) and type 2 (non-insulin dependent; NIDDM) diabetes can occur in older people. The prevalence of type 2 is much higher
- In overweight older people, diabetes is mostly due to peripheral tissue insulin resistance (type 2). Glucose-induced insulin release is normal
- Lean older people with diabetes often have impaired insulin release and may have islet cell antibodies more typical of type 1 diabetes. They respond poorly to oral hypoglycaemics
- There are ↑ numbers of older people with type 1 diabetes who developed the disease in early or mid-life and have survived decades on insulin, sometimes with no or few complications
- Many people with type 2 diabetes progress to require insulin to achieve acceptable glycaemic control. This group is insulin-requiring (hence IRDM) and are unlikely to develop ketoacidosis if insulin is withdrawn
- When assessing a patient on insulin, determine whether they are insulin-dependent (type 1; must always have background insulin infused) or insulin-requiring (type 2; in which insulin may safely be withheld for a time, without risk of ketosis)

## Secondary diabetes

More common in older people. Causes include:

- Drugs. Often steroids, sometimes high-dose thiazides, rarely other drugs
- Pancreatic disease, e.g. chronic pancreatitis
- Other endocrine diseases, e.g. Cushing's, hyperthyroidism

## Presentation

- Diabetes often presents atypically or late in older people
- Up to 50% of older people with diabetes are undiagnosed. This is at least partly due to physiological age-related changes, e.g. the renal threshold for glucose ↑ (glucosuria and polyuria occur later) and the thirst mechanism is impaired (polydipsia occurs later)
- The diagnosis is often made by screening blood or urine tests, or during intercurrent illness
- Think of diabetes in many clinical circumstances, e.g. coma, delirium, systemic stress (e.g. sepsis), oral or vaginal thrush (candida), vulval itch (subclinical candida), cellulitis and necrotizing fasciitis, weight loss, urinary incontinence, polyuria, malaise, vascular disease, or peripheral neuropathy
- Steroid administration may reveal a diabetic tendency—always monitor, especially when high doses are used

## HOW TO . . . Diagnose diabetes in older people

- Confirm the diagnosis with a random blood sugar or fasting sugar. Criteria are the same as for younger patients
- In general, the diagnosis is confirmed with a second measurement, unless the diagnosis is clear (e.g. severe hyperglycaemia with metabolic decompensation). A single high measurement in the absence of symptoms is not diagnostic
- In some older diabetic people, fasting sugars may be normal. This is more common in lean older people, who have only postprandial hyperglycaemia. If in doubt, do an oral glucose tolerance test
- Elevated HbA$_{1c}$ levels can now be used to make the diagnosis, but a normal level does not exclude the diagnosis
- Test annually in those with risk factors (e.g. family history, obesity)

*Diagnostic criteria*

At least one of the following criteria must apply:

- Symptoms + *random plasma glucose* >11.1mmol
- *Fasting plasma glucose* >7.0mmol
- 2h plasma glucose >11.1mmol during *oral glucose tolerance test* (75g anhydrous glucose or the equivalent volume of a proprietary glucose drink such as Lucozade)
- Elevated HbA$_{1c}$ levels (>48mmol/mol or 6.5%)

*Obtaining a fasting blood sugar*

- Give the completed request card to the patient
- The patient should make an early morning appointment with a phlebotomist or GP nurse
- There must be no caloric intake for at least 8h before the blood test
  - Tell the patient to go for the blood test before breakfast
  - Clear fluids (water; tea or coffee without milk or sugar) may be taken
  - Other beverages or food must be avoided

# Diabetes: treatment

- In all patients, aim to avoid symptoms of hyper- and hypoglycaemia
- In the more robust older patient, good glycaemic control probably reduces complication rates:
  - Aim for HbA$_{1c}$ levels of around 6.5–7.5% and fasting sugar of 5–7mmol/L
- Frail patients and the very old (>80 years) have not been included in most prospective treatment studies. There is therefore doubt whether tight glycaemic control improves long-term outcome
  - Balance the potential benefits of tight control with the risk of drug-induced symptomatic hypoglycaemia, confusion, falls, and fractures
  - Symptoms of hypoglycaemia may go unrecognized or be considered an ageing change by carers
  - Reasonable targets for the frail are HbA$_{1c}$ 7.5–8.5% and fasting sugar 7–10mmol/L
  - Vulnerable older patients are probably at higher risk of hypoglycaemia (e.g. causing confusion and falls) than hyperglycaemia. In some circumstances (e.g. where glucose levels appear very variable), it may be safest to accept very high ceiling levels (e.g. up to 20mmol/L), although persistent levels above 15mmol/L may predispose to infection

▶ In general, in frail older people, the approach is to reduce symptoms, not to normalize sugars.

## Diet

- Dietary change is often the only treatment needed in obese people with type 2 diabetes
- Wholesale changes to diet may not be accepted, but even small changes are worthwhile and, on their own, can result in much ↑ insulin sensitivity within weeks
- Full compliance may not be possible for the functionally or cognitively impaired, but an experienced dietician or nurse working with the patient and family is usually effective
- Severe dietary restrictions are often not appropriate, especially for the very old or very frail
- Beware the strict diet that takes enjoyment from (the last months of) life while giving little back

## Education

- Educate the family, carers, and nursing home staff continually
- Provide simple written information and instructions
- The approach must be tailored to the individual, taking note of cognitive and sensory impairments

## Other interventions

- Exercise, especially endurance exercise (e.g. walking, cycling), improves insulin sensitivity
- Weight loss. Even modest reductions are beneficial
- Reduction of other vascular risk factors, including smoking
- Home or pendant alarm systems in case of hypoglycaemia

## Disease surveillance

Patients should be encouraged to take control of their own diabetes and facilitated to monitor their own blood sugars. In addition, they should be reviewed at least annually. In the very frail or dependent, regular reviews remain vital, e.g. to ensure that treatments remain appropriate and that adverse effects have not occurred.

- Assess diet/drug adherence
- Check weight
- Optimize cardiovascular risk factors, including BP and lipids
- Assess glycaemic control. Blood glucose testing, supplemented by 6-monthly $HbA_{1c}$ estimation, is the preferred method. Urine glucose testing is less reliable, due to ↑ renal glucose threshold
- Examine for evidence of complications, including microalbuminuria, an early sign of nephropathy
- Ensure regular retinal screening is in place
- Check the feet and advise on their care (see ➲ 'The elderly foot', pp. 492–3)

▶ Utilize the advice and support of nursing staff with specialist knowledge of diabetes—either community nurses with a special interest or dedicated diabetes specialist nurses.

# Diabetes: oral drug treatment

### Biguanides

For example: metformin (start at 500mg od)

- Commonly used as first-line drug therapy in obese (BMI >25), elderly patients (where insulin resistance predominates)
- Do not cause hypoglycaemia
- Common side effects are nausea, diarrhoea, anorexia, and weight loss. These are less common if the drug is introduced slowly
- Can cause lactic acidosis in patients with hepatic or renal impairment, or where tissue hypoxia ↑ lactate production
  - Use cautiously in patients with kidney impairment (avoided if eGFR <30), hepatic impairment, or heart failure (even if treated). Age itself is not a contraindication
  - Stop in acutely unwell patients (especially with AKI, sepsis, respiratory failure, heart failure, or MI)
  - Discontinue before the administration of radiographic contrast media, restarting if/when renal function normalizes

### Sulfonylureas

For example: gliclazide (start at 40mg od)

- Commonly used as first-line drug therapy in lean elderly patients (where impairment in insulin release predominates)
- Can cause hypoglycaemia. This is uncommon if short-acting agents (gliclazide, glipizide, tolbutamide) are used. Avoid long-acting drugs (glibenclamide) which can cause prolonged and damaging hypoglycaemia. In patients taking these (often for years without problems), consider a switch to shorter-acting drugs
- Commonly cause weight gain

### Dipeptidyl peptidase-4 inhibitor (DPP-4)

For example: sitagliptin (start at 50mg od)

- Usually prescribed for people who have not responded to first-line agents; given as an intensification
- Effective in older people; do not cause hypoglycaemia

### Thiazolidinediones

For example: pioglitazone (start at 30mg od)

- Effective in older people; do not cause hypoglycaemia
- Usually used as part of triple therapy to avoid introducing insulin
- LFTs must be monitored, initially 2-monthly. Stop if dysfunction occurs
- Can be used in mild/moderate renal failure. Avoid in heart failure. Doubles the risk of bone fracture in women

### Other classes

For example: glucagon-like peptide-1 (GLP-1) mimetics, sodium–glucose co-transporter-2 (SGLT-2) inhibitors

- Should be initiated by diabetes specialists

## HOW TO . . . Manage older diabetic people in care homes

In care homes:
- The prevalence of diabetes is very high
- Individual diabetic patients are at great risk of complications
- Hypoglycaemia and other medication side effects are frequent

To enhance quality of care:
- Every resident should be screened for diabetes on admission to the home and each year thereafter. Blood sampling is far more sensitive than urinalysis
- Every resident with diabetes should have an individual care plan including at least: diet, medications, glycaemic targets, and monitoring schedule. Monitoring should be varied in time (pre-/postprandial; breakfast, lunch, evening meal, late evening), to provide a more complete picture of glycaemic control
- Diabetic diets should be available
- An annual diabetes review should be performed by either a nurse with specialist training in diabetes, a GP, or a specialist (geriatrician or diabetologist)
- An annual ophthalmic screening assessment should be performed. Rarely, domiciliary screening is available. Usually, the resident will need to leave the home to attend a specialist screening centre, but this is usually worthwhile as vision contributes significantly to quality of life
- There should be easy access to specialist services, including podiatry, optometry, diabetic foot clinic, dietetics, and diabetes specialist nursing
- Each home with diabetic residents should have a diabetes care policy. Staff should have received training in the identification and treatment of diabetic emergencies and the prevention of complications

## Further reading

Diabetes UK (2010). *Good Clinical Practice Guidelines for Care Home Residents with Diabetes.* London: Diabetes UK.

# Diabetes: insulin treatment

- Insulin is essential for the treatment of type 1 diabetes
- Insulin is started in type 2 diabetes when oral agents fail to achieve adequate control, if hyperglycaemia is severe (especially if the patient is lean, and insulin deficiency likely), if a patient is unwell, and if oral drugs are contraindicated (e.g. hepatorenal impairment)
- Side effects include:
  - *Weight gain*. Common. Lessened if an oral drug (especially metformin) is co-prescribed
  - *Hypoglycaemia*. Much more common with insulin than with any oral agent

## Insulin regimens

- Increasingly initiate treatment with long-acting insulins (insulin glargine and insulin detemir) which are effective if given just once daily. These are particularly helpful in those who:
  - Require assistance (relative, nurse) with injections
  - Are frequently hypoglycaemic on other regimens, especially at night
  - Would otherwise need twice-daily insulin injections plus oral drugs
- Alternative strategies, e.g. twice-daily insulin injections with pre-mixed insulins (e.g. Humalog® Mix 25) are rarely initiated now, but some older patients have been stable for years on such treatment, so there is no advantage in changing
- Daily long-acting insulin once daily can be supplemented by oral hypoglycaemics during the day
- If eating is very erratic, consider giving short-acting insulin after each meal, based on what has been eaten—a simple sliding scale
- Regimens based on rapid-acting insulin alone or a basal-bolus structure (the mainstay of management in younger patients with type 1 diabetes; provide an insulin profile as close to health as possible), are rarely appropriate in older people, unless lifestyle (meals and activity) are especially chaotic and the patient has the cognitive and physical ability to manage dosing

## Initiating insulin

- Involve the MDT (especially the diabetic nurse specialist)
- If the patient is likely to need professional support to administer insulin, then also involve community teams—insulin administration may be very time-consuming for them
- Patients may be very reluctant to begin, because of fears about injections, hypos, or learning new skills
- Remember insulin administration issues: cognition, dexterity, and vision
- Pre-mixed insulins avoid having to draw up multiple types of insulin
- Insulin pens make the measuring of doses much easier for patients, but syringes are more suitable when insulin is drawn up by a third party (relative or nurse)
- Pens have been adapted to make delivery easier for the less dextrous, e.g. preloaded vials, large dials for dosing

- Some patients are able to self-inject but cannot safely draw up insulin into syringes or use an insulin pen. In this case, doses may be drawn up in syringes by relatives or the community nurse and stored in a refrigerator until needed
- If insulin is given by a relative, what happens during family holidays?

## Changing insulin requirements

- Always consider whether your patient is on the correct insulin regimen (type and dose)
- Earlier in the course of the disease, insulin requirements often rise as disease severity ↑
- In advanced old age, insulin requirements often fall as appetite declines, body weight drops, and renal function deteriorates. Type 2 diabetic patients on insulin may get off insulin altogether. Stop insulin, maximize oral drug treatment, and monitor regularly
- Dying patients can often have treatment withdrawn (see ➋ 'HOW TO . . . Manage diabetes in the terminally ill patient', p. 434)

# Diabetes: complications

In general, these are more common in older people, especially vascular complications. Evidence for risk reduction in very old diabetic patients is weak. In practice, evidence from younger age groups is extrapolated to apply to older groups, except in the very frail and/or those with very poor life expectancy where a more conservative approach may be appropriate. Make an individual decision.

## Vascular

A very common cause of morbidity and mortality. The risk of MI is as high in diabetic patients without known coronary disease as it is in non-diabetic patients who have had an infarct.

- Improve glycaemic control to the extent that it is possible without inducing hypoglycaemia
- Treat hypertension if it is persistent despite lifestyle management:
  - Target BP <140/<80mmHg; lower if eye or kidney disease
  - In frail patients, target <150/<90mmHg
  - The drug class used is less important than the reduction in BP achieved. β-blockers are not contraindicated. ACE inhibitors and ARBs may have an important additional effect in preventing nephropathy
- Treat hyperlipidaemia, except in very elderly and frail patients. Statins are well tolerated. The Heart Protection Study demonstrated benefit in diabetic patients with cholesterol >3.5mmol
- Stop smoking. Health benefits begin in 3–6 months
- Low-dose aspirin should not be offered to all older patients with diabetes, unless there are other risk factors

▶ In older people, BP control is as important as glycaemic control in reducing cardiovascular risk.

## Neuropathy

This is more common in older diabetic people and is often asymptomatic, although may contribute to falls (see ➋ 'Balance and dysequilibrium', pp. 110–11). Annual screening is necessary—check pinprick, vibration sense, light touch (nylon monofilament), and reflexes.

- Classically and most commonly, a distal symmetrical polyneuropathy is seen. Consider other causes
- Mononeuropathy is usually of sudden onset and asymmetrical, and resolves over weeks or months. Often painful. May coexist with polyneuropathy, e.g.:
  - Third nerve palsy. Most common. Causes ophthalmoplegia
  - Diabetic amyotrophy. Pelvic girdle and thigh muscle weakness and wasting. Difficulty rising from chair
- Diabetic neuropathic cachexia. Painful peripheral neuropathy, depression, anorexia, and weight loss
- Autonomic neuropathy may cause orthostatic hypotension and gastroparesis

## Nephropathy

A major problem in older diabetic people.

- Microalbuminuria indicates a group at high risk of progression. Treat hypertension aggressively (preferentially with ACE inhibitors or ARBs), target BP 130/80, and optimize glycaemic control
- If renal function deteriorates rapidly, exclude papillary necrosis by obtaining emergency renal tract ultrasound

## Eyes

Retinopathy, glaucoma, and cataract are common (see ➜ 'The eye and systemic disease', p. 580). All diabetic people should have annual screening ophthalmic assessment that includes retinal examination (fundoscopy via a dilated pupil) and visual acuity testing. This is usually provided by ophthalmic specialist clinics or diabetologists (or other physicians) with particular expertise. Indications for urgent referral for specialist assessment include:

- Inadequacy of fundoscopic examination, e.g. due to cataract
- Diabetic maculopathy. Either exudates close (<1 optic disc diameter) to the macula or suspicion of macular oedema (nothing may be observed that is abnormal, but visual acuity is impaired)
- Preproliferative changes (many cotton wool spots, flame or blot haemorrhages, venous change (beading, loops))
- Proliferative changes (pre-retinal or vitreous haemorrhage, new vessels, retinal detachment)

▶ Preventing blindness depends on early diagnosis of diabetes, good glycaemic control, effective retinal screening, and early treatment of maculopathy and retinopathy.

## Ears

Malignant otitis externa, manifesting as severe ear pain, is more common in diabetes (see ➜ 'Osteomyelitis', pp. 490–1).

## Teeth

Gum disease and caries are more common. Good oral hygiene and regular dental assessment are essential.

## Erectile dysfunction

Predominantly due to vascular causes.

## Feet

Neuropathy and vascular disease lead to infection, injury, and ischaemia. Outcomes include pain, ulceration, immobility, and amputation. Impeccable foot care is essential (see ➜ 'The elderly foot', pp. 492–3).

# Diabetic emergencies

Although overall presentations with diabetic emergencies are diminishing, two are especially important—hypoglycaemia and hyperosmolar hypergly-caemic state (HSS). However, older patients can present with any diabetic problem, including diabetic ketoacidosis.

## Hyperosmolar hyperglycaemic state

- A complication of type 2 diabetes, and may be the first presentation
- Most common in older people
- Often severe. Mortality is very high (10–20%)
- There is often underlying sepsis, particularly pneumonia. Leucocytosis is common, with or without infection. Have a low clinical threshold to beginning antibiotics, after blood and urine cultures
- There is usually enough endogenous insulin to suppress ketogenesis, but not hepatic glucose output. Therefore, there is usually only a mild metabolic acidosis (pH >7.3), and ketonaemia is absent or mild. Blood glucose is often very high (>30mmol/L). Serum osmolality (measured or calculated) is usually over 320mOsm/kg
- Subacute deterioration occurs. Impaired thirst and an impaired 'osmostat', contributing to severe dehydration with high serum osmolarity, hypernatraemia, and uraemia. The fluid deficit is often around 10L
- Neurological problems are common and include delirium, coma, seizures, or focal signs, e.g. hemiparesis. Only a small proportion are in coma
- Treatment elements include:
  - *Fluid volume resuscitation*. Frequent and careful clinical assessment and fluid prescription are usually sufficient to determine rate and volume, but consider insertion of a central line in those with cardiac or renal disease or who are shocked. In general, fluid administration should be slower than in the younger patient with diabetic ketoacidosis. For the patient who is sick but not moribund, 2L in the first 3h and a total of 3–4L in the first 12h is often optimal. The exception is the shocked patient where filling should be more aggressive, with the advice and support of ITU colleagues if appropriate
  - *Correction of electrolyte abnormalities*. Initially give normal saline. If plasma sodium is very high (>155mmol/L), consider 5% dextrose when sugars are under control (e.g. <12mmol/L), but beware as sodium can rise with initial treatment. Maintain serum potassium in the range 4–5mmol/L. Give potassium with fluid, even if the patient is normokalaemic, as patients are usually total body potassium-depleted, and insulin will drive potassium into cells. Hypokalaemia is a major cause of dysrhythmias and sudden cardiac death
  - *Hyperglycaemia* often responds well to rehydration and treatment of an underlying cause (e.g. sepsis). iv insulin is often needed, but mod-est doses (e.g. 1–3 units/h) are usually enough. Patients with HSS are more insulin-sensitive than those with DKA

- *Thromboprophylaxis*. Low-molecular-weight heparin should always be prescribed; some advocate full anticoagulation because the thrombo-embolic complication rate is very high
  - *Pressure care*
- Although mortality rates are high, many patients recover promptly. The severity of presentation does not correlate closely with the severity of underlying disease, and in some, the diabetes may subsequently be controlled with diet alone

## Hypoglycaemia

Risk of severe hypoglycaemia ↑ hugely with age. In older people:

- The physiological response to hypoglycaemia is weaker (e.g. reduced glucagon secretion)
- Autonomic warning symptoms (e.g. sweating, tremor) are less marked
- Psychomotor response may be slow, even if symptoms are recognized

Other risk factors include frailty, comorbidity, renal impairment, care home residency, social isolation, and previous hypoglycaemia.

Clinical features are often not recognized or are atypical:

- Check sugar in any unwell known diabetic person (e.g. falls, confusion)
- Focal neurological signs or symptoms may be misdiagnosed as stroke. Signs may persist for some time after correction of blood sugar
- Acute severe or chronic hypoglycaemia can cause a dementia-like syndrome

### Prevention

- Assess each patient's risk of hypoglycaemia, and individualize therapy
- Balance the lifetime risk of hypoglycaemic attacks with reduction in long-term complications
- If altering medications, monitor sugars closely afterwards
- Educate the patient/carers about signs/symptoms and therapeutic response
- Put in place alarm systems—pendant alarms, 'check' telephone calls, neighbour visits, etc.
- Accept higher target glucose levels for those at high risk

### Treatment

- 'Hypos' can persist for hours or days and can recur late, especially if a long-acting insulin or oral drug is responsible. If severe, monitor closely (if necessary by admission) for 2–3 days
- Post-event, explore why the 'hypo' occurred. How might the next be prevented, or better treated? Many patients have lost weight or appetite and require a substantially reduced hypoglycaemic prescription

**HOW TO ... Manage diabetes in the terminally ill patient**

This includes end-of-life situations in all disease, not just cancer.

The sole aim of therapy is to minimize symptoms of hypo- and hyperglycaemia.

Ensure that the family and carers understand the changed aims of treatment and the rationale for medication changes.

Involve community nursing teams and diabetes specialist nursing teams early, particularly if you are planning a discharge from hospital to home.

*Drug treatment*
- As weight declines and oral intake falls, lower doses of insulin and oral drugs are usually needed
- Dose reductions will also be needed as renal function declines
- Make stepwise reductions in drug(s) and assess response
- In some cases, drugs may be phased out completely. For example, type 2 patients on insulin may now manage on oral drugs alone; those on oral drugs may be asymptomatic off them
- Type 1 patients require insulin until the very latest stages of dying (e.g. coma). Simplification of an insulin regimen (e.g. a move to once-daily insulin) is often helpful and may allow a patient to be cared for at home

*Diet*

Encourage food and fluid of whatever type is acceptable and attractive to the patient. Rigidly imposed diabetic diets are futile and unkind—it is usually better to encourage food of whatever type can be taken, and to accept the (usually modest) consequences for glycaemic control.

*Blood glucose monitoring*
- Monitoring should be tailored to the individual patient. In general, testing can be relaxed
- In all cases, test if symptoms suggest hypo- or hyperglycaemia
- In patients who are clinically stable (i.e. their condition is steady) or slowly deteriorating, testing can be infrequent (perhaps once on alternate days)
- In patients whose condition is deteriorating, or in those who have begun steroids, or where diabetes treatment has recently been changed, then testing should be more frequent
- In the patient who is moribund or comatose due to terminal illness, testing is pointless

## HOW TO . . . Interpret thyroid function tests

(See Table 15.1.)

- TSH is the most useful screening test. It can also be used to monitor treatment of thyroid disease. TSH takes 6–8 weeks to respond to changes in serum T3 and T4, so do not rush to repeat tests too often. If TSH is abnormal, check free T4
- Total thyroxine (total T4 and total T3) is affected by changes in thyroid-binding globulin (TBG). Some drugs influence TBG, e.g. glucocorticoids and androgens ↓ TBG levels while oestrogens, tamoxifen, and raloxifene ↑ TBG levels
- Free T4 (FT4) has replaced total thyroxine measurement in most centres, as it is less influenced by changes in TBG
- Free T3 (FT3) is useful to monitor thyrotoxicosis, especially if T4 is not elevated with a suppressed TSH

Table 15.1 Interpreting thyroid function tests

| TSH | FT4/FT3 | Most likely diagnosis | Other causes |
|-----|---------|----------------------|--------------|
| Low | High | Hyperthyroidism, e.g. toxic nodule | Graves' disease |
| | | | Thyroiditis |
| | | | Thyroxine overtreatment |
| | | | Post radioiodine treatment |
| | | | Thyroxine overdosage |
| Low | Low | Non-thyroidal illness | 2°/central hypothyroidism |
| High | Low | 1° hypothyroidism | Post-treatment (irradiation/surgery) |
| High | Normal | Subclinical hypothyroidism | Recovery from non-thyroidal illness |
| | | | Poor compliance with thyroxine |
| | | | Certain drugs* |
| High | High | Very rare | TSH-secreting tumour |
| | | | Assay error |
| | | | Variable compliance with thyroxine |
| Normal | Low | 2°/central hypothyroidism | Certain drugs* |

* Many common drugs cause abnormalities in TFT or change the effectiveness of treatment.

► Always consult the *BNF*.

## Further reading

Diabetes UK (2013). *End of life care.* ℘ https://www.diabetes.org.uk/end-of-life-care.
Joint British Diabetes Societies Inpatient Care Group (2012). *The management of the hyperosmolar hyperglycaemic state (HHS) in adults with diabetes.*

# Hypothyroidism: diagnosis

Common. Up to 5% prevalence in older men, 15% in older women. Incidence ↑ with age.

## Causes

1° autoimmune disease (Hashimoto's disease, usually without goitre) is by far the most likely cause, unless iatrogenic causes are present, e.g. drugs (amiodarone, antithyroid drugs), previous hyperthyroidism treatment (radioiodine or surgery), head/neck radiotherapy.

## Presentation

- Onset is usually insidious—over months, years, or decades
- Very variable presentation, often unmasked by intercurrent illness. In older people, symptoms and signs are more often mild and non-specific. None or all of the following may occur:
  - Hypothermia, cold intolerance
  - Dry skin, thinning hair
  - Weight gain or loss, constipation
  - Malaise
  - Falls, immobility, weakness, myalgia, arthralgia, elevated CK
  - Bradycardia, heart failure, pleural or pericardial effusion, non-pitting oedema of feet and hands (myxoedema)
  - Depression or cognitive slowing. Frank dementia is very rare
  - Hyporeflexia with delayed relaxation phase; ataxia or non-specific gait disturbance
  - Anaemia. Often normocytic; less commonly macrocytic or microcytic (reduced iron absorption)
  - Hyponatraemia, hypercholesterolaemia, hypertriglyceridaemia
- Symptoms of hypothyroidism are very common in the euthyroid older population. Often, only treatment reveals which symptoms were due to hypothyroidism

## Investigation

- *Have a low threshold* for thyroid function testing, in view of high disease incidence, poor sensitivity of clinical assessment alone, and the ease and effectiveness of treatment
- *Opportunistic screening* of older people in 1° care (e.g. at yearly health assessment) and 2° care (e.g. on presentation to acute medical take) is probably justified. But beware of abnormal TFTs due to sick euthyroid syndrome (see ➲ 'The ageing endocrine system', p. 420)
- *Overt 1° (thyroid gland failure) hypothyroidism* is confirmed when TSH is high and FT4 is low. TSH elevations may be less marked in older people
- *Subclinical or 'compensated' hypothyroidism* is suggested when TSH is high, but FT4 is normal (although often towards the lower end of the normal range). T3 production from T4 is stimulated by TSH, so may be well maintained. The patient is often asymptomatic. Only 2–5% per year will go on to develop overt hypothyroidism

- *Thyroid masses* are sometimes found on examination. Ultrasound scanning, isotope scanning ± fine-needle aspiration (FNA) will help characterize them. Malignant nodules are usually non-secreting ('cold'), so new single nodules in a euthyroid patient merit further evaluation
- *Antithyroid antibodies* have reasonable sensitivity and specificity in confirming autoimmune hypothyroidism and may help management in subclinical disease

▶ If patients have persistent lethargy despite successful treatment, consider alternative diagnoses, including other autoimmune disease, e.g. coeliac disease, Addison's disease, or pernicious anaemia.

# Hypothyroidism: treatment

- *Overt (or 'clinical') hypothyroidism*: this should always be treated. The patient might believe themselves to be asymptomatic but could feel much improved with treatment
- *Subclinical hypothyroidism*: trials of treatment in this group have revealed a complex balance of risk/benefit. Older patients with TSH of 4.5–8mU/L may suffer net harm from treatment. Consensus suggests that TSH >10mU/L warrants treatment. Thyroid autoantibodies may also help guide management—if they are positive, then the rate of transformation to overt hypothyroidism is much higher (25% compared with 5% per annum), so treatment is warranted

## Starting treatment

- Begin levothyroxine (T4) at low dose—usually 25 micrograms daily. More rapid initiation risks precipitating angina, insomnia, anxiety, diarrhoea, and tremor
- Dosing is optimized biochemically—symptoms and signs alone are very misleading
- Repeat TFTs monthly or 6-weekly, increasing the dose of T4 in 25 micrograms increments
- TSH levels guide dosage; T3 and T4 levels are not needed
- Aim for a TSH in the mid-range of normal, say 1–3mU/L
  - Overtreatment (TSH too low) risks AF and osteoporosis
  - Undertreatment risks physical and cognitive slowing, weakness, and depression
- Older people usually require slightly less T4—usually 50–125 micrograms daily is sufficient
- Heavier people require proportionately more T4 than lighter people
- T4 half-life is around 1 week. Therefore, if fine-tuning of dosing is needed, simply alternate higher and lower doses, e.g. 100/125 micrograms on alternate days

## Long-term management

- Tell the patient that treatment is for life
- Check thyroid function every year and if clinically indicated
- In the very long term, thyroxine requirements may rise, fall, or remain unchanged

## Administration

- Foods reduce absorption—take on an empty stomach, usually first thing in the morning
- If a dose is missed, take it as soon as remembered, and the next dose as normal
- If compliance is a problem, twice-weekly or weekly administration (of proportionately higher doses) gives acceptable control

## Thyroxine—interactions with other drugs

- *Antiepileptics* (phenytoin, primidone, and carbamazepine), *barbiturates*, and *rifampicin* ↑ thyroid hormone metabolism, so a higher T4 dose may be needed
- *Colestyramine, iron, calcium, and antacids (e.g. aluminium hydroxide)* reduce T4 absorption. Give T4 at least 2h beforehand
- *Amiodarone* has complex effects. Monitor TFTs regularly
- *β-blockers* may reduce conversion of T4 to T3

## Disease–drug interactions

As thyroid disease is controlled, dose changes of the following may be needed: *diabetic drugs (insulin and oral hypoglycaemics), digoxin, warfarin, theophylline, corticosteroids*.

# Hyperthyroidism: diagnosis

Subclinical hyperthyroidism is more common in older people (prevalence 3%), but severe disease is less common (incidence 0.1% per year in older women, 0.01% per year in older men).

## Causes

- *Toxic nodular goitre*. The most common cause in older people. There is often slow (years) progression from smooth goitre (euthyroid) to multinodular goitre (euthyroid). Then nodule(s) begin autonomous function, with subclinical and then clinical hyperthyroidism. It does not remit but may be relatively mild and indolent
- *Graves' disease*. The thyroid is stimulated by autoantibodies. Exophthalmos and diffuse goitre are less common than in younger people; 40% have no palpable goitre. Many remit within a year, perhaps more so than in younger patients
- *Exogenous levothyroxine*, i.e. overtreatment of hypothyroidism. This usually occurs insidiously when age-related slowing in T4 metabolism is not paralleled by reductions in the dose of T4
- Less common causes include:
  - Sources of excess iodine
  - *Subacute thyroiditis and Hashimoto's thyroiditis*. There is transient thyroid hormone excess due to gland destruction. Suspect if acute hyperthyroidism occurs with sore throat or tender neck. There may be an associated viral syndrome or upper respiratory tract infection
  - *Single autonomous nodule* (Plummer's disease)
  - *Malignant T4-secreting thyroid tumours and pituitary/non-pituitary TSH-secreting tumours*

▶ Distinguishing between the two very common causes (toxic nodular goitre and Graves' disease) is relatively unimportant, as treatment is similar. However, always consider the possibility of drugs (thyroxine or amiodarone) or acute thyroiditis where treatment is clearly different.

## Presentation

In older people with overt hyperthyroidism:
- Presentation may be more subtle, with fewer symptoms and signs
- Diagnosis is often delayed. Features are attributed to comorbidity or suppressed by β-blockers
- 'Negative' symptoms may dominate ('apathetic hyperthyroidism'), e.g. anorexia, weight loss, fatigue, weakness, and depression. Non-specific symptoms are more common, e.g. nausea, weakness, functional decline
- More classical symptoms of sympathetic overactivation may be absent, e.g. tremor, restlessness, sweating, tachycardia, and hypertension
- Cardiovascular complications are more common, e.g. angina, heart failure, AF (although ventricular response may be slow)
- Constipation is more common than diarrhoea
- ↑ bone turnover leads to hypercalcaemia and osteoporosis

# Hyperthyroidism: investigation

## Thyroid function tests
- Have a low threshold for testing in older people, especially if there is a personal or family history of thyroid disease
- Screening is recommended by some—at least every 5 years in women >60
- Low TSH is sensitive, but not specific, to hyperthyroidism
  - Drugs or non-thyroidal illness can suppress TSH below normal, but it usually remains detectable (0.1–0.5mU/L)
  - Very low TSH levels (<0.1mU/L), indicating total suppression of TSH secretion, are more specific to hyperthyroidism
- *Overt hyperthyroidism*:
  - In most cases, TSH is undetectable and both T4 and T3 are high
  - Elevated T3 without T4 ('T3 toxicosis') suggests toxic nodules or relapsing Graves', and is treated as hyperthyroidism
  - Elevated T4 but normal T3 (due to reduced peripheral conversion) suggests intercurrent illness
  - In severe hyperthyroidism, T4 may be normal (reduced binding globulin). FT4 remains high
  - Acute systemic illness in euthyroid people may cause transient (days) elevation of T4. TSH will be normal or moderately low
- *Subclinical hyperthyroidism*:
  - This is common: up to 5% point prevalence of ↓ TSH in healthy older people. TSH levels are low, with normal (often high normal) free T3 and T4
  - In most cases, TSH levels revert to normal within a year
  - Progression to overt hyperthyroidism occurs in <10% per year
  - Symptoms are few, but there is an ↑ risk of osteoporosis, AF, LVH, and possibly dementia
  - Consider the possibility that non-thyroidal illness (rather than thyroid hormone excess) may be suppressing TSH production

## Antithyroid antibodies
- Their presence supports a diagnosis of Graves' disease, especially if a smooth goitre is also palpable, but they are not wholly specific
- Antibody tests are usually negative in toxic nodular goitre
- Graves' and toxic nodular goitre are both common and can coexist. In that case, a nodular goitre may be palpable, with positive antibodies
- If Graves' disease is likely, screen for pernicious anaemia and coeliac disease (using relevant autoantibody tests and vitamin $B_{12}$ levels)

## Thyroid radioisotope scanning
This can help confirm the cause of hyperthyroidism and determine glandular size prior to radioiodine treatment.
- In thyroiditis, uptake is low or very low. Inflammatory markers are up
- In Graves', there is a diffuse pattern of ↑ uptake
- In toxic nodular goitre, there are multiple 'hot' nodules with surrounding 'cold' tissue
- A single autonomous 'hot' nodule is surrounded by 'cold' tissue

# Hyperthyroidism: drug treatment

Overt hyperthyroidism should always be treated, even if mild.

Several options are available for immediate and long-term treatment. Select on an individual basis, depending on the likely diagnosis, severity of illness, and patient characteristics and preferences.

## Drug treatment: thioamides (carbimazole or propylthiouracil)

- Suitable for initial management of Grave's disease or toxic nodular goitre
- In *Graves' disease*, this is an option for long-term therapy, as there is a greater probability of long-term remission than in younger people. Duration of treatment is usually 18 months, after which treatment is stopped and regular monitoring continues. Relapse risk is ~50% and is more likely if disease is severe, there is a large goitre, or antibody levels are high. If relapse occurs, begin thioamides again, and refer for definitive treatment (usually radioiodine)
- In *toxic nodular goitre*, long-term remission is less commonly achieved using thioamides. They are therefore used either:
  - Short-term, to achieve euthyroidism prior to definitive treatment (usually radioiodine)
  - Long-term, in the frail patient in whom life expectancy is short
- Initial daily dose: carbimazole 20–40mg, propylthiouracil 200–400mg (od or divided doses)
- Full thyroid suppression takes several weeks. Continue the initial dose for 4–8 weeks, until euthyroid. Measure FT4 every 2 weeks to assess when the euthyroid state is achieved, as TSH may be suppressed for months despite adequate treatment
- Once control is achieved, there are two options, with similar outcomes:
  - *Titration regimen*. Thioamide dose is reduced gradually, guided by TFTs, to a maintenance dose of carbimazole 5–15mg or propylthiouracil 50–150mg daily
  - *Block and replace regimen*. Thioamide dose is maintained high, entirely switching off thyroid synthetic function. Introduce levothyroxine once FT4 is suppressed
- Side effects include:
  - Skin rash or pruritus. Continue treatment. Try antihistamines. Try switching thioamides
  - Fever, arthralgia, headache, and gastrointestinal symptoms are usually mild
  - Agranulocytosis. This is uncommon, but more frequent in older people. Usually occurs early in treatment. Check FBC regularly (monthly until stable). It is vital to advise the patient and/or relative that the drug must be stopped and urgent advice sought if fever, sore throat, mouth ulcers, or other symptoms of infection develop

## Drug treatment: beta-blockers

- Used for rapid symptomatic treatment (tremor, anxiety, angina) and to reduce the risk of dysrhythmia. There is no effect on the hypermetabolic state itself
- May be especially useful in those with known structural or ischaemic heart disease or who are tachycardic, but should be introduced cautiously, with regular monitoring. Digoxin is ineffective in controlling AF in hyperthyroidism
- Check carefully for contraindications (e.g. asthma)
- All β-blockers are effective. Atenolol is a good choice, as it may be given od. Metoprolol and propranolol must be given tds or qds (↑ hepatic metabolism in hyperthyroidism)
- They have a role:
  - In Graves' or toxic nodular goitre, as an adjunct to thioamides
  - Where hyperthyroidism is only mild, β-blockers may be the only drugs needed prior to definitive treatment with radioiodine
  - In thyroiditis. The hyperthyroid state is transient, and β-blockers alone may be sufficient treatment until the disease moves onto euthyroidism or hypothyroidism

## Subclinical hyperthyroidism

- If due to excess T4 in a patient with treated hypothyroidism, reduce the dose by 25 micrograms and recheck TFTs in 6 weeks
- In other cases, in order to protect the bone, heart, and brain, consider treatment as for overt hyperthyroidism. This is especially indicated if:
  - There is osteopenia or heart disease, or significant risk factors
  - Suppressed TSH is persistent or severe, or T3/4 levels are at the higher limits of normality
- If treatment is not begun, reassess every 3–6 months

## Atrial fibrillation and hyperthyroidism

- Occurs in 10–15%. Most revert to sinus rhythm within weeks of becoming euthyroid, unless AF has been present for many months
- Digoxin is usually ineffective in controlling ventricular rate. β-blockade is more effective
- Consider cardioversion if AF persists for 4 months in new-onset AF
- Anticoagulate

See ➐ 'Atrial fibrillation', p. 274.

## Amiodarone and thyroid disease

Incidence of amiodarone-induced thyroid disease is high in older people because of this cumulative exposure and the drug's very long half-life.

- Clinical assessment alone is insensitive. Check TFTs before amiodarone treatment, and then every 3–6 months. If amiodarone is stopped, continue TFT monitoring for several years
- For clinical features and management of amiodarone-induced hypo- and hyperthyroidism

# Hyperthyroidism: non-drug treatment

### Radioiodine ($I^{131}$)

- Radioiodine is effective, well tolerated, safe, and simply administered. The sole contraindications are:
  - When safe disposal of radioactive body fluids after treatment cannot be guaranteed (e.g. home drainage is not into the main sewer). This can usually be overcome
  - In early treatment of hyperthyroidism, when administration of the iodine load can precipitate a thyrotoxic crisis
- Radioiodine is especially useful if there are drug intolerances, polypharmacy, or comorbidities
- Patients should be warned that physical contact with children and pregnant women should be avoided after treatment
- Give once initial symptomatic control has been achieved with drugs
- Thioamides must be stopped several days before administration of radioiodine (to permit uptake) and are usually restarted several days after (to prevent thyroid storm). Permanently discontinue thioamides after 3–4 months if TFTs are satisfactory
- Estimating the dose of $I^{131}$ required to render a patient euthyroid is difficult:
  - On average, larger doses are needed for patients with toxic nodular goitre (cf. Graves'), those with larger goitres, in severe disease, and in men
  - Most centres give a single larger dose (400–600MBq) that controls hyperthyroidism in most cases but leads to early hypothyroidism in up to 50%. A second dose is needed for a minority who remain hyperthyroid
- Post-treatment, TFTs should be checked every 4–6 weeks for the first year, and then lifelong at reduced frequency but at least every year for life
- 2° hypothyroidism may occur early (weeks, often transient) or late (years). Eventually, up to 90% become hypothyroid. There may be an early (weeks) rise in TSH that is transient and does not need treatment if there are no symptoms
- If the patient remains hyperthyroid at 6 months, then repeat $I^{131}$ dosing is usually needed

### Surgery

This is rarely performed in older people, considered only if both drug and radioiodine treatments are problematic or if a large goitre is especially troublesome. The patient must be euthyroid before surgery; β-blockade alone is not sufficient. Lifelong post-operative thyroid function monitoring is essential.

## Life-threatening thyroid emergencies

*Thyroid storm*

A rare, but life-threatening, manifestation of hyperthyroidism:

- Most commonly seen in patients with undiagnosed hyperthyroidism, often precipitated by non-thyroidal illness (including surgery, sepsis, or trauma) or administration of iodine-containing drugs
- Very rarely seen after radioiodine treatment
- Features include delirium, restlessness, coma, fever, vomiting, heart failure, tachycardia, and myocardial ischaemia
- The diagnosis is clinical—TFTs are often no worse than in typical hyperthyroidism
- Support failing organs, treat the underlying cause(s), and seek urgent specialist advice (ITU/endocrinology)
- Antithyroid drugs and iodide may be given iv to reduce thyroid hormone synthesis
- β-blockers and corticosteroids reduce the peripheral activity of thyroid hormones

*Myxoedema coma*

A rare, but life-threatening, manifestation of hypothyroidism:

- More common in older people, presenting as circulatory and respiratory failure and progressive drowsiness leading to coma, often with fits
- There is usually an acute precipitant (e.g. infection) in a patient with chronic hypothyroidism
- High mortality, requires specialist treatment
- iv T3 and hydrocortisone (to cover for possible coexisting adrenal insufficiency)
- Think of this also in patients who have stopped taking or absorbing levothyroxine

# Primary adrenal insufficiency

Also known as Addison's disease.

## Presentation

Usually insidious and often non-specific onset:

- Symptoms include fatigue (helped by rest), weight loss, anorexia, abdominal pain, nausea, constipation, hypotension (orthostatic and supine), depression, delirium, and ↓ functional status
- Skin and mucous membrane hyperpigmentation is common but is a late sign and may be absent. Pigmentation affects sun-exposed and unexposed areas, especially scars and pressure points
- Electrolyte disturbance (hyponatraemia and hyperkalaemia) and a mild acidosis (bicarbonate 15–20mmol) are usually present. Hypoglycaemia and mild anaemia may be present

▶ In some people with impaired adrenocortical function, there may be no symptoms when well, but acute stress (trauma, illness, psychological) leads to adrenal crisis with shock. If the possibility of adrenal insufficiency crosses your mind, then test for it, with a short ACTH stimulation test.

## Causes

- Mostly autoimmune. Often evidence of other autoimmune disease
- TB is relatively more common in older people
- Uncommonly due to: metastases, lymphoma, haemorrhage, or infarction. Very rarely due to drugs, e.g. ketoconazole

## Diagnosis

*Serum cortisol*

Cortisol is secreted episodically, so do not make or exclude a diagnosis on the basis of a single measurement.

- A very low cortisol level (<100nmol) makes adrenal insufficiency likely, especially if the patient is stressed/unwell at the time
- A moderately high (>300nmol) cortisol level makes adrenal insufficiency unlikely
- In Addison's, a random cortisol may be low or normal, i.e. a normal level does not exclude Addison's
- Early morning (6.00 to 8.00 a.m.) cortisol levels should be higher—a low level is more likely to be significant
- *Short ACTH stimulation test ('Synacthen® test')*. The only test that has good sensitivity and specificity (see ➔ 'HOW TO . . . Perform a short ACTH stimulation test (short Synacthen® test)', p. 411)
- *Adrenal autoantibodies* are positive in many autoimmune cases
- *AXR* and *CXR* may show signs of TB (e.g. calcification)
- *Adrenal CT* or *MRI* reveals a small gland in autoimmune disease, large if infection or tumour

If adrenal insufficiency is diagnosed, exclude 2° adrenal insufficiency (pituitary failure).

- *Check gonadotrophins* (follicle-stimulating hormone, luteinizing hormone, and *TSH*
- *ACTH* is elevated in 1° adrenal insufficiency, low in 2°

## Treatment

If the patient is unwell, do not delay treatment pending the results of tests—fluid-resuscitate with iv normal saline, normalize electrolytes, and give high-dose iv or im hydrocortisone (100mg tds). Improvement should occur quickly.

Long-term treatment includes oral glucocorticoids (usually hydrocortisone 20mg a.m., 10mg p.m.) and mineralocorticoids (usually fludrocortisone 0.1mg).

On treatment, older people are much more likely to develop hypertension that may require mineralocorticoid dose reduction and non-diuretic antihypertensive drugs.

Older people have a worse prognosis, due to more sinister causation (TB, malignancy) and possibly later presentation.

## Adrenal 'incidentalomas'

- An 'incidentaloma' is a tumour detected by scanning (ultrasound, CT, or MRI) that is unrelated to the indication for the scan
- Adrenal incidentalomas are relatively common (up to 4% of CT scans). Advances in imaging techniques have allowed better characterization/follow-up of these lesions
- They are more common in older people and the hypertensive. Key questions are '*Is it malignant?*' and '*Is it functional?*'
- If further investigation is warranted, there are complex investigation algorithms best undertaken by specialist MDTs

### Types of adrenal mass

*Adrenal adenomas* are very common and usually small (<2cm), benign, and non-functional. Signs of a functional nodule include hypertension and hypokalaemia. Fine-needle biopsy helps exclude malignancy if scan appearances are worrying, but usually only observation (periodic scanning) is needed. The larger the tumour, the higher the chance of malignancy. Large tumours should generally be excised, as biopsy may not identify foci of malignancy.

*Metastases* common (1°: breast, bronchus, bowel). Scan appearances are usually diagnostic. Adrenal insufficiency does not occur unless both glands are almost totally destroyed.

*Cysts and lipomas* make up most of the remainder.

*Benign adrenal cysts* are common in older people and may be due to cystic degeneration or local infarction.

*TB* may seed haematogenously, causing adrenal masses, often calcified.

Non-functional *adrenal carcinoma* usually presents late, with retroperitoneal spread and distant metastases.

# Hormone replacement therapy and the menopause

The menopause (cessation of menstruation due to ovarian failure) occurs typically between ages 45 and 55. The diagnosis can usually be made clinically. If the presentation is atypical, consider alternative diagnoses, e.g. hyperthyroidism. Following menopause, the risk of osteoporosis and vascular disease ↑ substantially. Symptoms can occur for several years before and after menopause and can be disabling. They include:

- Hot flushes
- Genitourinary atrophy
- Insomnia, depressed mood, and cognitive symptoms

HRT with oestrogen (plus progestogen in those with an intact uterus):

- Is an effective treatment for peri-menopausal symptoms
- Does not improve well-being in those with no symptoms
- Does not improve cognitive function or prevent dementia
- ↑ the risk of stroke, coronary events, PE, and breast, ovarian, and endometrial cancer. ↑ risk (cumulative serious events) is 1 in 1000 if treated for 1 year, 1 in 100 if treated for 5 years
- Reduces colon and rectal cancer and hip fracture by small amounts, but is no longer recommended for osteoporosis treatment in the absence of menopausal symptoms

In those with menopausal symptoms:

- Consider *non-systemic treatments*, e.g. topical oestrogens for atrophic vaginitis (vaginal cream or tablets, given daily for 2 weeks, then once or twice weekly for 6–8 weeks; sometimes needed long term). There is some systemic absorption; the risk of endometrial cancer is unknown. In those with reduced manual dexterity, consider a slow-release vaginal ring (replaced after 90 days)

*Other drugs* that can help but are less effective than systemic oestrogens include:

- Progestogens, e.g. medroxyprogesterone, megestrol
- Herbal remedies, some of which may have oestrogen-like activity
- Clonidine (an α-adrenoceptor stimulant; usual dose 50–75 micrograms bd) may reduce hot flushes. Side effects are often problematic. Watch BP

If symptoms continue, consider *HRT*, explaining the risks and benefits.

- Start treatment at low dose, increasing gradually until symptoms are controlled
- Explain that HRT is a short-term, and not an indefinite, treatment
- Every few months, taper the dose of HRT, assessing whether ongoing treatment is needed. Hot flushes usually cease after a few months to a few (<5) years

In women who have taken HRT for very prolonged periods, the risks and benefits of continuing must be assessed. In most cases, the advice will be to stop HRT:

- Risk is probably cumulative (dose and duration)
- Risk is probably multiplicative (non-HRT risk × HRT-related risk). As background risk of cancer and vascular disease rises exponentially in older people, so the net added risk of HRT is higher in older people
- In most cases, HRT may be withdrawn without recurrence of menopause symptoms
- In most cases, HRT will have been started (and the patient last advised) when the risks were not appreciated

▶ HRT is an effective treatment for symptoms but has potentially serious side effects.

## Male menopause

- There is a reduction in ♂ sex hormones with age, but not the abrupt cessation seen in women (unless there is ♂ gonadal failure for other reasons)
- This fall might cause a reduction in energy, sexual function, muscle mass, erythropoiesis, and bone density
- 2° hypogonadism (diabetes, obesity) should be considered
- HRT with testosterone cannot be routinely justified as risk (e.g. prostate cancer, thrombosis risk, gynaecomastia) exceeds potential benefits (which are unproven)
- Treatment should only be considered with serial confirmed low testosterone levels and attributable symptoms and counselling of risks. It should not aim to achieve the testosterone level of a young man
- Those on treatment must have clinical and prostate-specific antigen (PSA) monitoring on a regular basis

# Haematology

# The ageing haematopoietic system

There are very few changes as the bone marrow ages. Be very reluctant to ascribe changes seen on testing to age alone—pathology is much more likely.

## Haemoglobin

- Epidemiological studies show that population Hb concentration gradually declines from age 60
- There is debate as to whether the reference range should be adjusted since lower Hb levels are associated with ↑ morbidity and mortality, compared with older patients who maintain normal levels
- Thus, anaemia is common in old age (between 10 and 20% will have Hb <120g/L in ♀ or 130g/L in ♂), but this is due to disease(s), not ageing per se
- The decision about whether to investigate anaemia should be made not on the absolute value, but the clinical scenario. Consider symptoms, past medical history, severity of anaemia and rate of fall of Hb, MCV, and finally the patient's wish/tolerance of investigation
- A fit elderly man with no significant past history may merit investigation with an Hb of 115g/L (especially if his Hb was 130g/L last year or if the MCV is abnormal), while a patient with known rheumatoid arthritis, renal failure, and heart failure who has a normocytic anaemia with Hb 105g/L for years usually does not

## Erythrocyte sedimentation rate

- The height of the red cells in a standard bottle of blood, after being allowed to sediment for 60min
- This is a simple and non-specific test; however, it is inexpensive and remains useful for screening and monitoring disease in older people. CRP is often used in conjunction
- Red cells fall gradually because they are more dense, but the rate of fall ↑ where the cells clump together
- ESR rises with age and is slightly higher in women, so values up to 30mm/h for men and 35mm/h for women can be normal at age 70
- Anaemia can cause a mild elevation in ESR
- A high ESR occurs in disorders associated with elevated plasma proteins (fibrinogen and globulins). Numerous acute and chronic disorders can cause modest elevation
- Very high levels (>90) are commonly found with paraproteinaemias, GCA, and chronic infections such as TB

# Investigating anaemia in older people

A low Hb is a frequently encountered abnormality in geriatric practice. It is worth remembering the following:

- Other parameters, usually documented in the FBC report (e.g. MCV), will greatly assist in characterizing the anaemia and should be scrutinized
- Looking up old FBC results will often reveal a pattern, e.g. a frail older person may run a chronically low Hb because of chronic disease or marrow failure. If there is a recent change, this should prompt more urgent investigation
- Unwell older patients may have low Hb as a result of fluid overload or marrow suppression. Repeat FBC as they recover, and see if it persists
- Multiple aetiology is common, so check a full range of blood tests in all anaemic older patients
- It is very important to check that the laboratory has received the correct blood specimens for these tests before arranging blind replacement therapy or a transfusion—subsequent samples will be invalid for haematinics

Most anaemic patients will require:

- Blood film
- Ferritin, serum iron and total iron-binding capacity (TIBC), or transferrin saturation
- $B_{12}$, folate
- Renal, liver, and thyroid function testing
- Blood and urine electrophoresis, serum free light chains and look for Bence–Jones proteins in the urine if the ESR is raised

If the anaemia has been characterized (e.g. iron-deficient, macrocytic, etc.), then decisions can be made about the nature and extent of further testing (see ➲ 'Iron deficiency anaemia: diagnosis', pp. 454–5 for details).

If the picture is mixed, then there may be multiple contributing factors (e.g. CKD, minor gastritis, early myelodysplasia)—list these and address each in turn.

# Iron deficiency anaemia: diagnosis

This is the most common cause of microcytosis (but beware the occasional patient with lifelong microcytosis who has an inherited thalassaemia or sideroblastic anaemia).

## Causes

- The most common is occult blood loss in the gut, especially in patients taking NSAIDs (even 75mg aspirin)
- Malabsorption (e.g. coeliac disease, gastrectomy, achlorhydria due to atrophic gastritis, or use of PPIs)
- Malnutrition as a sole cause is very unusual

▶ Multifactorial aetiology is common, e.g. mild chronic blood loss, borderline dietary intake, and mild malabsorption syndromes.

## Diagnosis

History is vital (ask about weight loss and gut, kidney, urogenital, or ENT blood loss). Pallor (conjunctivae, nail beds) may be found. The emphasis of examination should be to find rectal or abdominal masses, hepatomegaly, and lymphadenopathy.

## Investigations

- Microcytosis usual, but not in combined deficiency or acute blood loss
- Low serum ferritin levels (<12 micrograms/L) are diagnostic. Moderately low levels (12–45 micrograms/L) may also point to the diagnosis, as ferritin levels rise with age. Ferritin is an acute phase reactant, so normal/high levels do not rule out deficiency
- Serum iron levels will be low with high iron-binding capacity, i.e. the ratio of iron/iron binding (transferrin saturation) will be low (<15%). This is a useful way of distinguishing anaemia of chronic disorder where both iron and iron binding are low (and the ratio will be normal) (see also Table 16.1)
- Low iron stores on a bone marrow trephine are diagnostic, but this investigation is painful and rarely required
- Faecal occult blood is of limited value in cases of established iron deficiency—it is usually positive and you may feel that further gastrointestinal tests are needed anyhow

**Table 16.1** Characteristic findings in iron deficiency and chronic disease

| Test | Iron deficiency | Chronic disease |
| --- | --- | --- |
| MCV | Microcytic | Normocytic |
| Iron | Low | Often low |
| Transferrin or TIBC | Normal or high | Low |
| Iron:TIBC ratio (transferrin saturation) | Low (<15%) | Normal |
| Ferritin | Low is diagnostic | Normal or high |

- Haematuria sufficient to cause anaemia is rare, and usually severe. Urinalysis may be indicated in patients with poor vision or cognition to look for renal tract blood loss
- Iron deficiency without anaemia should still be investigated, but the lower the Hb, the higher the likelihood of finding attributable pathology

---

## HOW TO . . . Investigate iron deficiency anaemia

The main dilemma is deciding how far to take investigations.

A *fit patient*, who would be a candidate for surgery, should have a minimum of an OGD and colon imaging (see ➔ 'How to . . . Image the older colon', p. 371). These should proceed, regardless of the degree of anaemia and whether there are symptoms. The finding of oesophagitis or an upper gastrointestinal ulcer should not stop a screening test for the colon to rule out a coexisting neoplasm. If these tests are negative, screen for coeliac disease and haematuria. Small bowel barium studies or capsule endoscopy are sometimes helpful. If there is intermittent overt gastrointestinal blood loss, mesenteric angiograms can demonstrate small angiodysplastic lesions if there is active haemorrhage.

At the other extreme, a *frail, bedbound nursing home patient* with dementia will probably merit empirical iron and PPI therapy without further investigations.

In *between these extremes*, physicians often adopt a 'halfway house'. Some examples of this compromise include:
- Not proceeding to lower gastrointestinal tests if upper gastrointestinal pathology is found
- Where NSAIDs are the likely problem, stop the drug, give iron and a PPI, and only investigate if anaemia or evidence of bleeding continues after a suitable therapeutic trial
- Not performing lower gastrointestinal tests if the patient is not fit for, or not consenting to, surgical intervention
- Performing a flexible sigmoidoscopy, rather than a full colonoscopy (80% of tumours can be excluded this way without complete bowel preparation and with less risk and discomfort)
- Using oral contrast-enhanced CT colonography to image the colon (better tolerated) will miss small lesions but excludes large tumours
- Assuming that very long-standing and stable iron deficiency (several years) presents low risk for a malignant source

There are *no hard rules* about making these decisions, but it is advisable that any risk-taking is shared with the patient and/or relative and that you record your discussions in the notes. Remember that:
- Investigations are often better tolerated than you would expect, e.g. OGD remains a very safe test, even in very old people
- Sometimes it is worth doing tests, even if definitive treatment is not available, e.g. for a frail patient with bloody diarrhoea, a sigmoidoscopy may yield an alternative diagnosis or guide future palliative therapy
- A second medical opinion may help

Most patients are highly persuadable—if you do want them to take an active part in decisions, you will need to give an unbiased view of their options—'You don't want one of those unpleasant dangerous endoscopies, do you?' does not present the patient with a fair choice.

# Iron deficiency anaemia: treatment

Treatment is often simple. Treat the underlying cause, and replenish iron stores. The underlying marrow is usually healthy. Hb should rise by about 5g/L/week.

Blood transfusion is expensive and usually unnecessary, and can be dangerous. It should be used only for severe symptoms (e.g. unstable angina) or where ongoing acute bleeding is present.

## Enteral iron

- Oral supplements (ferrous sulfate) are very effective, but compliance is often poor due to gastrointestinal side effects (constipation, nausea, diarrhoea)
- Sometimes a different preparation (i.e. ferrous gluconate or fumarate) is better tolerated
- Start with a low dose and ↑ as tolerated. It is better to take a lower dose for longer than abandon treatment after a few days due to side effects. Alternate day supplementation is often sufficient
- If stool is not greeny-black, adherence is poor
- Avoid slow-release preparations, as they are often poorly absorbed
- Remember that achlorhydria (atrophic gastritis or PPI administration) significantly reduces iron absorption
- Vitamin C may enhance absorption

### Failure to respond to enteral iron

This should prompt consideration of the following:

- Is there ongoing haemorrhage?
- Is the patient adherent with therapy?
- Are there other contributory factors (e.g. kidney disease)?
- Is the iron being absorbed?

## Parenteral iron therapy

- Use is ↑ with the development of safer preparations
- Consider if blood loss exceeds the ability of the gut to absorb oral iron (e.g. with angiodysplasia), the patient does not tolerate oral iron, or the oral iron is not adequately absorbed (e.g. with atrophic gastritis)
- Also used in renal patients on dialysis and those with inflammatory bowel disease (often intolerant of oral iron)
- iv infusions of iron sucrose, ferric carboxymaltose, or iron dextran can be given
- Risk of anaphylaxis, so test dose recommended, and there should be resuscitation facilities available
- Ferric carboxymaltose has a lower risk of anaphylaxis and can be infused quite quickly (over 15min) so is often preferred
- im preparations are rarely used

## Duration of iron therapy

Continue iron for 3 months after the Hb concentration has normalized (to replenish the iron stores), but do not leave the patient on life-long treatment, unless you are unable to trace or treat the cause of ongoing blood loss. Monitoring Hb off iron can guide management by telling you whether blood loss continues; iron overload is not without risk.

# Macrocytic anaemia

## Causes

- B$_{12}$ deficiency—usually malabsorption
- Folate deficiency—often dietary, but also consider coeliac disease
- Myelodysplasia
- Aplastic anaemia
- Hypothyroidism
- Myeloma
- Liver failure and alcohol excess
- Drugs, e.g. methotrexate, phenytoin, azathioprine, metformin
- Reticulocytosis

## Megaloblastic anaemia

- Caused by vitamin B$_{12}$ and folate deficiency
- Bone marrow shows big erythroblasts with immature nuclei due to defective DNA synthesis, while blood film may show hypersegmented neutrophils
- Can also cause suppression of white cell and platelet production (pancytopenia) and a mild jaundice with raised LDH due to low-grade haemolysis
- Lack of B$_{12}$ and/or folate also affects the brain (rare cause of reversible dementia) and nerve function (peripheral neuropathy and subacute combined degeneration of the cord). There is a poor correlation between the degree of anaemia and the presence of neurological sequelae which are often irreversible

## Pernicious anaemia

An autoimmune gastritis is present in 80% of B$_{12}$ deficiency cases, resulting in achlorhydria, the absence of intrinsic factor, and therefore B$_{12}$ malabsorption. It is more common in elderly ♀ with a history of autoimmune disease. Proving the diagnosis (gastric biopsy, Schilling's test to look for malabsorption and autoantibodies for intrinsic factor, and parietal cells) is fiddly and rarely undertaken. Treatment is empirical and pragmatic.

## Treatment

- In combined deficiency or blind treatment, always correct both deficiencies simultaneously, as treating one can precipitate acute deficiency of the other and worsen neurology (especially subacute degeneration)
- Folic acid 5mg od is very well tolerated
- Hydroxocobalamin loading is 1mg by im injection three times a week for six doses, then 1mg every 3 months indefinitely
- Those with low B$_{12}$ levels without anaemia can go straight to the 3-monthly regimen

# Anaemia of chronic disease

This is the most common cause of anaemia in older people. Illnesses such as infection, malignant disease, or connective tissue disorder may be accompanied by a moderate anaemia (90–100g/L). Frequent acute illness may have a similar effect.

## Diagnosis

Often a diagnosis of exclusion. Normocytic and normochromic. There is low serum iron and iron binding capacity (normal transferrin saturation) with a normal or raised serum ferritin concentration. Bone marrow aspiration is rarely indicated but will usually demonstrate ↑ iron stores.

This underlying condition may not always be apparent, even after a careful history and examination, and screening tests should include:

- Blood film, ESR, CRP, and immunoglobulins
- Liver and renal function tests
- CXR
- Autoantibody screen
- Urine analysis
- TFTs
- PSA

If no diagnosis is made at this stage, symptomatic treatment should be given and the patient should be kept under regular review.

## Treatment

- Hb will improve only after treatment of the underlying condition
- Patients should not be placed on long-term iron and/or folate supplements without evidence of deficiency (iron overload can occur and has theoretical risks)
- Symptomatic blood transfusion may be warranted
- Chronic disease often coexists with renal impairment; consider a trial of an erythropoiesis-stimulating agent (see ➋ 'Chronic kidney disease: complications', p. 392)

### Unexplained anaemia

It is common to find mild anaemia (usually <20g below threshold) in older patients, that is not readily explained by any single process.

It is likely that there are several subtle factors at play, e.g.:

- Mild kidney impairment
- Low-level chronic inflammation
- Serial acute events
- Androgen reduction
- Erythropoietin reduction
- In some cases low level marrow failure

Approach by excluding other causes and listing possible contributing factors. It is probably not unexplained—just complex.

# Paraproteinaemias

Abnormal expansion of a single line of plasma cells, which produce a mono-clonal immunoglobulin. This is a malignant, or potentially malignant, condition that ↑ in prevalence with advancing age.

▶ A polyclonal hyperglobulinaemia is a common benign reaction to many illnesses and infection and is not related to paraproteinaemias.

It is important to exclude paraproteinaemias in any older patient with an unexplained anaemia or raised ESR. This is easily done with:

- Serum immunoglobulin level
- Serum free light chain assay (kappa:lambda ratio). An abnormal ratio suggests more sinister pathology
- Serum and urine electrophoresis, including quantification of a monoclonal immunoglobulin
- Bone marrow aspirate/trephine if one is found

## Monoclonal gammopathy of undetermined significance (MGUS)

- This is the most common paraproteinaemia, occurring in 3% of over 70-year olds
- It is benign and usually has no clinical manifestations, although a minority may develop renal disease (known as monoclonal gammopathy of renal significance)
- There is a small/moderate monoclonal band (<20g/L), a low level of plasma cell expansion in the marrow (<10%), and a raised ESR, but no other clinical or laboratory features of multiple myeloma (MM)
- The paraprotein level should remain stable over time
- 'Smouldering myeloma' is sometimes diagnosed where the monoclonal band or plasma cell levels are higher than the thresholds listed here, but there are no other features of MM—this is treated in the same way as MGUS
- The importance of MGUS is that up to a quarter of the patients will eventually develop another haematological disease (usually MM). The median transformation time is 10 years and many patients die of unrelated illness during follow-up. There is no test which can predict which remain stable and which transform, so all should receive an annual clinical and laboratory review (FBC, serum electrophoresis with quantification of paraprotein level, kidney function, and calcium)

# Multiple myeloma

Incidence in people over 80 is 30 per 100,000 per year. The marrow plasma cell expansion is malignant and causes bone erosion and marrow failure. Bence–Jones proteins (light chains excreted in urine) may contribute to kidney failure. Plasma hyperviscosity syndrome can occur.

▶ Exclude MM in anyone with an unexplained high ESR or anaemia.

## Clinical features

- Malaise/fatigue (anaemia)
- Bone pain, pathological fracture, and cord compression (bone erosion)
- Thirst, confusion, and renal impairment (hypercalcaemia)
- Infections/fever (immunoparesis and neutropenia)
- Bleeding (thrombocytopenia)
- Hepatomegaly (20%) and splenomegaly (5%)
- Rarely neuropathy or amyloidosis can occur

## Investigations

- Serum immunoglobulins and electrophoresis show a monoclonal band (sometimes two), usually quantified as over 30g/L with suppression 'immunoparesis' of other immunoglobulins. Immunoglobulin G (IgG) paraprotein most common, then IgA and light chains
- Serum free light chain assay with kappa:lambda ratio
- Other blood tests:
  - High ESR—usually above 100
  - Normochromic normocytic anaemia
  - Neutropenia and thrombocytopenia occur late
  - Hypercalcaemia
  - Renal impairment
  - ALP—may be normal despite bone lesions and hypercalcaemia
  - Hypoalbuminaemia
  - High $\beta 2$-microglobulin levels
- Urine immunoglobulins—light chains occur as Bence–Jones protein in 75%.
- Plain X-rays—show lytic lesions or generalized osteopenia
- Isotope bone scans may be negative and are not recommended
- MRI may show non-specific, patchy high-signal marrow replacement
- Bone marrow aspirate and trephine—30% plasma cells

A confident diagnosis can be made with at least two of:

- >30% plasma cells in marrow
- Evidence of bone involvement
- A myeloma protein present in serum or urine, or both

Unfortunately, many cases are not this straightforward and cases are found with a normal ESR, no serum protein band (just Bence–Jones), or <30% plasma cells (where marrow expansion is patchy or occurring in a single plasmacytoma deposit).

## Management

Should involve a haematologist.

Most patients will receive *symptomatic treatment*:

- Blood product transfusion
- Analgesia for bone pain
- Radiotherapy for localized bone pain/pathological fracture and for spinal cord compression
- Treatment of hypercalcaemia—see ➔ 'HOW TO . . . Manage symptomatic hypercalcaemia', p. 633
- Social and psychological support

Disease-modifying options include:

- A regimen containing melphalan, prednisolone, and thalidomide (MPT) chemotherapy is often used as first line for those >65
- Treatment is given in cycles (4-day courses of melphalan and prednisolone every 6 weeks, with daily thalidomide)
- Treatment continues in cycles until a plateau phase is reached (monitor M-protein in blood and urine)
- In younger (usually under 65), fitter patients, a bone marrow transplant is often recommended after initial chemotherapy

## Prognosis

This is improving. Nonetheless, 5-year survival for patients aged 70–79 is 38%, dropping to 18% for those aged over 80, and palliative care should not be neglected at the end.

Severe anaemia (Hb <90g/L), kidney impairment, and hypercalcaemia are all associated with a poor prognosis.

# Myelodysplasia and myelodysplastic syndrome

A group of neoplastic disorders of the haematopoietic stem cell, characterized by ↑ bone marrow failure with qualitative and quantitative abnormalities of all three cell lines, resulting in varying degrees of:
• Anaemia (macrocytic or normocytic)
• Neutropenia (sometimes with a monocytosis)
• Thrombocytopenia

A single cell line may be affected, especially at presentation. The qualitative abnormalities mean that function may be poor, even with normal counts (e.g. susceptibility to infection without neutropenia).

Common and under-diagnosed, with peak incidence at age 80. Cause unknown (except a tiny proportion who have myelodysplasia 2° to previous cytotoxic therapy).

Usually a hypercellular bone marrow (some normocellular/hypocellular) with dysplastic changes and up to 20% of blast cells. Some patients have ring sideroblasts (iron deposits in a ring shape around the nucleus). Transformation to acute myeloid leukaemia where blasts >20% occurs in a significant proportion (up to 30% eventually)—especially those with a high blast count at diagnosis.

## Diagnosis

Around half of patients are asymptomatic at diagnosis (incidental finding on blood test). The rest present with anaemia, infections, or bleeding and may have splenomegaly (10%), hepatomegaly, and skin purpura.

First exclude $B_{12}$ and folate deficiency, alcohol excess, cytotoxics, and thyroid/liver/kidney failure. If characteristic features on blood film and mild disease, bone marrow examination may be unnecessary, but confident diagnosis/staging will usually require trephine and aspirate. Subclassification based on bone marrow morphology and karyotyping can be done by haematologists and aids prognostic precision.

## Management

• Asymptomatic patients require nothing more than monitoring with regular blood counts—often stable for many years
• Mainstay of symptomatic treatment is blood transfusions
• Recurrent infections and bleeding complications should be treated with antibiotics and platelet transfusions, respectively
• Younger patients (age <70) with poor-risk disease are sometimes suitable for bone marrow transplantation or cytotoxic treatment, but these have a very high morbidity and mortality in older patients
• Growth factors, such as erythropoiesis-stimulating agents or granulocyte colony-stimulating factor, are occasionally used
• Average survival ranges from 6 months (high risk) to 12 years (very low risk), and around one-third die of unrelated causes
• Transformation to acute myeloid leukaemia has a very poor prognosis—palliative treatment only

## HOW TO . . . Transfuse an older person

*Acute transfusions*

For example: haematemesis, post-operative blood loss.

- Speed of transfusion should be determined by the haemodynamic status (postural BP useful, remember elderly patients—especially those on β-blockers and with pacemakers—may not be able to mount an appropriate tachycardia)
- Furosemide not required in a volume-depleted patient
- Reassess fluid balance and repeat Hb frequently—it is very easy to under- or overestimate blood requirements, and older patients do not tolerate this as well

*When not to transfuse*

- Older people admitted acutely may have an alarmingly low Hb (often an unexpected finding on a screening blood test), but this should not automatically trigger urgent, fast, or large transfusion
- Most of these patients have a newly diagnosed chronic anaemia and can come to harm if transfused overenthusiastically—indeed many of these patients are better managed as an outpatient
- First assess the patient's haemodynamic status and symptoms (fainting, very breathless, new confusion, unstable angina, or severe peripheral ischaemia are indications to transfuse; simple tiredness/malaise are not)
- $B_{12}$ injections or oral iron therapy can cause Hb to rise by 5–10g/L per week and may avoid inpatient care and the risks of transfusion
- If you do elect to transfuse, 1U may be sufficient (even for an Hb of 60) to tide the patient over until other treatments work

*Routine/planned symptomatic transfusions*

For example, myelodysplasia.

- In general, transfuse only when Hb drops to below 80 (unless symptoms, e.g. angina, occur at higher levels)
- Outpatient transfusion is now frequently done in DHs, with the patient sitting in a chair, rather than bed-bound
- Some units now give up to 4U/day (2h), unless the patient has heart failure or previous reactions
- Usually with oral furosemide cover (20–40mg/bag of blood)
- A careful system for cross-matching in 1° care (e.g. some units send out a pack containing pre-labelled bottles, request cards, and patient bands to district nurses to collect at home or in the GP surgery) can minimize traumatic journeys to hospital

# Chronic lymphocytic leukaemia

Chronic lymphocytic leukaemia is the most common of the lymphoid leukaemias. Malignant proliferation of mature B-lymphocytes causes persistent lymphocytosis. Peak incidence age 60–80. ♀:♂ = 1:2.

## Clinical features

- Often picked up incidentally on blood film when asymptomatic
- Symmetrical, non-tender lymphadenopathy (also tonsillar enlargement)
- Splenomegaly and/or hepatomegaly (in later stages)
- ↑ susceptibility to infections (e.g. thrush, herpes zoster, bacterial) due to low immunoglobulins and/or neutropenia
- Bruising/purpura due to thrombocytopenia

## Investigations

Abnormal findings include:

- Lymphocytosis (>5 × $10^9$/L)—may be >100 × $10^9$/L
- Normocytic, normochromic anaemia and thrombocytopenia can occur
- Marrow trephine/aspiration replaced by lymphocytes (20–95% of cells)
- Reduced immunoglobulins develop with advanced disease
- LDH raised in some (indicating poor prognosis)

Staging systems use blood and marrow counts, chromosomal analysis, and degree of lymphadenopathy and organ involvement to predict survival and therefore guide management.

## Treatment

- Presentation and prognosis are highly variable, so management varies enormously and should be guided by a haematologist
- Asymptomatic patients with non-progressive, early-stage disease may be just observed/reviewed in haematology clinics
- Tailored chemotherapy is used. New treatments (e.g. ibrutinib, obinutuzumab) offer excellent early results in selected patients
- Prednisolone can help with anaemia, neutropenia, or thrombocytopenia and reduces hepatosplenomegaly
- Radiotherapy can be useful for bulky lymph nodes
- Most patients respond to treatment initially but relapse after time

## Prognosis

- Varies according to stage and prognostic factors but, in most patients, is a chronic, non-aggressive disease
- Many elderly patients are likely to die with, rather than of, the disease (as in myelofibrosis and prostate cancer)
- However, patients with aggressive disease have a life expectancy of 2–3 years

# Musculoskeletal system

# Osteoarthritis

Osteoarthritis (OA) is the most common joint disorder in older patients, causing massive burden of morbidity and dependency. It is not inevitable with ageing.

It is a disorder of the dynamic repair process of synovial joints, causing:
- Loss of articular cartilage (joint space narrowing)
- Vascular congestion
- New growth of cartilage and bone (osteophytes)
- Capsular fibrosis

Inherited factors determine susceptibility, but individual genes are not identified. ↑ age is the strongest risk factor. ♀ and those with high bone density are at higher risk. Obesity, trauma, and repetitive adverse loading (e.g. miners or footballers) are potentially avoidable factors. 'Burnt-out' rheumatoid arthritis or neuropathic joints (e.g. in diabetes), as well as congenital factors (e.g. hip dysplasia), can result in 2° OA.

## Clinical features
- Pain—assess severity, impairment, and impact on life. Usually insidious in onset and variable over time, worse with activity, and relieved by rest. Chronic pain may cause poor sleep and low mood
- Only one or a few joints are affected with minimal morning stiffness and often worsening of symptoms during the day
- Restricted movement, e.g. walking, dressing, rising from a chair
- Severe OA can contribute to postural instability and falls

## Examination
- Heberden's nodes (asymptomatic bony swellings on distal fingers) associated with inherited knee OA
- Limp with jerky 'antalgic' gait
- Deformity including:
  - Muscle wasting
  - Knees may be valgus (knees together, feet apart—'knock-knees'), varus (knees apart, foot inwards—'bow-legged'), or flexion deformity
  - Hip shortening/flexion (check on couch by flexing the opposite hip to see if the affected hip lifts off the bed—Thomas' test)
- Restricted range of movement
- Crepitus
- Effusions

## Investigations
▶ OA is a clinical diagnosis. Symptoms correlate poorly with radiological findings. The main role of X-ray is in assessing severity of structural change prior to surgery. Features include joint space narrowing, osteophytes, sclerosis, cysts, and deformity. Blood tests are normal, even when an osteoarthritic joint feels warm—reconsider your diagnosis if inflammatory markers are elevated.

# Osteoarthritis: management

OA is the most common chronic painful condition. Drug dependence and side effects can be a big problem.

▶ Always consider non-pharmacological treatments first.

## Non-drug treatments

- *Exercise*: aerobic and focal muscle strengthening. Swimming, yoga, and t'ai chi are particularly good. PT may help. Encourage the patient to exercise despite the pain—no harm will be done
- *Heat/cold packs*: but be very careful to avoid burns in patients who may have ↓ temperature awareness
- *Weight loss*: not a quick fix but influences other health outcomes
- *Sensible footwear*: soft soles with no heels. Trainers are ideal
- *Walking aids*, e.g. stick (in contralateral hand)
- *Education and support*: self-management programmes are helpful
- *Osteopaths or chiropractors*: help some patients but are expensive

## Drug treatments

Patients should be offered regular paracetamol in adequate dose before moving onto drugs with greater side effect profiles. Patients may need per-suading to try a regular prophylactic dose, perceiving it as a 'weak' drug.

- Topical NSAIDs can be helpful and are lower risk than oral
- The next step is to add a low-potency opiate—often combined with paracetamol. Beware constipation and sedation
- A short course of oral NSAIDs can be useful in acute exacerbations, but avoid long-term use. If NSAIDs are used for >1 week or in the presence of known dyspepsia or ulceration, reduce the gastrointestinal risk by co-prescribing, e.g. lansoprazole 15mg od. The cyclo-oxygenase-2 (COX-2) selective inhibitors have better gastrointestinal tolerability but have ↑ vascular adverse events and so have fallen out of favour. Both can worsen heart failure
- Intra-articular steroids can be rapidly effective, particularly if the joint is hot/very painful. There is a substantial placebo effect, but symptoms tend to recur after 4–6 weeks. Side effects limit use to four injections/joint/year. The cumulative systemic effect risks osteoporosis
- Counter-irritants, e.g. capsaicin cream, are safe and have some effect
- Oral chondroitin and glucosamine are available unlicensed over-the-counter, but there is little evidence of benefit

## Surgical treatment

Includes cartilage repair, osteotomy, and joint replacements. Arthroscopic debridement/lavage has limited evidence and should not be offered unless locking. Indications include pain, deformity, or joint instability where other treatments have failed. Outcomes can be excellent for fitter older people, but cases should be carefully selected.

## Further reading

National Institute for Health and Care Excellence (2014). *Osteoarthritis: care and management*. Clinical guideline CG177. ℗ http://www.nice.org.uk/cg177.

## HOW TO . . . Manage non-operative fractures

- Fractures that very rarely require operative intervention include the pubic rami, humerus, wrist, and vertebra
- Other fractures, often immobilized surgically in younger people, may be treated more conservatively in older patients to avoid perioperative risks (e.g. simple tibial plateau fractures may be immobilized by functional brace)
- Patients with these 'non-operative' fractures are often cared for by geriatricians, having been transferred either:
  - From A&E to medical, ortho-medical, or ortho-geriatric units
  - From orthopaedic wards for ongoing rehabilitation
- Minor fractures can result in significant functional impairment, e.g. a Colles' fracture, and plaster of Paris (POP) may prevent an older person from washing, dressing, and toileting. Even walking may not be possible (if a frame can no longer be used)

*General principles of management*
These include:
- *Pain control.* This allows earlier mobilization and reduces the risks of immobility (pressure sores, pneumonia, thromboembolism)
  - Consider novel treatments such as heat, TENS, calcitonin, bisphos- phonates, or vertebroplasty for vertebral fracture
  - A short course of NSAIDs is sometimes appropriate in low-risk patients, but remember to stop this as soon as possible
- Encouraging mobility and independence as early as possible. Best achieved in a rehabilitation environment. Patient and family often expect 'bed rest' after a fracture and may need to be educated
- Consider the mechanism of the fall and injury (see ➲ 'Assessment following a fall', pp. 102–3)—are there medical risks that could be reduced? For example, sedating medication, excessive antihypertensive use, undiagnosed illnesses (e.g. urinary infection or minor stroke), need for aids/adaptations
- Maintaining contact with orthopaedic colleagues. They can advise on when to replace/remove plasters and how much exercise/weight- bearing is appropriate. Ask for reassessment if progress is poor, e.g. ongoing severe pain, or apparent malunion—sometimes a diagnosis has been missed or an interval operation is needed
- A pragmatic approach to weight-bearing may be needed, e.g. in dementia (where concordance with non-weight-bearing is difficult) or where immobility causes an unacceptable rise in frailty
- Prescribing prophylactic heparin if there are multiple risk factors for thromboembolic disease or the patient is immobile
- Osteoporosis treatment (there is no current evidence that bisphosphonates reduce callus formation or delay bone union)
- Start to plan discharge early. Many patients can be managed at home with a care package and outpatient rehabilitation. Others may need transitional care beds (e.g. while they wait to be weight-bearing or for plasters to be removed), after which they can return to an active rehabilitation programme prior to going home

# Osteoporosis

Osteoporosis is the reduction in bone mass and disruption of bone architecture, resulting in ↑ bone fragility and fracture risk. Results from prolonged imbalance in bone remodelling where resorption (osteoclastic activity) exceeds deposition (osteoblastic activity).

Osteoporosis is very common and very much under-recognized and undertreated. In combination with falls (see ➔ 'Interventions to prevent falls', pp. 104–5), osteoporosis contributes to the high incidence of fractures in older people. In the UK, 50% of women aged >50 years have at least one osteoporotic fracture in their lifetime and 32% aged 90 will have had a hip fracture.

▶ If you make the diagnosis, do not delay initiating 2° prevention. Always think of osteoporosis when assessing post-operative orthopaedic patients or any patient who has fallen.

## Pathology

- Total bone mass ↑ throughout childhood and adolescence, peaks in the third decade, and then declines at about 0.5% per year
- Bone loss is accelerated after the menopause (up to 5% per year) and by smoking, alcohol, low body weight, hyperthyroidism, hyperparathyroidism, hypoandrogenism (in men), kidney failure, and immobility
- Steroids, phenytoin (and other antiepileptics), PPIs, long-term heparin, and ciclosporin cause 2° osteoporosis
- High peak bone mass reduces later risk. Determined by genetics, nutrition (optimal BMI and calcium/vitamin D, especially in childhood), and weight-bearing exercise
- Diagnosis is complicated by the common coexistence of asymptomatic osteomalacia (defective mineralization) in older people with low sunlight exposure

## Clinical features

- Osteoporosis itself is asymptomatic—it is the fractures that cause symptoms
- Often presents with a fragility (i.e. low-energy) fracture—wrist, femoral neck, or crush fracture of the vertebral body
- Wedging of vertebrae is caused because there is higher load-bearing by the anterior part of the vertebral body. This can present as:
  - An incidental asymptomatic finding (in around a third)
  - Acute painful fracture
  - Progressive kyphosis ('dowager's hump'). The bent-over posture is not just unattractive; it causes loss of height, protuberant belly, abdominal compression, oesophageal reflux, and impaired balance with further predisposition to falls and fracture. Restricted rib movements lead to restrictive lung disease

### Diagnosis

▶ Blood tests are normal (except after a fracture). If calcium or ALP is elevated, consider an alternative diagnosis, e.g. metastases or Paget's disease.

- X-rays may show fractures and give an idea of bone density
- The gold standard is dual-energy X-ray absorptiometry (DEXA) scanning (rarely employed in the elderly population, but useful in younger women). Usually two scores are quoted at the hip and spine. The T-score compares bone density to peak bone mass, while the Z-score compares it to age/sex/weight-matched sample. A T-score of <−2.5 defines osteoporosis, with scores of −1 to −2.5 indicating osteopenia
- Peripheral densitometry assessments can be done at the heel, wrist, and ankle, the advantage being that the required machine is more portable. Results correlate with formal testing, but there are concerns about reliability in the ♂ population
- Think of 2° causes:
  - TSH in all
  - Testosterone levels in men, coeliac, and myeloma testing

In patients aged >75 years, NICE guidelines allow the assumption that osteoporosis exists where there is a:

- Low-energy (a fall from standing height or less) fracture of the wrist, femoral neck, or vertebra OR
- Progressive kyphosis without features of malignancy

### Primary prevention of osteoporosis

- Sensible public health measures (e.g. diet, exercise, stop smoking, reduce alcohol) should be advised but generally affect peak bone mass, i.e. too late for older people
- Prophylaxis with a bisphosphonate should be started for those taking significant steroid therapy (>7.5mg/day for more than a month) (see ➔ 'Osteoporosis: management', p. 472)
- HRT is no longer recommended—post-menopausal bone loss returns after it is stopped; ↑ thromboembolic, cancer, and vascular risk
- In patients with falls, osteoporotic risk should be assessed and managed (e.g. using FRAX tool, ℘ http://www.shef.ac.uk/FRAX/tool.jsp)

# Osteoporosis: management

- In patients with good calcium intake and normal serum calcium, *vitamin D* alone should be offered, as additional calcium in this group may cause ↑ cardiovascular mortality
- *Oral calcium and vitamin D* is cheap and effective, especially in frail institutionalized people (possibly due to treatment of osteomalacia and associated myopathy as much as osteoporosis). Tablets containing calcium are large and chalky, and can be unpalatable. Effervescent tablets or granules may be better tolerated. Take 1200mg calcium and 800IU vitamin D daily
- *Bisphosphonates* are very effective and used as first line. NICE recommends in any patient aged >75 following a fragility fracture (without the need for DEXA scanning)
  - The weekly dose regimens (risedronate 35mg, alendronate 70mg once weekly) are easier to remember and to tolerate than daily dosing, but patients should still take daily vitamin D ± calcium
  - Use bisphosphonates cautiously when there is dysphagia or a history of dyspepsia. Upper gut ulceration occurs rarely. Risedronate is better tolerated. Must be taken on an empty stomach 30min before food or other medicines. Swallow the tablet whole with a full glass of water while sitting or standing. Remain upright for 30min after swallowing
  - Up to 15% of patients are 'non-responders' and continue to lose bone mass. Up to 50% will stop taking the medication within 6 months. In the event of treatment failure (a new fracture), consider adherence, bone turnover markers, and changing medication if indicated
  - Contraindicated in hypocalcaemia. Manufacturers advise avoiding in CKD (eGFR <35)
  - iv zoledronic acid is given once per year for 3 years and may be used for those patients who cannot tolerate oral preparations due to side effects or poor adherence
  - Osteonecrosis of the jaw is a very rare, but serious, side effect (↑ risk with cancer, steroid treatment, and poor dental hygiene). Stop the drug and refer to a maxillofacial surgeon
- *Denosumab* is a monoclonal antibody given s/c 6-monthly. Do not give if hypocalcaemia exists or if eGFR <15
- Less common drugs, usually advised only by specialist teams include: *teriparatide, raloxifene,* and *calcitonin*
- *Strontium ranelate* significantly ↑ the incidence of stroke, MI, and VTE. It is no longer widely used in the older population
- *Vertebroplasty* can be considered for severe pain after spinal wedge fracture where conservative measures are not effective

## Further reading

National Osteoporosis Guideline Group (2014). *Osteoporosis: clinical guideline for prevention and treatment.* ℬ http://www.shef.ac.uk/NOGG/NOGG_Executive_Summary.pdf.

# Polymyalgia rheumatica

PMR is a common inflammatory syndrome causing symmetrical proximal muscle aches and stiffness. It affects only older people (do not diagnose it under age 50). There is usually rapid (days) onset of shoulder, and then thigh, pain that is worse in mornings. Sometimes associated with malaise, weight loss, depression, and fever. Often quite disabling, with little to find on examination.

## Pathology

Pathogenetically similar to GCA (TA); the two conditions commonly coexist and may represent a spectrum of disease. Pain in PMR is thought to be due to synovitis and bursitis.

## Diagnosis

▶ A difficult diagnosis to make reliably—a significant number of patients are misdiagnosed. The following should be present for a firm diagnosis:
1. Age >50
2. Bilateral aching and morning stiffness (lasting 45min or more). The stiffness should involve at least two of the following three areas: neck or torso, shoulders or proximal regions of the arms, and hips or proximal aspects of the thighs
3. Raised inflammatory markers
4. Duration >2 weeks

The following should also be considered:
- Often have anaemia (usually normochromic normocytic), weight loss, and mild abnormalities of the liver (especially ALP)
- Clinical examination often normal—despite the name, muscle tenderness is absent and pain arises because of bursitis/synovitis. Rarely there may be palpable synovitis in peripheral joints (e.g. knee, wrist)
- Muscle enzymes and EMG are normal
- Temporal artery biopsy (TAB) is positive in <25% and is rarely required
- Exclude other causes (e.g. connective tissue disease, tumour, chronic infection, neurological diseases), particularly if a patient does not respond quickly to steroids

## Treatment

- Prednisolone 15mg usually produces a reduction in symptoms, with complete resolution in most within 1 week
- Treat until symptom-free for 3 weeks and ESR/CRP normalize, then reduce the dose quickly initially (e.g. 2.5mg/3 weeks), then more slowly below 10mg (1mg/month or slower), checking for relapse of symptoms or blood tests
- If symptoms recur with an associated rise in ESR/CRP, then put the steroid dose up until both settle, then restart tailing more slowly

- Some patients can be taken off steroids after 6–8 months, but most need long-term steroids (median duration 2–3 years)
- Always give bone protection (e.g. alendronic acid 70mg once weekly with calcium and vitamin D). If a treatment trial, wait until diagnosis clear
- Azathioprine or methotrexate may be used as steroid-sparing agents or as adjuvant therapy with specialist guidance
- Educate and involve the patient in monitoring disease

### Diagnostic dilemma and steroid 'dependency'

Some older patients who were diagnosed with PMR years ago no longer exhibit or remember their symptoms, and will be having steroid side effects. They may resist steroid withdrawal or experience symptoms as steroids are ↓ or withdrawn, even if the characteristic syndrome and inflammatory responses are not displayed.

Many other diseases (even simple OA) respond to steroids (although usually less dramatically). Steroid withdrawal itself can cause general aches, which some have called 'pseudo-rheumatism'.

Avoid this difficult situation by:

- Comprehensive assessment at onset with good record-keeping, so that others can reappraise the diagnosis if response to treatment is poor
- Ensuring that where the diagnosis is not clear, a treatment trial is reviewed early for impact—if the response is not convincing, then stop the steroids. ► Beware continuing steroids because the patient feels 'a bit better'
- Considering the differential diagnosis carefully
- Discussing diagnosis and treatment with the patient
- Agreeing with the patient a clear plan for reviewing steroid therapy
- Explaining that steroid withdrawal can cause muscle aches, but the blood tests help us distinguish between this and disease reactivation

# Giant cell arteritis

GCA, or TA, is a relatively common (18 per 100,000 over age 50) systemic vasculitis of medium to large vessels. Mean age of presentation 70 (does not occur age <50). More common in women and Scandinavia/northern Europe.

## Pathogenesis

- Chronic vasculitis, mainly involving cranial branches arising from the aortic arch. Similar pathology seen in PMR, but different distribution
- Possibly an autoimmune mechanism, but no antibodies/antigen isolated

## Clinical picture

- *Systemic*: fever, malaise, anorexia, and weight loss
- *Muscles*: symmetrical proximal muscle pain and stiffness as in PMR
- *Arteritis*: tenderness over temporal arteries—not so much a headache as scalp tenderness. Classically unable to wear a hat or brush hair. If an artery occludes, distal ischaemia or infarction occurs
  - *Severe headache* is present in 90% (due to ischaemia or local tenderness of facial or scalp arteries)
  - *Jaw claudication* (occlusion of maxillary artery)
  - *Amaurosis fugax*: blindness due to occlusion of the ciliary artery, which supplies the optic nerve—this causes a pale, swollen optic nerve, but not retinal damage (which is a feature of central retinal artery occlusion with carotid disease)
  - *Stroke* (carotid artery)
  - Any large artery, including the aorta, can be affected

▶ Always suspect GCA if amaurosis fugax involves both eyes (atheroma is more commonly unilateral).

## Investigations

- ESR usually >100
- CRP also very high and falls faster with treatment than ESR
- May have normochromic normocytic anaemia and renal impairment
- TAB is highly specific, and therefore the gold standard test. Because the vasculitis may be patchy, TAB is not always positive, i.e. the sensitivity is moderate. TAB becomes negative quickly (1–2 weeks) with treatment
- Ultrasound of the cranial arteries is an alternative to diagnosis
- Same-day ophthalmology assessment if visual symptoms

## Treatment

- Never delay treatment while waiting for a biopsy
- Prednisolone 40–60mg (higher doses and slower dose reduction are required than for PMR)
- Amaurosis fugax due to GCA is an ophthalmological emergency that can result in permanent visual loss. Give 60–80mg oral prednisolone or high-dose methylprednisolone iv (500mg to 1g daily for 3 days) and aspirin 75mg and gastric protection with a PPI
- Between a third and a half of patients are able to come off steroids by 2 years

- After stopping steroids, continue to monitor as relapse is common
- Osteoporosis prophylaxis should be started at initiation of steroids (usually a bisphosphonate with calcium and vitamin D)
- Azathioprine and methotrexate are sometimes used as steroid-sparing agents once therapy is established. Consider them if:
  - Steroid side effects are prominent
  - High steroid doses are required
  - There is slow tailing off
  - There is recurrent relapse off treatment

## HOW TO . . . Manage steroid therapy in giant cell arteritis

A suggested protocol for steroid treatment in complicated GCA (with visual symptoms or severe jaw claudication) is shown in Fig. 17.1.

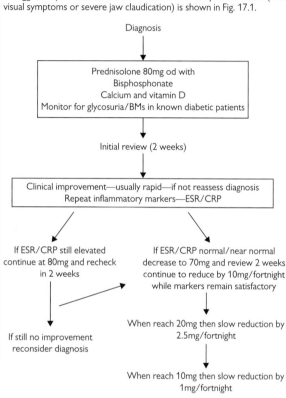

Diagnosis

Prednisolone 80mg od with
Bisphosphonate
Calcium and vitamin D
Monitor for glycosuria/BMs in known diabetic patients

Initial review (2 weeks)

Clinical improvement—usually rapid—if not reassess diagnosis
Repeat inflammatory markers—ESR/CRP

If ESR/CRP still elevated continue at 80mg and recheck in 2 weeks

If still no improvement reconsider diagnosis

If ESR/CRP normal/near normal decrease to 70mg and review 2 weeks continue to reduce by 10mg/fortnight while markers remain satisfactory

When reach 20mg then slow reduction by 2.5mg/fortnight

When reach 10mg then slow reduction by 1mg/fortnight

Fig. 17.1 A protocol for steroid treatment in giant cell arteritis.

- If rebound of symptoms or inflammatory markers occurs, then take two steps back on the reduction schedule. Wait 4 weeks before reducing again
- Beware a steroid withdrawal syndrome, which can occur without arteritis recurrence. ESR and CRP are normal (see ➋ 'Diagnostic dilemma and steroid "dependency"', p. 475)
- Other blood parameters (anaemia, impaired liver function) may help guide treatment

# Muscle symptoms

Muscular symptoms are common in older people and can arise from a range of conditions.

It should be possible to distinguish between the following:

- *True muscle weakness* due to:
  - UMN lesions (e.g. midline brain lesions such as tumours, subdural bleeds, degenerative brain disease, or cord pathology such as discs or vertebral collapse)
  - Anterior horn cell lesions (e.g. MND, polio)
  - Motor nerve root problems (spinal stenosis, malignant infiltration)
  - Peripheral motor nerve problems (inflammatory polyneuritis, thyroid disease, toxins, diabetes)
  - Neuromuscular transmission problems (myasthenia gravis, malignancy-related impairments, drug-induced problems)
  - Muscle abnormalities (dermatomyositis, inclusion body myositis, drug damage—especially steroids or statins, thyroid disease, vitamin D deficiency, electrolyte or pH imbalances)
- *Joint disease* with local pain and stiffness, reducing use with resulting weakness (e.g. OA)
- *Asthenia*—feeling of weakness, low energy and apathy as a result of systemic disease (e.g. cancer, heart disease, and chronic lung disease), confinement to bed, or psychological factors (anxiety, depression). Commonly present as feeling too tired/weak to participate in therapy

## History and examination

- Take a full history, including drugs and comorbidities
- Ask about muscle pain (rarely a feature of true myopathy—consider overexertion or fibromyalgia) and cramps
- Look for muscle wasting and abnormal movement (localized wasting indicates a problem with the relevant motor nerve or muscle body; fasciculation may indicate MND)
- Is the weakness generalized (usually due to cachexia or myasthenia gravis) or limited to specific tasks (more common with localized muscle weakness)?
- Grade muscle strength with standardized score (see ➲ 'HOW TO . . . Grade muscle strength', p. 481) for later comparisons
- A lack of demonstrable muscle weakness, despite symptoms, usually indicates asthenia
- Check for fatigability (may indicate myasthenia gravis)
- Ask about CNS disease and examine neurologically (brisk reflexes with upgoing plantars point to the CNS, whereas absent reflexes may indicate peripheral nerve disease)
- Check the joints for degenerative disease; ask about pain and stiffness
- Look for evidence of systemic disease (e.g. thyroid, malignancy)
- Assess mood

### Investigations

- Screening *bloods* should include: potassium (K), calcium (Ca), magnesium (Mg), urea, creatinine, LFTs, TFTs, autoantibody screen, FBC, ESR, CRP, serum electrophoresis, and haematinics. CK is elevated after prolonged lie, seizure, or an im injection, or with pathology of the muscle unit
- *Plain X-rays* can reveal joint disease
- *Ultrasound* can be used to assess joints and muscle
- *CT or MRI scans* can demonstrate CNS pathology, cord problems, and degree of muscle atrophy
- *Nerve conduction studies and EMG* are useful to demonstrate nerve pathology, problems with neuromuscular transmission, and intrinsic muscle disease. It can confirm the diagnosis in a number of conditions (e.g. chronic inflammatory demyelinating polyneuropathy)
- *Muscle biopsy* can sometimes be useful

---

### HOW TO . . . Grade muscle strength

The widely used Medical Research Council grading system allows sequential assessments to be compared. It involves assessing muscle activity in isolation, against gravity, and against resistance, and is scored as follows (see Table 17.1).

**Table 17.1** Medical Research Council grading system

| 0 | No muscle contraction |
|---|---|
| 1 | Flicker or trace of muscle contraction |
| 2 | Limb or joint movement possible only with gravity eliminated |
| 3 | Limb or joint movement against gravity, but not resistance |
| 4 | Power ↓ but limb or joint movement possible against resistance |
| 5 | Normal power against resistance |

Scores can be augmented if the category is not quite reached (−) or slightly exceeded (+), e.g. minor reduction in power against resistance may be described as 5−.

# Paget's disease

This is a very common bone disease of old age (up to 10% prevalence, more common in men). It is usually clinically silent—only about 5% are symptomatic.

The cause is unknown. There is abnormal bone remodelling. Most commonly affects the pelvis, femur, spine, skull, and tibia. The resultant bone is expanded and disordered and can cause pain and pathological fracture, and predisposes to osteosarcoma.

## Presentation
- Most commonly as asymptomatic elevated ALP
- Often an incidental finding on a pelvis or skull X-ray
- Less commonly as:
  - *Pathological fracture* (especially hip and pelvis)
  - *Bone pain*: constant pain commonly in legs, especially at night. The diseased bone itself can be painful, or deformity can lead to accelerated joint disease at, e.g. the hip, knee, or spine. Fracture or osteosarcoma can cause suddenly ↑ pain
  - *Deformity*: bowing of legs or upper arm is often asymmetrical. The skull can take on a characteristic 'bossed' shape due to overgrowth of frontal bones
  - *Deafness*: bone expansion in the skull compresses the eighth cranial nerve, causing conduction deafness, which can be severe
  - *Other neurological compression syndromes*, e.g. spinal cord (paraplegia), optic nerve (blindness), brainstem compression (dysphagia and hydrocephalus)

## Investigations
- ALP is constantly elevated
  - The bone isoenzyme is more specific and useful when liver function is abnormal
  - Rarely (e.g. if only one bone is involved), total ALP can be normal, but the bone isoenzyme is always raised
- Other markers of bone turnover, e.g. urinary hydroxyproline are raised
- X-rays show mixed lysis and sclerosis, disordered bone texture, and expansion (a diagnostic feature)
- Radioisotope bone scans show hot spots
- Immobile patients with very active disease can become hypercalcaemic, although this is rare. If calcium and ALP are raised, there is more likely to be another diagnosis (e.g. carcinomatosis, hyperparathyroidism)

## Management

As most cases are asymptomatic, often no treatment is required. Symptomatic cases may warrant referral to a rheumatologist

- Analgesia and joint replacement may be needed
- Fractures often require internal fixation to correct deformity and because they heal poorly
- Bisphosphonates (usually by iv infusion) are very useful. They have several effects:
  - Reduce pain
  - Reduce vascularity before elective surgery
  - Improve healing after fracture
  - Improve neurological compression syndromes
  - Reduce serum calcium in hypercalcaemia
- Calcitonin is now rarely used
- ALP, other bone turnover biochemical markers, and occasionally nuclear bone scans can be used to monitor the effectiveness of treatment

# Gout

Uric acid crystals deposit in and around joints and intermittently produce inflammation. Serum urate levels correlate poorly with the disease manifestations.

↑ incidence with age due to:
- Worsening renal function and impaired uric acid excretion
- ↑ hyperuricaemic drug use, e.g. thiazides, aspirin, cytotoxics
- Common acute precipitants, e.g. sepsis, surgery

## Presentation

- *Acute monoarthritis* in feet or hands is the most common but can also occur in large joints such as knee or shoulder. The joint is very painful, hot, and red. Patients often refuse to bear weight or move the joint. The patient can look unwell and sometimes has a fever
- *Chronic tophi* (usually painless) over finger joints and in ears can occur, associated with a chronic arthritis. Sometimes mistaken for other more common arthritides
- *Olecranon bursitis*
- *Uric acid kidney stones*

## Investigations

- During an acute attack, *serum uric acid* may be normal or high
- *WBC, ESR*, and *CRP* are usually high or very high
- *Joint fluid*:
  - May be cloudy or frankly purulent on visual inspection
  - Microscopy shows many inflammatory cells
  - Under polarized light, negatively birefringent uric acid crystals are seen in joint fluid or in phagocytes
- *X-rays* are usually normal (rarely see small punched-out erosions in fingers in chronic tophaceous cases)

The main aim is to exclude an infective arthritis.
▶ If in doubt, consider using iv antibiotics until cultures are negative.

## Treatment

- *For acute gout*:
  - Use *paracetamol* with a short course of NSAIDs with gastric protection
  - If you have ruled out infection, local steroid injections are often effective (e.g. methylprednisolone 40mg intra-articular)
  - When NSAIDs are contraindicated, use a short course of oral *steroids* (e.g. prednisolone 30mg od for 5 days)
  - *Colchicine* 0.5mg bd is also effective, but gastrointestinal side effects may limit use
  - *For chronic arthritis* with or without tophi: treat with allopurinol or febuxostat

## Prevention

One or two attacks of gout probably do not warrant prophylaxis (especially as such drugs can precipitate further attacks). Instead, try:

- Changing drugs (stop thiazides and aspirin)
- Lifestyle advice:
  - Reduce alcohol (wine is preferable to lager or beer)
  - Reduce dietary purines (meat/shellfish)
  - Lose weight
- Do not leave patients on long-term NSAIDs. Very early use of NSAIDs or colchicine can abort a severe attack of gout

Two or more attacks of gout in one year merit slow introduction of allopurinol (caution in CKD) or febuxostat.

Principles include:

- Start 1–2 weeks after acute inflammation settles
- Consider co-prescription of colchicine or steroids to prevent acute flare
- Dose-titrate to target uric acid level of <300 micromoles/L (associated with reduction in cardiovascular risk)

---

### HOW TO ... Aspirate/inject the knee joint

*Why?*

- Aids diagnosis of the swollen joint: infection, crystals, blood
- Useful skill often performed in clinic, DH, or as an inpatient. Hard to do harm
- Allows therapeutic interventions: ↓ pressure and/or injection of medication
- If preceding trauma, obtain X-rays before procedure
- Check clotting and platelets if concerns or on warfarin

*Procedure*

1. Obtain verbal consent explaining benefits (pain relief, diagnosis, improving mobility) and risks (pain, infection, bleeding, inability to locate joint space)
2. Lay the patient supine with the target knee slightly flexed (a rolled towel under the knee may help with this)
3. Using the parapatellar approach is the simplest; either the lateral or medial aspect of the midpoint of the patella, depending on where most fluid is felt to be
4. Clean and drape using aseptic technique
5. Infiltrate local anaesthetic to subcutaneous tissue if desired
6. Use a 21G (green) needle and 20mL syringe, and briskly insert into the joint, aspirating as you advance. Aim perpendicular to the femur and below the patella. Usual depth 1–2cm
7. Remove as much fluid as possible for relief and samples for analysis. If injecting treatment, keep the needle in place, remove the syringe, and attach a pre-prepared medicine syringe so to avoid repeated skin penetration
8. Withdraw the needle and apply a dressing

# Pseudogout

### Features

This is an acute, episodic synovitis closely resembling gout, except that:
- Calcium pyrophosphate, rather than uric acid crystals (with positive, rather than negative, birefringence), are found
- Large joints are more commonly affected (especially knees, but also shoulder, hips, wrists, and elbows)
- It is not associated with tophi, bursitis, or stones
- X-rays often show calcification of articular cartilage 'chondrocalcinosis' in the affected joint
- It does not respond to allopurinol—so consider this diagnosis where recurrent attacks persist despite allopurinol

As with gout, the patient has an acutely inflamed joint which is very painful to move. They may be systemically unwell with a fever and highly elevated inflammatory markers. Serum calcium is normal.

▶ Consider this diagnosis in the post-acute patient with a hot, swollen wrist.

### Management

Make a confident diagnosis. This usually involves immediate synovial fluid sampling and urgent microscopy to exclude infection and gout.

Effective treatment for acute pseudogout is the same as for acute gout and include:
- Intra-articular steroid injections
- Oral NSAIDs with gastric protection
- Oral corticosteroids
- Colchicine

Long-term preventative treatment is not available.

# Contractures

Contractures are joint deformities caused by damaged connective tissue. Where a joint is immobilized (through depressed conscious level, loss of neural input, or local tissue damage), the muscle, ligaments, tendons, and skin can become inelastic and shortened, causing joints to be flexed.

Common causes worldwide include polio, cerebral palsy, and leprosy; in geriatric medicine, common causes include stroke, dementia, and musculo-skeletal conditions, e.g. fracture. Contractures are under-recognized—they occur, to some degree, in about a third of nursing home residents and it is still not uncommon to find patients who are bed-bound and permanently curled into the fetal position.

## Problems

- *Pain*: on moving joint but can occur at rest due to muscle spasm
- *Hygiene*: skin surfaces may oppose (e.g. the hand after stroke or groins in abduction/flexion contractures), making it difficult for carers, and painful for the patient, to keep clean and odourless
- *Pressure areas*: abnormal posture ↑ risk
- *Aesthetics*: although the lack of movement causes most disability, the abnormal posture/appearance can be more noticeable
- *Function*: chronic bed-bound patients may become so flexed that they are unable to sit out in a chair

## Prevention

- Where immobilization is short term, e.g. after a fracture, passive stretching followed by exercise regimens should begin promptly
- All health-care staff should understand the importance of maintaining mobility (including sitting out of bed for short periods) and positioning of immobile patients
- Preventative measures are rarely successful at preventing contractures in joints with long-term immobility, e.g. in residual hemiparesis after stroke
- Splinting might help mould the position. Therapists often have expertise in this area

## Treatment

- Periodic injection of *botulinum toxin* is helpful where muscle spasticity is the major problem. There are no real adverse effects, but some patients develop an antibody response after repeated treatment, which renders therapy less effective. Newer preparations are less immunogenic
- There is little point using *muscle relaxants*, except to help with pain. Even then, drugs such as baclofen, dantrolene, tizanidine, and diazepam usually cause side effects of drowsiness before they reach therapeutic levels. Occasionally assist with PT stretches
- *Surgery*, e.g. tendon division, has a place in severe cases
- *PT* can, to some extent, reverse established changes, especially if of relatively recent onset and not severe

# Cervical spondylosis and myelopathy

Degeneration in the cervical spine causes neurological dysfunction with both radiculopathy (compression of nerve roots leaving spinal foramina) and myelopathy (cord compression). The resulting mixture of lower (nerve root) and upper (cord) nerve damage causes pain, weakness, and numbness. Progress is usually gradual but can be sudden (especially following trauma). The disease is unusual before the age of 50. Mild forms are very common in the elderly population.

## History

- Neck pain and restricted movement may be present but are neither specific nor sensitive markers of nerve damage. Pain may radiate to the shoulder, chest, or arm in a dermatomal distribution (see ➲ Appendix, 'Dermatomes', p. 700)
- Arms and hands become clumsy, especially for fine movements (e.g. doing up buttons). Weakness, numbness, and paraesthesiae can occur
- Leg symptoms usually occur later, with a UMN spastic weakness and a wide-based and/or ataxic gait, often with falls
- Urinary dysfunction is unusual and late
- Rarely can cause vertebrobasilar insufficiency symptoms

## Signs

- Arms have predominantly lower motor signs with weakness, muscle wasting, and segmental reflex loss. The classical 'inverted supinator' sign is due to a C5/6 lesion where the supinator jerk is lost but the finger jerk (C7) is augmented—when the wrist is tapped, the fingers flex
- Legs may have brisk reflexes, ↑ tone, clonus, and upgoing plantars. In severe cases, a spastic paraparesis with a sensory level can develop

## Differential diagnosis

This is wide and includes:
- Syringomyelia
- MND (look for signs above the neck and an absence of sensory symptoms/signs)
- Peripheral neuropathy (no UMN signs)
- Vitamin $B_{12}$ deficiency
- Other causes of spastic gait disorders

## Investigations

- *Plain X-rays* in older people almost always show degenerative changes, which correlate poorly with symptoms. They are only useful in excluding other pathology or in demonstrating spinal instability
- *MRI scanning* is the investigation of choice. Bone and soft tissue structures and the extent of cord compression are all well demonstrated
- *CT scanning* may be used where there are contraindications for MRI
- *Nerve conduction studies* can help confirm the clinical impression and exclude other pathology

## Management

*Cervical collars* do not influence progression but can sometimes help with radicular pain and may provide partial protection from acute decline following trauma. The only definitive treatment is *surgical*—laminectomy with fusion for stabilization.

Surgery is indicated for:

- Progressive neurology (especially if rapidly progressive—consider steroids while surgery is arranged)
- Severe pain unresponsive to conservative measures
- Myelopathy more than radiculopathy

Discuss the risks and benefits with the patient—function is rarely restored once lost, but pain improves and further damage is usually avoided.

# Osteomyelitis

Infection of the bone that is most common in the very young and the very old. It is important in geriatric practice because it complicates conditions that frequently occur in older patients, yet presentation is often non-specific and indolent, so the diagnosis may be missed.

### Vertebral osteomyelitis
- Usually affects the thoracolumbar spine
- Patients complain of mild backache and malaise and will often have local tenderness. When examining a patient with pyrexia of unknown origin (PUO), always 'walk' the examining fingers down the spine, applying pressure to find local bony pain
- Vertebral osteomyelitis (commonly T10–11) may lead to:
  - Perivertebral abscess with a risk of cord compression
  - Vertebral body collapse with angular kyphosis
- Discitis occurs when the infection involves the intervertebral disc. The patient is relatively less septic, and X-rays appear normal until disease is very advanced (at which point end-plate erosion can occur). Haematogenous spread may occur after surgery or disc space injections
- Haematogenous spread is most common, often after UTI, catheterization, iv cannula insertion, or other instrumentation
- Commonly due to *Staphylococcus aureus (consider MRSA)*, less commonly Gram-negative bacilli, rarely TB

### Osteomyelitis of other bones
- Generally more common in children but arise in older patients in some circumstances:
  - As a complication of orthopaedic surgery
  - As a complication of ulceration (venous or pressure ulcers)

▶ Always consider osteomyelitis in non-healing ulcers; may be present in as many as 25%.
  - In susceptible individuals (e.g. diabetic patients with vascular disease and neuropathy are prone to osteomyelitis in small bones of the feet)
- Organisms include *S. aureus, Staphylococcus epidermidis* (especially with prostheses), Gram-negative bacilli, and anaerobes

### Clinical features of osteomyelitis
- Pain is usual but may be missed if there is a pre-existing pressure sore, or the patient has peripheral neuropathy and foot osteomyelitis (e.g. diabetics)
- Malaise is common
- Fever may be absent

## Investigations

- Blood cultures should be taken in all and are positive in around half
- Leucocytosis is variable
- ESR and CRP are usually raised (although very non-specific)
- X-ray changes lag behind clinical changes by about 10 days. Initially normal or showing soft tissue swelling. Later develop classic changes: periosteal reaction, sequestra (islands of necrosis), bone abscesses, and sclerosis of neighbouring bone
- MRI is the investigation of choice, being both sensitive and specific, even in early disease
- Radioisotope bone scanning will show a 'hot spot' with osteomyelitis but will not distinguish this from many other conditions (e.g. fracture, arthritis, non-infectious inflammation, metastases, etc.)
- Biopsy or FNA of bone is required to guide antibiotic therapy—this may be done through the base of an ulcer or using radiological guidance (ultrasound is useful here)
- Wound swabs reveal colonizing organisms and are often misleading

## Treatment

- General measures such as analgesia and fluids if needed
- Obtaining tissue specimens permits bacterial culture and determination of antimicrobial sensitivity. Duration of therapy is usually long, and identification of the organism allows antibiotic precision to reduce side effects. After specimens are obtained, but prior to results, 'best guess' therapy may be started according to local guidelines and with microbiological advice
- Treatment is initially iv, often later converted to oral therapy
- Total treatment duration is usually many weeks or months (depending on sensitivity of organism and extent and location of infection)
- Surgical drainage should be considered after 36h if systemic upset continues or if there is deep pus on imaging

## Complications

- *Metastatic infection*
- *Suppurative arthritis*
- *Chronic osteomyelitis* infection becomes walled off in cavities within the bone, discharging to the surface by a sinus. Symptoms relapse and remit as sinuses close and reopen. Bone is at risk of pathological fracture. Management is long and difficult—this is a miserable complication of joint replacement. Culture organisms and use appropriate antibiotics to limit spread. Surgical removal of infected bone and/or prosthesis is required for cure. Involve specialist bone infection teams, if possible
- *Malignant otitis externa* occurs when otitis externa spreads to cause osteomyelitis of the skull base. Occurs particularly in frail, older diabetic patients. Caused by *Pseudomonas* and anaerobes. Facial nerve palsy develops in half, with possible involvement of nerves IX–XII. Requires prolonged antibiotics, specialist ENT input, and possible surgical debridement

# The elderly foot

Foot problems are very common (>80% of over 65s) and can cause major disability, including ↑ susceptibility to falls. A particular problem in older people because:

- Multiple degenerative and disease pathologies occur and interact
- Many older people cannot reach their feet—monitoring and basic hygiene (especially nail cutting) may be limited
- Patients think foot problems are a part of ageing or are embarrassed by them and do not seek treatment
- Health professionals often neglect to examine the feet and are too slow to refer for specialist foot care. It is common to find a patient naked under a hospital gown but still with thick socks on
- Inappropriate footwear may be worn—most older people cannot afford or refuse to wear 'sensible' shoes such as trainers
- Access to chiropody services is variable on the NHS (rationed to diabetic patients and those with peripheral vascular disease in most areas)

## Nails

- *Very long nails* can curl back and cut into toes
- Nails thicken and become more brittle with age. This is worsened by repeated trauma (e.g. bad footwear), poor circulation, or diabetes. Ultimately, the nail looks like a ram's horn (*onychogryphosis*) and cannot be cut with ordinary nail clippers
- Fungal nail infection (*onychomycosis*) produces a similarly thickened, discoloured nail
- *Ingrowing toenails* can cause pain and recurring infection

## Skin

- Calluses (hard skin)
- Corns (painful calluses over pressure points with a nucleus/core)
- Cracks and ulceration (see ➲ 'Leg ulcers', p. 593)
- Cellulitis

### Between the toes

Fungal infection ('athlete's foot') is very common. The skin maceration that results is a common cause of cellulitis.

### Bone/joint disease

- A *bunion* (hallux valgus) is an outpointing deformity of the big toe, which can overlap the second toe
- *Hammer toes* are flexion deformities of proximal interphalangeal (IP) joints
- *Claw toes* have deformities at both IP joints
- *OA or gout* of the metatarsophalangeal joint causes pain and rigidity
- *Neuropathic foot*: long-standing severe sensory loss in a foot (e.g. diabetics, tabes dorsalis), with multiple stress fractures and osteoporosis disrupting the biomechanics of the joints (*Charcot's joint*). The foot/ankle is swollen and red, but painless with loss of arches (*rockerbottom foot*)

### Circulation impairment

Common. Assess vasculature (including an ABPI; see ➋ 'HOW TO . . . Measure ABPI', p. 307) if there is pain, ulceration, infection, or skin changes.

### Sensory impairment

Touch, pain, and joint position sense are all important to maintaining normal feet.

---

### HOW TO . . . Care for the elderly foot

*Prevention*
- Inspect both feet frequently (at least every other day). A hand mirror assists inspection of the sole. ▶ If a patient cannot see, reach, or feel their feet, someone else should be helping them regularly
- Examine for swelling, discoloration, ulcers, cuts, calluses, or corns
- If these are identified, consult a health professional (podiatrist, nurse, or doctor) promptly
- Wash feet daily in warm water with mild simple soap. If feet are numb, check that the water temperature is not too hot with a hand or with a thermometer (35–40°C is best)
- After washing, dry feet thoroughly, particularly between the toes
- Change socks or stockings daily
- Dry, hard, or thick skin should be softened with emollients such as liquid and white soft paraffin ointment ('50:50')
- Footwear should be supportive but soft. Take particular care with new footwear, inspecting feet frequently after short periods of wear to ensure that no sores have developed
- Avoid barefoot walking
- Cut nails regularly, cutting them straight across and not too short

*Treatment*
- Qualified podiatrists or chiropodists will debride calluses/corns and use dressings and pressure-relieving pads to prevent them from recurring. Availability on the NHS has been severely restricted recently (only diabetics qualify in most regions), so cost may deter patients
- Treat athlete's foot (e.g. clotrimazole cream bd for 1 week)
- Distinguish between thick, discolored nails due to onychomycosis from simple onychogryphosis by sending nail scrapings for microscopy for fungal hyphae. Topical antifungal treatment is often not practical, and tablet treatment (e.g. terbinafine) can take months to be effective, so the vast majority of elderly patients remain untreated. If you do decide to use terbinafine, monitor liver function and be wary of drug interactions
- Surgery may be used to remove nails or correct severe bone deformity

# The elderly hand

Hand problems are common in older people and may lead to functional problems (finding it hard to perform necessary ADLs), as well as social and cosmetic problems (e.g. unable to wear a wedding ring). Hand function can be assessed by:

- Opening and closing the hand—looking for smooth and full movement
- Assessing grip strength
- Assessing ability to make a pincer grip
- Asking the patient to perform fine motor tasks (e.g. doing up a button)

## Hand deformity

- *Heberden's nodes* (at distal IP joint) and *Bouchard's nodes* (at proximal IP joint) are common in older hands and have X-ray appearances of OA. They are rarely painful, but hands may become clumsy or difficult to use
- *Mallet finger* is a flexion deformity of the distal IP joint, usually after trauma (due to tendon rupture). Splinting acutely can correct the problem
- *Trigger finger* arises because of digital tendinitis and tenosynovitis (inflammation of tendons and tendon sheaths of the hand, often with fibrosis). More common in people with diabetes. The finger may lock in flexion, suddenly extending with a snap. Treat with rest and splinting, and consider NSAIDs with gastric protection. Steroid injection may help, or surgical release can be done
- *Swan-neck deformity* occurs classically in rheumatoid arthritis (but also with other tendon problems) and involves hyperextension of the proximal IP joint with flexion of the distal IP joint. Can cause significant disability, and surgery may help
- *Boutonnière deformity* is flexion of the proximal IP joint and hyperextension of the distal IP joint, due to tendon rupture, dislocation, fracture, OA, and rheumatoid arthritis. Early splinting may help, but surgery is rarely useful
- *Dupuytren's contracture* is progressive contracture of the palmar fascial bands, producing flexion deformities of the fingers. Occurs mainly in older men, with diabetes, alcoholism, or epilepsy. Autosomal dominant inheritance (incomplete penetrance). Steroid injection may help early disease; advanced disease requires surgery

## Common hand symptoms

- *Cold hands* are commonly reported in older patients, and indeed hands may feel cold, despite good vascular supply. Reassure, and use simple measures (gloves, warm soaks) to provide relief
- *Numb hands* should prompt assessment for nerve entrapment or peripheral neuropathy, but symptoms may be present in the absence of these. Patients will describe intermittent pins and needles or just a lowered sense of touch and may be clumsier. Use of warm soaks, analgesia, stretching exercises, and reassurance can be helpful
- *Hand cramps* can be troublesome, especially at night. Try warm soaks, hand stretches, or calcium supplements to relieve
- *Dropping objects* in the absence of demonstrable pathology is common and may result from subtle changes in proprioceptive ability

## Repetitive strain injury

This is becoming more common in older people, often from excessive use of computers. Treatment is with rest, analgesia, and modification of the precipitating behaviour.

## Carpal tunnel syndrome

- More common with age, OA, rheumatoid arthritis, diabetes, hypothyroidism, obesity, smokers, or those who apply repetitive strain to the wrist
- Hand and wrist pain with paraesthesiae and numbness in the median nerve distribution
- The patient will often wake at night with burning or aching pain, numbness, and tingling; shaking the hand provides relief
- Reduced sensation in the median nerve distribution and weak thumb abduction are common and suggestive
- Check for Tinel's sign (tingling in the median nerve region, elicited by tapping the palmar surface of the wrist over the median nerve site in the carpal tunnel) or Phalen's test (flexion of the wrist for 1min)
- Thenar muscle atrophy occurs late
- Older patients will often have multilevel nerve entrapment (cervical as well as at the wrist)
- Treatment is initially with splinting and analgesia. Steroid injections can help; surgery is usually curative. Consider this even in frail patients in whom function (e.g. ability to hold their frame) is impaired

## Complex regional pain syndrome

- Also known as reflex sympathetic dystrophy or shoulder hand syndrome
- Occurs in the extremities, characterized by pain, swelling, limited range of motion, vasomotor instability, skin changes, and patchy bone demineralization
- Can occur following an injury, surgery, or a vascular event such as MI or stroke
- Pathophysiology poorly understood
- Think of the diagnosis where there is intense throbbing arm pain with an alteration in skin temperature
- Autonomic testing is abnormal, and bone scans show ↑ uptake early in the disease. X-rays may show osteopenia, and MRI may show skin and tissue changes later in the disease
- Early mobilization after a stroke helps prevent this condition
- Early disease can be treated with smoking cessation, topical counter-irritants (e.g. capsaicin), oral NSAIDs, and steroids. Bisphosphonates help prevent bone loss and provide pain relief
- More advanced disease may respond to regional sympathetic nerve blocks and generally require specialist pain team input

# The painful hip

▶ The important diagnosis not to miss in the frail elderly is *fracture*. Having a low threshold of suspicion and for investigation is key.

## Hip fracture

- The absence of a recent fall and ability to weight-bear should not put you off obtaining an X-ray
- In any bedbound patient after a fall, look for inability to lift the leg off the bed and pain on movement (especially rotation), even if they are not fit to stand. A shortened externally rotated leg is a useful sign but will occur in many who have replacement hips and is not seen in all
- Some patients can walk on a fractured hip
- Always:
  - Get anteroposterior pelvis and lateral hip X-rays
  - Have the X-rays reported by a radiologist—changes can be subtle
  - Check for pubic ramus fractures, as well as fractures of the femoral head and shaft
- If initial films are normal but clinical suspicion is high, an MRI should be obtained and is sanctioned in NICE guidance. It is important to make the diagnosis early—do not be afraid to argue your case with radiology

Almost all hip fractures require surgical repair no matter how frail the patient (conservative management with or without traction is painful and has a massive morbidity and mortality). By contrast, low-energy pelvic fractures in older people do not require surgery (see ➡ 'HOW TO . . . Manage non-operative fractures', p. 469). Even with surgery, the 30-day mortality for a fractured neck of femur is high (8–9%). Remember to initiate osteoporosis treatment.

## Osteoarthritis

- Pain is 'boring' and stiffness occurs after rest
- Restriction of movement occurs in all planes
- OA can significantly ↑ chance of falls
- Total hip replacement is now widely available and very effective
  - Consider referral for radiographic moderate/severe disease with ongoing pain or disability despite trial of conservative treatment
  - There is 1% mortality, but older people often have a good long-term result. Revision surgery is rarely needed because activity levels are lower than in younger people (and life expectancy less)

## Other causes of hip pain

- *Paget's disease*: also causes 2° OA
- *Radicular pain* referred from the spine
- *Metastases*
- *Septic arthritis*: rare and difficult diagnosis to make, but consider joint aspiration under ultrasound if your patient appears septic with a very painful hip, especially after recent hip surgery
- *Vitamin D insufficiency* may present with pelvic girdle weakness and pain
- *Referred pain* from the knee
- *Psoas abscess*
- *Avascular necrosis of the femoral head* (rheumatoid arthritis, diabetes, steroids)

# The painful back

## Assessment

- History should include position, quality, duration, and radiation of pain, as well as associated sensory symptoms, bladder or bowel problems, and a systems review
- Undress the patient and look for bruising and deformity
- Apply pressure to each vertebra in turn, looking for local tenderness
- Look for restriction of movement and gait abnormality
- Always check neurology and consider bowel/bladder function

▶ 'Red flags' for serious pathology include acute onset, leg weakness, fever, weight loss, and bowel and bladder dysfunction (including a new catheter).

## Causes

- *OA* of the facet joints becomes more common than disc pathology with advancing age (discs are less pliable and less likely to herniate)
- *Osteoporosis* and vertebral crush fractures can cause acute, well-localized pain, chronic pain, or no pain at all
- *Cervical myelopathy*
- *Spondylolisthesis* most commonly affects the lumbar spine and is worse on activity or standing
- *Metastatic cancer* should always be considered, especially if pain is new or severe, there are constitutional symptoms such as weight loss, or pain from an apparent fracture fails to improve
- *Vertebral osteomyelitis and infective discitis* should be considered in those with fever and raised inflammatory markers, especially if they are immunosuppressed (e.g. rheumatoid arthritis on steroids)

▶ Not all back pain comes from the spine. Differential diagnoses that should not be missed include pancreatitis or pancreatic cancer, biliary colic, duodenal ulcer, aortic aneurysm, renal pain, retroperitoneal pathology, PE, Guillain–Barré syndrome, or MI.

## Investigations

- FBC, ESR, myeloma screen, CRP, ALP, calcium, PSA (in men)
- MRI is good at identifying serious pathology, e.g. cancer, infection, compression syndromes
- CT can be done if unable to have MRI but has lower diagnostic yield
- Bone scan is sometimes useful if there are multiple sites of pain
- Plain X-rays may reveal diagnosis, but 'wear and tear' changes are very common and correlate poorly with pain. May miss serious pathology

## Treatment

Firstly, make a diagnosis to guide therapy.

*Specific therapies* include:
- Bisphosphonates, calcitonin, or vertebroplasty for osteoporotic collapse
- Radiotherapy and/or steroids are very effective for metastatic deposits
- Urgent surgery or radiotherapy should be considered for cord compression, with high-dose iv steroids while awaiting definitive treatment

*General therapies* for most diagnoses include:
- Standard analgesia ladder (see ➲ 'Analgesia', p. 136)
- PT is often helpful in improving pain and function or at least preventing deconditioning
- Exercise and weight loss (if obese) are difficult to achieve but will help
- TENS can help some and is without side effects
- Antispasmodics, e.g. diazepam 2mg, if muscular spasm is prominent
- Consider referral to a pain specialist for local injections, e.g. facet joints or epidurals
- Once serious pathology has been excluded, a chiropractor/osteopath can sometimes help

# The painful shoulder

The shoulder joint has little bony articulation (and hence little arthritis), but lots of muscle and tendon which is prone to damage. Many conditions become chronic, and examining elderly people will reveal a high prevalence of pain and restricted movement. Patients compensate (e.g. by avoiding clothes that need to be pulled over the head) and may not report symptoms.

Before diagnosing one of the conditions that follow, exclude systemic problems such as PMR and rheumatoid arthritis. Remember that neck problems, diaphragmatic pathology, apical lung cancer, and angina can also produce shoulder pain.

### Frozen shoulder/adhesive capsulitis

- Usually idiopathic but sometimes follow trauma and stroke
- More common in people with diabetes
- Loss of rotation (internal and external) and abduction
- Painful for weeks to months, then stiff (frozen) for further 4–12 months
- Mainstay of treatment is PT/exercise—avoid rest
- Intra-articular steroids may help pain and improve tolerance to early mobilization

### Biceps tendonitis

- Pain in specific area (anterior/lateral humeral head) aggravated by supination on the forearm while the elbow held flexed against the body
- Treatment is rest and corticosteroid injection, followed by gentle biceps-stretching exercises

### Rotator cuff tendonitis

- Dull ache radiating to the upper arm with 'painful arc' (pain between 60° and 120° when abducting the arm)
- Rest, occasionally with immobilization in a sling, and corticosteroid injection
- PT and exercises may help
- Arthroscopic decompression can sometimes relieve pain

### Rotator cuff tear

- May occur following trauma
- Reduced range of active and passive movements of shoulder
- Ultrasound and MRI diagnostic
- Treat with rest and corticosteroid injection
- PT and exercises may help
- Surgical repair possible in some cases

### Shoulder dislocation

- May occur after a fall (usually anterior) or seizure (may be posterior)
- Shoulder is painful and appears deformed, and X-rays will confirm
- Check for neurovascular damage; pain relief, and arrange joint reduction by manipulation

### Glenohumeral osteoarthritis

- Uncommon site for arthritis—there is usually previous trauma
- Presentation and examination similar to frozen shoulder
- Classic examination findings are of:
  - Local glenohumeral joint line tenderness and swelling anteriorly
  - Loss of range of motion of external rotation and abduction
  - Crepitation
- X-rays will confirm
- Initial treatment is with analgesia and mobilization
- Joint injection with steroids can be useful
- Failure to respond to conservative measures should prompt consideration of surgical referral for joint replacement—this is highly successful in appropriate patients

# Pressure injuries

# Pressure sores

Areas of skin necrosis due to pressure-induced ischaemia found on the sacrum, heels, over the greater trochanters, shoulders, etc. Also known as decubitus ulcers or bedsores. Incidence higher in hospital (new sores form during acute illness), but prevalence higher in long-stay community settings (healing takes months/years). Average hospital prevalence 5–10% despite drives to improve education and preventative strategies. The financial and staffing resource burden of pressure sores is huge. Forms a major part of nursing role, but important that the whole MDT prioritizes prevention and management.

## Grading

(Most sites use photographic images to guide classification.)
I.   Non-blanching erythema
II.  Broken skin or blistering (epidermis ± dermis only)
III. Full-thickness skin loss, subcutaneous fat or slough seen
IV.  Ulcer down to bone, joint, or tendon

Moisture lesions are a separate category—caused by excessive moisture from urine, faeces, or sweat. Not usually over bony prominence.

▶ Two hours of tissue ischaemia are sufficient for the subsequent development of an ulcer, and the causative insult often occurs just prior to, or at the time of, admission (on ED trolleys, intraoperative, at home). There is considerable lag between the ischaemic insult and the resulting ulcer. Grade I erythema often progresses to deep ulcers over days/weeks without further ischaemic insult. Inspect the sacrum and heels at least daily. If there is a lesion, classify and document carefully—measure the dimensions or consider photographing for medical record.

## Risk factors

Include age, immobility (especially post-operative), low or high body weight, malnutrition, dehydration, incontinence, neurological damage (either neuropathy or ↓ conscious level), sedative drugs, and vascular impairment.

Several scoring systems (e.g. Waterlow score) combine these factors to stratify risk. They aid/prompt clinical judgement of individual patient risk.

## Mechanisms

- *Pressure*—normal capillary pressure 24–34mmHg—pressures exceeding 35mmHg compress and cause ischaemia. This pressure is easily exceeded on simple foam mattress at pressure points, e.g. heels
- *Shear*—where the skin is pulled away from fixed axial skeleton, small blood vessels can be kinked or torn. When a patient is propped up in bed or dragged (e.g. during a lift or transfer), there is considerable shear on the sacrum
- *Friction*—rubbing the skin ↓ its integrity, especially at moving extremities, e.g. elbows, heels. Avoid crumbs, drip sets, and debris between the patient and sheets. Massage of pressure areas no longer recommended
- *Moisture*—sweat, urine, and faeces cause maceration and ↓ integrity

## Management

- *Prevention*—demands awareness—all patients should be risk-assessed within 6h of admission. Regular reassessment during hospital admission should occur, especially if condition of the patient changes
- *Turning and handling*—there is no evidence to suggest how often immobile, high-risk patients should be turned in bed. Two-hourly turns are historically based and rarely achieved. Frequency should be judged individually. Modern mattresses ↓ frequency but do not eradicate the need for turns. Avoid friction and sheer by using correct manual handling devices. Consider limiting sitting out to 2h. Encourage early mobilization; optimize pain control, and minimize sedative drugs
- *Pressure-relieving devices*—consider for beds, chairs, and localized body parts (e.g. heels). Wide variety available—balance pressure relief with cost and limitation to independent mobility
- *Promote a healing environment*:
  - Nutrition—protein and calorie supplements. There is no evidence to support the use of vitamins, e.g. vitamin C, or minerals, e.g. zinc, but they are unlikely to do harm
  - Manage incontinence (one of the few times that a geriatrician might recommend a catheter)
  - Good glycaemic control in people with diabetes
  - Correct anaemia (normochromic/normocytic anaemia common)
- *Debridement*—dead tissue should be removed with a scalpel (no anaesthetic required), maggots, or occasionally topical streptokinase or suction. Specialist tissue viability nurses can usually help with this at the bedside, but some patients require surgery, e.g. debridement, skin grafting, or myocutaneous flaps
- *Dressings*—enormous choice with little evidence to favour one type over another. Use gels to soften, hydrofibre/gels (often seaweed-based) for cavities, then a 2° dressing over the top. Tissue viability nurses will often visit to monitor progress and advise
- *Antibiotics*—all ulcers are colonized (surface swabs positive 100%); only 1% at any given time have active infection causing illness. Look for surrounding cellulitis and signs of sepsis; check blood cultures, or deep tissue biopsy for confirmation. Common organisms include mixed Gram-negatives (*Bacteroides*), Gram-positives (enterococci and staphylococci), and yeasts. If antibiotics are indicated, use wide-spectrum antibiotics, including anaerobic cover. Consider osteomyelitis where bone is exposed (see ➔ 'Osteomyelitis', pp. 490–1). MRSA colonization is a growing problem, is very difficult to eradicate, and often leads to a patient having prolonged isolation, which is detrimental to their psychological well-being and rehabilitation

## Further reading

National Institute for Health and Care Excellence (2014). *Pressure ulcers: prevention and management*. Clinical guideline CG179. ⌖ http://www.nice.org.uk.

# Compression mononeuropathy

- Where nerves are compressed against bone, they can be damaged
- This is usually a demyelination injury (neuropraxia) which resolves spontaneously in 2–12 weeks
- Alcohol, diabetes, and malnutrition ↑ susceptibility
- Any patient who has had a period of immobility on a hard surface is at risk, especially if they were unconscious
- Such injuries can be misdiagnosed as strokes but are LMN in one nerve territory only (see ➲ Appendix, 'Dermatomes', p. 700)
- Nerve conduction studies are rarely required to confirm diagnosis
- Treatment is supportive—many such patients are acutely unwell—but recognition becomes more important during rehabilitation (see Table 18.1)

**Table 18.1** Clinical features of common mononeuropathies

| Nerve damaged | Site/mechanism | Motor effects | Sensory effects |
|---|---|---|---|
| Radial | Upper arm—spiral groove on humerus | Wrist drop and finger extension weakness | Small area of numbness at base of thumb |
| Ulnar | Elbow—cubital groove | Little and ring finger flexors and finger abduction and adduction | Little and ring finger |
| Common peroneal | Knee—fibula head | Foot drop and failure of foot eversion and toe extension | Lateral calf and top of foot |
| Sciatic | Buttock or thigh | Knee flexors plus common peroneal as this table, above | Posterior thigh plus common peroneal as this table, above |

# Rhabdomyolysis

Following prolonged pressure (e.g. if the patient cannot get up after a fall or stroke or after a period of unconsciousness), muscle necrosis can occur, which releases myoglobin. High levels are nephrotoxic, precipitating to cause tubule obstruction with acute renal failure, especially as these patients are usually dehydrated.

▶ Remember to check U, C+E and CK in all patients who have been found on the floor after a 'long lie'. Many frail elderly patients with bruises after a fall will have raised CK levels without developing renal problems, but ensuring good hydration (often with 24–48h of iv fluids) and repeating renal function in such patients is good practice.

## Diagnosis

Suspect the full rhabdomyolysis syndrome in any patient with:

- Prolonged unconsciousness
- Signs of acute pressure sores of the skin
- CK levels at least five times normal

Urine may be dark ('Coca-Cola' urine), and urinalysis is positive to Hb but without red blood cells. Hyperkalaemia and hypocalcaemia can occur.

## Treatment

Treat with aggressive rehydration. Monitor urine output, electrolytes, and renal function closely—if renal failure occurs, consider temporary dialysis. Prognosis is good if the patient survives the initial few days.

Other causes of rhabdomyolysis include drugs (especially statins), compartment syndrome, acute myositis, severe exertion, e.g. seizures/rigors, heat stroke (see ⮊ 'Heat-related illness', p. 418), and neuroleptic malignant syndrome (see ⮊ 'Neuroleptic malignant syndrome', p. 167).

# Genitourinary medicine

# The ageing genitourinary system

### Changes in women

- Oestrogen levels fall following menopause (usually around age 50), leading to vaginal epithelium atrophy, ↓ vaginal lubrication, and acidification and greater vulnerability to vaginal and urinary infection
- The uterus and ovaries atrophy
- The vagina becomes smaller and less elastic

*HRT* improves menopausal symptoms but has other serious adverse effects that severely limit its use (see ➜ 'Hormone replacement therapy and the menopause', pp. 448–9).

### Changes in men

- There are gradual changes in anatomy and function, but no sudden change in fertility, and most older men remain fertile
- Testicular mass and sperm production fall as does semen quality
- The prostate gland enlarges and fibroses—benign prostatic hypertrophy (BPH)—but the volume of ejaculate remains similar
- Erection becomes less sustained and less firm, and the refractory period between erections lengthens. However, severe erectile dysfunction, i.e. inability to sustain an erection sufficient to have sexual intercourse, is usually the result of pathology or drug treatment, rather than ageing itself
- Testosterone levels remain stable or ↓ slightly. In a minority, more severe falls are seen and hypogonadism may become symptomatic, manifesting as fatigue, weakness, osteoporosis, muscle atrophy, declining sexual function, and impaired cognition

*Testosterone replacement* may be considered in those with low hormone levels and symptoms. This may have symptomatic benefit but risks serious side effects (e.g. rising haematocrit, prostatic hypertrophy). Low doses (delivered by patches or injection) may reduce this risk, but monitoring is probably needed. There are no good-quality long-term trials of replacement therapy.

### Changes in both sexes

Cross-sectional studies show much reduced frequency of sexual behaviour of all kinds in older people. However, longitudinal studies show much smaller changes, suggesting that many changes are due to cohort effects, e.g. changes in the prevailing social environment during early adulthood.

Other factors include physical and psychological illness (e.g. arthritis, depression), reduced potency, and social changes (e.g. lack of a partner due to bereavement). Most of these factors are modifiable.

**HOW TO . . . Examine the older female genital system**

This is an important part of the assessment for symptoms such as post-menopausal bleeding, urinary incontinence, and symptoms of prolapse. Approach tactfully—many older women will not be keen on pelvic examination.

Proceed as follows:

- Reassure the patient and position for examination—the standard position with the patient on her back and the legs spread may not be possible with hip disease; consider rolling the patient onto her side, drawing up the knees and inspecting from this position
- Inspect the external genitalia, looking for atrophy, erythema, infection, and abrasions. Severe prolapse may be immediately apparent
- Ask the patient to bear down, which may reveal smaller degrees of prolapse
- Perform a vaginal examination, remembering to use plenty of lubrication. Begin with a single digit if the vaginal opening is tight
- Some rectoceles are only detected by bimanual examination of the vagina and rectum
- Use a speculum if available and tolerated—a Sims speculum applied to the anterior, and then the posterior, vaginal wall, while the patient is in the lateral position, can reveal abnormalities

# Benign prostatic hyperplasia: presentation

BPH is characterized by non-malignant enlargement of the prostate gland and an ↑ in prostatic smooth muscle tone. The resulting bladder outlet obstruction leads to lower urinary tract symptoms (LUTS; 'prostatism').

Prostatism affects 25–50% of men over 65 years, although the histological changes of BPH are even more common—almost universal in those >70. The natural history is variable—some deteriorate, some stay the same, and some improve, even without treatment.

## Assessment

*Symptoms*

LUTS are variable and may be mostly either:

- *Obstructive*—weak stream, straining, hesitancy, nocturia, acute retention, or chronic retention with overflow incontinence, or
- *Irritative*—frequency, dysuria, urgency, and urge incontinence

Other presentations include haematuria (the prostate is hypervascular), UTI, and renal failure 2° to hydronephrosis. Obstructive symptoms may be worsened by drugs, e.g. sedating antihistamines. Tricyclic antidepressants may improve irritative symptoms but worsen obstruction.

Scoring systems (see Box 19.1) can help determine symptom severity, track progression, and response to treatment.

*Examination*

Include the genitals (phimosis or meatal stenosis), abdomen (palpable bladder), neurological system, and digital rectal examination (DRE).

In BPH, the prostate is usually smooth, firm, and enlarged. An irregular prostate can occur in BPH, calculi, infarction, or cancer.

*Investigations*

Tests may help confirm the diagnosis, exclude other pathology, and identify complications:

- *Urinary flow rate* confirms obstruction but is rarely needed
- *Blood glucose* to exclude diabetes, a common cause of urinary symptoms
- *U, C+E* (renal failure)
- *Urinalysis* (infection, haematuria)
- *Ultrasound scanning of renal tract* (hydronephrosis, high residual volume; see Box 20.1)
- *PSA.* Consider this, especially if the prostate is irregular. However, testing is not mandatory and, in general, should be guided by the patient's views, after a discussion of risks and benefits of further investigation and treatment (see ➲ 'Prostatic cancer: presentation', pp. 516–17 and ➲ 'Prostate-specific antigen', p. 518)
- *Cystoscopy and ultrasound scanning.* If haematuria is detected, to exclude renal and bladder cancer

**Box 19.1 International Prostate Symptom Score (IPSS)**
This is a well-validated, widely used assessment tool that can be either self-administered or given as part of a structured assessment by a health professional. Aggregate scores from the seven questions to give a total score range of 0–35 (see Table 19.1):
- 0–7: mildly symptomatic
- 8–19: moderately symptomatic
- 20–35: severely symptomatic

**Table 19.1** International Prostate Symptom Score

|  | Not at all | <1 time in 5 | Less than half the time | About half the time | More than half the time | Almost always |
|---|---|---|---|---|---|---|
| *Incomplete emptying.* Over the past month, how often have you had a sensation of not emptying your bladder completely after you finish urinating? | 0 | 1 | 2 | 3 | 4 | 5 |
| *Frequency.* Over the past month, how often have you had to urinate again <2h after you finished urinating? | 0 | 1 | 2 | 3 | 4 | 5 |
| *Intermittency.* Over the past month, how often have you found you stopped and started again several times when you urinated? | 0 | 1 | 2 | 3 | 4 | 5 |
| *Urgency.* Over the past month, how difficult have you found it to postpone urination? | 0 | 1 | 2 | 3 | 4 | 5 |
| *Weak stream.* Over the past month, how often have you had a weak urinary stream? | 0 | 1 | 2 | 3 | 4 | 5 |
| *Straining.* Over the past month, how often have you had to push or strain to begin urination? | 0 | 1 | 2 | 3 | 4 | 5 |

|  | None | 1 time | 2 times | 3 times | 4 times | 5 times or more |
|---|---|---|---|---|---|---|
| *Nocturia.* Over the past month, how many times did you most typically get up to urinate, from the time you went to bed until the time you got up in the morning? | 0 | 1 | 2 | 3 | 4 | 5 |

# Benign prostatic hyperplasia: treatment

Treatment choice is influenced by patient preference, severity of symptoms, presence of complications, and fitness for surgery.

## Conservative measures

'Watchful waiting' is reasonable if symptoms are mild or moderate and complications absent. Reassure the patient. Reassess clinically and check renal function at 6- to 12-monthly intervals. Advise reduction in evening fluid intake; stop unnecessary diuretics. The main risk is acute urine retention (1–2% per year).

## Herbal preparations

These are widely used by patients, bought 'over the counter'; always ask about non-prescription remedies. The most widely used is saw palmetto (*Serenoa repens*) extract, and there is some evidence that it works, especially in milder disease, perhaps acting as a 5α-reductase inhibitor (see ➲ 'Drugs', p. 514). PSA levels may therefore be reduced.

## Drugs

Suitable for mild, moderate, or severe symptoms without complications, especially if patient preference is strong. Patients with more severe symptoms benefit the most. Two drug classes may help:

- *α-adrenergic blockers* ('α-blockers', e.g. doxazosin, terazosin, tamsulosin). They relax prostatic smooth muscle, increasing urine flow rates and reducing symptoms in days. Side effects are common—the most important are hypotension, especially orthostatic hypotension, and syncope. Use cautiously, starting with low dose (e.g. doxazosin 1mg od, ↑ in 1mg increments at 2-week intervals to 4mg). Exercise great caution if prescribed with diuretics or other vasodilators, if there is a past history of syncope, and in the frail. Tamsulosin may be more prostate-selective than other α-blockers and may have fewer circulatory side effects

- *5α-reductase inhibitors* (e.g. finasteride). These inhibit prostatic testosterone metabolism, reducing prostatic size. Benefit occurs slowly (months) and is most likely if the prostate is large (>40mL); those with mild enlargement benefit little or not at all. Side effects are uncommon but include erectile dysfunction (<5%), gynaecomastia, and loss of libido. Given the absence of cardiovascular side effects, 5α-reductase inhibitors may be a better option in the frail older person. PSA levels fall by ~50%, so double the observed value to give an indication of prostate cancer risk

- *Combination treatment*. For patients with severe symptoms or who do not have adequate response to maximal monotherapy with an α-blockers, try combination treatment with both agents

## Alpha-blockers, prostatism, and hypertension

Many men have symptoms of prostatism and are also hypertensive. α-blockers can be an attractive option as the one drug may treat both. However, the evidence for α-blockers in the treatment of hypertension is inferior to that for several other drug classes. Assess the impact on each problem separately, and consider prescribing the most appropriate treatment for each individual condition. See ➔ 'HOW TO . . . Use anti-hypertensives in a patient with comorbid conditions', p. 269.

## Surgery

More effective than drugs or 'watchful waiting', but side effects are more common and usually irreversible. Indicated if:
- Symptoms are moderate or severe (with patient preference)
- There are complications (recurrent UTI or haematuria, renal failure)
- A trial of drug treatment has failed

*Transurethral resection of the prostate (TURP).* The (gold) standard procedure. Success rates are >90%. Adverse effects include retrograde ejaculation (most), erectile dysfunction (5–10%), incontinence (1%), and death (<1%); 10% need further surgery within a few years.

*Newer procedures.* Several have been developed. They are generally less invasive and probably have fewer adverse effects, but long-term outcome data are less good. Local availability and expertise are limited. For example:
- Transurethral incision of the prostate (TUIP). Effective in those with smaller prostate glands. Low incidence of side effects
- Transurethral microwave thermotherapy (TUMT), transurethral needle ablation (TUNA), transurethral enucleation, plasma vaporization, photoselective vaporization, and radiofrequency ablation are newer options that are well tolerated and require only local anaesthesia in an outpatient setting, often with less bleeding risk. However, some are time-consuming and difficult to learn; long-term results are less well known, and availability varies locally

*Open prostatectomy* is reserved for very large glands and where other interventions are needed, e.g. removal of bladder stones. It is very effective, but comorbidity is higher.

## Urinary catheterization

Urinary catheterization is an option where:
- Symptoms are severe, or significant complications have occurred (e.g. retention)
- Surgical mortality and morbidity would be high
- Drug treatment has not been tolerated or is unlikely to be effective

A long-term catheter may be required if the patient fails a trial (or trials) without catheter.

# Prostatic cancer: presentation

A very common cancer in men, much more so with age—median age at diagnosis is over 70. However:
- Most die *with* tumour, rather than *because* of it
- Most are asymptomatic or have only obstructive symptoms
- Many tumours do not progress, even without treatment

This leads to difficult management decisions, especially in older people where life expectancy for other reasons may be low, and expensive, unpleasant, or risky treatments may not be worthwhile.

## Assessment

Predictors of an adverse disease course (symptoms, local progression, metastases, and death) include more advanced stage (TNM classification) and histological grade (e.g. Gleason score; see ➲ 'Gleason score', p. 516).

*Localized cancer*—often detected when evaluating a man with lower tract symptoms due to BPH (by finding an elevated PSA), or incidentally, e.g. at TURP for BPH. The tumour remains within the gland capsule; the tumour focus may be very small and in no way responsible for symptoms. DRE may be normal. Prognosis is generally good, especially if the grade is favourable. Cure may be possible, although for more indolent tumours, attempts at cure (surgery, radiotherapy) may be worse than the disease.

*Locally advanced cancer without metastases*—usually detected in patients with urinary symptoms, or at DRE performed for other reasons. A much larger group now that PSA testing is more common. The tumour has broken through the capsule, and prognosis is more adverse. Cure is not usually possible, but survival may be prolonged.

*Metastatic cancer*—up to half of newly diagnosed patients have metastatic disease. Many are asymptomatic. Features (↓ frequency) include urinary symptoms, bone pain, constitutional symptoms (e.g. weight loss), renal failure, pathological fracture, and anaemia due to bone marrow infiltration. A minority have an indolent course and, with treatment, may survive many years.

## Gleason score

A histological grading system that correlates well with outcome and helps guide treatment choice. A composite of two scores (each range 1–5), therefore range 2–10:
- 2–4: well differentiated
- 5–7: moderately differentiated
- 8–10: poorly differentiated

## Screening

There is no good evidence that earlier detection through screening improves prognosis. This often requires careful explanation. Rectal examination is insensitive—tumours detected in this way are often large and locally advanced. PSA has its own drawbacks (see ➲ 'Prostate-specific antigen', p. 518).

**Tests**

These should be selected advisedly, after considering the patient's wishes, the implications of a negative or positive result, and any risks of the test.

- *PSA*. See ➔ 'Prostate-specific antigen', p. 518
- *FBC*. Evidence of marrow infiltration
- *Serum calcium, LFTs*. Evidence of metastases
- *U, C+E*. Evidence of post-renal renal failure
- *Transrectal ultrasound and biopsy*. Provides tissue for histological diagnosis and grading. Risks haemorrhage and infection
- *Bone scan or X-rays*. If there are symptoms or bone biochemistry is suggestive. Metastasis to bone is common; appearance is sclerotic much more commonly than lytic
- *CT/MRI scan*. For tumour staging where surgery is contemplated

# Prostate-specific antigen

PSA is made in the prostate and blood levels reflect prostatic synthesis.

## Using PSA

It has two definite useful roles:
- In very early detection of localized prostate cancer when treatment may be curative
- In tracking tumour progression: changes in PSA usually reflect changes in tumour mass

## Screening with PSA

PSA is produced by both benign and malignant prostatic tissue, and there is no single useful cut-off point that separates those with cancer from those without:
- Two-thirds of men with a high PSA do not have prostate cancer
- One-fifth of men with prostate cancer have a normal PSA

The higher the PSA level, the more likely is cancer. However, even at moderately high levels (>10 micrograms/L), the positive predictive value is only 65%. Specificity is even less in older people, as the benign causes of elevated PSA are more common.

Combining this with the limitations of treatment, any screening programme utilizing PSA yields:
- Many people with high PSA, but no cancer is found after further tests
- Many people with locally advanced prostate cancer for whom early treatment is not known to improve prognosis
- Public Health England states that the low specificity of the PSA test has led to harms of over-diagnosis and overtreatment in up to 50% of men

*Non-malignant causes of increased PSA*

PSA ↑ with age and with:
- BPH
- Prostatitis
- UTI
- Rectal examination (up to 7 days)
- Prostatic biopsy (6 weeks)
- Urethral catheterization
- Urethral instrumentation, e.g. cystoscopy
- Vigorous exercise (48h)
- Ejaculation (48h)

(Figures in brackets are approximate durations of elevation.)

*Age-specific PSA values*

The following have been suggested as cut-off points to reduce unnecessary referral and investigation of patients with benign prostate disease:
- 50–59 years: ≥3.0 micrograms/L
- 60–69 years: ≥4.0 micrograms/L
- ≥70 years: ≥5.0 micrograms/L

PSA reduces with some drug treatment (e.g. 5α-reductase inhibitors; herbal remedies such as saw palmetto) and may therefore reduce the thresholds given for referral.

# Prostatic cancer: treatment

- *Localized cancer*—there are several treatment options, including 'watchful waiting', hormonal treatment, radiotherapy, and surgery. Cure can often be achieved
- '*Watchful waiting*'—usually reserved for those with modest life expectancy (<10 years) and lower-grade (Gleason score 2–6) localized tumours where progression is rare within 10 years. Check PSA every 4–6 months. Start treatment (usually hormonal) if symptoms or if PSA rises
- *Active surveillance*—is an option to men with low-risk localized prostate cancer for whom radical prostatectomy or radical radiotherapy would be suitable (involves serial PSA and rectal examinations, with repeat biopsy at a year)
- *Hormone treatment*—there is doubt whether early hormone treatment improves outcome, compared to 'watchful waiting'
- *Radiotherapy*—the most usual choice for high-grade localized tumours. Probably as effective as surgery, but better tolerated. Side effects include erectile dysfunction, irritative urinary symptoms, and radiation proctitis
- *Surgery*—radical prostatectomy is a major procedure, usually indicated only for those with long life expectancy, high-grade tumours, and in good health. Major side effects are incontinence, impotence, and haemorrhage. Robot-assisted surgery has better results
- *Locally advanced disease without metastases*—key treatments are radiotherapy (also discussed here) and/or androgen deprivation (also discussed here). The relative benefits are unclear. Surgery probably offers no benefit, other than TURP to relieve outflow symptoms
- *Metastatic disease*—androgen deprivation ('hormone treatment') is the linchpin of treatment. This can be achieved by castration (bilateral orchidectomy, usually under local anaesthesia) but is usually chemical, largely for reasons of patient preference. Treatment should not be delayed, even if there are no symptoms. Luteinizing hormone-releasing hormone (LHRH) agonists are used commonly and are usually effective for 12–18 months. If disease progresses despite LHRH agonists, patients occasionally respond to antiandrogens. Surgery offers no benefits
- *LHRH agonists* (e.g. goserelin)—given as injections or implants, these cause initial (2 weeks) stimulation and then sustained depression of testosterone release. The initial ↑ can cause tumour growth ('flare') with adverse effects, e.g. urinary outflow obstruction, spinal cord compression, or bone pain. If anticipated, antiandrogens may help. Continuous therapy is not needed—survival appears similar if therapy is stopped when PSA levels are normal and restarted when they rise
- *Antiandrogens* (e.g. bicalutamide, flutamide)—useful in inhibiting tumour flare after LHRH agonist initiation, in tumour refractory to LHRH agonists, if LHRH agonists are not tolerated or accepted (e.g. because of erectile dysfunction), or where oral drugs are preferred. There is no evidence that combined antiandrogens and LHRH agonists are helpful

Side effects of LHRH agonists and antiandrogens include hot flushes, erectile dysfunction, bone mineral loss and gynaecomastia.

## Late-stage prostate cancer

Eventually, prostate cancer may become resistant (refractory) to hormone treatment, manifesting as a rising PSA and/or worsening symptoms while on treatment. Other treatments (e.g. oestrogens, docetaxel) may be tried but are rarely very effective. Death follows, often in months.

Common complications, usually in more advanced disease, include:

- Bone pain:
  - A major cause of reduced quality of life
  - Optimize oral analgesia: combinations of paracetamol, opiates, and NSAIDs are effective
  - Local pain is helped by radiotherapy
  - Bisphosphonates or steroids may also help
- Pathological bone fracture:
  - Usually requires surgical fixation
- Acute urine retention:
  - Catheterize
  - Intensify anti-tumour treatment if appropriate (e.g. hormone treatment, radiotherapy)
  - Consider TURP
- Post-renal renal failure—determine site of obstruction by ultrasound:
  - Prostatic obstruction: catheter, TURP, intensify anti-tumour treatment
  - Ureteric obstruction: stenting or nephrostomy
- Spinal cord compression:
  - An emergency, as early decompression improves neurological outcome
  - Confirm with CT or MRI
  - Steroids, radiotherapy, or surgery help decompress the cord

# Post-menopausal vaginal bleeding

Defined as bleeding from the genital tract over 1 year after onset of menopausal amenorrhoea. The time criterion reflects the fact that menstruation is often irregular and infrequent around menopause, and investigations for sinister pathology are not then worthwhile.

Most cases are 2° to benign pathology, but treatment of the few cases of cancer (largely endometrial) is far more effective if identified early, so do not delay assessment. Malignancy is more likely if bleeding is significant and recurrent—investigate vigorously if no cause is apparent.

## Causes of post-menopausal vaginal bleeding

In approximate order of frequency:

*Atrophic vaginitis*

Inflammation results as the thinner, less cornified epithelium is exposed to a more alkaline vaginal environment colonized by a broad microbial flora.

*Endometrial hyperplasia*

2° to:
* Exogenous oestrogen (e.g. HRT)
* Unopposed endogenous oestrogen (especially in older, obese women where peripheral conversion of steroid hormones to oestrogens by fat cells is higher)
* Benign tumour, e.g. cervical or endometrial polyps
* Vaginal prolapse and ulceration

*Vaginal infection*

*Carcinoma*
* Endometrial
* Cervical
* Vulval
* Vaginal
* Ovarian

*Spurious*

Other relatively common causes of 'vaginal' bleeding are haematuria and rectal bleeding. Drugs causing endometrial disease (hyperplasia, polyps, and cancer) include:
* HRT (with cyclical replacement: investigate if bleed at unexpected times; for continuous oestrogen and progestogen: investigate if irregular bleeding persists for >12 months after treatment initiation)
* Tamoxifen (via a paradoxical endometrial oestrogen-like effect)

After hysterectomy, bleeding is commonly due to atrophic vaginitis or overgrowth of post-surgical granulation tissue.

## Assessment

- *History*—assess the amount and frequency of bleeding, if necessary by discussing with carers. Consider other possible sources of blood, e.g. urinary, rectal. Take an accurate drug history
- *Examine*—examine the genitalia, perineum, and rectum to exclude tumour, trauma, and bleeding from atrophic sites. Obesity or OA may make examination difficult; the left or right lateral positions are usually more successful
- *Investigation*—FBC to exclude severe anaemia. Urine dipstick for haematuria is unlikely to be specific to blood of urinary tract origin, especially if bleeding is recurrent or ongoing

Further tests are usually guided by expert gynaecological advice but may include:
- Cervical smear
- Vaginal ultrasound to assess endometrial thickness (<5mm effectively excludes cancer and may prevent the need for more tests)
- Hysteroscopy—can be done under local or general anaesthetic
- Dilatation and curettage
- Consider investigation of the urinary and gastrointestinal tract (cystoscopy, sigmoidoscopy)

## Treatment

Is directed to the underlying cause, e.g.:
- *Atrophic vaginitis*: topical oestrogens (see ⊃ 'Hormone replacement therapy and the menopause', pp. 448–9)
- *HRT*: used if topical oestrogens fail. Review the balance of risks and benefits, and consider stopping the drug. Consider change of preparation, e.g. reduction of oestrogen dose, ↑ in progestogen dose
- *Endometrial carcinoma*: total abdominal hysterectomy and bilateral salpingo-oophorectomy and/or radiotherapy are the usual interventions. In those unfit for surgery, progestogens (e.g. medroxyprogesterone) may control the tumour

# Vaginal prolapse

A prolapse is a protrusion into the vagina by a pelvic organ (bladder, bowel, or uterus) caused by:

- Weakness of pelvic connective tissue and musculature due to cumulative effects of childbirth trauma, ageing, and oestrogen deficiency
- ↑ abdominal pressure, e.g. constipation, obesity, and coughing
- Depending on which structures are weak, the following may be seen (see Fig. 19.1):
  - Cystocele: the bladder protrudes through the anterior vaginal wall
  - Rectocele: the rectum protrudes through the posterior vaginal wall
  - Enterocele: herniation of the peritoneum and small bowel (the pouch of Douglas) through the posterior vaginal wall
- Uterine prolapse: descent of the cervix and uterus down the vagina
  - First degree: the cervix lies within the vagina
  - Second degree: the cervix protrudes from the vagina on standing/straining
  - Third degree (procidentia): the cervix lies outside the vagina

## Assessment

Often asymptomatic. Most commonly, there is a sensation of heaviness, fullness or bearing down, a palpable mass, or a dull pelvic ache or backache. Symptoms may be abolished by lying down.

- Cystocele may cause stress or overflow urinary incontinence, UTI, or bladder outflow obstruction
- Rectocele may cause faecal incontinence or difficulty in defecation—manual evacuation or digital reduction of the prolapse may be needed
- Enterocele causes pelvic fullness and discomfort
- Third-degree uterine prolapse may cause ulceration and bleeding, and bladder symptoms e.g. difficulty in urinating

Examination should include an abdominal and pelvic assessment (see ➲ 'HOW TO . . . Examine the older female genital system', p. 511).

## Treatment

This is dictated by symptoms, prolapse severity, the organs involved, general fitness, and patient preference. Urodynamic testing and imaging may be needed prior to treatment.

- Mild symptoms: topical oestrogen cream and pelvic floor exercises
- Moderate or severe symptoms: pessary or surgery
  - Surgery is now generally well tolerated and effective. Usually via a transvaginal approach, weakened structures of the pelvic floor are strengthened and fixed in place. Hysterectomy is sometimes necessary
  - Pessaries—fitting of a pessary is indicated for reasons of patient preference, when the risks of surgery are unfavourable, and as a temporary measure prior to surgery. They come in many shapes and sizes, but the most commonly used is the ring pessary. An oestrogen-releasing ring pessary will also treat atrophy and associated recurrent UTIs. Other shapes may be used, commonly for severe disease, but can be difficult to insert and remove

### HOW TO . . . Care for a vaginal pessary

Every 4–6 months:
- Remove and clean the pessary
- Examine the vagina for evidence of ulceration
- Replace a damaged pessary
- Reinsert if all is well

*Complications*
- If vaginal ulceration occurs, the pessary should be removed for several weeks, until complete healing has occurred. Local oestrogen creams assist healing and may prevent recurrent ulceration. Try a different shape or size of pessary
- Pessaries can embed in inflamed vaginal mucosa and become stuck. Topical oestrogens and treatment of infection (e.g. *Candida*) may reduce inflammation and assist removal. If the pessary remains stuck, refer for specialist gynaecological assessment

# Prolapse: illustrations

Fig. 19.1 shows the types of prolapse.

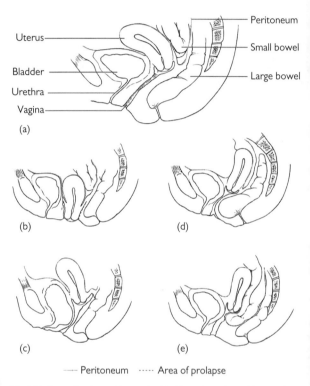

**Fig. 19.1** Types of prolapse: (a) normal pelvis, (b) uterine prolapse, (c) cystocele, (d) rectocele, (e) enterocele.

Reproduced with permission from Impey L, *Obstetrics and Gynaecology*, Wiley-Blackwell Publishing, 1999.

# Vulval disorders

Most non-malignant vulval disorders are worsened by local irritants (e.g. soap, deodorant, perfume) and improve if avoided. Good perineal hygiene also helps, e.g. wiping front-to-back after urination or defecation, keeping the area dry, and wearing loose-fitting non-synthetic clothing.

## Vulvitis

*Symptoms*
Itching, discharge, burning discomfort.

*Causes*
These include:
- *Candida* ('thrush'). The most common cause, especially in diabetes and obesity. Vaginal infection almost always coexists
- Local dermatitis. Often exacerbated by soap and deodorants
- Sexually transmitted pathogens (rare), e.g. *Chlamydia*

*Treatment*
- Treat candidiasis with antifungal cream to the vulva (e.g. clotrimazole 1% cream) and pessaries or cream inserted high into the vagina (e.g. clotrimazole 200mg pessary daily for 3 days). Single-dose pessaries (e.g. clotrimazole 500mg pessary once) are effective and may be better tolerated. Oral treatment is also effective, e.g. fluconazole 150mg once
- Recurrent candidal infection is common, especially in diabetes and in those receiving repeated antibiotics. Consider longer-term treatment, e.g. weekly clotrimazole (500mg pessary) or fluconazole (100mg po)
- Treat irritant dermatitis by removing the cause and regular application of topical steroid cream (e.g. hydrocortisone 1%) for 7–14 days
- If vulval itch persists without obvious cause, consider systemic disease, e.g. iron deficiency, thyroid disorders. Use emollients and a low-potency topical steroid to break the itch–scratch–itch cycle. Antihistamines are not effective (see ➲ 'Pruritus', pp. 596–7)
- If obvious vaginal atrophy, consider local oestrogen replacement.

## Vulvodynia

A chronic pain syndrome manifesting as burning, pain, or tenderness of the vulva. There are often psychological contributors, and a sensitive life-long sexual history may be useful. Infection, dermatitis, and epithelial disorders (neoplastic and non-neoplastic) should be excluded. Refer for specialist assessment, and consider treating depression and empirical treatment with topical steroids or oestrogens.

## Non-neoplastic epithelial disorders

*Lichen sclerosus*
Common in middle aged and older women. Asymptomatic or else causes itching or soreness or dyspareunia. Seen as white or pink/purple macules or papules resembling thin parchment paper and often in a figure-of-eight distribution around the vulva. Biopsy to exclude neoplasia. Treat with potent topical steroids, tapering the potency and frequency as symptoms improve. Progression to carcinoma can occur. Long-term follow-up is sensible.

*Squamous hyperplasia*
Raised white keratinized lesions that may be very localized. Biopsy may be needed to exclude malignancy. Treat with medium-potency topical steroids, tapering to a stop as symptoms improve.

*Other disorders*
For example, psoriasis and chronic dermatitis can usually be diagnosed clinically, but biopsy permits more confident management.

## Malignant epithelial disorders

*Vulval cancer*
- Easily treated in its early stages and often preceded by a pre-malignant stage
- Late presentation is more common with age
- Commonly asymptomatic and an incidental finding, but may itch, discharge, bleed, or cause pain
- Appearance is variable—may be raised or ulcerated, or else appear as white or coloured macules. If in any doubt that a lesion may be malignant or pre-malignant, then refer for biopsy
- Treatment depends on the size and invasiveness of the tumour, the presence or absence of metastases, and the condition of the patient
- Options include topical cytotoxic creams, resection under local anaesthesia, wide local excision, or radical vulvectomy
- Extensive vulval surgery is relatively well tolerated in older people

▶ If any vulval lesion does not respond as expected to treatment, re-consider the possibility of malignancy.

# Sexual function

Studies show that most older people desire some sexual contact. Up to 30% of men in their eighties and 15% of women remain sexually active. However, the frequency of sexual intercourse, both penetrative and non-penetrative, falls with age. This decline is multifactorial, including:

- Lack of partner, e.g. death of spouse
- Physiological changes of ageing, e.g. ↓ vaginal secretions, less sustained penile erections
- Physical comorbidity and medication, e.g. circulatory disease, β-blockers
- Psychological comorbidity, e.g. low self-esteem, depression
- Societal expectations and judgements
- Lack of privacy, especially in institutional care

The clinical response to a patient's report of sexual dysfunction involves addressing each of these factors in a supportive and understanding way.

## Erectile dysfunction

Erection requires intact neurological, circulatory, hormonal, and psychological processes. In older people, several factors more commonly contribute to erectile dysfunction or impotence. A solely psychological cause is uncommon. Common contributors are drugs, vascular disease (arterial > venous), and neurological disease (stroke, autonomic neuropathy, local surgery, e.g. prostatectomy).

### History

Assess onset and progression, circumstances, and associated psychological issues. Erectile dysfunction is common, yet is rarely asked about. Older men may volunteer the symptom, but many will accept it as part of 'normal ageing'. Do not assume that an older man is not sexually active, and always warn about impotence as a potential side effect of relevant drugs.

### Drugs causing erectile dysfunction

Along with vascular disease, drugs are the most common cause in older people:

- Antihypertensives (especially β-blockers and diuretics; ACE inhibitors less so)
- Alcohol
- Antiandrogens, LHRH agonists, oestrogens, progestogens
- Antidepressants (all classes, except trazodone)
- Less commonly: cimetidine, spironolactone

### Examination

Of mental state (depression, anxiety). Presence of 2° sexual characteristics. Vascular disease. Genitourinary examination. Neurological examination to include perineal and perianal sensation.

*Investigations*
Exclude systemic illness with FBC, U, C+E, and glucose. Diagnostic tests to determine an underlying cause of erectile dysfunction do not often alter management and are rarely performed. Hypogonadism is an uncommon cause of erectile dysfunction, so checking testosterone level is not usually necessary. If libido (rather than erectile dysfunction) is the problem, then exclude hypogonadism by checking testosterone, luteinizing hormone, TSH, and prolactin.

*Treatment*
Where possible, stop incriminated drugs. Treat underlying disease, including anxiety/depression. Recently developed drug treatments are highly effective.

*Phosphodiesterase type-5 inhibitors*
For example, sildenafil. Cause smooth muscle relaxation and ↑ blood flow; they are easily used (take po before intercourse), effective, and safe. Contraindications include patients on nitrates; exercise caution in those with coronary or cerebrovascular disease. Side effects are gastrointestinal and vascular (flushing, headache).

*Alprostadil (prostaglandin E1)*
Is usually given as an intraurethral pellet, is absorbed locally, and causes local smooth muscle relaxation. There is no significant systemic absorption, so systemic side effects are rare and vascular disease is not a contraindication.

*Other options*
Include intracavernosal injections (the most effective treatment) and non-drug options such as vacuum devices (effective, but often discontinued due to discomfort).

## Hypersexuality

- Sexually disinhibited behaviours may occur in people with dementia and frontal lobe pathology, e.g. stroke. It can present practical and ethical problems to the caregiver. Assessment of the behaviours, the contexts in which they arise, and any possible risk is essential. Environmental modification and carer education are needed. Medication may help (e.g. antipsychotics), but none are licensed
- A small proportion of patients with Parkinson's disease (particularly if treated with dopamine agonists) may develop impulse control disorders which can include hypersexuality

# HIV in older people

### Prevalence
- ↑ in the over 50s

### Reasons for this include
- Prolonged survival on antiretroviral therapy (one in four diagnosed with HIV now live beyond 50)
- Wider scope of HIV testing
- ↑ transmission due to ↓ awareness of HIV in older adults

### Risk factors
- Broadly similar to younger group, except less likely to be due to iv drug use
- In men, the biggest risk factor is homosexual intercourse. US data looking at homosexual men >50 reveals less frequent sexual activity, but still multiple partners (>9 in the last 12 months for 25%)
- In older women, heterosexual intercourse is the biggest risk factor. They may be less likely to use barrier contraception, as there are no risks of conception. Also, age-related changes to the ♀ genital tract (e.g. atrophic vaginitis) may make transmission more likely

### Testing
Delay in testing and diagnosis common (50% of >50s, compared with 30% of younger patients) because:
- Clinicians are less likely to suspect HIV infection in older patients
- Patients may mistake early symptoms for other age-related disorders and not seek help

▶ It is important to take a sexual history and bear the diagnosis in mind as for younger patients, particularly if there is an opportunistic infection such as TB.

### Clinical features
In older patients:
- Mortality is higher, although this may relate to delayed diagnosis—in one study, 75% of those over 50 diagnosed with HIV/acquired immune deficiency syndrome (AIDS) were dead within a year
- Antiretroviral therapy has equivalent efficacy as in younger patients, improves survival, and drug concordance may be better
- Comorbidity more common, causing greater overall disability and possible problems with drug treatments
- There may be an ↑ risk of HIV-associated dementia, although studies are small
- Risk of cardiovascular disease is high—may be effect of HIV or the antiretrovirals, plus accumulation of other risk factors (hypertension, smoking, high cholesterol, etc.)

# Incontinence

# Urinary incontinence: causes

▶ Incontinence has a major adverse impact on quality of life and has significant associated morbidity (it may be the last straw leading to institutionalization). Even long-standing cases may be reversible, so always explore continence issues, even if everyone else is complacent.

It is very common (around 30% of elderly at home, 50% in care homes) but is not a natural consequence of ageing. Most incontinence in older people is multifactorial, so think of all the possible contributing factors and address each in turn. They can be divided as follows.

## Age-related changes
- Diminished total bladder capacity, but ↑ residual volume
- Diminished bladder contractile function
- ↑ frequency of uninhibited bladder contractions
- Reduced ability to postpone voiding
- Excretion of fluid later in the day with less concentrated night-time urine
- Atrophy of vagina and urethra in ♀
- Loss of pelvic floor and urethral sphincter musculature
- Hypertrophy of the prostate in ♂

## Comorbidity
- Diminished mobility—may have an urge to urinate, then not be able to get to the toilet in time
- Prescribed medications affect the lower urinary tract, conscious state (e.g. sedatives), or ability to get promptly to the toilet (e.g. antihypertensives causing postural drop)
- Constipation
- Impaired cognition— a continent person needs to be able to recognize that they need to urinate, locate and reach a toilet, then undress in time to pass urine in the right place. Confusion can cause inappropriate micturition (initially failure to find an appropriate receptacle, then in later dementia, they may be unaware altogether of urination). There may also be interference with UMN input into continence pathways

## Reversible factors
- UTI (see ➐ 'Urinary tract infection', p. 621)
- Delirium
- Drugs e.g. diuretics cause polyuria, anticholinergics such as tricyclic antidepressants cause retention, sedatives can reduce awareness or mobility
- Constipation—may cause voiding difficulty and ↑ residual volumes in both sexes
- Polyuria (e.g. poorly controlled diabetes, hypercalcaemia, oedema resorption at night can cause nocturnal polyuria, psychogenic polydipsia)
- Urethral irritability (e.g. atrophic vaginitis, *Candida* infection)
- Prolapse (women)
- Bladder stones and tumours

### Irreversible (but treatable) factors

- In ♂, prostatic hypertrophy or carcinoma causes outflow obstruction, overactive bladder (OAB) syndrome, or 'overflow' incontinence
- OAB syndrome (symptom diagnosis)/detrusor overactivity (urodynamic diagnosis)—spontaneous contractions of the bladder muscle causes urgency and frequency ± incontinence
- In ♀, outlet incompetence (stress incontinence)—usually due to pelvic muscle and ligament laxity (which supports the urethra) following childbirth—any rise in intra-abdominal pressure causes small leaks, e.g. with cough, hoisting
- Mixed symptoms—suggesting the presence of both overactivity and stress incontinence
- Fistula (connection between the bladder and vagina) can occur after pelvic malignancy and irradiation, causing constant wetness

### Environmental factors

- Being bedbound and reliant on assistance with toileting makes continence a challenge. While nurses will endeavour to promptly attend to a request for toileting, there is an inevitable delay
- In ♂ with reduced mobility, a lack of manual dexterity and/or small penile size can make the use of bottles a challenge
- In hospitals, the toilet may be further away than at home, or difficult to find. In addition, the acute illness may mean that mobilizing is difficult
- At home, access to a toilet may become harder with reducing mobility (e.g. if there is only an upstairs toilet)

# Urinary incontinence: assessment

Much is written in the literature of the different symptoms in different diagnostic groups.

- *Urgency symptoms*. Frequent (>8 times per day) and/or precipitant voiding—strong urge and ↓ time to reach the toilet. If incontinence occurs, this is termed wet OAB. Urge alone while maintaining continence is termed dry OAB and may be a precursor to the wet form. Nocturnal incontinence is common. Urge symptoms are commonly due to detrusor muscle overactivity where the residual volume is small but can also occur in obstruction
- *Stress symptoms*. Small-volume leaks during coughing, laughing, lifting, walking, and other exercise. Often coexist with urge symptoms in women
- *Obstructive symptoms* in men include ↓ force of urinary stream, hesitancy, and intermittent flow

Older patients are often unable to give precise descriptions, and the different symptom complexes can overlap. Even where a 'pure' symptom complex exists, you may get the diagnosis wrong, e.g. prostatic outflow symptoms where incontinence is actually detrusor overactivity or symptoms of urgency as a presentation for retention with overflow. Additional factors such as reduced mobility, dexterity, and cognition also interact to produce the syndrome of incontinence.

A more pragmatic approach is often required.

- *Take a history*—a bladder or voiding diary can help, especially if you are relying on carers for information. Ask questions such as:
  - 'Do you know when you need to go to pass urine?'
  - 'Do you get much time between getting the urge and when the urine comes?'
  - 'Do you sometimes leak urine when you cough or run?'
- *Examination*—include vaginal, rectal, and neurological examination
- *Exclude a significant residual volume* (see Box 20.1)
- *Investigations*—urinalysis and MSU, general screening blood tests, cytology, and cystoscopy if haematuria. Urodynamics can be helpful if the patient's incontinence cannot be explained or they are not responding to treatment, and essential if surgical intervention is contemplated

## Bladder diaries

It is helpful to ask patients and/or carers to complete a bladder diary to aid assessment. This should include the timing and volume of all urine voided, along with details of any symptoms and episodes of incontinence. An example is shown in Table 20.1.

Analysis of this will allow correct assessment of:

- 24h urine volume
- Number and severity of incontinence episodes
- Maximum and minimum voided volumes
- Diurnal variation

### Box 20.1 Residual volume

Normal young people have only a few millilitres of urine post-micturition, but normal elderly people can have up to 100mL and intervention is rarely required under 200mL.

Causes of raised residual volume include:

- Prostatic hypertrophy, carcinoma
- Urethral stricture
- Bladder diverticulum
- Large urinary cystocele and other pelvic organ prolapse (♀)
- Hypocontractile detrusor
- Neurological disease, e.g. multiple sclerosis, Parkinson's disease, spinal cord disease, disc herniation
- Bladder tumour
- Drugs, e.g. tricyclic antidepressants, anticholinergics

Acute retention is usually painful but can present atypically with delirium, renal failure, etc.

Chronic bladder distension is usually painless, presenting with infection, abdominal distension/mass, or incontinence (continuous dribbling due to overflow or urge incontinence due to detrusor instability).

Persistently elevated residual volume ↑ the risk of infection.

If pressure is elevated, this can cause dilation of the urinary tract and eventually hydronephrosis and renal failure.

Residual volume can easily be estimated using a simple ultrasound bladder scan or a diagnostic (in/out) catheterization after attempted micturition.

**Table 20.1** Bladder diary

| Date | Time | Voided volume | Symptoms | Incontinence episodes and cause |
|------|------|---------------|----------|---------------------------------|
|      |      |               |          |                                 |
|      |      |               |          |                                 |
|      |      |               |          |                                 |

# Urinary incontinence: management

- Depends on the cause, so try to make a diagnosis first
- Incontinence is multifactorial in most elderly, so combining treatments may be necessary, e.g. a man with obstructive prostatic symptoms and detrusor hyperactivity may benefit from an α-blocker and an anti-muscarinic (e.g. tolterodine) (see Table 20.2)

**Table 20.2** Management of urinary incontinence

| Treatment | Indication | Notes |
|---|---|---|
| Bladder retraining (gradually ↑ time between voiding) | OAB syndrome/detrusor overactivity | |
| Regular toileting (taking to toilet every 2–4h) | Dementia OAB syndrome | ↓ likelihood of incontinence episodes |
| Pelvic floor exercises | Stress incontinence | Effect wears off when exercises stop |
| Vaginal pessaries | Stress incontinence due to prolapse | |
| Topical oestrogens | Urgency/incontinence due to vaginal atrophy | Reduces atrophy and urinary infection |
| Anticholinergics, e.g. tolterodine, solifenacin, oxybutynin | OAB syndrome/detrusor overactivity | May precipitate urinary retention<br>Side effects of dry mouth, constipation, and postural hypotension may limit effectiveness<br>Titrate the dose up slowly. Use for 6 weeks before maximal effect<br>Anticholinergics cause confusion and in long-term use (>3 years) predispose to cognitive impairment<br>Reassess risk/benefit before 3 years |
| β3-agonists, e.g. mirabegron | OAB syndrome/detrusor overactivity | Avoids anticholinergic side effects but may precipitate hypertensive crisis—use with caution in vasculopaths |
| Surgery—♀ | Tension-free vaginal tape (TVT) or colposuspension (for stress)<br>Urethral collagen injection (for stress)<br>Intravesical botulinum toxin (for OAB) | Refer for urodynamics prior to surgery |

URINARY INCONTINENCE: MANAGEMENT

**Tabel 20.2** (*Contd.*)

| Treatment | Indication | Notes |
|---|---|---|
| *Surgery*—♂ | For outflow tract obstruction TURP | |
| Antiandrogens finasteride | For prostatic hyperplasia Improves flow and obstructive symptoms | Slow onset of action ↓ libido/impotence |
| α-*blockers*, e.g. doxazosin, tamsulosin | Smooth muscle relaxant for BPH—improves flow and obstructive symptoms | Titrate dose slowly—watch for hypotension (especially postural) and syncope/falls Useful for co-treatment of hypertension |
| *Double micturition* (ask patient to repeat voiding) | Sometimes helps reduce large residual volumes and ↓ UTI | |
| *Intermittent catheterization* | Atonic/hypotonic bladder—removing residual volumes daily can aid continence and reduce renal damage and infection. Also used to dilate stenotic urethras | Surprisingly well tolerated in 'flexible' elderly people |
| *Synthetic vasopressin* either oral or intranasal | Useful for nocturnal frequency | Main troublesome side effect is dilutional hyponatraemia—unlicensed for >65s in the UK Caution in patients with comorbid conditions, likely to be exacerbated |

# Catheters

A catheter is indicated for:
* Symptomatic urinary retention
* Obstructed outflow associated with deteriorating renal function or hydronephrosis
* Acute renal failure for accurate urine output monitoring
* Intensive care settings
* Sacral pressure sores with incontinence
* Where other methods of bladder management cause undue distress to a frail older person
* Occasionally to facilitate discharge home by reducing care needs (especially overnight) where non-catheter options have failed

▶ A catheter is NOT usually indicated for:
* Immobility—even from stroke
* Heart failure—just because you are giving furosemide
* Monitoring fluid balance in a continent patient
* Convenience of nursing—at home or in hospital
* Asymptomatic chronic retention—refer to urology for assessment

## Catheter selection
* Long-term catheters should be either silicone, Silastic, or silver-impregnated (expensive but reportedly fewer blockages and infections)
* Catheter size should be as small as practical
* Catheters should be changed at least every 3 months
* Consider the use of a catheter valve (like a beer keg tap), rather than a drainage bag
* If duration is likely to be more than a year, consider suprapubic placement to preserve urethral sphincter function

## HOW TO . . . Manage urinary incontinence without a catheter

In spite of correct diagnosis, investigation, and treatment of reversible causes, there will still be patients who will be permanently or intermittently incontinent of urine.

▶ An indwelling catheter is not always the best solution. They have been shown to ↑ morbidity (infection, stones, urethral erosion) and even mortality.

Suggesting that catheters are removed is one of a geriatrician's most important jobs in post-acute care. If in doubt, involve a specialist continence nurse/team.

Other options for continence management include:

- *Environmental modifications*: urinals (available for both ♂ and ♀) or commodes by the bed, easy access clothing, etc. can minimize or prevent accidents
- *Regular or individualized toileting programmes*: this can be very successful in patients with dementia but is labour-intensive
- *Pad and pants*: can be very effective but is quite labour-intensive for very immobile patients
- *A drainage sheath* or *condom catheter* (Conveen® is a manufacturer) for men: like a catheter but held onto the penis with a plastic sheath like a condom. Particularly useful for isolated nocturnal incontinence, as it can be removed by day. Main problem is displacement and leakage which can be a problem with small or unusually shaped penises
- *Intermittent catheterization*: for those with obstruction or atonic bladders. Consider in agile, cognitively intact patients. Can be supported by district nursing services

## HOW TO . . . Treat catheter complications

*Blocked catheters*
- Consider the possibility of stones, infection, sediment, encrustation, constipation, or bladder tumour
- Renew the catheter if necessary
- Maintain good fluid intake
- Blockage due to sediment can be prevented with regular saline bladder washouts
- Catheter encrustation occurs with *Proteus* infection; acidic irrigations instilled into the bladder may dissolve these (e.g. Suby G®)

*'Bypassing'*
- Catheters can irritate the bladder causing contractions—resulting leak of urine past the catheter can render them useless and occasionally causes very painful spasms
- This is particularly common where detrusor overactivity was the cause of incontinence
- Can be induced or aggravated by infection
- Exclude catheter blockage (presents with spasms and leaks)
- If no residual volume, reduce catheter diameter
- Anticholinergic drugs can sometimes help
- Longer-term catheters can cause urethral sphincter incompetence, so urine will leak continuously. This may be temporarily helped by passing a larger-gauge catheter but is a difficult problem to manage— avoid by using suprapubic catheters earlier

*Catheter infections*
- All catheters become colonized after a few days; all catheter urine will dipstick positive, and most catheter specimens of urine will grow bacteria. ▶ This alone is not an indication for antibiotics
- Bad-smelling, dark-coloured, and cloudy urine is more commonly due to dehydration and is not an indication for antibiotics per se
- There are now some trials of cranberry juice/capsules that suggest there is a minor effect on reducing recurrent infections
- Only treat clinically significant infections (fever, malaise, delirium, pain, abnormal inflammatory markers, etc.) or you will just promote resistant organisms
- If you believe a catheter is a source of significant infection:
  - Send a catheter specimen of urine to guide antibiotic choice
  - Remove the catheter where possible. If not possible, change the catheter, with a single shot of im gentamicin (80–120mg)
  - Ensure adequate hydration
  - Choose a narrow-spectrum antibiotic if sensitivities allow
- For repeated significant infection, consider if the catheter is really necessary
- Low-dose continuous antibiotic prophylaxis are advocated by some, but there is little evidence

## HOW TO . . . Manage trial without catheter ('TWOC')

*Avoid insertion if possible*
- Consider other options such as condom catheters for men
- Manage incontinence with containment if skin integrity is not threatened

*Treat precipitant before removing*
- Consider why the catheter was inserted, as this will guide management
- Treat precipitants, e.g. infection, constipation, immobility
- Consider routinely giving an α-blocker to men presenting with retention 48h prior to a TWOC

*When?*
- For a prolonged admission, TWOC during the inpatient stay is sensible, to allow adjustment to toileting needs
- For brief admissions, or where retention is the only problem, TWOC can occur in the community
- Balance the convenience of a catheter for continence against the possible harm—always aim to remove catheters if possible

*What time of day?*
- For inpatients, remove the catheter at midnight, so that if retention occurs, it is likely to be during the day
- For community TWOC, early morning catheter removal may be better

*What to do if it fails?*
- Have all precipitants been considered and treated?
- For men, add an α-blocker, then try again after at least 48h
- Consider urology referral for repeated episodes of ♂ retention

# Faecal incontinence: causes

Defined as the involuntary passage of faeces in inappropriate circumstances. The importance of situational factors means there is potential for anyone to be incontinent in some circumstances.

- Incontinence of faeces is always abnormal, and often curable
- It is much less common than urinary incontinence, but more distressing
- There is gross under-referral for diagnosis and treatment
- Prevalence—10% of care home residents incontinent at least once per week

## Continence mechanisms

- *The sigmo-rectal 'sphincter'*—the rectum is usually empty. Passage of faeces into the rectum initiates rectal contraction (and anal relaxation), normally temporarily inhibited. The acute angle in the pelvic loop of the sigmoid may be important in causing temporary hold-up
- *The ano-rectal angle*—the pubo-rectalis sling maintains an acute angle between the rectum and anus, preventing passage of stool into the anal canal
- *The anal sphincters*—the external sphincter (striated, voluntary muscle), internal sphincter (smooth muscle), and anal vascular cushions which complete the seal
- *Ano-rectal sensation*—sensation in the anus and rectum is usually sufficiently accurate to distinguish gas from faeces, permitting the passage of flatus without incontinence. Good sensation may be particularly important when diarrhoea is present

## Causes of faecal incontinence

- Disorders of the anal sphincter and lower rectum: sphincter laxity (from many causes), severe haemorrhoids, rectal prolapse, tumours, constipation
- Any cause of faecal urgency (occasionally associated with reduced mobility): constipation (with spurious diarrhoea), any cause of diarrhoea (inflammatory bowel disease, drugs, etc.)
- Disorders of the neurological control of the ano-rectal muscle and sphincter: LMN lesions (neuropathic incontinence), spinal cord lesions, cognitive impairment (neurogenic incontinence)

The most common cause (>50%) is faecal impaction. This is important because 95% are curable. The second most common cause is neurogenic incontinence where cure is still possible.

# Faecal incontinence: assessment

Most patients can be helped by asking a few questions and performing a rectal examination.

Effective treatment is directed at the underlying cause, so adequate assessment is vital.

## History

- The duration of symptoms is not helpful: impaction is just as common in those who have been incontinent for >3 months as in those in whom the incontinence is recent
- Having the bowels open regularly (e.g. every day) is usual in elderly patients with impaction
- Complete constipation (not having the bowels open at all) is unusual in impaction
- A feeling of rectal fullness with constant seepage of semi-liquid faeces is almost diagnostic of impaction, but rectal carcinoma may also present in this way
- Where there is a combination of urinary and faecal incontinence, consider impaction as the cause of both
- Soiling without the patient being aware of it suggests neuropathy

## Examination

- *Inspect the anus*—and ask the patient to strain as if at stool. Look for inflammation, deformities, large haemorrhoids (internal or external), and prolapse
- *Rectal examination*—assess anal tone by the pressure on the finger after asking the patient to 'tighten'; feel for faeces and tumour; it is easy to miss even large internal haemorrhoids, unless proctoscopy is performed
- *Abdominal examination*—feel for the descending colon. Work proximally to assess colonic faecal loading (this may be misleading)
- *Neurological examination*—look for signs of a peripheral neuropathy and other neurological damage. Check perianal sensation (sacral dermatomes). Include a mental status assessment if you think neurogenic incontinence is likely

## Investigations

A plain abdominal radiograph may be necessary to detect proximal faecal loading of the colon (see → 'Faecal incontinence: management', p. 546). Investigation of the anal sphincter tone and neurological control of the rectum and anus is in the province of the proctologist and may occasionally be needed for neuropathic incontinence.

# Faecal incontinence: management

The two common treatments in old age are for constipation and neurogenic incontinence. In addition, specialist proctology clinics can perform ano-rectal physiology assessment prior to the use of biofeedback techniques and surgery (e.g. sphincteroplasty, colostomy).

## Treatment of constipation

*Faecal impaction, faecal retention, faecal loading*

▶ In hospitalized older people, constipation is by far the most common cause of incontinence; assume that any incontinent patient is constipated until proven otherwise, and do not exclude it until after adequate bowel care for high faecal impaction.

See ➋ 'Constipation', pp. 368–9 for definition, diagnosis, causes, prevention, and treatment of constipation, and ➋ 'HOW TO . . . treat "overflow" faecal incontinence', p. 547.

## Mechanism

Passage of faeces from the sigmoid into the rectum (often soon after a meal—the gastro-colic reflex) produces a sensation of rectal fullness and a desire to defecate. If this is ignored, the sensation gradually habituates, and the rectum fills up with progressively harder faeces. At this stage, some leakage past the anal sphincter (incontinence) is almost inevitable. Impaction of hard faecal material produces partial obstruction, stasis, irritation of the mucosa with excessive mucus production, and spurious diarrhoea. Emptying the colon of faeces has two main effects—it prevents spurious diarrhoea, and therefore urgency, and it permits normal colonic motility and habit to be restored.

## Treatment of neurogenic faecal incontinence

Loss of control of the intrinsic rectal contraction caused by passage of normal faecal material from the sigmoid into the rectum results in the involuntary passage of a normal, formed stool at infrequent intervals, and usually at a timing characteristic of that patient (typically after breakfast).

It is a syndrome analogous with the uninhibited neurogenic bladder and usually only occurs in the context of severe dementia. However, note that incontinence in patients with dementia is commonly due to constipation.

Since the diagnosis is usually one of exclusion, it is reasonable to treat most patients as though they have impaction, particularly if you cannot exclude high impaction by radiology. Once impaction has been excluded, there are three strategies:

• In patients with a regular habit, toileting at the appropriate time (perhaps with the aid of a suppository) may be successful. This requires an attendant who knows the patient well
• Arrange for a planned evacuation to suit the carers, by administering a constipating agent (e.g. loperamide) combined with a phosphate enema two or three times weekly
• If the patient has no regular habit and refuses enemas, the situation may have to be accepted and suitable protective clothing provided

## HOW TO . . . Treat 'overflow' faecal incontinence

- *General*—rehydration (possibly iv), regular meals, and help with toileting are important
- *Enemas*, e.g. phosphate enema given od or (occasionally) bd. Continue until there is no result, the rectum is found to be empty on DRE, and the colon is impalpable abdominally. This may take a week or more
- *Complete colonic washout*, e.g. using bowel prep such as Picolax®. This is rather an extreme method but is sometimes required. Ensure the patient is well hydrated before you start
- *Manual evacuation of faeces*—can cause further damage to the anal sphincters and is almost never necessary
- *Laxatives*—generally less effective than enemas but can be used in addition, for milder cases and in the very frail. If the stool is hard, use a stool-softening laxative such as lactulose—stimulant laxatives (e.g. senna) may produce severe pain. Stimulant laxatives or suppositories may be appropriate for those with soft faecal overloading.
  A combination of stool softener and stimulant is sometimes used, or try a laxative with dual mechanism (e.g. macrogols). While extra fibre is useful in prophylaxis, stool-bulking agents such as methylcellulose are of limited value in treating constipation, as they ↑ the volume of stool being passed and may ↑ your problems

▶ After treatment, think prevention (see ⟳ 'Constipation', pp. 368–9).
   If, despite these measures, a patient has impaction for a second time (without an obvious and removable cause), then regular (say once or twice weekly) enemas should be prescribed. Progress can only be satisfactorily monitored by examining the patient abdominally and rectally.

# Ears

# Deafness and the ageing ear

Deafness is a common, debilitating complaint that ↑ with age; 6% of adults, 33% of retired people, and 80% of octogenarians in the UK have impaired hearing. Deafness is often ignored ('part of getting older'), yet it prevents communication, causes social isolation, anxiety, and depression, and can contribute to functional decline.

Around half of sufferers could be helped by a hearing aid, yet less than a quarter have one. Generally patients with unilateral, mild bilateral, or profound bilateral deafness do not benefit from conventional hearing aids.

▶ Be alert to hearing loss. A quick assessment directs appropriate referral to audiology or ENT when necessary.

## Normal ageing

*Presbyacusis*

- Describes the decline in hearing that commonly occurs with age—'degenerative deafness'
- ♂ > ♀
- Usually detectable from age 60–65
- Both the sensory peripheral (cochlea) and central (neural) components of the auditory system are affected, with peripheral degeneration being accountable for at least two-thirds of the clinical features of presbyacusis
- A variety of possible mechanisms exist—cellular degeneration gives rise to a reduction in the numbers of hair cells, particularly at the basal end of the cochlea (the part responsible for high-frequency sound appreciation). *Circulatory* changes such as atherosclerosis, microangiopathy, and atrophy of the stria vascularis contribute
- The relative contributions of 'normal ageing' and cumulative exposure to noxious stimuli (noise, toxins, oxidative stresses, otological disease, poor diet, vascular disease) are unclear, but not all older people have hearing problems
- The high frequencies are lost first—usually noticed when high-pitched ♀ voices become hard to hear. As consonants are high frequency, the patient can often hear noise, but not understand, feeling that everyone is 'mumbling' (loss of discrimination)
- 'Recruitment' is a common problem where the thresholds for hearing and discomfort are very close ('Speak up . . . don't shout')
- Busy, noisy environments make hearing harder, so patients may avoid social situations
- There is no treatment to halt progression, but hearing aids may help

*Other ear changes with age*

These include:

- Thinner walls to the external auditory canal, with fewer glands, making it dry and itchy
- Drier wax due to ↓ sweat gland activity, making accumulation (a cause of reversible hearing impairment) more common. Ear syringing is no longer recommended—try olive oil or sodium bicarbonate drops. ENT can provide microsuction for resistant cases
- Degenerative changes of the inner ear and vestibular system contributing to ↑ in deafness, vertigo, and tinnitus

## Classifying deafness

### Conductive

A disturbance in the mechanical attenuation of sound waves in outer/middle ear, preventing sound from reaching the inner ear.

- It can be caused by outer ear obstruction (e.g. wax, foreign body, otitis externa), some types of tympanic membrane perforation, tympanosclerosis, or middle ear problems (effusion, otosclerosis, ossicular erosion 2° to infection or cholesteatoma)
- It may be surgically correctable and can be helped by a hearing aid

### Sensorineural

A problem with the cochlea or auditory nerve, so impulses are not transmitted to the auditory cortex.

- Caused by genetic or perinatal factors in children
- In adults, may be traumatic, infective (viral, chronic otitis media, meningitis, syphilis), noise-induced, degenerative (presbyacusis), ototoxic (e.g. aminoglycosides, cytotoxics), neoplastic (acoustic neuroma), or others such as Ménière's disease
- Usually irreversible
- The appropriate hearing aid can be helpful
- Cochlear implants can be considered in severe sensorineural deafness but seem less effective than in younger patients, perhaps due to limitations in cerebral processing

### Mixed

A combination of both conductive and sensorineural—probably the most common cause in older people.

---

### HOW TO . . . Communicate with a deaf person

- Ensure hearing aids are inserted correctly, are turned on, and have working batteries
- Speak clearly and at a normal rate
- Use sentences, not one-word answers—this gives contextual cues to lip readers
- ↑ the volume, but do not shout
- Lower the pitch of the voice
- Minimize background noise
- Maximize face-to-face visual contact—look straight at the person, and ensure there are not bright lights behind you that will dazzle
- Use visual cues when talking (e.g. hand gestures)
- Be patient—repeat things if asked, changing the sentence slightly if possible
- If confusion arises, write things down—do not give up

**HOW TO . . . Assess hearing**

*General*

Conversation will give an informal idea of hearing ability.

Clarify by performing free field speech tests by asking the patient to repeat words spoken in a whispered voice, conversation voice, and shouted at 60cm from the ear. The non-test ear is masked by pressing the tragus backwards and rotating it with the index finger. Sit the patient next to you, so that lip reading is not possible.

*History*

- Rate of onset and progression (witnesses will often be more accurate than patients)
- Unilateral or bilateral
- History of trauma, noise exposure, or ear surgery
- Family history of hearing problems or hearing aid use
- History of ototoxic drugs, e.g. aminoglycoside antibiotics (gentamicin, streptomycin, etc.) and high-dose furosemide
- Associated symptoms (pain, discharge, tinnitus, vertigo)

*Examination*

- External ear and canal (looking for wax, inflammation, discharge, blood, abnormal growths, etc.)
- Drum (perforations, myringitis, retraction, bulging of drum, etc.)
- Tuning fork tests (with a 512kHz fork) may be helpful. Both are based on the principle of improved bone conduction perception with a conductive hearing loss
  - *Rinne's*—compares air and bone conduction. Hold the tuning fork in front of the ear, then place on the mastoid, to compare air and bone conduction. Air > bone is normal. Bone > air implies defective middle and outer ear function
  - *Weber's*—assesses bone conduction only. Hold the tuning fork at the vertex of the head, and ask which ear hears the sound most loudly. With conductive deafness, it is heard loudest in the deafer ear; with sensorineural deafness, it is heard most loudly in the normal ear

*Who to refer?*

Patients with sinister features should be referred to an ENT surgeon:

- Recent or abrupt hearing loss
- Unilateral hearing loss or tinnitus
- Variable hearing loss
- Ear pain

▶ Sudden-onset sensorineural deafness is an ENT emergency and requires urgent referral (causes include infection, vascular event, tumour, leaking canals, etc.)

All other patients with suspected hearing loss should be referred routinely to an audiologist for further assessment and management.

# Audiology

The majority of patients with hearing impairment are managed by audiologists and hearing therapists. They do the following.

## Specialized hearing tests

- *Audiometry*—quantifies the degree and pattern of loss. May be 'pure tone' (using signals at varying frequencies and intensities) or 'speech' (discriminating spoken words at differing intensities). The hearing thresholds are charted on an audiogram and interpreted by the audiologist (indicates conduction or sensorineural deafness, which frequency, and which ear)
- *Impedance tympanometry*—indirectly measures the compliance of the middle ear, identifying infection and effusion in the middle ear and Eustachian tube dysfunction
- *Evoked response audiometry*—measures action potentials produced by sound. No conscious response is required by the patient and so tests are less open to bias. (Before MRI, this was the main diagnostic test for acoustic neuromas)

## Recommend and fit hearing aids

Many types. Help patients to have realistic expectations about their hearing aids (rarely a 'miracle cure') and train them how to use them optimally (e.g. minimizing background noise). Programme digital hearing aids.

## Offer practical advice

About assistive listening devices such as:
- *Alternative signals*—buzzers and flashing lights, instead of doorbell or telephone ring; vibrating devices that attach to the wrist and alert the wearer to environmental noises. Hearing dogs can also be used
- *Television*—subtitles, or devices that connect to the hearing aid allowing the television signal to be amplified
- *Telephones*—with high-/low-volume control and 'T' settings that amplify the telephone noise without the background noise
- *Transmitter and receiver devices* (infrared or FM radio wave) for use in theatres, etc. with transmission from the sound source. The listener can adjust the volume in their receiver
- Advise about better *communication*

## Aural rehabilitation

Age-matched group sessions that help with adjustment to the sudden reintroduction of noise with a hearing aid (after what is usually a gradual hearing loss), teach skills (e.g. blocking out background noise, lip reading), and share practical tips (e.g. eating in a booth at a restaurant to limit background noise).

## Other

- Train people to *lip read*
- Help manage *tinnitus*
- *Counsel* about psychosocial implications of hearing impairment

# Hearing aids

The past decade has seen many advances in hearing aid technology and performance. Modern hearing aids offer improved fidelity, greater amplification, and frequency-specific amplification. Patients who have tried hearing aids in the past and not found them beneficial should be encouraged to try them again.

## What do hearing aids do?

Generally consist of a microphone that gathers sound, an amplifier that ↑ the volume and a receiver that transmits amplified sound. Most hearing aids also include circuitry that filters and processes sound prior to amplification.

## Whom do they help?

- Help many to some degree, but not all
- Does not restore normal hearing—the wearer needs to learn to interpret the new auditory input efficiently
- Conductive hearing loss is helped more than sensorineural loss

## What are the different types?

*Different sizes*

- Smaller units (e.g. completely-in-the-canal devices) are cosmetically more appealing and give good reception for mild to moderate hearing loss, but are fiddly and expensive
- Medium-sized units (e.g. in-the-ear devices) are more visible and have more feedback, but can be used for worse hearing loss
- Larger units (e.g. behind-the-ear) provide the most amplification and are easier to handle, but suffer from feedback if the ear mould deforms

*Monaural versus binaural*—binaural hearing aids yield a subjective improvement in sound clarity, but monaural may be considered for unilateral loss.

*Analogue devices*

- Cheapest, with least processing of sound
- Set to hearing loss at the time of fitting
- Audiologist adjusts amplification and tonality settings at time of fitting, but these are then fixed
- Patient can adjust the volume manually (turn the device volume up when the noise is quiet, and down when it is loud)

*Digitally programmable devices*

- More expensive, with moderate sound processing
- Analogue circuit that can be adjusted at the time of fitting by a computer programme to best fit the patient's needs
- Automatic volume control

*Digital devices*
- Most health authorities now fit digital hearing aids for all new referrals and exchange old analogue aids. All but the most expensive are funded by the NHS where clinically indicated
- Programmable with flexible digital circuits that manipulate each sound according to pitch and volume to give the clearest sound for that individual
- Higher clarity of sound, less circuit noise, faster processing, and automatic volume control

*Disposable devices*
- 'One size fits all'—actually fit around 70% of patients
- Widely available, e.g. in pharmacies
- Not individually tailored, so less good
- No need for battery changes, low breakdown costs
- Last about 40 days, so expensive in the long term

*Cochlear implants*
- Unilateral cochlear implantation is recommended as an option for people with severe to profound deafness who do not receive adequate benefit from acoustic hearing aids
- Requires MDT assessment prior to insertion
- Simultaneous bilateral implants may be considered where there is coexistent blindness, making the patient more reliant on aural input

## HOW TO . . . Use a hearing aid

*To check a hearing aid*
- Put a new battery in
- Turn to the 'M' setting
- Turn the volume up as far as it will go
- A working hearing aid will whistle

*Putting it in*
- The audiologist will take an impression of the ear to make an ear mould that fits snugly
- This should be inserted, so that it fits correctly and comfortably

*Turning it on*
- Most hearing aids have three settings: 'O' = off; 'M' = microphone (use this setting for normal conversation); 'T' = telecoil (use this setting with listening equipment such as loop devices. These transfer sound direct to the hearing aid and cut out background noise)
- In addition, there will often be a volume wheel, which can be adjusted as needed

*What to do if there is no sound*
- Check the hearing aid is not switched to 'O' or 'T'
- Check the batteries are not dead, or put in upside down
- Check the mould is not clogged with wax
- Check the tubing is not wet (dry with a hairdryer) or twisted

*What to do if there is a whistling or squealing noise (feedback)*
- Occurs when the ear mould is not snug, allowing sound to escape into the microphone
- Worse at high volumes
- Check that the ear mould is a good fit (return to the audiologist if not) and is inserted correctly
- Ensure there is not excess earwax impeding fit
- Try turning the volume down

*Maintaining the hearing aid*
- Handle carefully
- Keep the hearing aid dry, away from strong heat or light
- Use a clean, dry tissue to clean, never a damp cloth
- Use wax remover on a regular basis

If the ear mould is separate (e.g. behind-the-ear), then periodically remove and wash with warm soapy water, ensuring it is totally dry before reconnecting it.

# Tinnitus

The perception of a sound in one or both ears, without an external stimulus. Intermittent or continuous. Varying kinds of noises (ringing, humming, buzzing, occasionally other noises) and at varying pitches. Large spectrum of disease. More common in men than women, and incidence rises with age. Up to a quarter of older people may experience intermittent symptoms, but only 1 in 20 will be disabled by it. A quarter of patients will get worsening symptoms with time.

Tinnitus can be due to actual sounds that are generated by local structures:

- *Vascular structures* (aneurysmal vessels, vascular tumours, etc.—generate a pulsatile or humming noise that may worsen with exercise)
- *Muscle spasms* (palatal or middle ear muscles—generate a clicking noise. Usually indicates underlying neurological disease)
- *Eustachian tube* may be patulous (can occur after dramatic weight loss), resulting in a roaring sound
- *Joints* (e.g. temporomandibular joint, cervical spine joints)

More commonly, the noise is generated from somewhere within the auditory pathway (cochlear organ, nerve, brainstem, or auditory cortex) after some sort of damage or injury. The following are associated with tinnitus:

- *Hearing loss*—a very common cause in older people. Mechanism unclear—may be akin to phantom limb pain. Note tinnitus may precede deafness. May be associated with conductive (e.g. wax accumulation) or more commonly sensorineural deafness (including presbyacusis). Treatment of deafness (with hearing aid or occasionally cochlear implant) often results in improvement of tinnitus
- *Drugs*—many commonly prescribed drugs in older people can either cause or exacerbate tinnitus (see Box 21.1)
- *Vascular disease*—microvascular damage to the auditory system, or a stroke affecting the auditory cortex. Modify vascular risk factors to limit progression
- *Infection*, e.g. chronic otitis media. Treat the cause, but may have residual problems
- *Other*—Ménière's disease, diabetes, thyroid disease, Paget's disease, brain tumour (intracanalicular and cerebello-pontine), trauma, and autoimmune disease. Treat underlying cause

## History

- Obtain a description of tinnitus. This may indicate the cause, e.g. pulsatile noise is often vascular; clicking noise is often due to palatal muscle spasms; high-pitched continuous noise is usually due to sensorineural hearing loss; low-pitched continuous noise is more commonly seen (but not exclusive to Ménière's disease)
- Screen for possible causes (drug history, ear disease, noise exposure, injury, etc.)

## Examination

Should include full head and neck examination, cranial nerve examination, auscultation for bruits, and inspection of the auditory canal.

## Box 21.1 Drugs causing or exacerbating tinnitus

- Aspirin (high dose)
- Other NSAIDs
- Loop diuretics
- ACE inhibitors
- Calcium channel blockers
- Doxazosin
- Aminoglycoside antibiotics
- Clarithromycin
- Quinine and chloroquine
- Carbamazepine
- Tricyclic antidepressants
- Benzodiazepines
- PPIs
- Some chemotherapy agents

### Investigation

Check FBC, glucose, and thyroid function. Refer to specialist for full audio-metric assessment and possible imaging, especially if unilateral (MRI ± angiography).

### Treatment

- Difficult and frustrating—often best done in specialist clinics with MDT support
- Stop all ototoxic medication and avoid in future
- Assess whether caffeine, aspartame sweetener, alcohol, nicotine, and marijuana worsen tinnitus and avoid if so
- Treat the cause wherever possible
- Strong association with insomnia and depression, both of which worsen the suffering and should be treated. Some evidence to suggest that antidepressants (SSRIs) may help, even when there is no overt depression
- Many other treatments have been tried (e.g. lidocaine, magnetic and ultrasonic stimulation, melatonin, *Ginkgo biloba*, niacin, and zinc), but limited evidence they work and adverse effects common
- Hearing aids are useful if the ↑ hearing loss—the ↑ awareness of the background sound tends to make the noise less apparent
- Masking techniques involve wearing a 'white noise' generator, rather like a hearing aid that aims to distract the patient from the tinnitus by reducing the contrast between the tinnitus signal and background noise, improving the plasticity of the central auditory cortex and thereby facilitating a reduction in perception of the sound
- Mainstay of treatment is aimed at adjusting patients' perception of the tinnitus, trying to habituate them to the noise and limiting the negative emotions it generates. Includes tinnitus retraining therapy, biofeedback, stress reduction techniques, and cognitive and behavioural therapy
- Tinnitus support groups can be helpful (⅌ http://www.tinnitus.org.uk)

# Vertigo

### Definition

Vertigo is the hallucination of movement. A sensation of rotatory motion either of the patient with respect to the environment ('it's like being on a roundabout') or the environment with respect to the patient ('the room is spinning'). The key element is a feeling of motion, without which a clinical diagnosis of vertigo should not be made.

### Understanding vertigo

The vestibular system comprises the temporal bone labyrinths (composed of the semicircular canals, the saccule, and the utricle), the vestibular nerve, and the central vestibular structures in the brainstem. Normally, there is a constant input from both ears updating the central structures on head position. In the brainstem, they are integrated with inputs from the visual cortex and from proprioceptive receptors (most important are the neck and ankles). Any interruption of this input leads to an excess of information from the good side, and so an acute feeling of dizziness and nausea (vertigo), along with disruption of the vestibulo-ocular reflex (which will cause nystagmus). This situation continues until either input is restored or the vestibular system adapts to the altered balance of signals.

Adaptation means that:

- Vertigo is not a chronic condition. Multiple recurrences may occur, but a complaint of long-standing continuous dizziness is not vertigo
- Vertigo rarely occurs with slowly progressive conditions (e.g. acoustic neuroma), as adaptation occurs along the way
- All vertigo is made worse by head movement—if not, then seek an alternative diagnosis
- The use of vestibular sedatives, e.g. prochlorperazine, should be limited to the acute phase for symptom relief only—prolonged use will delay adaptation

▶ There is no indication for long-term use of vestibular sedatives.

### Causes

(See Table 21.1.)

- Many patients complaining of dizziness will have vertigo (see ➋ 'Dizziness', p. 112)
- Over all ages, 80% of vertigo arises from peripheral structures (the ears) and 20% from central structures (the brain)
- Peripheral vertigo is due to benign positional paroxysmal vertigo in up to 50%
- Central vertigo is usually due to stroke
- The proportion of central vertigo ↑ with age, because of the ↑ incidence of stroke

Table 21.1 Common causes of vertigo

| Condition | Features | Cause | Treatment |
|---|---|---|---|
| Benign paroxysmal positional vertigo (BPPV) | Mild episodes lasting less than a minute, recurring frequently over weeks to months | Calcium debris in semicircular canal Usually idiopathic May be preceded by minor head trauma | Resolves spontaneously but may recur Epley's manoeuvre may help (see ➔ 'HOW TO… Perform Epley's manoeuvre', p. 564) |
| Acute vestibular failure (labyrinthitis) | Acute onset of severe vertigo, lasting hours to days Associated nausea, vomiting, and postural instability Patient in bed, refuses to move head | Ischaemia of vestibular apparatus, often preceded by a viral respiratory tract infection | High-dose steroids acutely may speed recovery Treat with vestibular sedatives only while vomiting, then allow adaptation to occur May have recurrent (milder) episodes |
| Ménière's disease | Recurrent episodes of violent vertigo, vomiting, tinnitus, ear fullness (lasting up to 12h), and fluctuating hearing loss | Dilation of endolymphatic space in the canals—primary cause still unknown | Symptomatic treatment of acute attacks Betahistine is a labyrinthine vasodilator Diuretics may reduce attack frequency Surgical options include grommet insertion, transtympanic gentamicin, endolymphatic decompression, and vestibular nerve sectioning |
| Vertebrobasilar stroke | TIAs cause stuttering symptoms (see Box 5.1). Stroke will cause abrupt onset, prolonged symptoms Vertigo is most common symptom, usually associated with other neurology (e.g. ataxia, diplopia, visual loss, slurred speech, motor or sensory impairment) Cerebellar stroke can cause vertigo alone | | After stroke, slow improvement is normal, but often residual defects Modify vascular risk factors (see ➔ 'Vascular secondary prevention', p. 310) to prevent recurrence |

# Vertigo: assessment

## History

- This is the most important diagnostic tool in vertigo. Use open questions with clarification
- Describe the dizziness—is it a sensation of movement of self or the room (likely vertigo)? Or a light-headed feeling (less likely vertigo)? A non-specific description does not exclude vertigo
- Establish if likely peripheral (abrupt onset and cessation with nausea, vomiting, and tinnitus) or central (more prolonged, less severe, less positional episodes; usually with other neurological symptoms and signs)
- Ask about onset, severity, duration, progression, and recurrence to narrow down the cause (see Table 21.1)
- Ask about provoking factors—may be spontaneous or brought on by changes in middle ear pressure (sneezing, coughing) or head/neck position (question carefully to distinguish this from orthostatic symptoms)
- Ask about associated symptoms, e.g. tinnitus and hearing loss (is it worse during an attack?)
- Ask about predisposing factors, e.g. vascular risk factors, recent infections, headache, ototoxic drugs, ear discharge, deafness, tinnitus, etc.
- Ask about psychiatric symptoms (e.g. low mood)—these are rarely offered spontaneously

## Examination

- General examination (including cardiovascular examination)
- Postural BP measurements
- Neurological examination
- Examine eye movements for pursuit and saccades. Abnormalities in a patient with balance complaints suggests a cerebellar origin
- Head and neck examination, including otoscopy (to assess auditory canals and tympanic membranes)
- Gait assessment
- Hearing test (see &#10137; 'HOW TO . . . Assess hearing', p. 552)
- Vestibular assessment (see &#10137; 'HOW TO . . . Examine the vestibular system', p. 563)

## HOW TO . . . Examine the vestibular system

This is hard to do directly—it largely relies on testing the integrity of the vestibulo-ocular reflex.

- Test eye movements with the head still, looking for nystagmus (the eyes drift slowly *towards* the bad side, and the rapid correction phase is towards the good side). Visual fixation may suppress a peripheral nystagmus, but not a central. Peripheral lesions cause horizontal nystagmus in both eyes; central lesions cause nystagmus in any direction that is more prolonged and severe
- Try to provoke vertigo and nystagmus by asking the patient to gently flex, extend, rotate, and laterally bend the cervical spine
- Check visual acuity with a Snellen chart, both with the head still and with the patient slowly shaking their head. If acuity is >4 lines worse with head shaking, this suggests impairment
- Head thrust test—ask the patient to fix the gaze on the examiner's nose, while the examiner turns the head rapidly to one side or the other. The patient should be able to keep the gaze fixed. If there is a peripheral vestibular problem, the gaze may drift during rotation to that side, which is manifest by a catch-up saccade back to the point of fixation. When done properly, this test has a better than 80% sensitivity and specificity for vestibular hypofunction
- Ask the patient to shake their head, and then check for nystagmus—if it is present, this implies unilateral impairment
- Nystagmus after 30s of hyperventilation can be an indicator of a vestibular schwannoma

*Hallpike manoeuvre*
- Tests for BPPV (50–80% sensitive)
- Sit the patient up, and stand behind them
- Hold their head turned 45° to one side
- Keep holding the head at this angle, and rapidly lie the patient down so the head is 30° below the level of the couch, looking down to the floor (steps 1 and 2 of the Epley's manoeuvre; see ➍ 'HOW TO . . . Perform Epley's manoeuvre', p. 564)
- Ask about symptoms, while watching for nystagmus (towards the floor)
- BPPV can be diagnosed confidently when the nystagmus is *latent* (occurs after a few seconds), *transient* (stops after <30s), and *fatigable* (lessens with repeat testing)
- If any of these features are absent, the vertigo is likely to be due to another cause
- Repeat with the head turned in the other direction

# Vertigo: management

Some specific treatments depending on the cause (see Table 21.1).

Symptomatic relief in the short term can be achieved with vestibular sedatives:

- Anticholinergics (e.g. hyoscine patch)
- Antihistamines (e.g. cyclizine, cinnarizine)
- Phenothiazines—usually sedating (e.g. prochlorperazine)
- Benzodiazepines (e.g. diazepam) if unable to take anticholinergics

May also benefit from antiemetics (e.g. metoclopramide).

These drugs are not for long-term use, and rarely beneficial in BPPV as attacks are so short-lived. Most vertigo will resolve with vestibular adaptation, leaving only brief feelings of imbalance on rapid head turns.

Some, however, will develop chronic dysfunction, in which case management is directed towards facilitating adaptation and development of coping strategies—*vestibular rehabilitation*. This is done by PTs or ENT specialist nurses and adopts a holistic approach. It involves a series of habituating exercises performed regularly to enable adaptation via compensation to occur. In addition to vestibular rehabilitation, consider spectacles to improve visual acuity, exercise to improve muscle strength, and a walking stick to aid peripheral balance.

Specific manoeuvres (see ➔ 'HOW TO . . . Perform Epley's manoeuvre', p. 564) and exercises are used for BPPV.

---

**HOW TO . . . Perform Epley's manoeuvre**

(See also Figs. 21.1–21.6.)

- Aims to clear debris from the posterior semicircular canal
- Requires the patient to be fairly flexible (modified version is available for more immobile patients)
- Stand behind the patient, firmly holding the head between your hands
- Make movements quickly and smoothly, holding each position for at least 30s
- The procedure takes approximately 3–5min:
  1. With the patient upright, turn the head 45° to the affected side
  2. Lie the patient down, with the head still turned, until they are reclined beyond the horizontal (as in the Hallpike manoeuvre)
  3. With the patient still reclined beyond horizontal, rotate the head through 90°, with the face upwards
  4. Keeping the head still, ask the patient to roll on to their side
  5. Rotate the head so the patient is facing downwards
  6. Keep the head at this angle, and raise the patient to the sitting position
  7. Finally, rotate the head so it faces the midline with the neck flexed (looking forward and downwards)

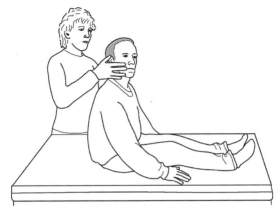

**Fig. 21.1** With the patient upright, turn the head 45° to the affected side.

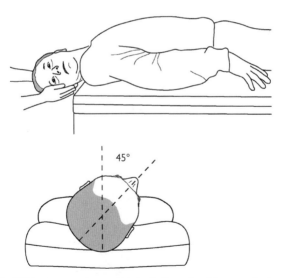

**Fig. 21.2** Lie the patient down, with the head still turned, until they are reclined beyond the horizontal (as in the Hallpike manoeuvre).

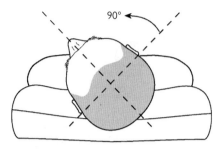

**Fig. 21.3** With the patient still reclined beyond horizontal, rotate the head through 90°, with the face upwards.

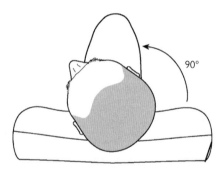

**Fig. 21.4** Keeping the head still, ask the patient to roll on to their side.

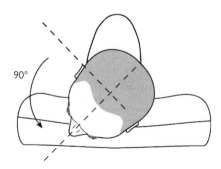

**Fig. 21.5** Rotate the head so the patient is facing downwards.

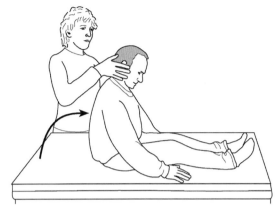

**Fig. 21.6** Keep the head at this angle, and raise the patient to the sitting position. Finally, rotate the head so it faces the midline, with the neck flexed (looking forwards and downwards).

# Chapter 22

# Eyes

# The ageing eye

Vision is a complex activity which involves eye function, cognition, reasoning, and memory. With ↑ age, the chance of visual impairment ↑ because of:
- Changes due to senescence
- Changes due to cumulative exposure to environmental toxins
- Changes in associated functions (cognition, hearing, etc.)
- ↑ incidence of many eye diseases

Visual impairment is not inevitable—there is considerable diversity both in visual decline and in compensatory adaptations. There is a tendency for patients to blame failing vision on age, and so not to seek help. However, some changes may be age-related (but corrective action may be available, e.g. glasses), or else impairment may herald the onset of treatable disease. Prompt identification and treatment may make all the difference between independence and dependence. Distinguishing what is 'normal' and when to refer to a specialist is key.

## Changes in vision with age

### Visual acuity often decreases
- Multifactorial—changes in macula, lens, and cornea
- May be corrected (e.g. glasses)
- Consider eye disease if deterioration is rapid

### Visual fields—peripheral vision less sensitive
- Although formal field-testing normal—consider cerebrovascular disease if distinct homonymous field defect
- Multifactorial—pupil smaller, lens cloudier, and peripheral retina less sensitive

### Near vision decreases
- Accommodative power diminishes due to increasingly rigid lens
- Presbyopia (a lack of accommodation range) is part of normal ageing, begins in middle age, and can be corrected with glasses

### Colour vision
- Retinal receptors unchanged
- Alterations in colour perception may relate to yellowing of the lens, altering the light reaching the retina

### Light adaptation slower
- Rods and cones may be slower to react to changes in illumination, and the pupil may let in less light, requiring brighter lighting for good vision
- Causes difficulty with night driving in particular
- Glare may be a problem as the lens, cornea, and vitreous become less clear and minute particles scatter light

### Contrast sensitivity decreases
- Due to changes in cornea, lens, and retina

### Floaters
- Due to aggregation of collagen fibrils in vitreous
- Usually normal, but if sudden onset or large quantity, may indicate retinal detachment or vitreous haemorrhage

# Visual impairment

One in five people over 75 years of age in the UK has visual impairment not amenable to correction by glasses alone. There is considerable social and psychological impact, yet it is underreported and optimal help is often not delivered.

## Causes
- Macular degeneration (by far the most common)
- Glaucoma
- Cataracts
- Diabetes
- Hypertension and stroke disease

## Interventions
Include:
- Low vision clinics are available in most hospitals
- Change glasses prescription (benefits 10–20%)
- Explain the disease (often does not cause total blindness, e.g. with macular degeneration; improve understanding of future)
- Psychological support (often combined with hearing loss in older people—beware social withdrawal. Acknowledge problem; discuss fears)
- Discuss blind registration
- In some cases, consider guide dogs and learning Braille
- Take specific history of certain activities and provide practical advice:
  - *Reading*—what do they actually need to read? Advise about good light, magnifiers, large-print books, photocopy recipes to larger size
  - *Writing*—use black pen on white paper; consider a writing frame or bold-line paper; discuss specific tasks such as cheques and pension books
  - *Television*—sitting closer, black and white sets may improve contrast
  - *Telling the time*—talking watches and clocks
  - *Cooking*—improving lighting in the kitchen by removing net curtains, tactile markers for cookers, electronic fullness indicators on cups
  - *Telephoning*—large-button telephones
  - *Social interaction*—sit with back to the window to improve light on a visitor's face; discuss accessible holidays

## Further reading
Royal National Institute of Blind People. ℘ http://www.rnib.org.uk. Sense. ℘ http://www.sense.org.uk.

# Blind registration

Done by ophthalmologists. Copy of the form goes to social services, the GP, and the Office for National Statistics.

Generally there is under-registration—probably due to stigma and a sense that this is the end of the fight, rather than the start of new help and opportunity.

## Definitions
- *Partially sighted* <6/60 in both eyes or reduced fields (e.g. homonymous hemianopia)
- *Blind* need not mean no vision. Statutory definition is that the person should be 'so blind as to be unable to perform any work for which eyesight is essential'. Pragmatically it is vision <3/60 or very diminished fields

## Benefits to individual
- Financial—including personal income tax allowance, personal independence payment, attendance allowance, pension credit, extra housing or council tax benefits, carers' allowance, help towards care home fees, free NHS sight test, free NHS prescriptions, lower television licence fee, and car parking and public transport concessions
- Easier access to help from social services
- Loan of talking books and newspapers (also available without registration)

---

**HOW TO . . . Optimize vision**

*Bigger*
- Magnifiers (glasses or contacts, hand magnifiers, stand magnifiers, illuminated magnifiers, reading telescopes). Consider portability, cosmetic aspects, and posture required to use
- Larger print (books, enlarge frequently used items with photocopier)

*Bolder*
- Contrasting colours, e.g. black on white
- Helps emphasize written word, door handles, stair edges, etc.
- Use white cups for dark drinks
- Put contrasting strips round light fittings

*Brighter*
- Remove net curtains
- Use high-power lamps
- Use directable light sources (e.g. angle-poise lamps)

---

# Visual hallucinations

Management varies with the cause.

## Organic brain disease

- Lewy body dementia (occurs in 50–80%; usually well formed,
  e.g. animals). Also occurs in dementia of Parkinson's disease. Can
  respond dramatically to cholinesterase inhibitors
- Anoxia, migraine, and delirium—treat the underlying cause
- Focal neurological disease, e.g. stroke or tumour (especially occipital and
  temporal lobes—range from unformed lines and lights, etc. to complex)
- Occipital lobe seizures—treat with anticonvulsants

## Drugs

- Common with dopamine agonists and anticonvulsants (usually mild and
  unformed). Try reducing the dose, watching for rebound in symptoms
- Overdose of anticholinergic drugs such as antihistamines or tricyclic
  antidepressants
- Use of amphetamines and LSD
- Alcohol withdrawal

## Psychiatric disease

Visual hallucinations occasionally occur with schizophrenia (auditory more
common)

## Charles Bonnet syndrome

- Diagnosis of exclusion
- No other psychiatric symptoms or diseases present
- Occurs with bilateral visual loss (typically 2° to cataracts or glaucoma) as
  a 'release phenomenon'
- These are usually well formed and vivid, and occur in clear
  consciousness
- Insight is usually present
- Duration is usually seconds to a minute or so
- May be simple (flashes, shapes) or complex (recognizable images)
- Non-threatening—the patient's reaction is often one of curiosity or
  amusement
- Probably underestimated, as patients reluctant to tell doctors for fear of
  being labelled as 'mad'
- Not related to psychiatric problems
- Reassurance is often all that is required, but symptoms may be improved
  by enhancing vision

# Cataract

Term used to describe any lens opacity. The most common cause of treatable blindness worldwide. In the UK, it is largely a disease of the older population—65% of people in their 50s and everyone >80 have some opacification. This is probably caused by cumulative exposure to causative agents, rather than senescence per se.

## Causes
- Exposure to environmental agents (e.g. ultraviolet (UV) light, smoke, blood sugar)—more exposure with ↑ age
- Ocular conditions (trauma, uveitis, previous intraocular surgery)
- Systemic conditions (e.g. diabetes, hypocalcaemia, Down's syndrome)
- Drugs (especially steroids—ocular and systemic)

## Symptoms
- Painless visual loss which varies depending on whether unilateral/bilateral and severity/position of the opacity
- Commonly begins with difficulty in reading, recognizing faces, and watching television
- May be worse in bright light or be associated with glare around lights

## Signs
- Reduced visual acuity—usually gradual
- Diminished red reflex on ophthalmoscopy
- Change in the appearance of the lens (appears cloudy brown or white when viewed with direct light)
- Beware coexisting conditions—pupil responses are normal, and the patient should be able to point to the position of a light source

## Management
- Optimizing visual conditions

▶ New glasses prescription may delay need for surgery.
- Surgical removal of opacified lens
- No effective medical treatment

## When to treat?

Tailor treatment to the individual. Depends on visual requirements of the patient, severity of cataract, and presence of other ocular disease (worsens outcome from surgery). Roughly speaking <6/18 in both eyes is likely to benefit from surgery, but an elderly person who does not read much may be quite content with this visual level. Conversely, someone who wishes to continue driving or needs precise vision for other reasons may wish for surgery much sooner. Consider as part of falls risk reduction. Previously, surgeons waited for the cataract to 'ripen' to aid extraction—this is no longer the case. Have a frank discussion about risks and benefits with each individual.

## What the surgery involves

- Usually done as a day case under local or topical anaesthesia
- Patient must be able to lie fairly flat and still. Patients with dementia may need sedation or general anaesthesia (altering risk/benefit); consider heart failure, chest disease, and spinal deformity—can they lie flat? If not, then the surgeon may be able to adapt the procedure
- It is not necessary for patients to discontinue medications. The procedure may be done safely while a patient is taking aspirin, and even anticoagulation
- Generally a safe and well-tolerated procedure; takes 15–20min
- Phacoemulsification is most commonly used in the UK (a small cut in the eye to access the lens that is then liquefied with an ultrasonic probe). A replacement lens is then folded into the empty lens capsule. Sutures are not usually needed
- Other methods (extracapsular and intracapsular extraction) are less commonly used
- Post-operatively, the patient will wear an eye shield (usually at night) for a period, and use steroid and antibiotic eye drops
- May experience sticky/itchy eye with mild discomfort for 1–2 days
- Surgery is done on one eye at a time. The poorer-seeing eye is usually done first. Second eye surgery may be done once outcome from the first eye is assessed

## Outcome

With no ocular comorbidity, 85% have a visual acuity of >6/12 at discharge. Outcome is worse with other eye diseases, e.g. glaucoma, and in patients with diabetes and cerebrovascular disease.

As the replacement lens has a fixed focus and is usually chosen to allow clear distance vision, the patient will usually require glasses for reading. A new prescription should be made up a few weeks after surgery, once post-operative inflammation has settled. If second eye surgery is planned, then glasses are usually issued once both surgeries are completed.

# Glaucoma

Second most common cause of blindness worldwide.

▶ Leading cause of *preventable* blindness in the UK. Early detection can slow/halt progression.

## Definition

Visual loss due to a combination of loss of visual fields and cupping of the optic disc. Usually associated with a rise in intraocular pressure sufficient to cause damage to the optic nerve fibres (either direct mechanical damage or by inducing ischaemia).

## Intraocular pressure

- Ciliary body (posterior) makes aqueous, which flows anteriorly through the pupil and drains via the trabecular network in the anterior chamber angle of the eye
- Balance of production and drainage determines pressure
- Wide range of pressures seen in normal adults (detected with tonometry)—average 15.5mmHg, normal <21mmHg
- The pressure at which ocular damage occurs is probably highly variable between people
- Can develop glaucoma with 'normal pressure–normal tension glaucoma' (may be high for that person/other factors such as ischaemia may be relevant). More common in older patients. Fluctuating BP may be contributory
- Can have 'high' pressures without glaucoma—'ocular hypertension'
- Symptoms depend on rate and degree of rise in pressure. Generally asymptomatic unless advanced or acute

## Primary ('chronic') open-angle glaucoma

- Most common
- Failure of outflow of aqueous causes slow rise in pressure, allowing adaptation, so subtle symptoms
- No pain, corneal cloudiness, or haloes
- Slow loss of visual field, typically in an arc shape ('arcuate scotoma'), with preservation of central vision (macula has more nerve cells so is relatively protected). Progresses to tunnel vision, and then blindness

*Risk factors*

- Age (1% in fifth decade, rising to 10% in ninth decade)
- African-Caribbean origin (four times risk)
- Blood relatives with glaucoma

*Screening*

- Target those at higher risk
- Combination of ophthalmoscopy (looking for disc 'cupping'), automated perimetry testing (for minor field defects), and tonometry (for intraocular pressure) is best
- Newer non-invasive ocular imaging techniques are available which provide less user-dependent quantitative data
- Most cases picked up by optometrists
- Encourage regular eye tests and include careful fundoscopy in physical examination

*Treatment*

- Topical treatments (eye drops): β-blockers, e.g. timolol (↓ aqueous secretion, can cause systemic β-blockade); prostaglandin analogues, e.g. latanoprost (improve drainage, may darken iris); α-agonists (↓ aqueous production); carbonic anhydrase inhibitors, e.g. dorzolamide (↓ aqueous secretion); parasympathomimetics, e.g. pilocarpine (constrict pupil so will reduce visual field—not commonly used)
- Oral treatments: carbonic anhydrase inhibitors, e.g. acetazolamide, very powerful, with many side effects including electrolyte imbalance and paraesthesiae of extremities
- Surgical treatment: trabeculectomy—operation to improve aqueous outflow. Argon laser trabeculoplasty (applied to the trabecular meshwork) may be effective. Cyclodiode laser to the ciliary body (↓ production) is used in refractory cases
- Support group: International Glaucoma Association (➲ https://www.glaucoma-association.com/)

## Acute angle closure glaucoma

▶ Emergency sight-threatening condition—requires urgent referral and treatment.

- Apposition of the lens to the back of the iris prevents outflow of aqueous, with a rapid rise in pressure
- Causes red, painful eye with vomiting, blurred vision, and haloes around lights (due to corneal oedema)
- May be precipitated by pupil dilation, e.g. at dusk. Pupil constricts when asleep, so episodes at night may be aborted by sleep
- Very rarely can be precipitated by anticholinergic drugs
- More common in older patients, those with a family history, women and long-sighted individuals—beware of the vomiting older woman with a red eye
- On examination, the cornea is usually cloudy and visual acuity significantly reduced (e.g. counting fingers)
- Refer immediately to ophthalmology for treatment with iv acetazolamide, topical glaucoma treatment, and laser iridotomy to restore flow. Treat the other eye prophylactically with laser iridotomy to prevent pupillary block

# Age-related macular degeneration

Age-related macular degeneration (AMD) is the most common cause of adult blind registrations in the UK and USA.

▶ New treatments for early stages make detection crucial.

### Definition

As it sounds—age-related degenerative changes affecting the macula (central part of the retina responsible for clear central vision).

Two types:

- 90% *dry* with gradual onset of symptoms (drusen and atrophy of the retinal pigment epithelium)
- 10% *wet* where symptoms relate to leaking vessels causing distortion or sudden loss of central vision due to sub-macular haemorrhage (choroidal neovascularization—new vessels can leak, bleed, and scar, causing visual loss in a few months)

### Prevalence

- ↑ with age
- 25–30 million worldwide
- Up to 30% of >75s may have early disease, and 7% late disease

### Risk factors

- Cause unknown
- Age, smoking, and family history are strongly associated
- ♀ sex, Caucasian race, hypertension, blue eyes, other ocular conditions (lens opacities, aphakia), and low dietary antioxidants

### Symptoms

- Asymptomatic in early stages, progressing to loss of central vision
- May also have ↓ contrast and colour detection, flashing lights, and hallucinations
- Distortion of straight lines is a feature of wet AMD
- Peripheral vision is normal in absence of other pathology

### Detection

- Regular ocular examination
- Use of Amsler grid in high-risk patients (see Fig. 22.1)

### Prognosis

- Dry AMD progresses slowly and rarely causes blindness
- Wet AMD may progress rapidly (blind in under 3 months) and accounts for 90% of AMD blind registrations. Sudden onset of distortion of central vision should prompt urgent referral
- Bilateral disease—42% with wet AMD will develop this within 5 years

### Prevention

- Smoking is the most important modifiable risk factor
- A diet rich in fruit and vegetables may reduce risk of progression
- Systematic reviews have not supported the use of antioxidant/dietary supplements

## Management

- Appropriate for subset of wet AMD only
- Halts progression, so early treatment is desirable
- Fluorescein angiography should be done within a few days of onset of symptoms to determine the type and location of neovascular areas

Treatment options for neovascular AMD include:

- *Photodynamic therapy*—this targets sub-foveal neovascular areas (while preserving normal retina) by using photosensitive drug (verteporfin) along with a non-thermal activating laser. Used in early disease, this therapy can slow or halt progression
- *Anti-angiogenic therapy*—recombinant humanized monoclonal antibodies that neutralize all active forms of vascular endothelial growth factor A are available. NICE recommends their use for wet AMD under certain conditions. Various agents are available, e.g. ranibizumab
- *Laser photocoagulation* is sometimes used for extra-foveal lesions

---

**HOW TO . . . Use an Amsler grid to detect macular pathology**

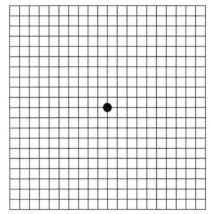

**Fig. 22.1** Amsler grid.

- Test one eye at a time
- Usual reading glasses should be worn, and the grid held at comfortable reading distance
- Ask the patient to look at the central spot, and not to look away
- Assess the following:
  - Can all four corners of the grid be seen?
  - Are any of the lines missing, wavy, blurred, or distorted?
  - Do all of the boxes appear the same size and shape?
- Any abnormalities may indicate macular pathology and should prompt referral to an ophthalmologist

---

# The eye and systemic disease

Two of the top four causes for blind registration are due to systemic disease—diabetes and vascular disease. Eye disease develops as a late complication of prolonged poor control in both cases, and the important message is to strive to prevent these problems in the first place.

## Diabetes

Causes retinopathy, cataracts, and 'microvascular' cranial nerve palsies.

*Retinopathy*
- Associated with ↑ duration of diabetes—at 20 years, 80% will have some retinopathy
- All patients with diabetes require dilated annual screening (either photographic, or by an appropriately trained professional). Direct ophthalmoscopy alone is inadequate
- Appearance: microaneurysms, haemorrhages (background retinopathy) progressing to cotton wool spots, blot haemorrhages and tortuous vessels (pre-proliferative retinopathy), then new vessels (proliferative retinopathy). Exudates and macular oedema are indicators of maculopathy
- Early detection of problems (especially when near the macula) should prompt referral to an ophthalmologist. Sight-threatening retinopathy requires laser treatment to limit progression

▶ A diabetic person diagnosed at age 70 may well live 20 years, so tight control is desirable. Meticulous control of diabetes and hypertension has been shown to reduce microvascular complications.

## Vascular disease
- Affects the eye directly with hypertensive retinopathy, and more indirectly when stroke disease impacts on vision. Associated with 'microvascular' cranial nerve palsies
- Early detection and control of risk factors for vascular disease will ameliorate this problem (see ➔ 'HOW TO . . . Protect your patient from another stroke', p. 193). Tight BP control, smoking cessation, lipid lowering, diabetic control, and appropriate antiplatelet/anticoagulant use should all be targeted at the older age group as aggressively as the younger patients
- There is little in the way of treatment for the disease once it is established
- Appearances of hypertensive retinal disease: silver wiring, arteriovenous nipping, and arteriolar narrowing progressing to exudates, cotton wool spots, haemorrhages, and papilloedema

## Giant cell arteritis

See ➔ 'Giant cell arteritis', pp. 476–7.

# Drugs and the eye

Many drugs that are frequently used in the older patient can cause ocular side effects. Older people are more vulnerable to developing side effects but are least likely to report them (attributing it to part of getting older).

### Direct toxicity

- Chloroquine and hydroxychloroquine (used in treatment of rheumatoid arthritis and other connective tissue diseases, as well as malaria) cause a toxic maculopathy in large, prolonged doses
- Phenothiazines used for a long time (to treat psychosis) may cause retinal damage
- Tamoxifen (for breast cancer treatment) may cause maculopathy
- Amiodarone (for arrhythmias) may cause cataracts
- Ethambutol (anti-tuberculous) can cause optic neuritis and red/green colour blindness

### Altering accommodation

Causes blurred vision.
- Antihistamines
- Antihypertensives, e.g. $\alpha$-blockers

### Decreasing pupil size

Causes less light accommodation.
- Opiates
- Miotic drops used for glaucoma

### Steroids

- Oral steroids over time can cause cataracts
- Topical and oral steroids may raise the intraocular pressure

## HOW TO . . . Assess a red eye in an older person

*Assessment*
- Ask about trauma, pain, vision loss/blurring, and headache
- Examine the eye, including pupillary responses and (usually) fundoscopy

*Ophthalmology referral needed if*
- History of penetrating ocular trauma
- Vision loss
- Ocular pain (itch is ok)
- Pupillary reflexes altered
- Fundus blurred
- Redness centred around the pupil

*Benign causes include*
- Allergic conjunctivitis—occurs in allergy season, often associated with rhinorrhoea. Manage with antihistamines
- Bacterial conjunctivitis—usually itchy and sticky; tends to be bilateral and peripheral with central sparing. Treat with topical antibiotics/eye cleaning
- Conjunctival haemorrhage—there is localized haemorrhage with a posterior limit (a 'blotch'). Can look very dramatic if the patient is on antiplatelet/anticoagulants. NO pain and vision unaffected. Reassure the patient. Condition is self-limiting
- Corneal scratch—occurs after trauma/foreign body. Remove foreign body (may need referral). Antibiotic drops often given to avoid infection

*Other causes (needing referral)*
- Episcleritis—unilateral and segmental
- Acute iritis—redness in one eye, around the cornea, with small irregular pupils
- Glaucoma—redness in one eye around the cornea, pupils do not react to light
- Corneal ulcer—redness in one eye in the cornea

# Eyelid disorders

### Entropion

In-turning of the (usually) lower lid. Occurs as the orbicularis muscle weakens with age (or with conjunctival scarring distorting the lid). Lashes irritate the eye and may abrade the cornea, causing red eye. Lubricants and taping of the eye may relieve symptoms. Surgery (under local anaesthesia) provides definitive correction.

### Ectropion

Eversion of the eyelid. Occurs with orbicularis weakness, scarring of the periorbital skin, or seventh nerve palsy. Distortion prevents correct drainage of tears and tear film, leading to watery eye with conjunctival dryness. Use ointment to protect the conjunctiva. Surgery (local anaesthesia) corrects.

### Ptosis

Drooping of the upper eyelid. If severe, can cover pupil and impair vision.

Causes: aponeurotic (defects in levator aponeurosis), mechanical (lid lesion, lid oedema), neurological (third nerve palsy—look for pupil and eye movement problems, Horner's syndrome), myogenic (congenital levator dystrophy, muscular dystrophies, myasthenia gravis, chronic progressive external ophthalmoplegia).

▶ Do not ignore ptosis in older people—it may not be long-standing; look for signs of underlying disease.

### Dry eyes

Common with age as tear secretion diminishes. Eyes feel gritty but are not red. Diuretics may exacerbate. Most common cause is blepharitis (inflamed lid margins with blocked Meibomian gland orifices and crusting); usually worse in those with rosacea, eczema, and psoriasis.

Treat blepharitis with hot compresses (5min bd), lid massage (upwards towards lid margin lower lid, downwards towards lid margin upper lid), and eyelid cleaning targeting the base of eyelashes at the lid margin (warm water ± baby shampoo on a cotton wool bud). Antibiotic ointment not usually required unless staphylococcal infection suspected. Treat dry eyes with artificial tears or ointment (gives considerable relief).

### Eyelid tumours

Most common (90%) is basal cell carcinoma. Slow-growing, non-metastasizing, but locally invasive. Often ignored by the patient. More common in fairer skins after chronic sun exposure. A waxy nodule with telangiectatic vessels on the surface and a pearly rolled border (rodent ulcer) is the usual appearance. Treatment is with surgical excision or radiotherapy.

### Varicella-zoster infection

Facial shingles. Involvement of the ophthalmic division of the trigeminal nerve will cause vesicles and crusting periorbitally (see ➲ 'Varicella-zoster infection', pp. 624–5).

# Skin

# The ageing skin

Skin changes with age are universal, but many changes we associate with ageing are actually due to cumulative sun exposure (photoageing) and could be largely prevented by protecting the skin from the sun (compare an older person's facial skin to their buttock skin).

Intrinsic ageing does occur, however (see Table 23.1), and there are several skin diseases that are age-related (e.g. pruritus, pemphigoid, lichen sclerosus).

## Hair changes

- 50% of the over 50s will have grey hair, as melanocyte numbers drop
- ♂ pattern baldness (affecting the vertex and temples) starts in the late teens and progresses—80% of ♂ pensioners are balding
- Women may be affected after the menopause, but it is rarely as severe
- Diffuse hair loss occurs in both sexes with advancing age (consider checking for iron deficiency, thyroid dysfunction, renal impairment, hypoproteinaemia, inflammatory skin conditions, use of antimetabolite drugs, etc.)
- As hair follicles age, their function may be disrupted, leading to longer, tougher hairs growing in eyebrows, ears, and noses, in both sexes
- Post-menopausal hormonal changes may cause women to develop hair in the beard area and upper lip

**Table 23.1** Age-related changes and their clinical implications

| Age-related change | Clinical implications |
|---|---|
| Epidermis thins, with flattening of the dermo-epidermal junction, limiting transfer of nutrients and making separation of layers easier | ↑ tendency to blistering<br>↑ skin tearing |
| Slower cell turnover | Slower healing of wounds |
| Less melanocyte activity, with slower DNA repair | ↑ photosensitivity, with ↑ tendency to skin malignancy |
| Altered epidermal protein binding | Dry, rough, and flaky skin more common<br>Abnormal skin barrier, so more prone to irritant contact dermatitis |
| Altered connective tissue structure and function | Reduced elasticity and strength of skin |
| ↓ blood flow through dermal vascular beds | Skin appears cooler and paler<br>Thermoregulation is less efficient<br>Hair and gland growth and function slows |
| Subcutaneous fat ↓ in volume and is distributed differently (e.g. more abdominal fat) | Thermoregulation is less efficient<br>Protection against pressure injury lessens |
| Number of cutaneous nerve endings ↓ | Cutaneous sensation blunts (e.g. fine touch, temperature, proprioception)<br>Pain threshold ↑ |
| Fewer cutaneous glands | Thermoregulation is less efficient |
| Nail bed function ↓ | Nails become thick, dry, brittle, and yellow, with longitudinal ridges |
| Immune functioning of the skin ↓ | ↑ propensity to skin infections and malignancies |

# Photoageing

The dermis thickens with tangled elastic fibres; the epidermis is variable in thickness with regions of both hypertrophy and atrophy—leading to considerable skin changes:

- The skin becomes wrinkled (coarse and fine), rough, yellowed, and irregularly pigmented—these changes are all exacerbated by smoking
- The skin may develop actinic (solar) elastosis—thickened, yellow skin with rhomboid pattern and senile comedones
- Actinic (solar) purpura is a non-palpable rash often on the forearms, due to red cell extravasation from sun-damaged vessels (the platelet count is normal)
- Lesions include brown macules, multiple telangiectasia, actinic (solar) keratoses (scaly, rough hyperkeratotic areas on sun-exposed skin), as well as a tendency to skin tumours

Prevention is better than cure for these changes, but topical retinoids may reduce the appearance of wrinkles and pigment, and certain plastic surgery techniques are employed (e.g. chemical peels and injections of collagen and botulinum toxin).

## Sun protection

- Avoid unnecessary sun exposure
- Stay out of the sun during the hottest time of the day (11 a.m.–3 p.m.)
- Wear appropriate-factor sun screen (↑ sun protection factor for fairer skins)
- Areas that are often forgotten include balding heads (wear a hat) and the tops of ears (apply sun screen)

## Photosensitizing drugs

Several drugs may interact with UV or visible light to cause adverse cutaneous effects. These may be phototoxic or photoallergic reactions. Possible agents include:

- Amiodarone
- Phenothiazines
- Diuretics (including bumetanide and furosemide)
- Antibiotics, e.g. tetracyclines (especially doxycycline), isoniazid, ciprofloxacin
- Quinine
- Hydralazine

# Cellulitis

Deep infection of the skin and subcutaneous tissues with oedema, often on the lower leg. More common with ↑ age, immunocompromise (e.g. diabetes), and with a predisposing skin condition (leg ulcer, pressure sore, lymphoedema, toe web intertrigo, trauma).

## Organisms

Usually *Streptococcus* (group A, commonly *S. pyogenes*) and/or *Staphylococcus*. With open wounds (e.g. leg ulcers, pressure sores) and lymphoedema, colonization is broader, so infecting organisms may be more diverse, including highly resistant bacteria, e.g. MRSA (see ➲ 'Disease caused by MRSA', p. 612).

## Clinical features

- Red, hot, tender, raised area, often with poorly demarcated margins; blistering may occur
- Bilateral, non-tender, cool, red legs rarely are cellulitic (usually chronic changes, e.g. haemosiderin, poor circulation)
- Portal of entry for bacteria often evident (e.g. trauma)
- Systemic upset may follow (fever, malaise)
- May present non-specifically, so always examine the whole skin
- Spread can cause lymphangitis with tender nodes
- Risk of bacteraemia (up to 80% in nursing home residents with pressure sores; treat aggressively as mortality is as much as 50%)

## Investigations

- FBC: elevated white cell count in around 50%
- Blood cultures: take in all before antibiotics
- Local culture, e.g. wound swab, injection and aspiration of saline in the dermis, skin biopsy

## Treatment

- If the cellulitis is mild, and the patient well, then oral therapy can be used to start. Oral options include penicillins, macrolides, and lincosamides (clindamycin) and should be guided by local policy
- Draw around the cellulitis with a water-resistant pen to allow accurate subsequent assessments, and arrange early review (at 24–48h)
- Elevate the limb—oedema with blistering may cause ulceration
- If more extensive, with systemic upset, lymphangitis, and worsening on oral therapy, then rest, elevation, and parenteral therapy is needed in an appropriate environment
- Parenteral options depend on local policy and likely organism (e.g. vancomycin if MRSA likely)
- Continue iv until clinical response, then switch to oral; total treatment may be needed for up to 14 days (treat each case individually)
- If cellulitis complicates ulcers, pressure sores, or lymphedema, then broader-spectrum antibiotics are needed at outset
- Look for, and treat, toe web intertrigo in all (with topical antifungals)
- Cellulitis can be painful—ensure adequate analgesia
- Older patients will often become dehydrated with bacteraemia— assess clinically (pulse, BP, general condition) and biochemically (urea, creatinine, and electrolytes), giving iv fluids in the acute phase if needed

# Other bacterial skin infections

### Erysipelas
- S. pyogenes infection of the dermis and hypodermis
- Occurs on the face (bridge of nose and across cheeks), and less commonly on legs, arms, and trunk
- Flu-like prodrome
- Well-demarcated edge with erythema, oedema, and pain
- Progresses to vesicles that rupture and crust
- Portal of entry may be unclear, especially with facial erysipelas
- Bacteraemia in 55%; mortality of 10% without treatment
- Requires parenteral therapy unless mild—48h of iv benzylpenicillin, followed by 12 days of oral phenoxymethylpenicillin
- Recurs in 30% at some point

### Necrotizing fasciitis
- Rare and serious infection
- Affects soft tissues (usually arm/leg); spreads rapidly along fascial planes with severe pain
- Commonly due to S. pyogenes, but polymicrobial infection also occurs (e.g. staphylococci, Pseudomonas, Bacteroides, diphtheroids, coliforms)
- Patient feels and looks unwell with a high fever
- Area of swelling, redness, and tenderness enlarges rapidly and becomes purple and discoloured. Haemorrhagic bullae develop, followed by necrosis
- Prompt parenteral antibiotics and early surgical debridement essential

▶ Key to management is early recognition. Review a patient with cellulitis frequently if they are unwell, looking for rapid spread.

### Intertrigo
- Common complaint, almost exclusively in older patients, when there is superficial inflammation of skin surfaces that are in contact, e.g. flexures of limbs, groins, axillae, submammary
- Due to friction in a continually warm, moist environment
- May be underlying skin disease (e.g. seborrhoeic dermatitis, seborrhoeic eczema, irritant contact eczema (urine, faeces), psoriasis)
- 2° infection with yeast is common

*Treatment*
- Improve hygiene
- Wash carefully, and always dry the skin thoroughly
- Use powder to keep areas dry
- Apply topical antifungal (e.g. clotrimazole cream plus 1% hydrocortisone cream)
- Separate skin surfaces where possible (barrier creams can be used)

# Fungal skin infections

There are two main groups of fungi that cause infection in humans.

## Dermatophytes, e.g. *Tinea* species ('ringworm')

- Infect the feet, groin, body, hands, nails, and scalp
- Suspect if there is a distinct edge to an itchy lesion
- Confirm diagnosis with skin scrapings, or trial treatment
- Topical imidazoles, e.g. clotrimazole, are effective. Terbinafine is more effective, but more expensive
- Oral terbinafine will work for more resistant infection but should only be used if topical treatment fails and the diagnosis confirmed

## Yeasts, e.g. *Candida albicans* ('thrush')

- Normal commensal of the mouth and gastrointestinal tract
- Produces infection in certain circumstances, e.g. moist skinfolds, poor hygiene, diabetes, and use of broad-spectrum antibiotics—many of these commonly occurring in older patients
- Common sites include genital (associated with catheter use; see ➲ 'Vulval disorders', pp. 528–9), intertrigo (see ➲ 'Intertrigo', p. 590), around the nail (chronic paronychia), and umbilical and oral thrush (especially if dentures fit poorly; see ➲ 'The elderly mouth', pp. 352–3)
- Topical imidazoles, e.g. clotrimazole, are effective for skin infection. Preparations that include hydrocortisone will also reduce inflammation and help to break the itch/scratch cycle
- Nystatin, amphotericin, or miconazole lozenges, suspension, or gel can be used for oral infection
- More widespread infection (e.g. oesophageal candidiasis) or those with severe immunodeficiency may require systemic therapy—fluconazole is effective

## Seborrhoeic dermatitis

- Chronic inflammatory condition with erythematous scaly eruptions
- Possibly due to hypersensitivity to *Pityrosporum*—a yeast skin commensal
- Classic distribution—face (eyebrows, eyelids, nasolabial folds, post-auricular, beard area), scalp (dandruff), central chest, central back, and, in older patients, flexural (axillae, groins, submammary)
- May cause otitis externa or blepharitis
- ↑ prevalence and severity in older patients, exacerbated by poor skin care
- Associated with parkinsonism and HIV
- Scalp is treated with ketoconazole shampoo
- Elsewhere, use ketoconazole shampoo as a wash, and apply miconazole combined with 1% hydrocortisone cream
- Blepharitis is treated with warm compresses, cleaning eyelids with cotton buds and diluted baby shampoo, and steroid eye cream
- Difficult to treat—recurrence is common, and repeated treatments are often required. Aim to control, not cure

# Chronic venous insufficiency

Common, ranging from minor cosmetic problems to debilitating leg ulcers.

More common after phlebitis or DVT (25% with a history of DVT will develop venous insufficiency at 20 years; 4% will eventually develop leg ulcers), after leg injury, in obese patients, in women, and with advancing age.

## Pathogenesis

Due to failure of the venous pump in the legs. Commonly caused by deep vein occlusion (although only half will show signs of this on venography). Retrograde blood flow in the deep veins, valvular incompetence, and progressive pericapillary fibrin deposition also contribute to the process.

## Clinical changes

*Varicose veins*

- Initially there may be no symptoms, just venous dilation (starts with submalleolar venous flares and progresses to dilated, tortuous, palpable varicose veins)
- Problems may include itch, ache, thrombophlebitis, or bleeding from varicosities. Treatment at this stage is largely cosmetic and includes surgical management (injection/stripping of superficial veins). Ache may be relieved by use of support hosiery

*Oedema*

- May initially be unilateral and wax and wane with position (classically occurring at the end of a day of standing up)
- A feeling of leg heaviness is common
- Low-dose thiazide diuretics (e.g. bendroflumethiazide) may help, but as the patient is not fluid-overloaded, beware of volume depletion

*Skin changes*

- Haemosiderin pigmentation due to red cell extravasation
- Telangiectasia
- Lacy white scars
- Eczematous changes with itchy, weepy skin exacerbated by many topical treatments—improve with topical steroid application
- Lipodermatosclerosis occurs when fibrosis of the tissues leads to induration. May become circumferential and girdle the lower leg, causing an inverted champagne bottle appearance

*Venous ulcers*

Venous ulcers arise in the context of these skin changes, often precipitated by minor trauma.

# Leg ulcers

Common condition, afflicting 1% of adult population at any time; 50% are venous ulcers, 10% arterial, 25% mixed venous and arterial, and the remainder due to other causes (diabetes, infection, malignancy, blood disorders, vasculitis, drug eruptions, etc.).

Associated with high morbidity and health-care expenditure.

## Clinical features of common ulcers

*Venous ulcers*
- Occur on the medial ankle, along the course of the saphenous vein
- Shallow and tender, with irregular edges that are not undermined
- The base is usually red but may be sloughy
- Associated skin features of chronic venous insufficiency

*Arterial ulcers*
- Occur at sites of trauma or pressure—commonly the malleoli, toes, ball of the foot, heel, and base of the fifth metatarsal
- Deep, punched-out, and painful, with regular edges
- Associated features of peripheral arterial disease (↓ pulses; slow capillary refill; pale, cool, hairless skin; see ➲ 'Peripheral vascular disease', pp. 306–7)

*Diabetic ulcers*
- Occur at pressure points
- May be painless (due to diabetic neuropathy)
- Often infected, with undermined edges

*Malignant ulcers*
- Painless, with a raised edge
- Be suspicious if an ulcer fails to heal or has an atypical appearance

## A general approach to leg ulcers

- Establish cause—usually possible on clinical grounds. May need to consider Doppler ultrasound (looking for deep venous occlusion, valvular incompetence, and venous pressures), ABPI (diagnoses arterial disease; see ➲ 'HOW TO . . . Measure ABPI', p. 307), biopsy (looking for malignancy, or for tissue culture if infection suspected), or blood tests (FBC, glucose, ESR, CRP, autoantibody screen)
- Treat the cause where possible, e.g. compression bandaging for venous disease, revascularization for arterial disease
- Keep the ulcer clean and avoid irritant topical applications. Many available products will cause contact dermatitis. Keep it simple
- Ensure there is adequate pain relief
- Re-evaluate regularly. If the ulcer is not healing, then reassess the original diagnosis
- Avoid antibiotics unless there is cellulitis or osteomyelitis. Colonization is inevitable, and swabs usually unhelpful
- Do a patch test in any patient with a long-standing ulcer to exclude an allergic contact dermatitis

# Management of venous leg ulcers

Chronic and debilitating condition, with serious psychological and social implications. Median duration is 9 months, although 25% will still be present at 5 years. Correctly treated, 70% can be healed within 3 months, but 75% are recurrent.

## General measures

- Encourage mobility—this strengthens the muscle pump and helps prevent deep vein occlusion. If bed-bound, then exercises, such as toe and ankle wiggling and quadriceps movements, can help
- Stop smoking

## Limb elevation

- Raising the legs above the level of the heart improves venous return, reduces oedema, and assists healing of venous ulcers
- Unfortunately, this is rarely practical—many older patients cannot tolerate such a position owing to comorbidity (cardiac failure, COPD, arthritic hips, obesity, etc.) and even if they can, it is difficult to sustain
- Balance benefits against risks of immobility and complications (thrombosis, deconditioning)—usually only used for very resistant ulcers when admission to hospital may be required
- Elevating the foot of the bed mattress at night is helpful (easiest with electronic hospital beds; otherwise use a wedge under the mattress)
- During the day, sitting with the feet on a stool is better than nothing, although it fails to raise the legs high enough
- Elevation should *not* be used when peripheral arterial disease predominates—first check pedal arterial pulses and ABPI (see ➋ 'HOW TO . . . Measure ABPI', p. 307)

## Ulcer care

- Tissue viability/district nurses can advise
- Clean the ulcer by irrigation with saline
- Debridement of dead tissue may improve healing (no trial evidence):
  - Scalpel (local anaesthetic cream helps with pain)
  - Maggots (consume only dead tissue, leaving behind the healthy)
  - Facilitating the body's own system by creating a moist environment
  - Chemical agents are not recommended (can harm healing tissue)
- No single wound dressing has been shown to improve healing
- An ideal dressing keeps the wound moist with exudate, but not macerated, at an ideal temperature and pH for healing without irritants, excessive slough, or infection
- Simple, low-adherent, and low-cost dressings are the mainstay
- Impregnated dressings (e.g. with antiseptic, antibiotic, debriding enzymes, growth factors, or silver sulfadiazine) can cause contact allergic or irritant dermatitis (up to 85% of patients), worsening the ulcer, so avoid in routine use
- Occlusive or semi-occlusive dressings can aid with pain relief
- Gel and hydrocolloid dressings can be useful to remove exudates
- Metronidazole or charcoal dressings can be used for odour control

## Compression bandaging

- Mainstay of treatment for venous ulcers—when correctly applied, leads to healing for 70% in 3 months
- Ensure that the ABPI is >0.8 (see ➲ 'HOW TO . . . Measure ABPI', p. 307)
- When mixed aetiology ulcers are present, some compression is often required, but this has to be carefully moderated to compensate for the arterial insufficiency
- Provides an active counter-pressure to venous BP and enhances the function of the muscle pump
- Graduated four-layer compression from the ankle to the knee (wool bandage, crêpe bandage, elasticated bandage, and finally a self-adhesive elasticated bandage)
- Should be comfortable, allow the patient to continue with daily life (e.g. wear shoes as usual), and last a week (unless highly exudative)
- Should be applied by an experienced practitioner, as incorrect bandaging can cause more harm than good
- Intermittent pneumatic compression therapy may be useful for patients for whom standard compression stockings may be ineffective or not tolerated (e.g. morbid obesity, severe oedema)

## Oral agents

- *Diuretics*. Short courses may reduce oedema
- *Antibiotics*. Most ulcers are permanently colonized (commonly staphylococci, streptococci, *Escherichia coli*, *Proteus*, and *Pseudomonas*) and routine use of oral antibiotics will only promote resistance. Wound swabs will only grow these colonizing organisms and are not indicated. Treat with systemic antibiotics only if there is evidence of spreading infection (rapidly ↑ size, ↑ pain, surrounding erythema, tracking up the lymphatic system, or systemic upset)
- *Other agents*, e.g. pentoxifylline. May have a role in ulcer management, but evidence is not robust

## Surgery

- Skin grafts may be helpful. Pinch or punch skin grafts may stimulate healing
- Surgical correction of deep vein incompetence is considered where bandaging has failed. Involves ligation of superficial veins and valvuloplasty

# Pruritus

Intense itching. Common condition in older patients, often causing considerable distress. Threshold for itch affected by neurological and psychological factors—exacerbated by social isolation, sensory impairment (blind, deaf), and depression. Often ignored, yet simple measures can make a big difference.

## Causes

Often associated with *dry skin* (xerosis), common with ageing, and frequently worst on lower legs, forearms, and hands. Skin is dry and scaly, and may develop inflamed fissures when severe (asteatotic dermatitis).

*Contact dermatitis* may show few skin changes if mild, yet cause troublesome itching. Limited to areas exposed to allergen (e.g. under clothing if due to washing powder).

*Systemic disease* causes up to half of pruritus in older people, including:
- Liver failure (may be mild jaundice—itch caused by bile salts)
- Chronic renal failure
- Iron deficiency—even before anaemic
- Coeliac disease
- Haematological disorders (lymphoma, polycythaemia—itch may be exacerbated by water)
- Infections (including fungal infection, scabies and lice infestations, gastrointestinal parasite infections)
- Metabolic disorders including: thyroid disease (affects 10% of hyperthyroid patients, and many hypothyroid patients because of dry skin); diabetes mellitus
- Malignancy

Many *drugs* can cause a pruritic rash as an adverse drug reaction (usually allergic), but some cause itch without a rash (e.g. morphine, allopurinol, and benzodiazepines) or because of cholestasis.

## Assessment

- *History* should include full systems enquiry looking for underlying disease, drug history, and specific enquiries about possible irritants (e.g. biological washing powder, new bath products). Ask if anyone else is itching
- *Examination* should include inspection of all skin and thorough general examination (looking for, e.g. burrows or other signs of scabies, lymphadenopathy, hepatosplenomegaly, thyroid enlargement, etc.)
- *Investigations* should include: FBC, iron and ferritin, ESR, U, C+E, LFTs, TFTs, coeliac screen, and blood glucose. May include other tests, guided by history, e.g. stool examination for ova, cysts, and parasites, abdominal ultrasound if organomegaly felt, etc.

## Treatment

- Treat the underlying cause wherever possible
- Iron supplements if stores low (even if FBC normal)
- Stop any drugs that may be causing or exacerbating the condition

- Apply emollients— greasier preparations, e.g. 50:50 liquid paraffin, white soft paraffin, prevent moisture loss from the skin. May be mixed with 0.5% menthol, which has a cooling action
- Urea-containing emollients are used where the skin is scaly, and are often useful in the elderly (e.g. Balneum® plus, E45® itch relief cream, etc.)
- Avoid excessive bathing—no more than daily; avoid hot water and prolonged soaking
- Use preparations such as aqueous cream or emulsifying ointments, instead of soap. Emollient bath additives can be added to the water. Brand names such as Oilatum® and E45® are sold as both ointments and bath oils, and there are many others available
- Avoid exacerbating factors such as heat (especially hot baths), alcohol, hot drinks, and vasodilating drugs
- Wear loose, cotton clothing
- Keep nails short to limit skin damage from scratching
- Consider short-term bandaging where excoriation severe, to allow healing
- Antihistamines may be useful—sedating preparations, such as hydroxyzine hydrochloride, at night can help sleep. Less sedating agents can be used during the day (e.g. chlorphenamine, cetirizine, loratadine)
- Colestyramine is used to ↓ itch in biliary obstruction and 1° biliary cirrhosis
- Light therapy (phototherapy) may help—normal sunlight, or a course of UVB therapy, can be arranged

# Pruritic conditions

### Lichen simplex

- Local patch of pruritus which, when scratched, leads to skin damage with thickening, discoloration, and excoriation
- Worse in times of emotional stress
- Treat with steroids (topical or intralesional) and avoidance of scratching (bandaging may help). Capsaicin cream may alleviate itching by ↓ substance P levels in the skin

### Pruritus ani

- Common complaint
- Occasionally due to infection (streptococci, candidiasis, threadworms)
- Exclude allergic contact dermatitis, seborrhoeic dermatitis, lichen sclerosus (see ➔ 'Vulval disorders', pp. 528–9), or psoriasis
- Usually due to soiling of the perianal skin, which is worse with loose stool and difficulty in wiping effectively (e.g. with arthritis)
- Mainstay of treatment is improving hygiene after bowel movement (assist with wiping if physically difficult; consider wiping with a damp cloth, etc.)
- Use aqueous cream as a soap substitute
- Once developed, the itch may be self-perpetuating—break the cycle with steroids ± topical antifungals or antiseptics
- Patch test to exclude allergy

## HOW TO index . . . Recognize and manage scabies

▶ Thinking of this diagnosis is the first step.
- Caused by *Sarcoptes scabiei* mite
- Spread by skin-to-skin contact
- Outbreaks can occur within institutions (e.g. nursing homes, hospital wards)
- Occasionally serious, even fatal

*Symptoms and signs*
- Intense itch (worse at night)
- Widespread excoriation
- Examine the patient carefully for burrows and/or erythematous papules that are found:
  - Between fingers and toes
  - On the wrist flexor surface
  - Around the nipples and umbilicus
  - In the axillae and groin

*Treatment*
- Isolate the patient in a side room
- Barrier nurse (gloves, aprons)
- Apply topical pesticidal lotions or creams, e.g. permethrin, malathion
- Apply to the whole body, including the scalp, neck, and face. Ensure the interdigital webs are well covered
- Treat all household members (or all others in close contact in an institution) simultaneously, including asymptomatic contacts
- Wash clothes and bedding
- Repeat treatment after a week
- Applying after a hot bath is no longer recommended
- Antibiotics may be needed for 2° infection
- Itch may persist for weeks after treatment has eradicated the mite but should slowly diminish. Topical steroids and sedating antihistamines to aid sleep can be helpful
- Persistent itch may indicate treatment failure

*Norwegian scabies* occurs in immunosuppressed and frail older patients. A heavy load of mites produces hyperkeratotic lesions. Highly contagious. May require additional oral treatment (e.g. ivermectin—not licensed).

# Blistering diseases

There are many disorders causing skin blistering in older people (see Table 23.2 for a differential). Common causes include blistering 2° to cellulitis or rapid-onset oedema. Bullous pemphigoid is significant in that it occurs almost exclusively in the elderly population.

## Bullous pemphigoid

Chronic autoimmune bullous eruption.

### Clinical features

- Patient is systemically well
- Skin becomes erythematous and itchy
- Large, tense blisters then appear, usually on the limbs, trunk, and flexures (rarely mucous membranes)
- Blisters then heal without scarring
- May appear in normal-looking skin or at the site of previous skin damage (e.g. ulcer, trauma)
- Chronic and recurrent condition

### Diagnosis

- Confirmed by skin biopsy that shows linear IgG deposited at the basement membrane
- Circulating autoantibody (anti-BPAg1 and anti-BPAg2) is found in the serum of up to half of patients

### Treatment

- Should be managed by a dermatologist
- Responds well to steroids
- Mild, local disease can be treated with strong topical steroids
- More widespread disease requires oral prednisolone
- Topical or intralesional steroids are used for resistant lesions
- Remember to monitor for, and protect against, steroid side effects
- Consider steroid-sparing agents for longer-treatment courses (e.g. azathioprine)

### Prognosis

- 50% have self-limiting disease
- The majority will be off medication within 2 years

## Causes of blistered skin

(See Table 23.2.)

**Table 23.2** Overview of blistering disorders

| Blistering disorder | Clinical features |
|---|---|
| Blisters 2° to cellulitis | Features of cellulitis present (see ➔ 'Cellulitis', p. 589) |
| Blisters 2° to oedema | Occurs when onset is rapid, e.g. heart failure |
| Traumatic blisters | Due to friction, pressure, or knocks to skin<br>Localized to site of insult, e.g. heel blister with ill-fitting shoes |
| Pressure blisters | Due to prolonged pressure that causes skin ischaemia<br>Can occur after 2h of immobility<br>Risk factors include advancing age, immobility, dehydration, and extremes of body size<br>Classified as pressure sore (see ➔ 'Pressure sores', pp. 504–5) |
| Fixed drug eruption | Itch, erythema, and blistering that appears and reappears at the same site after ingestion of a drug (e.g. furosemide)<br>Reaction usually within 6h |
| Eczema | Blisters may occur in eczema, especially if there is 2° infection (e.g. eczema herpeticum, staphylococcal infection) |
| Infections | Herpes simplex—usually cause blisters on the face or genitals<br>Herpes zoster—shingles is common in older patients (see ➔ 'Varicella zoster infection', pp. 624–5)<br>Staphylococci and streptococci may cause 1° infections (e.g. impetigo—facial blisters that rupture to leave a yellow crust; erysipelas—well-defined area of redness and swelling that later blisters, usually on face or lower leg) or 2° infection of, e.g. a leg ulcer or wound. Either may result in blistering |
| Bullous pemphigoid | See ➔ 'Bullous pemphigoid', p. 600 |
| Pemphigus | Serious autoimmune blistering disease<br>Rare disorder, mainly affecting young or middle-aged patients<br>Widespread flaccid, superficial blisters that rupture early<br>Patients are systemically unwell |
| Dermatitis herpetiformis | Symmetrical extensor surface tense blisters, associated with coeliac disease. Rare, with peak incidence in the fourth decade |

# Skin cancers and pre-cancers

All ↑ in frequency with ↑ age and sun exposure. They are most common on sun-exposed areas, especially the head and neck, and are diagnosed by biopsy. Any suspicious skin lesion should be referred to a dermatologist for consideration of this after discussion with the patient.

## Actinic keratoses
- Rough, scaly patches
- Vary from skin-coloured to red, brown, yellow, and black (often patchy)
- Pre-malignant, with a small risk of becoming squamous cell carcinoma over years. Some resolve spontaneously. Treat established lesions
- Removal with destructive therapies, topical medications, chemical peels, or photodynamic therapy

## Bowen's disease
- Intraepidermal carcinoma, with small risk of transformation into squamous cell carcinoma
- Typically occurs on the lower leg of elderly women
- Caused by sun exposure, arsenic exposure, or human papillomavirus infection
- Pink or reddish, scaly plaques with well-defined edges
- Histology should be confirmed
- Watchful waiting may be appropriate, but most lesions are removed by cryotherapy, topical fluorouracil, curettage, or excision

## Lentigo maligna
- Irregular, pigmented macules that can be brown, black, red, or white
- Usually over 1cm in size, they occur in areas of sun exposure
- 1–2% become invasive with time
- Excision is required, although watchful waiting may be appropriate if the patient is frail

## Basal cell carcinoma
- Most common, accounting for 75% of all skin cancers
- Other risk factors include irradiation or chronic scarring
- Slow-growing and usually only locally invasive (metastasis virtually unknown), but facial tumours left untreated can cause erosion of cartilage and bone, with significant disfigurement
- Begins as a pearly papule that then ulcerates, characteristically with a rolled everted edge and surface telangiectasia (so-called rodent ulcer)
- Most lesions need excision with a 5mm margin; Moh's microsurgical method involves inspecting histology during the procedure to limit tissue loss; radiotherapy can be used where surgery is not an option or in cases of recurrence. Intralesional interferon or photodynamic therapies are newer options
- Recurrence in 5% at 5 years, so follow-up is required

## Squamous cell carcinoma

- Second most common skin cancer
- Other risk factors include irradiation, chronic ulceration or scarring, smoking, or exposure to industrial carcinogens
- 5–10% will metastasize, usually to local lymph nodes initially
- Begins as an erythematous, indurated area that becomes hyperkeratotic and scaly, and may then ulcerate
- Removal is by surgical excision with 5mm margins. Radiotherapy can be used for recurrence, or in older patients if excision would be hard (e.g. on the face)

▶ May develop in the edge of a leg ulcer.

## Malignant melanoma

- Most lethal of skin tumours, readily metastasizing
- Different subtypes include superficial spreading melanoma (most common; plaque with irregular border and uneven pigmentation), nodular melanoma (dark pigmented nodule), lentigo maligna melanoma, and acral lentiginous melanoma (pigmented macule in nail beds, palms, and soles)
- Suspect if a pigmented lesion has changed in size or colour, become irregular in shape, bleeds, itches, or looks inflamed
- Early detection is key as the thicker the lesion, the worse the outlook, and once metastasized, the disease is fatal—older men often ignore suspicious-looking skin lesions
- Removal is by surgical excision with wide margins. PD-1 inhibitors can be used for inoperable or metastatic melanoma

# Other skin lesions

### Campbell de Morgan spots

- Small, bright red papules on the trunk
- Benign capillary proliferations
- Occur from middle age onwards, almost universal by old age in Caucasians

### Skin tags

- Pedunculated, benign fibroepithelial polyps
- Occur in older patients
- Benign, usually multiple, cause unknown
- Removal for cosmetic reasons by snipping the stalk with scissors, or cryotherapy (liquid nitrogen)

### Seborrhoeic warts

- Also called basal cell papilloma
- Not infectious
- Oval papules (1–6cm in diameter) occurring on the face and trunk of older patients
- Initially yellow, become darker and more warty in appearance
- Seem to be 'stuck-on', usually multiple
- Removal can be done (usually for cosmetic reasons) by cryotherapy or curettage
- Where concerns exist about more serious pathology, excision biopsy is performed

# Infection and immunity

# The ageing immune system

The immune system ages in a complex manner:
- Some activities ↑ (e.g. production of memory T lymphocytes, IgA, and autoantibodies)
- Other activities diminish (e.g. production of some interleukins, antibodies in response to foreign antigens, macrophage clearance of antigens, and complement during acute infection)
- Overall, immune responses become less efficient, less appropriate, and occasionally harmful with age
- The immune system does not wear out—it becomes dysfunctional
- This is an insidious process, often unnoticed until times of physiological stress (e.g. acute illness)
- It is more marked in older people with chronic disease, multiple comorbidities, and significant genetic and environmental factors

This immune dysfunction alters the response to infection in older people:
- Infectious disease is a more significant cause of morbidity and mortality in older people (up to ten times more likely to be the cause of death)
- Impaired cellular immunity predisposes older people to reactivation of certain diseases e.g.:
  - Shingles (see ➔ 'Varicella zoster infection', pp. 624–5)
  - TB (see ➔ 'Tuberculosis: presentation', p. 336)
- Altered antibody production ↑ fatality from pneumonia, influenza, bacterial endocarditis, and hospital-acquired infections
- ↓ levels of lymphokines ↑ susceptibility to parasitic infections
- Age-related immune dysfunction probably has a negative impact on the course of AIDS in older patients (see ➔ 'HIV in older people', p. 532)

▶ Investigations may not show characteristic changes associated with infection, or these changes may develop more slowly (e.g. rise in white cell count, CRP, and complement).

It also has other clinical consequences:
- ↑ autoantibody production does not lead to an ↑ in autoimmune disease (this peaks in middle age) but may contribute to degenerative diseases
- Response to vaccination may be less good
- Falling immune surveillance may contribute to higher cancer incidence
- T lymphocyte dysfunction may contribute to the ↑ incidence of monoclonal gammopathy with age (see ➔ 'Paraproteinaemias', p. 459)
- Immunoglobulin E (IgE)-mediated hypersensitivity reactions are less frequent, so allergic symptoms tend to improve with age

# Overview of infection in older people

*Susceptibility* to infection is ↑ by:
• Immune senescence (see ➲ 'The ageing immune system', p. 606)
• Altered skin and mucosal barriers
• Acute and chronic illnesses (cause relative immunosuppression)

*Blunted response* to infection may occur in those with:
• ↓ cardiac adaptation to stress
• Comorbid conditions and frailty
• ↓ lean body mass or malnutrition
• Multiple previous hospital admissions or residence in a long-term care facility

## Presentation
• Frequently atypical, e.g. global deterioration, non-specific functional decline, delirium, falls, incontinence
• May initially give no clue to the site of sepsis, e.g. chest infections may present with falls, rather than cough
• Fever is often absent, reduced, or delayed (due to senescent hypothalamic and other responses)
• Often indolent with a slow deterioration over several days

▶ By the time sepsis is obvious, the patient may be very unwell.

## Investigations
Obtaining samples can be difficult, e.g. delirious uncooperative patient, urinary or faecal incontinence, inability to expectorate sputum, etc.
    Misleading results are common:
• Positive urine dipstick often does not indicate symptomatic infection (see ➲ 'Near-patient urine tests', pp. 618–19)
• Urine samples from a catheterized patient will usually be heavily colonized; dipstick tests will be positive and culture results difficult to interpret
• Ulcers will usually be colonized and swab results should be interpreted with caution (see ➲ 'Leg ulcers', p. 593)
• Abdominal ultrasound scan will often reveal gallstones in older patients—these are usually asymptomatic and do not necessarily imply biliary sepsis
• Classical markers of infection (leucocytosis, elevated CRP, ↑ complement) may be absent or delayed in older patients. Repeating them after 24h improves sensitivity. Procalcitonin is a new blood test that may prove useful (more specific for infection)

## Treatment
Because of the difficulties in making an accurate diagnosis:
• Therapy is often empirical
• Antibiotic failures are more common
• Antibiotic resistance frequently develops

In addition, treatment may be difficult to administer in delirious patients.

## HOW TO . . . Accurately diagnose infection in an older patient

Making an accurate diagnosis with evidence to support it is important to allow tailored antibiotic therapy. Have a low threshold for considering sepsis as a cause for decline of any sort, but conversely do not assume that all problems stem from infection.

*Investigations*

- *FBC*—white cell count may be elevated, suppressed (poor prognostic indicator), or unchanged
- *ESR, CRP*—often become elevated early on in infection, but this is very non-specific and they may take 24–48h to rise or remain normal. Serial measurements advised
- *U, C+E*—septic older patients are prone to AKI
- *Blood and urine cultures*—send before antibiotics are started and even in the absence of fever
- *CXR*—a patch of consolidation on an X-ray may be the first indicator that a global deterioration is due to pneumonia
- *Consider stool analyses* (if diarrhoea)

If the source remains unclear, repeat basic tests, then consider:

- *Skin*—check carefully for cellulitis and/or ulceration (see ⊃ 'Cellulitis', p. 589)
- *Bones*—osteomyelitis (particularly vertebral, after joint replacement, or where there is chronic deep ulceration of the skin) may present indolently. Check for bony tenderness and consider X-rays, bone scans, or MRI (see ⊃ 'Osteomyelitis', pp. 490–1)
- *Heart valves*—bacterial endocarditis can be very hard to diagnose. Consider in all with a murmur, and actively exclude in those with prosthetic heart valves
- *Biliary tree*—asymptomatic gallstones are common in older patients, but if an ultrasound also shows dilatation of the gall bladder or biliary system with a thickened, oedematous wall, then infection is likely. There is usually (but not always) abdominal pain. Send blood cultures. ERCP may be needed to remove any obstruction
- *Abdomen*—diverticulosis is common, and abscesses may present atypically. Examine for masses and consider abdominal ultrasound or CT if there is a history of diverticulae or abdominal pain
- *Brain*—meningitis, brain abscess, and encephalitis may present indolently in older patients, and the usual warning signs (confusion, drowsiness) may be misinterpreted. Headache and photophobia may be late or absent, and neck stiffness difficult to interpret. Consider CT head followed by CSF analysis if a septic patient has focal neurology, headache, photophobia, or bizarre behavioural change
- *TB*—may reactivate in older people and cause chronic infection. If there is known previous TB (clinical or CXR evidence), then look very carefully for reactivation. Consider early morning urines, sputum culture (induced if necessary), bronchoscopy, or biopsy of any abnormal tissue (e.g. enlarged lymph nodes)

▶ Remember that fever and raised inflammatory markers can also be due to non-infectious conditions (e.g. malignancy, vasculitis, etc.)

# Antibiotic use in older patients

Antibiotics are among the most frequently prescribed drugs, and their wide-spread use is promoting ↑ antibiotic resistance.

This is a particular problem in older patients where infections are more common, yet accurate diagnosis can be more difficult.

### Antibiotic resistance
Resistance is encouraged by:
- 'Blind' antibiotic therapy (where likely microbe and sensitivities are not known)
- Inappropriate antibiotic therapy (e.g. for viral respiratory infections)
- Inadequate treatment courses
- Poor adherence with therapy
- Transmission of resistant strains within healthcare settings

### Sensible antibiotic prescribing
Helps to limit the problem nationally. Applies to all ages but may be more of a challenge in older patients:
- Make a diagnosis—identify the source of sepsis (and so possible pathogens), which will guide therapy before microbiological confirmation is obtained
- Avoid antibiotics for infections that are likely to be viral, e.g. pharyngitis, upper respiratory tract infection
- Where practicable, send samples for culture and sensitivity before initiating antibiotics
- Local variations (e.g. diagnostic mix, local sensitivities) should be considered. Use local antimicrobial guidelines
- Choose the dose based on the patient (allergies, age, weight, kidney function, etc.) and the severity of the infection. Inadequate doses promote resistance
- Choose the route—aim for oral wherever possible, and convert iv therapy to oral as soon as feasible; im antibiotic therapy is uncomfortable but can be useful (e.g. cognitively impaired patients who refuse oral medication)
- Choose the duration based on the type of infection, e.g. simple UTI can be adequately treated in 3 days, whereas bacterial endocarditis can require many weeks of therapy. Unnecessarily long treatment courses will promote resistance, ↑ the risk of side effects and complications (e.g. CDAD), and ↑ cost
- Change empirical broad-spectrum antibiotics to narrow-spectrum alternatives as soon as sensitivities are known

### Further reading
*British National Formulary (BNF).* Section 5.1 Antibacterial drugs.

# Meticillin-resistant *Staphylococcus aureus*

Meticillin was introduced in the 1960s to treat staphylococcal infections. It was used widely (including spraying solutions into the air on wards) and initially successfully. Meticillin has now been discontinued and replaced by flucloxacillin, but the term MRSA persists.

Resistance to meticillin gradually emerged—firstly small numbers within hospitals, but the problem slowly ↑ and spread into the community, until globally dispersed epidemic strains emerged.

All staphylococci are easily transmissible and virulent (capacity to cause disease), and have capacity to develop further antibiotic resistance.

## The problem today

- Varies enormously, e.g. >9% of invasive *S. aureus* isolates are resistant in the UK, compared with <1% in Scandinavia
- However, rates peaked in 2005/6 and are now reducing—deaths where MRSA was mentioned on death certificates have ↓ from >1600/year to <300/year by 2012
- MRSA reduction continues to be a political target in the UK

## Contamination and transmission

- Anything coming into contact with an MRSA source can become contaminated, i.e. MRSA will exist for a short time on that surface
- Transient carriage on the gloves or hands of healthcare workers is likely to represent the main mode of transmission to other patients
- Up to 35% of environmental surfaces in a room being used by an MRSA patient will culture positive (role in transmission is unclear)
- Decontamination involves cleaning. Good hand hygiene and the use of alcohol hand gel after patient contact reduce transmission significantly

## Colonization

- This is asymptomatic carriage of MRSA. Patients and families often need reassurance that this rarely has implications for the patient
- Common sites are the anterior nares, perineum, hands, axillae, wounds, ulcers, sputum, throat, urine, venous access sites, and catheters
- Duration of colonization varies from days to years
- Transmission from a colonized person is more likely if there is a heavy bacterial load with abnormal skin (e.g. ulcers, eczema), devices (e.g. catheters, cannulae), or sinusitis/respiratory tract infection
- Many healthcare workers are colonized (usually nasal) and are a potential reservoir, but usually colonization is short-lived so that screening healthcare workers is only useful for investigating specific outbreaks
- Screening for MRSA colonization is now routine practice prior to elective procedures and for most hospital admissions, especially inter-hospital transfers. Eradication of MRSA may follow; treatment regimens include the application of nasal mupirocin, antimicrobial soaps, and sometimes oral antibiotics (e.g. fusidic acid, rifampicin)

# Disease caused by MRSA

The most common sites of infection are:
• Wounds—the most common cause of post-operative wound infections
• Intravenous lines—often leading to bacteraemia
• Ulcers—including pressure, diabetic, and venous ulcers
• Deep abscesses—infection can seed to many sites, e.g. lungs, kidneys, bones, liver, and spleen
• Bacteraemia—there is compulsory reporting

Thirty to 60% of hospital patients colonized with MRSA will go on to develop infection. This is more likely if there has been:
• Recent prior hospitalization
• Surgery or wound debridement
• Invasive procedures (including venepuncture and venous cannulation)

Infections due to MRSA cause ↑ morbidity and mortality, longer hospital stays, and ↑ cost, compared with a susceptible organism.

## Management

Infection control measures to reduce the reservoir and lower the rate of transmission are crucial (see ➔ 'HOW TO . . . Control MRSA', p. 613).

Antibiotic treatment is necessary when there is active infection—do not use for colonization, as this will promote drug resistance. Opposing responsibility to the patient (use the best drug available) and the community (do not promote antibiotic resistance) must be weighed up. The choice of drug will depend on local resistance patterns and the severity of the infection. Where possible, wait for sensitivities from microbiology.

Options include:
• Glycopeptide antibiotics (e.g. vancomycin, teicoplanin)—must be given iv; resistance is emerging
• Co-trimoxazole—useful for susceptible skin, soft tissue infections
• Fusidic acid, rifampicin, and doxycycline—can be effective, usually given in combination
• Clindamycin—used for deeper infections, but most UK strains are resistant
• Fluoroquinolones, e.g. ciprofloxacin. Resistance is rapidly emerging
• Linezolid—an oxazolidinone antibiotic with equivalent potency to vancomycin. Can be given po or iv. Use with caution because of high cost and less certain side effect profile (bone marrow toxicity common, especially with prolonged use)

## HOW TO . . . Control MRSA

### Identify the MRSA type
During an outbreak, the microbiology laboratory will be able to determine if this is a cluster of unrelated cases or a series of infections by a single strain—the latter indicating either high transmission rates or an ongoing reservoir.

### Identify the reservoir
- Commonly a patient with a heavily colonized or infected wound
- Healthcare workers may also act as reservoirs
- During an epidemic, it is usual to attempt to eradicate MRSA from likely reservoir sources (using nasal mupirocin, antimicrobial soap, and oral antibiotics)

### Reduce transmission rates
Transmission usually occurs from patient to patient via a healthcare worker. This is often when hands or gloves are transiently contaminated.
- Hand hygiene is the single most important factor in infection control. Good handwashing technique and bedside alcohol-based hand gels should be used by staff, visitors, patients, therapists, volunteers, and service personnel after touching a patient
- Known MRSA patients should be isolated where possible
- Gloves should be worn on entering and removed before leaving the room
- Gowns/aprons should be used if contact with the patient or environment is anticipated, or if the wound is open
- Masks may reduce nasal acquisition by healthcare workers
- Patients should be moved about the hospital as little as possible. Radiological investigations should be done at the end of a list to allow cleaning after the test
- Minimize the use of foreign devices (e.g. catheters, NGTs)
- Use dedicated equipment (e.g. stethoscopes, BP cuffs, thermometers), or clean carefully after use
- Active surveillance for MRSA colonization allows these procedures to be put in place earlier

▶ By following these guidelines, it is estimated that 70% of transmission can be prevented.

### Problems in geriatric care
- Isolation can cause problems with depression and lack of social stimulation
- Patients and carers may feel stigmatized or scared by the diagnosis
- Rehabilitation may be restricted (e.g. if the patient is confined to a side room and cannot visit the PT gym or practise mobilizing about the ward)
- It may be difficult to enforce isolation in patients with dementia
- Moving to nursing homes or community facilities may be delayed (e.g. while waiting for a side room)

# *Clostridium difficile*-associated diarrhoea

*C. difficile* is a Gram-positive, spore-forming, anaerobic bacillus. It was rarely described before the late 1970s but is now a major hospital-acquired infection. CDAD causes a huge burden of morbidity, mortality, and cost, but incidence has diminished in response to more focused antimicrobial therapy and effective infection control measures (annual death rate from CDAD in the UK fell from around 6000/year to under 2000/year between 2008 and 2012).

## Pathogenesis

- Asymptomatic *C. difficile* carriage occurs in <5% of population
- Spores persist for months to years in the environment and are resistant to many traditional cleaning fluids. Vegetative forms and spores can be transmitted from patient to patient
- Gastrointestinal carriage is ↑ in the hospital population, with advancing age, other bowel disease, cytotoxic drug use, and debility (e.g. recent surgery, chronic kidney impairment, cancer)
- Most antibiotics reduce colonization resistance of the colon to *C. difficile*.
- CDAD occurs when toxins (A and B) elaborated by *C. difficile* bind to the colonic mucosa, causing inflammation
- Outbreaks in hospital can occur from cross-infection and can affect patients never exposed to antibiotics

## Features

There is a wide range of manifestations from asymptomatic carriage to fulminant colitis. Most commonly presents with:

- Foul-smelling watery diarrhoea (mucus common, but rarely blood)
- Abdominal pain and distension
- Fever

In severe cases, can mimic an 'acute abdomen'. Occasionally causes chronic diarrhoea.

▶ Beware that an acute decline in a patient's condition (e.g. fever, delirium, or metabolic disturbance) can precede prominent diarrhoea; have a low threshold of suspicion in patients with multiple risk factors.

## Investigations

- Raised white cell count and inflammatory markers (following treatment of another infection, differential diagnosis includes relapse of the original infection)
- *C. difficile* toxin detection by enzyme-linked immunosorbent assay (ELISA) is both sensitive and specific for CDAD colitis. The test can remain positive for weeks after resolution, so is not useful in diagnosing recurrence
- Positive stool culture helps with the diagnosis of current infection (although culture positive/toxin negative indicates carrier status)

- X-ray or CT may show distended, thick-walled large bowel
- Sigmoidoscopy is often normal in mild disease or where colitis affects the proximal bowel. In more severe cases, a characteristic colitis with pseudomembrane formation is seen (also known as pseudomembranous colitis)

## Complications

Rarely occur and include toxic megacolon, paralytic ileus, perforation, and bacteraemia. Older patients requiring surgery have at least 50% mortality.

## Relapse

Defined as a second event within 2 months. Occurs in around 20%. Only rarely due to antibiotic resistance but can be difficult to treat. Patients with recurrence are then more prone to further repeated infection.

For repeated infection and recalcitrant CDAD, options include:

- Further oral antibiotics, e.g. metronidazole, vancomycin, bacitracin
- Fidaxomicin is an emerging drug with a role in recurrent disease
- Adjuvant therapy with colestyramine
- There is very limited evidence that probiotics, such as yeast or *Lactobacillus*, help induce and maintain remission
- iv immunoglobulins and steroids have been used in severe recalcitrant colitis

**HOW TO . . . Manage C. difficile infection**

*Prevention*

Use antibiotics wisely (see ➲ 'Antibiotic use in older patients', p. 610):
- Only when good evidence of infection. Always try to obtain a microbiological diagnosis, and only treat where you have diagnosed infection or if the patient is gravely ill and conservative management is judged unsafe
- Use the smallest number of antibiotics with the narrowest-spectrum possible. Some antibiotics are less likely to cause CDAD
- Use the shortest course possible: 3 days for a simple UTI, 5 days for bronchitis, 10 days or longer for septicaemia, abscess, etc.

*Treatment*

▶ Have a high index of suspicion—if the patient is ill, commence treatment without waiting for confirmatory tests.
- Stop antibiotics unless there is very good evidence they need a longer course
- Suspend concomitant PPIs, iron, and laxatives
- Aggressive rehydration—patients can become very hypovolaemic even before they start to get diarrhoea
- Start antimicrobials according to local policy, e.g. vancomycin (must be enteral to obtain high intraluminal levels) or metronidazole. If unable to swallow, consider NGT or metronidazole per rectum (pr); iv therapy may be added if septicaemia is suspected
- Fidaxomicin may be considered in recurrent, resistant, or severe cases
- Continue 7–10 days or until a formed stool
- Stool chart will indicate if diarrhoea frequency is improving
- Use of loperamide (2mg with each loose stool) is controversial—it may mask response to treatment and ↑ chances of complications. However, proponents suggest if the diagnosis is secure and treatment initiated, it can reduce debilitating symptoms and speed recovery
- Faecal transplant is an option
- Surgical complications may require colectomy

*Infection control*
- Nurse in a side room where possible
- Alcohol gels do not kill spores
- Use gloves and aprons for all contact. Wash hands well with soap and water
- Clean the environment thoroughly, especially after bed moves
- Patients are much less infectious once diarrhoea has resolved
- Where possible, avoid moving infected patients between wards

# Near-patient urine tests

UTI is a common problem in older people, but there is an even higher prevalence of asymptomatic bacteriuria and positive urinalysis without infection. In general, UTI is overdiagnosed.

▶ It is important to know how to diagnose a UTI correctly and when to initiate treatment appropriately.

### Near-patient urine tests (dipsticks)

Quick, cheap test that is commonly performed. Should only be done on urine that is collected as described in ❥ 'HOW TO . . . Sample urine for dipstick, microscopy, and culture', p. 619.

### Urinary nitrite

- Positive result has a high predictive value for UTI
- Many bacteria causing UTI convert urinary nitrate to nitrite, which is detected on dipstick
- False negatives occur with dilute urine
- Certain bacteria (e.g. *Pseudomonas, Staphylococcus, Enterococcus*) may not convert urinary nitrate, so the dipstick will be negative

### Leucocyte esterase

- Positive result has a high predictive value for UTI
- Lysed white cells release esterase, which is detected on dipstick
- Corresponds to significant pyuria—may not detect low levels
- False-negative results also occur when there is glucose, albumin, ketones, or antibiotic in the urine
- False positives ('sterile pyuria') occur with vaginal contamination, chronic interstitial nephritis, nephrolithiasis, and uroepithelial tumours. 'Sterile' pyuria can indicate renal TB and STD (e.g. *Chlamydia*)—consider testing if history suggestive

### 'Blood'

- Positive result for blood has a low predictive value for infection
- Dipstick does not distinguish red cells from Hb or myoglobin
- Detects red blood cells (blood in the renal tract), Hb (after haemolysis), and myoglobin (rhabdomyolysis)
- Causes of a positive 'blood' dipstick are varied and may be pre-renal (e.g. haemolysis), renal (e.g. tumours, glomerulonephritis), ureteric (e.g. stones), bladder (e.g. tumours, occasionally infection), urethral (e.g. trauma), or contamination (e.g. bleeding from the vaginal vault)
- Always repeat to ensure the haematuria has resolved with treatment
- Management of persistent isolated dipstick haematuria without apparent cause is difficult. In a fitter patient, referral for renal tract investigation by a urologist may be appropriate

## Protein
- Positive result has a low predictive value for infection
- Commercial dipsticks generally only detect albumin, and a positive result implies proteinuric renal disease
- False positives occur in very concentrated or contaminated urine

▶ The combination of nitrites and leucocyte esterases on urine dipstick has the highest positive predictive value for infection. If these are negative and clinical suspicion is high, proceed to urinary microscopy and culture.

---

### HOW TO . . . Sample urine for dipstick, microscopy, and culture

*Do not sample*
- Stale urine
- Urine that has been contaminated with faeces
- Urine from a catheter bag

*MSU sample*
- Ideal sampling method, but may be difficult in confused or immobile patients
- The external genitalia should be cleaned, a small amount of urine voided, then the middle portion caught cleanly in a sterile container
- Analysis should be performed while the urine is fresh

*In–out catheter sample*
- Carries a small risk of introducing infection (around 1%)
- Often well tolerated by older patients
- Discard the first urine, and sample the middle portion drained

*Suprapubic aspiration of urine*
- Rarely done, but will provide a clean specimen
- Clean the skin, and percuss to identify the bladder
- Aspirate with a green needle and 10mL syringe in the midline

*Samples from catheterized patients*
- These should be sent only if the patient is symptomatic, as the prevalence of positive dipstick is almost universal and bacterial colonization of urine is common
- Clamp the catheter for a period, then collect an MSU sample directly from the draining tube sampling port
- Do not use stale urine that has collected in the bag

---

# Asymptomatic bacteriuria

Defined as a positive urine culture in the absence of symptoms of urinary tract disease.

• It becomes more common with ↑ age (5% of community-dwelling ♀ under the age of 60, rising to 30% over the age of 80)
• It is less common in men but again ↑ with age (<1% of those under 60, rising to 10% over the age of 80)
• Up to 50% of frail institutionalized patients and almost all catheterized patients will have bacteria in their urine (see ➲ 'Catheters', p. 540)
• Other risk factors are as for UTI (see ➲ 'Urinary tract infection', p. 621)
• Associated diseases include renal stones, diabetes, and chronic prostatitis in men

### What does it mean?

• Probably represents urinary colonization, rather than infection
• No ↑ in mortality directly associated with asymptomatic bacteriuria
• Seems to be transient in most—only 6% will grow the same organism over three sequential cultures; however, it is estimated that around 16% will go on to develop symptomatic UTI

### Treatment

No treatment is required for isolated bacteriuria. The use of antibiotics:

• Does not impact on morbidity and mortality
• Does not improve continence
• Promotes antibiotic resistance

In addition, recurrence after antibiotic treatment is common.

▶ Avoid treating patients unless they have symptoms.

# Urinary tract infection

Major cause of morbidity and mortality in the older population. UTIs account for a quarter of infections in healthy older patients and are the most common hospital-acquired infection. They are the most frequent cause of bacteraemia in older patients. The annual incidence is up to 10% for older adults (but many are recurrent).

## Risk factors

- Advancing age
- ♀ sex (although the gap narrows with age)
- Atrophic vaginitis and urethritis in women
- Incomplete emptying (e.g. urethral strictures, prostatic hypertrophy or carcinoma, neuropathy)
- Abnormalities of the renal tract (e.g. tumours, fistulae, surgery)
- Foreign bodies (e.g. catheter, stones)
- Chronic infection (e.g. renal abscess, prostatitis)

## Organisms

- *Escherichia coli* is the most common, as in younger adults
- Older patients are more prone to UTI caused by other pathogens, including other Gram-negative organisms (e.g. *Proteus, Pseudomonas*) and some Gram-positive organisms (e.g. group B *Streptococcus*, MRSA)
- Catheter-related UTI is often polymicrobial and antibiotic-resistant

## Presentation

The presence of symptoms is essential to make the diagnosis. Urinary frequency, dysuria (stinging or burning sensation on urinating), and new urinary incontinence are clear indications of urinary infection, but symptoms may be vague or atypical, and include:

- Fever and general malaise
- Nausea and vomiting
- Confusion or delirium
- Deterioration in physical or functional ability

Infection may be:

- Uncomplicated UTI (normal renal tract and function)
- Complicated UTI (abnormal renal tract, patient debility, virulent organism, development of complications such as impaired renal function, bacteraemia, pyelonephritis, and perinephric or prostatic abscess)
- Recurrent UTI (see ➲ 'Recurrent urinary tract infection', p. 623)
- Catheter-associated UTI (see ➲ 'HOW TO . . . Treat catheter complications', p. 542)

## Investigations

- Urinalysis—collect sample and perform dipstick (see ➲ 'HOW TO . . . Sample urine for dipstick, microscopy, and culture', p. 619), and send for microscopy and culture

▶ A negative dipstick does not exclude the diagnosis if clinical suspicion is high. In such cases, send urine for culture.

- If the patient is unwell, consider checking blood tests, including kidney function (risk of impairment), blood cultures (risk of bacteraemia), FBC, and inflammatory markers

# Urinary tract infection: treatment

Treatment involves more than just antibiotics. Consider the following:
- Adequate hydration (oral often sufficient; sicker or more confused patients may require iv fluid)
- Medication review (consider suspending diuretics or drugs that are potentially nephrotoxic such as NSAIDs or ACE inhibitors)
- Management of symptoms (e.g. confusion or immobility may necessitate ↑ care at home, or even admission to hospital)
- Assessment for complications (e.g. pyelonephritis, bacteraemia, abscess formation). Older patients are at high risk for dehydration and renal impairment. Consider admission for iv antibiotics and hydration
- Prevention of recurrence with measures such as ensuring good fluid intake and avoiding catheters if possible. Topical oestrogens (vaginally) may be useful in post-menopausal women

## Antibiotic choice

Be guided by local sensitivity patterns and local guidelines.
Uncomplicated UTI can be treated empirically as follows:
- Trimethoprim (if local resistance is <20%), *or*
- Co-amoxiclav, *or*
- Nitrofurantoin
- Ciprofloxacin is effective, but there are concerns about emerging resistance and CDAD

## Duration of treatment

- Younger women with uncomplicated UTI can be successfully treated with a short course of antibiotics (3 days, or even a single dose)
- There is limited evidence for the duration required in older patients, but it is likely that a longer course (5–7 days) is needed

## Treatment failure

*Resistant organisms*
- Review the results of the urine culture and pathogen sensitivities
- *E. coli* resistant to ampicillin and sulfonamides is widespread, and trimethoprim resistance is ↑. Most are susceptible to nitrofurantoin and fluoroquinolones (e.g. ciprofloxacin) at present, although fluoroquinolone resistance is ↑
- Pathogens are more varied in older patients, and these may not be susceptible to empirical treatment
- MRSA UTI may occur in older patients (especially with indwelling catheters), which may require iv therapy (e.g. vancomycin)
- *Candida* in the frail, catheterized older patient (seen on microscopy)
- If no culture result is available, and the diagnosis is secure, try an empirical second-line agent such as co-amoxiclav or ciprofloxacin

*Incorrect diagnosis*
- Delirium and a positive urine dipstick may be misleading. Could the patient have another pathology?

# Recurrent urinary tract infection

Defined as >3 symptomatic UTIs in a year, or >2 in 6 months. May represent either a relapse (recurrent infection caused by the original infecting organism) or a reinfection (infection with different species or strain). Urinary culture is indicated.

## Recurrent infection

This may be due to:
- An ongoing source of infection (e.g. chronic prostatitis, renal abscess)
- Urological abnormality (e.g. stones, tumour, residual volume >50mL, cystocele)
- Catheterization
- Poor hygiene (e.g. faecal soiling)
- Impaired immunity (e.g. diabetes, chronic disease)
- Genetic susceptibility

## Treatment of recurrent infection

- Repeat treatment with up to a week of antibiotics
- Remove catheter if possible (see ➲ 'HOW TO . . . Manage urinary incontinence without a catheter', p. 541)
- General measures include ↑ fluid intake and treating constipation
- Arrange renal tract ultrasound to look for residual volume and any urological abnormalities (investigate ♂ after a single unprovoked UTI)
- Consider blood tests (e.g. glucose, renal function, FBC, serum electrophoresis, PSA in men)

## Prevention of recurrent infection

- In post-menopausal women, topical oestrogens (cream, pessary, oestrogen-releasing vaginal ring) are effective
- Maintain good hydration
- There is some evidence that cranberry juice reduces symptomatic UTI
- Prophylactic antibiotics are rarely indicated. Consider when there are multiple recurrences despite general measures or significant renal damage. Consider low doses of trimethoprim, nitrofurantoin, or amoxicillin, dependent on local resistance patterns
- Pre-emptive treatment can be useful in cognitively intact patients. A short course of antibiotics is held in reserve by the patient, to be taken when symptomatic

# Varicella-zoster infection

Initial exposure usually occurs in childhood, causing chickenpox. The virus lies dormant in the sensory dorsal root ganglia of the spinal cord and can be reactivated later in life to cause shingles.

*Shingles* is a painful, self-limiting, unilateral eruption of vesicles in a dermatomal distribution. It occurs in 20% of the population at some time but is most common in older people (probably due to a decline in cell-mediated immunity with age). Vaccination is now given in the UK to people aged 70–78 and will reduce the incidence, severity, and duration of shingles.

## Clinical presentation

- Prodrome of fever, malaise, headache, and sensory symptoms (pain, tenderness, or paraesthesiae) in the dermatome to be affected
- Rash follows after a few days, initially with a cluster of vesicles that spread across the dermatome and then become pustular
- 50% affect thoracic dermatomes (T5–T12), 16% lumbosacral, and 15–20% cranial nerve distribution
- Usually affects a single dermatome but may involve several adjacent ones
- Can rarely affect motor nerves, with focal weakness
- Acute herpetic pain is often a feature—may precede the rash by days and often described as sharp
- Crusting occurs after about a week, then the patient is no longer infectious (prior to this, susceptible individuals may catch chickenpox)
- Healing generally occurs within a month but may leave scars
- Recurrence in around 5%

## Treatment

- General measures include adequate oral fluid intake, simple analgesia (e.g. paracetamol), and topical agents such as calamine lotion
- Antiviral therapy (e.g. famciclovir, valaciclovir, aciclovir) should be given within 72h of rash onset to all patients over 50 years old, for a week. It reduces attack severity, promotes rash healing, and reduces the incidence of post-herpetic neuralgia
- Prednisolone (e.g. 40mg tailing down over a week) can be given with antiviral therapy to reduce the severity of the attack, but has limited value and possible drawbacks (e.g. ↑ bacterial superinfection, causing significant side effects) and should only be used where the infection is severe
- Analgesia for neuralgia should be given early where indicated

## Ophthalmic shingles

- More common in older patients
- Occurs when the ophthalmic division of the trigeminal nerve is involved, resulting in a rash on the forehead and around the eye
- Ocular involvement commonly occurs, causing a red, painful eye. Inflammation of the iris and cornea can cause vision loss, and topical steroid eye drops are used to limit the inflammatory response
- Prompt use of antivirals may limit the disease

## Ramsay–Hunt syndrome

- Shingles of several adjacent cranial nerves cause vesicles in the ear canal, ear pain, and an LMN facial droop
- May also cause vertigo, deafness, and disturbance of taste plus lacrimation

▶ Always look in the ears for vesicles when a patient presents with a facial palsy.

- Facial paralysis is less likely to fully recover than in Bell's palsy
- Treat with antivirals

## Post-herpetic neuralgia

- Distressing sensory symptoms that persist months beyond rash onset
- Occurs in up to 10% of cases
- More common in older patients (up to a third of those >60) who have sensory symptoms at prodrome and a more severe initial infection
- Subsides in the majority by a year; may become chronic and disabling
- Usually a deep, steady burning sensation, sometimes exacerbated by movement or touch. Occasionally paroxysmal and stabbing
- Can cause significant psychological symptoms (low mood, poor sleep, loss of appetite, etc.)
- Treatment is with opioids, anticonvulsants (e.g. gabapentin, carbamazepine, phenytoin), or tricyclic antidepressants (e.g. amitriptyline)
- Topical treatments with lidocaine or capsaicin are also effective
- Other options are used in specialist pain clinics such as iv lidocaine, intrathecal steroids, or local nerve blocks

## Other complications

All the following are more common in older patients:

- *Bacterial superinfection* (around 2%, can delay rash healing; treat with a topical antiseptic or antibiotic initially—more severe cases require systemic treatment)
- *Motor neuropathy* (occurs when the virus spreads to the anterior horn; symptoms depend on the segment affected, e.g. C5/6 may cause diaphragmatic paralysis; the majority will recover spontaneously)
- *Meningeal irritation* (causes headache; occurs in up to 40%; the CSF shows reactive changes—lymphocytosis and elevated protein)
- *Meningitis and encephalitis* (rare; diagnosis enhanced by MRI imaging and CSF PCR. Usually occur with the rash but may be up to 6 months later)
- *Transverse myelitis* (rare; occurs with thoracic shingles)
- *Stroke* (rare and serious; due to cerebral angiitis)

# Malignancy

# Malignancy in older people

Cancer is a disease of the elderly population, being relatively rare in people under 35 years of age, and ↑ in incidence with each decade.

## Why is there more cancer in older people?

- As more people avoid death from infection and vascular events, so they remain alive to develop cancer
- Some cancers are caused by cumulative exposure to environmental agents. A good example would be sunlight and skin cancer, or smoke and lung cancer, but dietary factors and exposure to other carcinogens are also likely to contribute over time
- The process of cell replication may senesce, increasing the chance of malignant change

## Is cancer different in older people?

- Development of metastases may appear to be slower, the cancer overall having a more indolent course, possibly due to altered immune or hormonal responses
- In contrast, some cancers appear to be more aggressive in older people (e.g. acute myeloid leukaemia, Hodgkin's disease, ovarian carcinoma)
- Overall, age itself has limited influence over disease progression and prognosis—factors such as comorbidity and performance status (see Table 25.1) are much more important
- The impact of cancer may be different in an older person. Non-cancer deaths are common in frail elderly people with malignancy, so cancer control by non-invasive means (e.g. tamoxifen for breast cancer) may be a better option than cancer cure by more unpleasant treatments (e.g. surgery)
- Never underestimate the psychological impact of a cancer diagnosis, whatever the age. Heart failure carries a worse prognosis than many cancers, yet news of its diagnosis rarely has such an impact. Whatever your assessment of a person's quality of life, they may see things very differently—you will not know until you ask. The adverse reaction to the diagnosis is often tied up with fears about a slow and painful death (rather than death itself), and careful explanation about symptom control measures may allay some concerns

---

**HOW TO . . . Describe performance status**

See Table 25.1.

Table 25.1 Performance status scoring

| | |
|---|---|
| 0 | Active, no limitations |
| 1 | Active, but unable to carry out strenuous or heavy physical work |
| 2 | Active, spending less than half the day in bed or resting |
| 3 | Spend over half the day in bed or resting, but still able to get up |
| 4 | Bedridden |

# An approach to malignancy

## Make the diagnosis

- Even if no curative treatment is possible, a diagnosis allows targeted symptom control and gives an idea about the likely course of the disease and the expected prognosis
- Many people find 'not knowing what is wrong' very hard and may find a diagnosis a relief, as it allows the future to be planned
- Sometimes a frail patient is obviously dying, and investigations can be an additional burden, without hope of finding reversible pathology. In this case, blind palliation of symptoms is the best course. This should be combined with careful explanation to the patient and family
- There are many shades of grey in between these two extremes. In some cases, finding multiple metastases on a scan may be enough to plan management. In others, a histological diagnosis by biopsy is required to fully balance risks and benefits of treatment. Each individual should have benefits of diagnosis weighed up against discomfort (and cost) of investigation

## Once diagnosis is made, attempt to stage the disease

This allows accurate prognostication and gives the patient better information on which to base treatment decisions. Again, there are exceptions to this (e.g. the very frail who are likely to die from other causes), and each individual should be considered separately.

## Assess patient factors that will influence outcome

▶ Age is not one of these factors
- Comorbidity will adversely affect both disease prognosis and tolerance to treatment
- Functional status is the other main predictor—is the patient active and asymptomatic, active but with symptoms, slowed down by symptoms or incapacitated by them? Oncologists use performance status (see Table 25.1) as an indicator of functional ability and survival prediction. Geriatricians have a role in optimizing performance status

## Utilize a specialist multidisciplinary approach

Cancer care changes rapidly, and it is hard for the generalist to keep up-to-date, so specialist referral is needed. Many different specialists work together in MDTs to provide cancer management, determining the best options individually. Specialist nurses often perform a coordinating role in the patient's journey through the system, providing consistent, non-threatening support, allowing fears to be discussed and providing practical help (e.g. arranging additional help at home).

## Discuss decisions carefully with the patient

Some patients who have led a long and healthy life (and so would potentially do well from therapy) may wish simply to die without being 'messed about'. Other patients with multiple problems and poorer outlook may take any chance at a prolongation of life whatever the cost.

# Presentation of malignancy

In a cognitively intact and physically fit older patient with a malignancy, presentation is often typical, e.g. a breast lump, a thyroid nodule, altered bowel habit with iron deficiency anaemia. In these cases, there is little dilemma—management is as for all patients with such a complaint.

In the frail older person, the presentation is often less clear. Cancer may be found incidentally (e.g. a mass on a routine CXR), or there may be a highly suggestive clinical scenario. Judging how hard to look and to what end is a common challenge in geriatric practice.

## Common presenting scenarios include

*Weight loss without apparent cause*

- Always check a dietary history (and corroborate it with family or friend); measure thyroid function; screen for depression, and assess cognitive state
- If there are no localizing symptoms or signs on careful history or examination, then check screening investigations (see ➊ 'HOW TO . . . Screen for malignancy', p. 631)
- If these are normal, then malignancy is relatively unlikely, and dietary support with reassessment at an interval may be appropriate (see ➊ 'HOW TO . . . Manage weight loss in older patients', p. 355)
- Following up hints offered in a systems enquiry (e.g. admits to occasional loose stool) will depend on the individual patient—whether they would tolerate bowel investigation, whether they would be fit for treatment if malignancy is found and, crucially, what they wish to do

*Elevated inflammatory markers (ESR, CRP)*

- Begin with the screening history, examination, and investigations
- An important differential diagnosis is sepsis, and this should be actively sought with cultures and appropriate tests such as echocardiogram; procalcitonin and white cell scans have a role
- Consider giving the patient a thermometer and temperature chart
- Look at joints and bones as a possible source (gout, septic arthritis, discitis, osteomyelitis)
- Have a low threshold for thinking of endocarditis (see ➊ 'Overview of infection in older people', p. 608)
- Vasculitides (especially see ➊ 'Giant cell arteritis', pp. 476–7) should be considered (PET scans can be useful). A trial of steroids may be appropriate, even if the history is not convincing, but remember to check response and rethink the diagnosis if the blood results do not normalize
- A CT scan of the thorax, abdomen, and pelvis (looking for lymphadenopathy and sub-diaphragmatic abscesses) may be justified if the patient is otherwise fit and has significantly abnormal tests
- Chasing mildly elevated markers in the frail older person is often unrewarding and can be very distressing for the patient. If initial assessment is unhelpful, watchful waiting may be a valid approach

*Anaemia*
- Iron deficiency anaemia should always raise the query of gastrointestinal malignancy, and investigation tailored to the individual situation (see ➲ 'Iron deficiency anaemia: diagnosis', pp. 454–5)
- A normochromic normocytic anaemia with normal haematinics is rather more difficult—it may represent anything from mild myelofibrosis or renal failure to disseminated malignancy
- Screening history, examination, and tests should be performed. If normal, then a decision about suitability for bone marrow biopsy needs to be made on an individual patient basis. Does the patient have a reasonable life expectancy? Would treatments (e.g. chemotherapy) be appropriate if haematological malignancy was confirmed?

---

### HOW TO . . . Screen for malignancy

*History*
Should include:
- Dietary history
- Mood assessment
- History of fevers and night sweats
- Travel history
- HIV risk factor assessment
- Full systems enquiry (especially meticulous enquiry into gastrointestinal symptoms and post-menopausal bleeding)

*Examination*
Full examination required, including:
- Lymphadenopathy
- Skin nodules or rashes (expose the patient fully)
- ENT
- ♂ external genitalia (testicular masses)
- ♀ breast and pelvic examination
- Rectal examination
- Thyroid examination

*Investigations*
- FBC with film, and haematinics
- Urea and electrolytes
- LFTs
- Calcium and phosphate
- Glucose
- TFTs
- ESR and CRP
- Urine and blood electrophoresis
- Urinalysis (dipstick for blood)
- CXR
- Faecal occult bloods (if anaemic)
- PSA in men

▶ Tumour markers have a role in monitoring of established disease but are controversial in screening—false-positive rates are high.

---

# Treating malignancy in older people

Overall, the response to treatment is as good in fit elderly people as in younger patients. Frailty and comorbidity will alter tolerance to treatments more than age. There are specialist MDTs for cancer care that will help to ensure that the most appropriate treatment modalities are considered. Any treatment should be discussed (where possible) with the patient, outlining benefits, potential harm, and practical considerations (such as travelling daily to the hospital for a course of treatment or supplying support for ADLs when weakened by therapy).

▶ Decisions about cancer treatment should not be based on chronological age, rather on biological age, functional status, and the presence of comorbid conditions.

The patient should be at the centre of the decision-making process—decisions are rarely clear-cut and require balancing of the side effects of therapy against potential benefits. Frank discussion of what to expect should facilitate patient-led decisions, and there will be a wide variety of choices. Some older people will wish to avoid interventions, while others will accept a high level of discomfort for the chance of a few extra months of life. Ask the patient.

- *Surgery* can be well tolerated if the patient is pre-selected and receives optimal attention before, during, and after an operation. Curative operations should always be considered, regardless of age and even palliative surgery may be appropriate, e.g. in a frail octogenarian, defunctioning colostomy for a sigmoid tumour may be preferable to constant diarrhoea that causes skin breakdown
- *Radiotherapy* is well tolerated by fit older people, and side effects may be acceptable to even the less fit if the benefits are sufficient. It is often pragmatic issues such as prolonged daily travel to the hospital that is the most difficult for an older person, perhaps worse than the treatment itself. Hospital transport may mean an early start, a late finish, and an uncomfortable journey. These problems should be discussed prior to treatment and psychosocial support offered where possible
- *Hormonal therapy* is often very useful in older people, being well tolerated and effective. It forms the mainstay of treatment for post-menopausal women with breast cancer and for men with prostate cancer. Its role is in disease control, not cure, until they die from another cause
- *Chemotherapy agents* are improving all the time, being better tolerated and more effective. Cardiac comorbidity can cause problems with the amount of fluid that is required. Social isolation can make transport to and from treatments and managing the side effects difficult. Recognition of this and provision of support are essential if treatment is considered

## HOW TO . . . Manage symptomatic hypercalcaemia

Older patients often present with acute confusion and constipation; the classical symptoms of thirst, itch, and bone pain may be less prominent.

▶ Important to check serum calcium for any unexplained confusion or constipation.

▶ Beware hypoalbuminaemia which can mask a high calcium—always check the corrected calcium level.

If the corrected calcium is high, send off a PTH level and screen for tumours. The most common malignant causes include myeloma and carcinomatosis with bone 2° (e.g. prostate or breast) and squamous carcinoma of the lung (where calcitonin-like substances are excreted). The most common benign cause is hyperparathyroidism.

*Management*

1. Rehydration with iv fluids—aim for 3L/day (but more cautious in heart failure)
2. Once the patient is rehydrated, give low-dose furosemide with each bag, as this promotes urinary calcium excretion and helps prevent fluid overload
3. Monitor calcium daily and adjust treatment

In *malignant disease*, consider:

- iv bisphosphonates, e.g. pamidronate
- Steroids, e.g. prednisolone or dexamethasone. Work by slowing tumour turnover. Can cause confusion or hyperglycaemia
- Specific tumour therapy (e.g. antiandrogens for prostate carcinoma, radiotherapy for myeloma), but localized therapies seldom influence serum calcium levels
- There is a group of patients with malignant hypercalcaemia who respond to treatment but relapse as soon as iv fluids are stopped. If all avenues of treatment have been tried, a palliative approach is sometimes appropriate in which calcium is allowed to rise and only symptoms are treated
- In *hyperparathyroidism*, consider parathyroidectomy
- Management of the *confused hypercalcaemic patient*:
  - Can be particularly difficult, especially as patients often pull out iv cannulae; s/c calcitonin may be useful here, rapidly reducing calcium levels to allow standard treatment
  - Consider opiate analgesia (there may be bone pain which the patient cannot tell you about)
  - Benzodiazepine sedation may be required

# Cancer with an unknown primary

Cancer with an unknown 1° makes up around 2% of all malignancy diagnoses, but this proportion ↑ with age because older patients may have less specific and less aggressive presentation. They also tend to seek medical attention less promptly. Presentation is with metastases, usually in the liver, lungs, bones, or lymph nodes.

Finding metastases during investigation for vague symptoms or when looking into more specific problems (such as bone pain, abnormal LFTs, breathlessness, enlarged lymph nodes, etc.) is a commonly encountered problem in geriatric practice, and a structured approach to management is essential.

## Aetiology

- After biopsy, 70% of cancers with an unknown 1° are found to be adenocarcinoma, 15–20% poorly differentiated carcinomas, and 10% poorly differentiated adenocarcinoma
- The 1° becomes clear in only 20% after investigation
- At post-mortem, 40–50% are found to be pancreatic, hepatobiliary, or lung, and most of the remainder are from the gastrointestinal tract, while 20–30% still do not have a 1° identified

## Approach to investigation

Sometimes, once metastatic cancer is identified, no further investigations are appropriate, e.g. if the patient is frail and asymptomatic, or if death is very near. In most cases, however, there is something to be gained by determining the 1° and extent of metastases—ranging from (very rare) cure, through prolongation of life (e.g. for hormonally sensitive tumours), to the targeted palliation of symptoms.

Arrange the following:

- Careful history and examination (including thyroid, breast, and pelvis in women and a rectal examination), looking for hints of the 1°
- Blood tests, including FBC, U, C+E, LFTs, calcium, phosphate, LDH, and PSA
- Tumour markers (CEA, CA 15-3, CA 19-9, CA125, α-fetoprotein, β-human chorionic gonadotrophin) are not useful in diagnosis or prognosis but may be used to monitor response to any treatment
- Urinalysis
- Faecal occult bloods (×3)
- CXR
- Consider thyroid ultrasound, mammogram, and abdominal CT scan

▶ Further radiological or endoscopic investigation is rarely helpful, often uncomfortable, and a poor use of resources.

## Biopsy specimens

- Should usually be obtained if possible (radiology may show the best site). Information from biopsy assists greatly in further management
- Occasionally there will be histological hints as to the 1° source (e.g. signet rings in the glandular cells indicating gastric cancer), but more commonly there is not enough differentiation to allow diagnosis

- Highly specific immunohistochemical stains and molecular profiling have helped considerably in identifying the likely 1°
- Combinations of less specific stains (e.g. CEA, CA 19-9, CA125, cytokeratins, breast cancer antigen) may reveal patterns that suggest the 1°, but these are less helpful

## Prognosis

Prognosis is better if:
- Fewer metastases
- Metastases only in lymph nodes and soft tissues (less good if bones or liver involved)
- Certain histological subtypes
- ♀ patient, with few comorbidities and a good performance status
- Normal serum LDH level

▶ It is unrelated to age.

## Common presentations and treatment options

*Women with peritoneal metastases*
- Usually ovarian or other gynaecological cancer
- Some show extremely good response to chemotherapy, with 15–20% long-term remission in papillary serous carcinoma

*Women with axillary lymph node metastases*
- Usually breast cancer
- Investigate with mammogram and MRI breasts if negative
- Even if no breast lesion found, treat as breast cancer in the standard way
- Involvement of axillary nodes only means potentially curable disease (by mastectomy, node clearance, and radiotherapy)

*Bone metastases*
- In men, these are usually from prostate cancer (especially if sclerotic or blastic metastases), and elevated PSA may confirm this. Standard hormonal treatment for prostate cancer often provides effective palliation
- Lung cancer is the other common cause, with liver, kidney, thyroid, and colon being rarer 1° sources

*Single metastatic focus in brain, lung, adrenal, liver, bone, or lymph node*
- Occasionally actually an unusual 1°
- Usually will metastasize to other sites fairly quickly
- Consider surgical resection
- Radiotherapy for a solitary brain metastasis can occasionally produce long-term survival

*None of the above*
- Empirical chemotherapy (based on histology, molecular typing, and clinical syndrome) produces some response in around 40%, and a good response in around 10%
- Overall, there is up to 20% 3-year survival with treatment (median survival around 10 months)

# Death and dying

# Breaking bad news

Geriatricians frequently break bad news. No matter how old and frail the patient, the news can always come as a devastating blow. Equally, news that may seem bad may be taken well—someone who has felt unwell for ages may welcome an explanation, even if it means a terminal diagnosis. Sometimes they will have been expecting worse ('I've had a stroke? Thank God it isn't cancer').

▶ Each case needs to be considered individually and carefully modified as reactions become apparent.

## Who should be told bad news?

- Information about a patient's diagnosis and prognosis belongs to the patient, and that individual has a right to know. The paternalistic tendency to 'protect' a patient or their relatives from bad news is now largely obsolete, but some patients and relatives still believe this exists and this may need to be corrected
- Very often, fears that an older person will not cope with bad news are unfounded. They may not have asked questions because they are not culturally used to quizzing doctors but will often have an idea that something is wrong. Anxieties about remaining family members (particularly spouses) can be addressed once everyone knows a patient's diagnosis and management plan. Open dialogue may ease distress
- Equally, there are some older people who simply do not wish to know details about diagnosis and prognosis, preferring to trust others to make decisions for them. It is inappropriate to force information on such patients and crucial to identify them. Approaches range from blunt questioning—'If you turn out to have something serious, are you the sort of person who likes to know exactly what is going on?' to a more subtle line—'We have some test results back, and your daughter is keen to talk to me about them. Would you like to know about them too?' The response to this is usually informative—either 'Yes, of course I want to know' or 'Oh, well I'd rather let my daughter deal with all that'
- Well-meaning relatives (usually children, who are more used to challenging authority) may be more proactive in seeking information than the patient and then try to shield their relative from the truth, believing that they would not be able to cope. In such situations, try to avoid giving information to relatives first—explain that you cannot discuss it with them without the patient's permission. Be sympathetic— these wishes are usually born from genuine concern. Explore why they do not want news told, and encourage reality—the patient knows that they are unwell and must have had thoughts about what is wrong. Point out that it becomes almost impossible to continue to hide a diagnosis from a patient in a deteriorating condition and that such an approach can set up major conflicts between family and carers. Be open—tell the relative that you are going to talk to the patient, and promise discretion (i.e. you will not force unwanted information). A joint meeting can be valuable if the patient agrees. They may be right, and the patient does not want to be told, but establish this for yourself first and always get permission from the patient before disclosing details to anyone else

## HOW TO . . . Break bad news

1. Make an appointment and ensure no interruptions
2. Ensure that you are up-to-date on all the latest information—about the disease itself and the latest patient condition. (Have you seen them that morning?)
3. Talk in pleasant, homely surroundings, away from busy clinical areas
4. Ensure that you are appropriately dressed (e.g. not covered in blood from a failed resuscitation attempt)
5. Suggest that family members or friends come along to support
6. Invite other members of the MDT (usually a nurse) who are involved in the patient's care
7. Begin with introductions and context ('I am Dr Brown, the doctor in charge of your mother's care since arriving in the hospital. This is Staff Nurse Green. I already know Mrs Jones but perhaps I could also know who everyone else is?'). It is sometimes useful to make some 'ice-breaking' non-medical comments (e.g. 'How was the journey?'), but do not be flippant
8. Establish what is already known ('A lot has happened here today—perhaps you could begin by telling me what you already know?' or in a non-acute setting 'When did you last speak to a doctor?')
9. Set the scene and give a 'warning shot'. ('Your mother has been unwell for some time now, and when she came in today, she had become much more seriously ill' or 'I'm afraid I have some bad news')
10. Use simple jargon-free language to describe events, giving 'bite-sized' chunks of information, gauging comprehension and response as you go
11. Avoid euphemisms—say 'dead' or 'cancer' if that is what you mean. Avoid false reassurances and platitudes
12. Allow time for the news to sink in—long silences may be necessary; try not to fill them because you are uncomfortable
13. Allow time for emotional reactions, and reassure in verbal and non-verbal ways that this is an acceptable and normal response
14. Encourage questions
15. Do not be afraid to show your own emotions, while maintaining professionalism—strive for genuine empathy
16. Summarize and clarify understanding if possible. If you feel that the message has been lost or misinterpreted, ask them to summarize what they have been told, allowing reinforcement and correction. Complex medical terms are usefully written down to take away and show to relatives or look up
17. Someone should stay for as long as is needed, and offer opportunity for further meeting to clarify questions that will come up later
18. Document your meeting carefully in the medical notes

# Bereavement

Common experience in older people—causes huge psychological morbidity. A quarter of older widowers/widows develop clinical anxiety and/or depression in the first year.

▶ The grieving process is amenable to positive and negative influences, so awareness of those at risk can help target care.

## Normal stages of grief

Not linear—often go back and forth between stages.

- *Shock/denial*: lasts from minutes to days. Longer if unexpected death. Resolves as reality is accepted
- *Pining/searching*: feel sad, angry, guilty, vulnerable; urge to look back and search for the dead person; restless, irritable, and tearful. Loss of appetite and weight. Poor short-term memory and concentration. Resolved by feeling pain and expressing sadness. May be hampered by social or cultural pressures to behave in a certain way
- *Disorganization/despair*: feel life has no meaning. Tend to relive events and try to put it right. Common to experience hallucinations of the deceased when falling asleep (reassure that this is normal). Resolves as adjust to the new reality without the deceased
- *Reorganization*: begin to look forward and explore a new life without the deceased. Find things to carry forward into the future from the past. May feel guilt and need reassurance. Period of adjustment
- *Recurrence*: grief may recur on anniversaries, birthdays, etc.

## Abnormal grief

Hard to define as everyone is different (both individual and cultural variability) and the process cannot be prescribed. In general, weight is regained by 3–4 months, interest is regained after several more months, and the beginnings of recovery have usually been recognized by 2 years.

### Risk factors for abnormal grief

These include:

- Sudden or unexpected loss
- Low self-esteem or low social support
- Prior mental illness (especially depression)
- Multiple prior bereavements
- Ambivalent or dependent relationship with the deceased
- Having cared for the deceased in their final illness for >6 months
- Having fewer opportunities for developing new interests and relationships after the death

Although older people are generally more accepting of death than younger people, they commonly have a number of these risk factors (e.g. an 80-year-old man who has cared for his demented wife for 3 years prior to her death is likely to have had an ambivalent relationship as well as being her carer. He may have limited social support and opportunity for alternative social contacts).

▶ Older widowers have the highest rate of suicide among all groups of bereaved persons.

**HOW TO . . . Promote a 'healthy bereavement'**
- Identify those at risk of abnormal grief (see ➲ 'Risk factors for abnormal grief', p. 640)
- Encourage seeing the body after death if wished
- Encourage involvement in funeral arrangements
- A visit by the GP after death to answer questions, or a meeting with the hospital team, can be very helpful
- Good social support initially is crucial, and professional/voluntary groups (e.g. CRUSE at ⌖ http://www.crusebereavementcare.org.uk) or counsellors can be helpful if family/friends are not present
- There needs to be permission for 'time out' and reassurance that they are experiencing a normal reaction
- As time goes on, setting small goals for progressive change can structure recovery

For the *confused, older patient*, repeated explanations and supported involvement in the funeral and visiting the grave have been shown to reduce repetitive questioning about the whereabouts of the deceased.

# Palliative care

Death is inevitable. Physicians should acknowledge their limitations, not seeing every death as a personal or system failure. Society has a misperception that medical technology can always postpone death—this should be addressed, and death portrayed when appropriate as a natural and inevitable end.

Palliative care is concerned with the holistic management of a patient in whom death is likely to be soon and where curative treatments are no longer possible. It aims to help the patient (and relatives) come to terms with death, while optimizing the quality of the time left. It involves an MDT approach, with attention to relief of physical symptoms and to social, psychological, spiritual, and family support. The UK government published its National End of Life Care Strategy (2008) with the aims of improving the number of people who experience a 'good death'.

Traditionally used in cases of incurable cancer (where a diagnosis has often been made and a prognosis given), the approach is valuable in many other situations. Death from, e.g. end-stage heart failure is as predictable as death from cancer, yet application of palliative care measures is less frequent. Discussing impending death with a patient is often difficult for doctor and patient, but it allows the goals to shift from hopeless (patient cure) to realistic and achievable (planning a good death). With the complexity of illness in older people, deciding when death is inevitable can be difficult and there is often a degree of uncertainty—not least about timescale—but the rewards to the patient and carers are many.

In the UK, very few people die in a hospice, with around half of patients dying in hospital and the rest split between community-based facilities (e.g. a community hospital or care home) and their own home. The challenge that health professionals often face is to deliver the more desirable characteristics of hospice care in a less specialist setting. That is usually achievable—1° and 2° care teams have huge experience and skills in caring for the dying patient, reinforced when necessary by specialist palliative care teams. But patients and families often need reassurance that exemplary end-of-life care can be delivered outside the hospice setting, in all but the most challenging cases.

## General principles of palliative care

- All symptoms should be evaluated and a diagnosis made, based on probability and pattern recognition
- Explanation of cause and planned treatment empowers the patient and keeps expectations realistic
- Treatment involves correcting what can be corrected (e.g. treating oral candida that is contributing to anorexia), counselling to help patients accept the limitations imposed by the disease (e.g. a patient with COPD may never be able to walk in the garden, but supplying a wheelchair will allow them to be taken), and drugs to control symptoms
- Treatment is planned for each individual with careful attention to detail. Effects are monitored closely, and treatment discontinued if ineffective

## At the very end

- Basic care should always be continued (warmth, comfort, shelter, freedom from pain, cleanliness, symptom control, offer of oral nutrition, and hydration)

- 'Artificial' nutrition and hydration (i.e. that which bypasses swallowing) is considered by many to be a treatment and, as such, may be withheld
- Simplify medications. Use s/c routes where appropriate
- Communication with the patient and family becomes even more important—continue regular visits, even if there is no apparent change
- Ask nurses and family about concerns they have (e.g. pain on turning)
- Enlist help from specialist palliative care teams if symptom control is difficult
- A proactive, positive approach at this time can transform the experience of losing a relative

### The principle of double effect

Sometimes treatments given to relieve symptoms can worsen the underlying disease, or even hasten death, e.g. opiates given for pain also cause respiratory depression.

It is not a duty of the physician to prolong life at all costs. The British Medical Association states: 'A single act having two possible foreseen effects, one good and one harmful, it is not always morally prohibited if the harmful effect is not intended.' In other words, if the 1° aim of morphine is to relieve pain, and a 2° (foreseen) consequence of this is respiratory depression and death, then the 1° aim justifies the 2° consequence.

Doctors should not be so concerned about the risk of doing harm that they are inhibited from providing effective symptom control. Good communication with family and other members of the team ensures that everyone understands the rationale behind a treatment plan.

### National End of Life Policy

The first UK End of Life Care Strategy was published in 2008 with the aims of improving the number of people who experience a 'good death'. The report promoted:

- Identification of dying patients, e.g. Gold Standard Framework
- Obtaining and supporting the patient's preferred place of death. Usually this is home, but as age ↑, a preference to die at home ↓. Preferences for home death in one study ranged from 45% (age 75+) to 75% (age 25–34)
- Coordinating and commissioning care across boundaries
- Planning final days care, including 24/7 provision

Although the original strategy supported the widespread use of the Liverpool Care Pathway (LCP), this received a lot of negative press publicity (around accusations of overzealous application of sedation and fluid withdrawal, inadequate communication with patient and family on a background of financial incentives for hospitals to improve percentages of patients dying on LCP). It has been phased out by the government, and local, more patient-centered pathways are now encouraged.

### Further reading

Department of Health (2008). *End of Life Care Strategy: promoting high quality care for adults at the end of their life.* ℜ https://www.gov.uk/government/publications/end-of-life-care-strategy-promoting-high-quality-care-for-adults-at-the-end-of-their-life.

Public Health England. *Cost-effective commissioning of end of life care.* ℜ http://www.endoflifecare-intelligence.org.uk/home.

# Symptom control in the terminally ill

▶ Is delivered usually by general 1° and 2° care teams, not by palliative care specialists.

## Pain

- Use the analgesia ladder, starting with non-opioids (paracetamol, NSAIDs)
- Next, add weak opioids (codeine, dihydrocodeine, tramadol); escalate the dose, then replace with strong opioids (e.g. morphine slow-release). Give regularly and treat all side effects (nausea, constipation)
- Aim to give po if possible, but consider s/c bolus/infusion, or transdermal or rectal routes if necessary
- Identify likely cause(s)—there may be different pains with different causes in one individual—and target treatment to cause
- Neuropathic pain is often opioid-responsive, but antidepressants and anticonvulsants can be added
- Treat muscle spasm with PT, heat, antispasmodics, and benzodiazepines
- Treat nerve compression pain with steroids

## Nausea and vomiting

- Identify the cause—is it reversible (e.g. medication, hypercalcaemia, bowel obstruction)?
- Give small portions of palatable food; avoid strong smells
- Use regular antiemetics:
  - Metoclopramide is indicated when there is gastritis, stasis, and functional bowel obstruction
  - Cyclizine is used with raised intracranial pressure and functional bowel obstruction
  - Haloperidol treats chemical causes such as hypercalcaemia
  - Domperidone
  - Ondansetron

## Constipation

- Start with a stimulant laxative (e.g. senna) or a stool softener if not on opiates, depending on stool characteristics
- Opiates cause ↓ peristalsis; a stimulant laxative is usually appropriate
- Danthron-containing stimulant laxatives are banned in all but terminal care, as they may be carcinogenic. They also cause skin burns so are usually avoided in incontinent patients
- Suppositories, enemas, or digital evacuation may be needed

## Anorexia

- Normal in advanced cancer and other conditions as death approaches
- Family concerns may be the main problem—they may feel their relative is giving up
- Deal with this directly—eating more will not alter the outlook and pressurizing the patient can make them miserable
- ↓ medications that cause nausea or anorexia (opiates, SSRIs)
- Give good mouth care
- Help with feeding if weak
- Offer frequent small meals
- Prokinetics (e.g. metoclopramide) or steroids (prednisolone, medroxyprogesterone) may help

## Dyspnoea

- Treat the cause (transfuse for anaemia, drain effusion, etc.)
- A terrifying symptom—plan the approach for how to deal with an attack without panicking
- Oxygen can help, as can an anxiolytic or opiates, fresh air or fans, and PT if mucus retention is an issue

## Confusion

- Identify the cause (infection, drugs, withdrawal from alcohol, electrolyte imbalances)
- Nurse in a calm, well-lit environment. Relatives can often help with reorientation
- Drugs (e.g. haloperidol, benzodiazepines) should be used only when non-drug measures have proven ineffective

## Dehydration

- Dying patients drink less (weakness, nausea, ↓ level of consciousness) but often do not feel thirsty
- Good mouth care is all that is required where the ↓ intake is part of the dying process and the patient is not distressed by thirst
- Reassure relatives (and staff) that it is the disease that is killing the patient, not the dehydration

## 'Death rattle'

- The patient is usually unaware. Reassure the family of this
- If excess secretion is causing distress or discomfort to the patient or the family, use hyoscine butylbromide, hyoscine hydrobromide, or glycopyrronium (available s/c or as patches)

## Further reading

British National Formulary. ℘ https://www.evidence.nhs.uk/formulary/bnf/current/guidance-on-prescribing/prescribing-in-palliative-care.

### How To . . . Prescribe a subcutaneous infusion for palliative care

#### Is the subcutaneous route appropriate?

- Use regular oral route where possible
- Consider when:
  - Vomiting/nausea/malabsorption
  - Difficulty swallowing, eg near the end or if semi-conscious

⇩

#### Is the patent already on an opiate?

- Calculate the current total dose given per 24her (including prn administration)
  - Has this been adequate? (Ask nurses, family, and patient)
- Convert the oral opiate dose to an equivalent parental dose (see *BNF*), eg morphine sulfate MR 20mg bd is equivalent to diamorphine 15 mg s/c per 24hr
- If starting strong opiates *de novo*, start low (eg 1mg/hr morphine with allowances on the prn side for breakthrough pain)
- Morphine is cheaper and more readily available, but diamorphine is more soluble so can be given in a smaller infusion volume and is less likely to precipitate with multiple other drugs. Morphine has about 2/3 potency of diamorphine

⇩

#### Are there any other symptoms?

- Other agents can be a added to the pump
- Eg metoclopramide for nausea (30–60mg/24hr)
  - Hyoscine hydrobromide for respiratory secretions (0.6-2. 4mg/24hr)
  - Haloperidol for nausea, restlessness and agitation (5–15mg/24hr)
  - Midazolam for sedation (10–60mg/24hr)

⇩

#### Write the prescription

- How large are the infusion pumps on the ward? (Usually 10mL or 50mL)
- Are the components compatible with each other, and water for injection eg diamorphine 30mg + haloperidol 5mg made up to 10mL with water for injection, run in s/c syring driver over 24hr

⇩

#### Reassess every 4–6hr

- Do not wait for 24hr
- Check whether there has been good symptom control–if not, increase the dose
- Check for side effects (eg drowsiness)—consider decreasing the opiate or benzodiazepine dose
- Check whether any prn doses have been used—add these to the next total dose you prescribe.

# Assisted dying

Forms of medically assisted dying (active euthanasia) are available in countries such as Holland and the USA, but it is illegal in the UK for doctors to encourage or support patients with terminal illnesses to end their lives (Suicide Act 1961). A paper issued in 2010 clarified the circumstances in which relatives who assist their loved ones with suicide are likely to be prosecuted, but this makes it very clear that any healthcare professional caring for a patient would be likely to face prosecution, regardless of their motives.

This is an emotive and divisive issue. While a majority of the general public supports assisted dying (around 80% support change to the law), doctors and their representative organizations have historically opposed any change in the law. In 2014, a Royal College of Physician survey showed that only 42% of doctors supported change to the law, with only around 20% of physicians being content to be involved personally with assisted suicide if that became legal.

In 2012, Lord Falconer led a privately funded, but independent, commission which determined that it was possible to put into place a legal framework that would provide for controlled assisted dying while still protecting frail older people. This led to the Assisted Dying Bill which was overwhelmingly rejected in a parliamentary free vote in 2015. While campaigns continue, the law relating to assisted suicide is now most unlikely to change in the next few years.

**Further reading**

*Assisted Dying (No. 2) Bill 2015–16.* ℘ http://services.parliament.uk/bills/2015-16/assisteddyingno2.html.

Campaign for Dignity in Dying. ℘ http://www.dignityindying.org.uk/.

# Documentation after death

### Verification of death

This is the confirmation that death has occurred and may be performed by an appropriately trained doctor, nurse, or paramedic before a body can be moved to the mortuary. It is recommended that you look for:

- Absence of response to pain/stimulation
- Fixed dilated pupils
- Absence of a pulse, heart sounds, respiratory movements, and breath sounds (examine for at least a minute)

Some of these tests can be done simultaneously to save time. Always record your findings in full, along with the time of death, persons present, and the time of verification.

### Certification of death

This is the writing of a medical certificate of cause of death (MCCD) or death certificate. It is an important duty and legal requirement of the doctor that has recently been looking after the patient—it allows the family to arrange a funeral and provides very important statistics for disease surveillance and public health.

- Inexperienced doctors tend to record the mechanism of death, rather than the underlying cause, which may lead to under-representation of the real pathology in national statistics. Patients die of dementia and stroke, although their complications, e.g. aspiration pneumonia, may be the last thing that was treated
- Always record as much information as possible, e.g.:
  Ia Aspiration pneumonia
  Ib Left total anterior circulation infarction
  Ic Non-insulin-dependent diabetes, atrial fibrillation
  II Parkinson's disease, peripheral vascular disease

  is more informative than:
  Ia Pneumonia
  Ib Stroke
- Be as precise as possible, e.g.:
  - When stating cardiac/renal/liver 'failure', qualify it with a more precise cause (e.g. heart failure due to ischaemic heart disease)
  - When a patient died of a septicaemic syndrome, where possible, state the causative organism and source (e.g. '*Escherichia coli* bacteraemia due to ascending urinary tract infection')
- Old age is an acceptable cause of death in the very elderly person who has had a non-specific decline and reasonable assessments to exclude serious treatable disease
- Use section II to record other diagnoses, which are often multiple in older people. Multiple causes can be stated on one line

- You must have seen the patient alive during their recent illness (usually in the last 2 weeks) to write a certificate—sometimes the GP writes a certificate for a hospital patient and vice versa if the patient has recently moved between sites
- The process of death certification is currently being reformed in the UK to incorporate a medical officer who will issue all certificates in a locality. Once the system is introduced, cremation forms will no longer be required

## Cremation forms

There are two parts to a cremation form, completed by different doctors who should not be related or work on the same team. You must have looked after the patient in their terminal illness to complete Part I. If you do not know the patient well, examine the body, the CXR, and the ECG for evidence of a pacemaker.

In contrast, a Part II doctor should not have known the patient and is required by law to be an impartial examiner of the case before the evidence (the body) is cremated. You must be a senior doctor (2 years post-MRCP/FRCS) to complete Part II. Ensure that you have seen the medical notes and have personally questioned the Part I doctor and one other person who knew the deceased (another doctor, nurse, or relative). If there are problems with the certificate or Part I, they can be corrected or reissued. Sometimes you may need to suggest the case is discussed with the coroner.

Following the UK scandal surrounding Dr Shipman in which cremation forms did not highlight a problem, the government is reviewing the protocols surrounding death and cremation. Cremation forms in their current iteration are likely to disappear.

# Other issues after death

### Bereavement services

- Most hospitals now have a bereavement office that coordinates the paperwork required after a death and provides the family with information about registration and funeral arrangements
- Bereavement officers provide a friendly, easily accessible interface between the hospital and relatives and can refer to voluntary bereavement support groups
- Consent for hospital post-mortem may be obtained or coordinated by bereavement officers
- If no family comes forward or if they are incapable/unwilling to arrange a funeral, the hospital (usually via the bereavement office) will arrange and pay for a low-cost cremation

### Post-mortems

- The coroner may initiate a post-mortem for legal reasons or where no doctor is able to write a certificate—the family cannot veto this
- Consented hospital post-mortems (at the family's discretion) are useful for education and audit, especially in unusual or difficult cases. The rate of hospital post-mortems is declining, but careful discussion with relatives (often coordinated by the bereavement services team) ↑ the likelihood of consent. A limited examination (e.g. restricted to the torso or one organ) is sometimes more acceptable
- After the Alder Hey scandal (retention and disposal of organs from children without parental consent; Liverpool, UK, 1990s), the new laws require a separate, explicit consent for retention of tissue for examination/teaching

### The registrar

- The registrar is responsible for recording all births and deaths
- The relatives have to register the death within 5 working days and this usually involves making an appointment
- The death must be registered before a funeral can be arranged
- If there is an error on the death certificate, they can refuse to register the death and will refer the case back to the certifying doctor

# The coroner

Coroners are officers appointed by the Council to investigate any sudden or unexplained death. They are independent of both local and central government. The police, a doctor, or the registrar may report a death to the coroner. The registrar must await the outcome of the coroner's enquiries before registering the death, so families should delay making funeral arrangements.

Under UK law, the following must be reported to the coroner:

- Death occurred in police custody or in prison
- No doctor has treated the deceased during the last illness
- The attending doctor did not see the patient within 14 days of death
- Death occurred during an operation or before recovery from anaesthesia
- Death was sudden and unexplained or in suspicious circumstances
- Death may be due to an industrial injury or disease, or to accident, violence, neglect, or abortion, or to any kind of poisoning (this may include injurious falls and head injuries)
- Some coroners also like to be informed when death occurred <24h after admission to hospital, but this is not a legal requirement

Although there is an obligation to report to the coroner deaths in the circumstances listed, the coroner might be happy to issue a 'Part A' certificate, which permits the doctor to write a death certificate. Only a minority of deaths that are reported will end up with a coroner's post-mortem or an inquest.

Consider discussing:

- Cases of pressure sores or severe malnutrition at home (neglect is possible)
- Cases of falls, especially where the incident is not fully explained or where injury from the fall contributed to death
- Post-operative cases
- Mesothelioma and occupational disease (compensation may rely on a post-mortem)
- Have a low threshold for reporting deaths when relatives are unhappy with social care or pre-hospital or hospital care, or are overtly litigious

The coroner's officers can advise you about acceptable causes of death on a certificate but are not medically qualified. A 'Part A' certificate records that you have discussed the case with him/her, but more commonly informal telephone advice is given—if you feel the case is at all contentious, ensure that a 'Part A' is issued to protect you.

▶ If in doubt, discuss your case with the coroner.

Following the Shipman murders (Dr Harold Shipman was a GP and a serial killer of his patients), the documentation after death and the role of the coroner is likely to be substantially revised by Parliament.

▶ The information given here applies to the UK only—local guidance should be sought in other countries.

# Chapter 27

# Ethics

# Capacity

- A patient with capacity is intellectually able to make a decision for themselves
- Capacity and competency are equivalent terms, but the UK Mental Capacity Act has ↑ the use of the former
- It is a fundamental human right and a basic ethical principle that individuals can make autonomous decisions. However, society also accepts that some of its members, e.g. children and adults with severe cognitive problems, sometimes do not have the ability to make decisions for themselves, and mechanisms are in place to protect them
- Older people and ill patients (matched for age) are much more likely to lack capacity than the general population and it is important that a geriatrician should be familiar with capacity and its assessment (see Table 27.1)
- Capacity may be impaired by permanent, temporary, or intermittent/ fluctuant cognitive impairment or communication difficulties
- Best English practice has now been enshrined in law by the Mental Capacity Act 2005 (Adults with Incapacity Act 2000 in Scotland)

▶ Always remember that in declaring someone without capacity, you may be robbing them of the ability to be involved in important decisions about their health and lifestyle—however benevolent your motives, such decisions should never be taken lightly or inexpertly.

Table 27.1 Assessing capacity

| | |
|---|---|
| Capacity is *decision-specific*. Questions which are more complex and/or more important demand a higher level of capacity | Assess capacity for each relevant question individually. Global tests, e.g. mental test scores, are not a substitute and can be misleading |
| Capacity is *assumed* for adults | The burden of responsibility is with the assessor to prove a lack of capacity |
| Capacity levels may *fluctuate*. Some types of dementia and delirium can cause transient, reversible incompetence | Ensure the patient is functioning at their best before assessing capacity. If in doubt, repeat the assessment later |
| *Ignorance* is not the same as a lack of capacity | Patients should be educated about a subject before being asked to make a decision (just as you would expect a surgeon to explain an operation before asking you to sign a consent form) |
| A patient with capacity may make an *unwise* or unconventional decision | Patients with capacity can make decisions which lead to illness, discomfort, danger, or even death. Carers/relatives often need education and support when the patient chooses an unwise option |

## HOW TO . . . Assess capacity

- *Trigger*—doctors should be alert to the possibility of a lack of capacity, but it is often people closer to the patient (relatives/carers) who highlight a problem. In real life, a capacity assessment is usually only employed where there is conflict or where an important step (such as a will or a change in discharge destination) is being considered. Previous assessments of capacity for other decisions, or at other times, are not a substitute for the latest assessment
- *Education*—the patient should be given ample time to absorb and discuss the facts/advice. Several education sessions may be needed. Maximize your chance of successful communication, e.g. hearing aids. Encourage other health professionals and relatives to discuss the topic with the patient as well
- *Assessment*—probe the patient to assess retention, understanding, and reasoning. The UK Mental Capacity Act outlines a functional test of capacity. Does the person have the ability to:
  - Understand the information?
  - Retain information related to the decision?
  - Use or assess the information while considering the decision?
  - Communicate the decision by any means?

The patient can fail at any step, most commonly the first.

In borderline or contentious cases, employ a second opinion (often from a psychogeriatrician).

- *Action*—document the results of the assessment using observations and patient quotes. If the patient lacks capacity, state how the substituted decision will be made, e.g. medical decision in best interests, involvement of carers, case conference, etc.

For examples of documented capacity decisions, see Boxes 27.1, 27.2, and 27.3.

## Further reading

The British Medical Association (http://www.bma.org.uk) and the General Medical Council (http://www.gmc-uk.org) provide extensive guidance on consent and capacity.

The UK Mental Capacity Act 2005 gives a legal framework. Available at: http://www.opsi.gov.uk/acts/acts2005/ukpga_20050009_en_1.

# The Mental Capacity Act 2005

Legislation covering England and Wales that provides a framework to empower and protect people who may lack capacity to make some decisions for themselves. Prior to the Act, decisions were often made guided by case law, and although this statutory law has not dramatically affected the way in which geriatricians function, it has clarified who can take decisions, in which situations, and how they should go about this. It also allows people to plan ahead for a time when they may lack capacity by creating a lasting power of attorney (LPA) which is a legally binding advance directive (AD) (see ➲ 'Advance directives', pp. 664–5).

The Act covers a range of decisions, from major (e.g. concerning property and affairs, healthcare treatment, and where the person lives) to more minor everyday decisions (e.g. what the person wears), where the person lacks capacity to make those decisions themselves.

There are five key principles in the Act:

- Every adult has the right to make his or her own decisions and must be *assumed to have capacity* to make them unless it is proved otherwise
- A person must be *given all practicable help* before anyone treats them as not being able to make their own decisions
- Just because an individual makes what might be seen as an *unwise decision*, they should not be treated as lacking capacity to make that decision
- Anything done, or any decision made, on behalf of a person who lacks capacity must be done in their *best interests*
- Anything done for, or on behalf of, a person who lacks capacity should be the *least restrictive* of their basic rights and freedoms

### Independent mental capacity advocates

Provision of independent mental capacity advocates (IMCAs) was a requirement of the UK Mental Capacity Act 2005.

An IMCA should be appointed where the following apply:

- The patient lacks, or has, borderline capacity
- There is no legal proxy, close relative, or other person who is willing or able to support or represent the patient
- There is a major decision to be made (e.g. serious medical treatment or a change of habitation)

The IMCA will have authority to make enquiries about the patient and contribute to the decision by representing the patient's interests, but cannot make a decision on behalf of the patient.

# Deprivation of Liberty Safeguards

The DoLS are described in the Mental Health Act (2007) which updates the UK Mental Capacity Act (2005). They aim to protect people in care homes and hospitals from being inappropriately deprived of their liberty. The safeguards have been put in place to make sure that a care home or hospital only restricts someone's liberty safely and correctly, and that this is done when there is no other way to take care of that person safely. The safeguards apply to vulnerable adults who lack capacity, but not those who are detained under the Mental Health Act (1983). More recently, the Care Act (2014) includes statutory safeguarding policies and procedures for social care in all settings.

## What is deprivation of liberty?

As there is no single legal definition of 'deprivation of liberty', it can sometimes be difficult to establish whether it is taking place. Restrictions of a person's activity can range from minor (e.g. not allowing choice of clothing) to extreme restriction (e.g. refusing to allow a person to see family or friends). Whether the restriction is great enough to amount to a deprivation of liberty will depend on the individual circumstances. Case law is growing in this area.

## When should the safeguards be used?

People should be cared for in hospital or a care home in the least restrictive way possible, and those planning care should always consider other options. However, if all alternatives have been explored and the institution believes it is necessary to deprive a person of their liberty in order to care for them safely, then strict processes must be followed. These are the DoLS, designed to ensure that a person's loss of liberty is lawful and that they are protected.

The safeguards provide the person with a representative, allow a right of challenge to the Court of Protection against the unlawful deprivation of liberty, and require that the decision be reviewed and monitored regularly.

If there is concern that a person is being deprived of liberty, then the institution should be approached and concerns addressed; this is often facilitated by the Adult Safeguarding team. If the institution believes that the restrictions are necessary for safe care of the patient, then a DoLS authorization must be sought via the relevant body (see ➲ 'Compulsory detention and treatment', pp. 228–9).

# Making financial decisions

### Power of attorney (POA)

This is a simple legal document that allows an adult who is competent to nominate another person to conduct financial affairs on their behalf. It is only valid while the person donating the attorney remains competent to do so. It is widely misunderstood by the general public to have wider application than it actually does.

### Lasting power of attorney for property and financial affairs

- This was introduced in the Mental Capacity Act (2005) and is often, but not always, combined with a health and welfare LPA (see ➲ 'Making medical decisions', p. 660)
- It enables nomination of an attorney to make decisions about property and financial affairs—usually trusted family member(s)
- Powers include paying bills, collecting income and benefits, or selling property, subject to any restrictions or conditions that might have been included in the LPA
- It can only be used once it has been registered at the Office of the Public Guardian, but this can be done before the donor lacks capacity, so the attorneys can carry out financial tasks under the supervision of the donor
- A registered LPA can be revoked by the donor if they have capacity

### Enduring power of attorney (EPOA)

- Before October 2007, people could grant an EPOA so a trusted person could act for them if they could no longer manage their finances. This has now been replaced by property and affairs LPA (see ➲ 'Lasting power of attorney for property and financial affairs', p. 658)
- Any EPOA remains valid whether or not it has been registered at the Court of Protection, provided that both the donor of the power and the attorney/s signed the document prior to 1 October 2007
- An EPOA can be used while the donor has mental capacity, provided they consent to its use
- Once capacity to manage finances is lost, the attorney/s are under a duty to register the EPOA with the Office of the Public Guardian
- An EPOA/POA does not cover anything other than financial decisions

### Patients who lack capacity

- An LPA/EPOA cannot be made once the patient is incompetent to understand the principles of the document (although it is not necessary for them to be fully competent to run their financial affairs)
- If an LPA/EPOA is not available for incompetent patients, sometimes the finances can be managed informally, e.g. the pension can be paid out and joint bank accounts can continue
- To formally take over financial management in these circumstances (especially for large estates or where conflict exists), an application to the Court of Protection must be made
- Since the Mental Capacity Act 2005, this court can appoint deputies to manage financial, health, and welfare decisions

## Testamentary capacity

This refers to the specific capacity to make a will. Solicitors and financial advisors can help draw up a will and occasionally request a doctor's opinion about competence. Legal guidelines are well established (see ➲ 'Making a will', p. 678).

## Signing an LPA

Patients should generally avoid making an LPA while unwell or in hospital, as this would make it harder to prove that the patient had capacity if the validity of the document was ever challenged.

Before an LPA is valid, there must be a certificate of capacity drawn up by an independent third party called a Certificate Provider. The Certificate Provider could be a solicitor, a doctor, or another independent person whom the donor has known personally for at least 2 years. In some cases (e.g. after a stroke), it may be most appropriate to ask a doctor to carry out the assessment.

If a capacity assessment is required, check that the patient understands that once registered, the LPA allows the attorney complete financial control; this power extends into the future and they will be unable to revoke the power if they lack capacity. Document carefully, as shown in Box 27.1.

The signing of an LPA must also be witnessed by an independent person (often a friend or in hospital by an administrator or manager). This should not be confused with the role of a Certificate Provider.

### Box 27.1  Assessment of capacity to complete an LPA

I interviewed Mrs Jones today. She indicated she wished to make an LPA in the favour of her husband and did not appear to be under duress from another person. She explained her health was deteriorating and she wanted her husband to manage the 'bills and things' if she did not feel up to it in the future. She was able to tell me that she owned a current account, a savings account, some premium bonds, and that the mortgage had been paid off on their house. She understood that an LPA would allow her husband to do as he wished with her money, without necessarily consulting her, both now and in the future. She knew that this power would continue even if she was too ill to be consulted. She confirmed that 'he has always sorted that sort of thing out and I don't want him to be stopped from doing it because I can't sign my cheques—I trust him to do the right thing'.

I believe Mrs Jones has capacity to give lasting power of attorney to her husband.

Dated _____

Signed _____

# Making medical decisions

## Lasting power of attorney for health and welfare

- This was introduced in the Mental Capacity Act (2005)
- It enables nomination of an attorney to make decisions about personal welfare—usually trusted family member(s)
- A personal welfare LPA can only be used once the form is registered at the Office of the Public Guardian and the patient has become mentally incapable of making decisions about their own welfare
- It can include the power for the attorney to give or refuse consent to medical treatment if this power has been expressly given in the LPA (a proxy medical decision-maker)
- Also includes power to make some social decisions, e.g. where the donor lives

## Patients who clearly lack capacity

- Unless a valid LPA is available in the UK, no one can make a decision about medical treatment for another adult without capacity
- It is always worth enquiring if an LPA is completed or if there is a written or verbal AD made by the patient prior to them becoming incompetent (see ➋ 'Advance directives', pp. 664–5)
- Doctors are required by the Mental Capacity Act to make decisions in the 'best interests' of their incompetent patients, and this holds true even if there is a valid LPA
- In America, a hierarchy of next of kin can legally make substitute decisions. Relatives are often surprised, and occasionally angry, to find that they have few rights in the UK
- In practice, doctors should routinely consult the next of kin where important or contentious medical decisions are made for patients without capacity. The human rights legislation, through its support of 'family life' as a basic human right, will reinforce the social shift towards increasing power for relatives. Relatives can help doctors to decide what the patient might have wanted under the circumstances, assisting decisions about best interest
- If there is conflict between the medical team and relatives about what is in the best interests of the patient that cannot be resolved, the doctor involved may wish to seek a second medical opinion, consult with the hospital legal team, an IMCA, or refer to the courts

## Patients who may or may not have capacity

- Patients' views should always be sought about medical treatments
- Often these views will concur with those of the medical professional, or they are happy to be guided by the doctor
- Rarely, a patient will express a view at odds with either the medical team or their family, in which case a careful assessment of capacity to make their own decision is required
- Assess capacity in line with the principles outlined previously, and document meticulously in the notes (see example in Box 27.2)

See ➋ 'Making complex decisions', p. 667.

### Box 27.2 Assessment of patient refusing a colectomy for cancer

Miss Joseph has told me she will not consent to a colectomy. I have explained the procedure that is being recommended, including the benefits and risks, and she has been able to remember and understand this information without difficulty. She explains that in view of her age and lack of current symptoms, she would rather not put herself through a major operation. She said 'I am 79 years old and I don't want to be mucked around'. She understands that by refusing surgery she might be shortening her life and that she may become ill in the future as the tumour grows but feels that this is a 'lesser evil' than an operation at the moment. I believe she has capacity to make this decision and we have agreed to discuss it again in 2 weeks' time during an outpatient appointment after she has spoken to her family.

Dated _____

Signed _____

# Making social decisions

The legal position for social decisions for patients without capacity (e.g. where a patient should live) is the same as for medical decisions. Unless an LPA is in place, the healthcare team should consult with the family to try to ensure that the patient's best interests are met.

If making a decision against the expressed wishes of a patient without capacity, involve an advocate. Where there are no family members, or there is a lack of support for the patient, an IMCA may be appropriate (see ➲ 'The Mental Capacity Act 2005', p. 656). The DoLS should be followed (see ➲ 'Deprivation of Liberty Safeguards', p. 657) and these demand that decisions are made 'the least restrictive'.

It may be necessary to apply to the Court of Protection for a court-appointed deputy to supervise welfare decisions.

A very common challenge for the geriatric MDT is the patient who wants to continue to live alone in their own home after they have developed physical or cognitive problems which means they are at risk in that environment (see ➲ 'HOW TO . . . Manage a patient insisting on returning home against advice', p. 662).

---

#### HOW TO . . . Manage a patient insisting on returning home against advice

First assess whether the patient has capacity to make the decision:
- Patients with capacity should accept that they are at risk and reason that they prefer to take this risk than accept other accommodation
- In borderline or contentious cases, a second opinion, often from a psychogeriatrician, can be helpful

If the patient *has capacity*, then they cannot be forced to abandon their home or accept outside help, although the healthcare team and family can continue to negotiate and persuade.
- It is worth determining what motives lie behind the patient's insistence; sometimes misconceptions can be corrected
- Patients will sometimes agree to a trial period of residential care or care package, and this often leads to long-term agreement

Where the patient *lacks capacity*, decisions should be made in the patient's best interest and be the least restrictive option. While the patient should not be discharged to an environment where they will be at unreasonable risk, the team should still attempt to accommodate the patient's wishes and steps may be taken to reduce risk (e.g. disconnecting or removing dangerous items, alarm systems, or regular carer visits, etc. may still allow a patient to return home). There is no such thing as a 'safe' discharge—only a safer one.

Finally record your capacity assessment clearly as per the following example.

### Box 27.3 Assessment of patient insisting on returning home against advice

Mr King has been a patient of mine for 2 years. He has a progressive dementia which is now severe, and concern has been expressed by his son and the carers that he is at risk to himself in continuing to live alone at home. He was admitted to hospital on this occasion after a small house fire (he left an unattended pan on the stove). He has had three other admissions since Christmas with falls and accidents. Over the last 2 weeks, I have had several discussions with him about why his family is concerned about him. The nurses, his son, and his home carers have also had such discussions. When I spoke to him today, he was disoriented in person and place (believing he was in a police station and that I was a policeman). He expressed a wish to go home to be with his wife (who died 12 years ago) but could not tell me his address. He did not believe that there were any risks involved in going home and did not accept that there was a possibility of falling over again, saying 'I am a very strong man, you would be more likely to fall over than me.' When I discussed the fire, he started talking about his war-time experiences and would not accept that there was a risk of fires in the future. At present I believe that Mr King lacks capacity to make a valid decision about his social circumstances. I have no reason to believe that his level of competency will improve with further education or time. A multidisciplinary best interests meeting has been arranged for next week to discuss if it is practical to continue to support him in his own home or whether placement should be sought.

Dated _____

Signed _____

# Advance directives

- An AD (also known as advance decision) is a patient-led medical decision, made when the patient is competent, which is designed to come into force if a patient becomes incompetent
- ADs were developed to promote personal autonomy
- They may be verbal statements but are more commonly written (sometimes known as a living will)
- ADs are usually employed by patients to refuse aggressive treatment but could, theoretically, be used to request or direct treatment. However, ADs cannot be used to request treatment which would not usually be offered or to withdraw 'basic care' (e.g. nursing or analgesia)
- A valid AD holds the same weight in law as a contemporaneous patient decision, and doctors who provide a rejected treatment could be sued for battery. However, a doctor must first assess whether an AD is valid and applicable (see ➲ 'HOW TO . . . Assess whether an AD is valid and applicable', p. 665)
- A template AD can be downloaded from the Compassion in Dying charity website (⅋ http://www.compassionindying.org.uk)

The UK Mental Capacity Act clarifies the legality of ADs. In an emergency, if an AD is not provided, or if there is doubt about the legitimacy of an AD, then clinically appropriate treatment should be provided. Where a healthcare professional has a conscientious objection to implementing a valid AD, the care should be handed to another practitioner. Despite the theoretical advantages of ADs for patients, relatives, and the medical team, they are still rarely seen in clinical medicine. There are several barriers to their successful implementation:

- Patients are often unaware of ADs or their legal validity
- Patients and doctors are often reluctant to confront these distressing topics or feel that the other party should initiate discussions
- The transfer of AD from 1° care, family homes, and solicitors (where they are often composed and lodged) to hospital (where they are most commonly designed to be implemented) is often poor
- Concern that views might change in future altered states of health
- ADs may be too vague to inform physicians, e.g. a refusal of 'life-sustaining treatment' may not help with decisions about iv fluids
- A high level of competence is required to complete an AD. Patients with conditions such as Alzheimer's disease have commonly lost the ability to make one by the time of diagnosis

Ideally an AD forms part of the wider process of advance care planning between a patient and healthcare professionals, being promoted by the UK Gold Standards Framework (⅋ http://www.goldstandardsframework.org.uk/advance-care-planning).

ADs are most likely to be useful when there is a predictable course of illness (disease-specific ADs have been used in AIDS, cancer, MND, and COPD).

## HOW TO . . . Assess whether an AD is valid and applicable

If a patient retains capacity, then you should discuss management decisions with them in the usual way. An AD is not an excuse for avoiding, often emotionally difficult, discussions with patients or relatives. Contemporaneous decisions always outweigh a previous AD.

As long as an AD is valid and applicable, it should usually guide treatment. This was true under common law before the Mental Capacity Act, but the conditions of validity and applicability are now more clearly defined.

*Validity*
- Verbal statements are theoretically valid, but it is much harder to ensure that they are correctly relayed and refusal of life-sustaining treatment must be written
- Ensure that the AD was not given under duress or pressure from a third party
- It is necessary to assess if the patient had capacity at the time the AD was created (both capacity to make an AD and capacity in terms of understanding the pros and cons of the medical treatment they are refusing), and this can be very difficult to assess

*Applicability*
- If the AD is applicable, then the circumstances should be the same as those defined in the AD, e.g. 'if I had a stroke, I don't want to be tube-fed' may not legally constrain management in other situations

The Mental Capacity Act now defines when an AD is *legally* enforceable. The following conditions must be met:
- The AD must be valid and applicable
- Written statements must be signed and dated
- Must have at least one signature from a witness who is not a relative, an LPA, or a beneficiary of the will
- If the AD refuses life-sustaining treatment, there must also be a statement to verify that the decision applies to treatment 'even if life is at risk'
- If a health and welfare attorney has been appointed under an LPA, this attorney should also be involved in discussions about the person's treatment, and doctors should take information provided by him or her into account.

## Further reading

British Medical Association (2017). *Advance decisions and proxy decision-making in medical treatment and research.* ℘ https://www.bma.org.uk/advice/employment/ethics/mental-capacity/advance-decisions-and-proxy-decision-making-in-medical-treatment-and-research.

General Medical Council (2010). *Treatment and care towards the end of life: decision making.* ℘ http://www.gmc-uk.org/guidance/ethical_guidance/end_of_life_care.asp.

# Diagnosing dying and estimating when treatment is without hope

A high percentage of elderly patients admitted to hospital are destined to die despite best medical care. A great deal of financial and human resources, and most importantly patient suffering, could be avoided if this death was predictable. The art of applying treatment aggressively when appropriate but backing off compassionately in other circumstances is one of the most common and challenging tasks in geriatric medicine.

There has been a lot of discussion about DNACPR orders, but decisions about less dramatic lifesaving technologies are just as hard (e.g. whether to admit a patient from a nursing home for iv antibiotics and fluids or selecting patients for renal replacement therapy; see ➔ 'Renal replacement therapy: dialysis', pp. 394–5) or when to initiate artificial nutrition (see ➔ 'The ethics of clinically assisted feeding', pp. 358–9).

Unfortunately, predicting futile treatment is fraught with difficulty—experienced doctors never underestimate the power of some older people to make a miraculous recovery. The following tips may help:

- Attempt to make a diagnosis (which usually requires some investigations and minor procedures) before estimating the prognosis
- Consider a trial of treatment, but constantly monitor the clinical response and be willing to up- or downregulate how aggressively to treat (e.g. a 2-week trial of NG feeding)
- Sometimes it is helpful to define a 'ceiling of care' at the onset of treatment (e.g. oral, but not iv, therapy, a 20 unit maximum transfusion for acute gastrointestinal bleeding)
- Decide about each intervention separately—every procedure and patient will have different risk/benefit and tolerability ratios
- If there is doubt or disagreement about the appropriateness of treatment, seek a second medical opinion
- Remember that medical decisions are not made in isolation—relatives, nurses, therapists, and community carers are ultimately affected by such decisions, and open dialogue will help everyone

The patients' wishes are paramount, but many severely ill patients do not have capacity to make decisions. Beware patients who reject treatment out of ignorance, misconceptions, or fear. Likewise patients or relatives who continue to demand treatment which is clearly not effective (or inappropriate) require education and support.

Deciding that treatment is futile is not the same as 'giving up'—a positive decision for end-of-life care allows a change in the therapeutic goal from 'cure' to 'keeping comfortable' and ensuring a dignified death. While in some branches of medicine, this shift can involve a change in environment (e.g. to hospice) and medical team (to community or palliative care team), in geriatric medicine, the line is often blurred (see ➔ 'Palliative care', pp. 642–3).

# Making complex decisions

All complex decisions should be made with the following in mind:
- The patient should be presumed to have capacity unless proven otherwise and, as such, should be at the centre of the process
- Efforts should be made to optimize decision-making capacity
- All decisions should be in the patient's best interests
- Wide communication avoids misunderstanding at a later date

Use the flow chart in Fig. 27.1 as a guide.

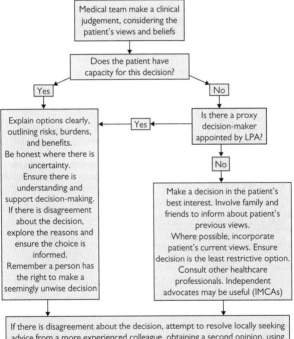

Fig. 27.1 Flow chart for making complex decisions.

# Cardiopulmonary resuscitation

Cardiopulmonary resuscitation (CPR) was first described in 1967 and is now widely applied both in and out of hospital. Around 20% of those who die in hospital in the UK will have at least one attempt at CPR during their terminal admission. Although the principles of CPR decisions are the same as for other medical decisions, they demand special attention because:

• Cardiac arrest often occurs unpredictably
• Withholding CPR in a cardiac arrest will lead to death
• There is an assumption that all patients will receive CPR in hospital—unlike most treatments, a decision is required to withhold it
• CPR is a highly emotive subject

CPR is undoubtedly a lifesaving procedure (in hospital, around 20% will recover a pulse, and half of these patients will survive to leave hospital). Those who survive CPR have a reasonable life expectancy, but a small percentage (1–2%) will be left with permanent hypoxic brain damage.

### Predicting outcome for CPR

(See Table 27.2.)

• Highest success rates are obtained treating arrests due to cardiac arrhythmia on coronary care units, lowest on general medical wards in frail patients with multiple pathologies
• Older patients have lower survival rates, but this is probably a feature of their multiple pathologies, and a good outcome is possible if older patients are carefully selected
• Individual pre-arrest factors are not sensitive or specific enough to be useful in predicting outcome. Morbidity scores combine several variables to attempt to predict outcome of CPR more accurately but are not in common use

**Table 27.2** Factors that predict outcome after CPR

|  | Worse survival rate | Better survival rate |
|---|---|---|
| Pre-arrest | Hypotension<br>Uraemia<br>Malignancy<br>Heart failure<br>Pneumonia<br>Homebound lifestyle | MI |
| Peri-arrest | Out-of-hospital arrest<br>Unwitnessed arrest<br>Asystole or electromechanical dissociation (EMD) | In-hospital arrest<br>Witnessed arrest<br>VF |
| Post-arrest | Long duration of CPR<br>Slow to waken | Short duration arrest<br>Quick to regain consciousness |

### Further reading

Gold Standards Framework. ℛ http://www.goldstandardsframework.org.uk/.

# The process of CPR decision-making

In some circumstances, it is appropriate to decide against doing CPR in the event of a cardiopulmonary arrest. These decisions are known as do not attempt CPR, or do not attempt cardiopulmonary resuscitation (DNACPR), or allow natural death (AND) decisions.

There has been much discussion about the best way of approaching this, with sometimes conflicting views from those in favour of patient autonomy and those who feel this is a medical decision, with many guidelines published. The UK General Medical Council guidance '*Treatment and care towards the end of life: decision making*' offers a sensible balance (⅋ http://www.gmc-uk.org).

## When to consider a DNACPR order

- Where attempting CPR will not restart the patient's heart and breathing (medical futility)
- Where there is no benefit in restarting the patient's heart and breathing (quality or length of life)
- Where the expected benefit is outweighed by the burdens of CPR
- Where a patient with capacity has decided this is what they want

It may be reasonable to only make decisions for those patients in whom arrest seems likely (e.g. critically unwell, actively dying), although facilities with limited out-of-hours cover may make more prospective decisions. Where no DNACPR decision is made, the presumption is that resuscitation should be attempted.

## Where CPR is clearly futile

- A doctor cannot be compelled to provide a futile treatment, and so this is a largely medical decision, although remember that 'futility' is rarely clear-cut
- Following the Tracey case (2014), it is clear that doctors have a legal duty to inform patients or their relatives (for a patient lacking capacity) using unambiguous language that this decision has been made. It is only appropriate to withhold this information from a competent patient where it is considered that it would harm them to have such a discussion

## Where CPR may be successful

- If CPR may be successful, but outcome may be poor (e.g. quality of life), then a decision made in the best interests of the patient should involve their personal view of that outcome
- For patients with capacity, a careful discussion should be had, outlining the risks, burdens, and benefits of CPR (see ➔ 'HOW TO . . . Manage DNACPR decisions', p. 671)
- For those who lack capacity, their views should be approximated from family and friends. Other healthcare professionals should be consulted and an independent advocate (IMCA) may occasionally be useful

## HOW TO . . . Manage **DNACPR decisions**

Ensure you know the local guidelines. Hospitals vary in how this decision is made and recorded, and who is authorized to make DNACPR. Busy physicians need to make time for DNACPR decisions, although they often prove to be easier than anticipated:

- Although it could take 30min to get an elderly patient to make a fully informed decision (many have not even heard of CPR), you can often get a fairly accurate idea from a competent patient with a few quick questions like 'Have you ever considered your views about resuscitation?'
- Never ignore patient cues, e.g. 'I don't suppose I will come out of this?' or 'I've had my time'. These are ideal times to discuss end-of-life issues and such patients are often relieved by this
- Experienced nurses will often provide helpful guidance

In reality, the majority of DNACPR decisions on geriatric wards will not involve the patient (because of incapacity), so a meeting with relatives may ensue to establish best interest:

- When sensitively handled, there is rarely conflict and many are relieved to be consulted or happy to be guided by the doctor
- Try to use the time to discuss general management (emphasizing positive management steps first—even if that is just maintaining dignity and comfort), so that the family does not perceive the only medical priority is avoiding CPR
- Where conflict does arise, it can be best to leave the patient for CPR and re-address the question later. Relatives often take some time to trust the doctors, to come to terms, or to consult other family/ friends, and often the conflict melts away. Remember, CPR is only a small fraction of the patient's care and it may distract from other more important things. While this might lead to a rise in unsuccessful CPR attempts (with consequent reduction in morale of resuscitation teams and resource implications), it does protect patient autonomy and doctors from complaints/litigation
- No one can be forced to provide a treatment which they feel is inappropriate, so if there is conscientious objection to providing CPR, consider moving the patient to a different doctor/ward

### Recording a DNACPR decision

- Write the decision prominently in the medical notes
- Many institutions have a specific form to record these decisions, but ensure that any relevant discussion is fully documented
- Sign, date, and time clearly
- Document the rationale for the decision and the names of those consulted in making the decision
- If the patient/relatives were not consulted, document the reason
- The responsible consultant should endorse a DNACPR order made by a junior doctor as soon as possible
- Ensure the duration of the decision is clear and if ongoing at time of discharge that it is communicated into the community

▶ Ensure that nurses are aware as soon as a DNACPR order is made.

# Rationing and ageism

## Rationing

- This has been present in the NHS since its inception in 1948, but the ever increasing cost of modern specialized, technological, and pharmacological medicine, along with the growing sophistication of patients, has meant that recently rationing has become more explicit and contentious
- No UK government has ever openly admitted to rationing, although 'efficiency saving' and 'commissioning' are thinly disguised ways of handling difficult rationing decisions
- The level at which rationing decisions are made has gradually moved up from physicians themselves (which led to considerable inequality) to hospital managers (which did not remove regional inequality). The introduction of NICE in 1999 was designed to help make rationing decisions at a national level by setting guidelines
- Some initial NICE recommendations that treatments should not be funded (e.g. interferon beta in multiple sclerosis) led to significant lobbying and the development of risk-sharing schemes (allowing government and drug manufacturers to share the cost in certain cases)
- In other cases, funding has been advised, but this has not led to widespread implementation
- So-called 'postcode prescribing' refers to the variable availability of drugs, depending on locality-based clinical commissioning groups

## Ageism

This is rationing applied by age criteria. Although the 2001 UK National Service Framework has banned explicit rationing (standard 1 states 'NHS services will be provided, regardless of age, on the basis of clinical need alone'), it is still widespread.

It is accepted that some medical interventions, e.g. ITU, may be less effective when applied to older people, but remember:

- Some older people are physiologically younger (i.e. chronological age does not correlate well with biological age)
- Some treatments (e.g. thrombolysis in MI) save more lives in an older age group (number needed to treat is lower because untreated death rate is higher than in younger groups)

Disability and dependence costs the state dearly. Preventing strokes, operating on severely osteoarthritic hips, etc. are often highly cost-efficient interventions if they enable patients to stay at home, rather than go into costly institutional care. There is good evidence that the average patient uses the majority of healthcare resources in the last year of their life, but it is rarely possible to predict prospectively when patients are entering their terminal year, nor is there evidence that voluntary restriction of medical treatment by ADs (see ➲ 'Advance directives', pp. 664–5) has any cost-cutting effect.

There is a more fundamental ideological principle that sectors of the population who are perceived to have less social worth are less likely to complain and are largely politically inactive, and should not be discriminated against—whether those sectors are defined by age, sex, or race. The commonly quoted 'fair innings' argument suggests that after a certain age, you have had your 'share' of world resources and younger patients should therefore take precedence. Older people commonly hold to this philosophy. This method of rationing assumes that everyone uses equal resources and enjoys equal quality of life up until the point that it 'runs out'. The logical consequence is that high users of resources (e.g. people with diabetes) should have had their fair innings at a much younger age. In reality, society accepts that some of its members will take more than they give to the system—it is prejudice that allows us to accept rationing for older patients, but not for a child with cerebral palsy.

## Further reading

Grimley Evans J. The rationing debate: Rationing health care by age: the case against. *BMJ* 1997; **314**: 822.

Williams A. The rationing debate: Rationing health care by age: the case for. *BMJ* 1997; **314**: 820.

# Elder abuse

Defined as any act, or lack of action, that causes harm or distress to an older person. Under-recognized, with few prevalence studies. One estimated around 5% of community-dwelling older people have suffered verbal abuse, and 2% physical abuse. Probably more prevalent within care homes, but precise extent unknown.

## Types of abuse

*Psychological*
- Bullying, shouting, swearing, blaming, etc.
- Look for signs of fear, helplessness, emotional lability, ambivalence towards caregiver, withdrawal, etc.

*Physical*
- Hitting, slapping, pushing, restraining, etc.
- May also include inappropriate sedation with medication
- Look for injuries that are unexplained, especially if they are different ages, evidence of restraint, excess sedation, broken glasses, etc.

*Financial*
- Inappropriate use of an older person's financial assets
- Includes using cheques, withdrawing money from an account, transferring assets, taking jewellery or other valuables, failing to pay bills, altering wills, etc.

*Sexual*
- Forcing an older person to participate in a sexual act against their will
- Look for genital bruising or bleeding, or sexual disinhibition

*Neglect*
- Deprivation of food, heat, clothing, and basic care
- Occurs in situations where an older person is dependent
- Look for malnutrition, poor personal hygiene, and poor skin condition
- Easier to spot in situations where a certain standard of care is anticipated (e.g. patients from care homes being admitted to hospital who are unkempt, dirty, or inappropriately dressed may raise concerns)

## Who abuses?

- Commonly someone in a caregiver role
- Often arises because of carer anger, frustration, and lack of support, training, or facilities, along with social isolation
- Relationship difficulties between carer and recipient, and carer mental illness or substance misuse (e.g. alcohol) exacerbates the situation
- Sleep deprivation or dealing with faecal incontinence may also precipitate abuse

▶ Most are under extreme stress ('at the end of my tether') and extremely remorseful afterwards.

## HOW TO . . . Manage suspected elder abuse

The UK Government's Care Act (2014) guidance provides a structure for local safeguarding policies and procedures. The term 'safeguarding' means a range of activities aimed at upholding an individual's fundamental right to be safe.

If abuse is suspected, then early referral to the local social services adult safeguarding team will trigger and coordinate a multi-agency investigation. Key features include:

- Involvement of all agencies involved in the patient's care (GP, home carers, etc.)
- Investigation will be detailed and individually tailored
- As abuse is usually as a result of caregiver stress, a common approach is to attempt to relieve that stress (e.g. providing home care, day care, respite care, health support, advice about sleep or continence, financial help, rehousing, etc.), while maintaining the patient at home
- Close multidisciplinary supervision is essential until the situation improves
- Removal of the patient from an abusive situation may occasionally be done using laws designed primarily for other purposes, e.g. the Mental Health Act (provision to act in the best interests of patients with mental illness)
- Police involvement may occasionally be necessary where there are no remediable factors or a very high risk for future harm
- Further information is available from the following UK charities:
  - *Action on Elder Abuse*, ℘ http://www.elderabuse.org.uk
  - *Age Concern*, ℘ http://www.ageuk.org.uk

# Finances

# Making a will

- Everyone over 18 should make a will. This need not be complicated—there are cheap will writing 'kits' available to buy, and forms can be downloaded from the Internet even more cheaply
- The will should be kept in a safe place, and family members informed
- Wills that are more complex should be made through a solicitor
- It is common for the question of wills to arise for the first time when someone becomes ill, often in hospital
- Doctors may become involved where there is doubt about the patient's capacity to make a will
- Capacity (competence) is covered in detail elsewhere (see ⊃ 'Capacity', pp. 654–5). It is decision-specific so must be reassessed for each important decision a person makes

## Testamentary capacity

This is defined in England and Wales by a specific set of legal criteria. These criteria were established in the 1870 court case of *Banks* v *Goodfellow*.

A person drawing up a will must:

1. *Understand the nature of the act and its effect*—i.e. know that they are choosing to whom to give their property after death
2. *Understand the extent of the property being willed*—this need not be precise, but the person should know roughly what they are willing (e.g. a house and savings), along with details of any joint ownership and debts. The larger the estate, the clearer this understanding should be
3. *Understand the nature and extent of claims on them*—both included and excluded parties. This means the person should be able to say who might reasonably expect to benefit from their will (spouse, children, etc.) and if people are excluded, give reasons why
4. *Have no mental disorder directly influencing points 1–3*—this does not mean that a will cannot be made if someone has a mental disorder—rather that this is not colouring his or her specific testamentary capacity. This can be hard to prove, but an example may be where a patient with dementia develops paranoid delusions about a caring spouse and excludes him or her from the will as a result
5. *Be under no undue influence from third parties*—this again may be hard to prove, except in very overt circumstances

It is sensible to assess capacity at the time the will is drawn up, and then to briefly check at signing (these can be some time apart).

A doctor asked to assess testamentary capacity should question the person with direct reference to *Banks* v *Goodfellow* criteria and make clear contemporaneous notes (with direct quotes) that support the conclusions drawn.

It is probably better to avoid being a witness to a will signing for patients in your care (this can be done by anyone), as this may be confused with a formal capacity assessment.

# Taxation

- Most income received by older people in the UK is taxed, although the universal tax-free allowance applies and has risen to over £10 000
- Some income is not taxed, e.g. attendance allowance, winter fuel payments, pension credit, council tax and housing benefit, and war pensions
- Some lump sums are also not taxed, e.g. from certain private pension schemes. Good financial advice will help to optimize an older person's resources
- The rate of tax then depends on the total income, ranging from 10% at lower incomes up to 45% for incomes over £100 000 per annum

# Pensions

As life expectancy extends, many older people can now look forward to long periods in retirement. Although there is a shift away from being totally financially dependent on the state towards financial planning and personal pensions, there is still a real risk of poverty for many very elderly people. Fuel poverty is one marker (defined as spending >10% of disposable income on fuel).

Pensioners with savings in the UK have been hit hard by low interest rates since 2008. New legislation permits the majority of pensioners with occupational or personal pensions greater autonomy with release of capital, but this requires careful consideration and sound financial advice.

## UK state pension

- Paid when pensionable age is reached (currently 60 for women, and 65 for men, but will change to 65 for both sexes by 2018, rising further to 68 in the future)
- Age of retirement was originally decided on economic grounds, based on life expectancy after stopping work, with little relation to physical ability to work. As people live longer, it becomes less economically viable (see ➲ 'Demographics: population age structure', p. 5)
- It is not automatically given under the age of 80—a person must qualify by making enough National Insurance (NI) contributions during their working lives
- Since 1975, all workers and their employers have made these contributions via NI payments as a percentage of earnings (prior to this, a weekly stamp was paid)
- Credits are awarded if a person cannot pay NI because of sickness, disability, or being a carer
- The full basic state pension is paid if enough NI contributions have been made (in 2015, this about £116 per week for a single person)
- A spouse qualifies for a state pension based on his or her partner's contributions—around half the full pension if they are still living together, but this amount rises if divorced or widowed
- If contribution conditions are not met, then a proportion of the pension may be paid, but some do not qualify at all
- The 'additional state pension' is an earnings-related top-up to the basic state pension for low and moderate earners who are not involved in occupational or private pension schemes
- Over the age of 80, a pension is paid, regardless of NI contributions if the person has been resident in the UK for 10 years since the age of 60
- State pensions are now paid directly into an account
- This money is often supplemented by income from other pensions or investments, or in lower-income households by benefits

## Occupational pensions

- Schemes set up by employers to provide pension and life assurance benefits for employers (e.g. tax-free lump sum on retirement)
- May be contributory (where around 5% of earnings are taken, in addition to an employer contribution) or non-contributory (employer makes all the payments)
- The employer pays most of the administrative costs of the scheme and there are also some tax benefits

## Personal pensions

- Schemes designed to provide an income after retirement (includes stakeholder pensions which have more flexibility)
- Individuals set these up for themselves, often with the help of a financial adviser
- Major tax incentives to save in this way in the UK

## War pensions

Paid to people injured (either in the forces or as a civilian) during a war, and to their dependants.

## Further reading

Age UK. ℘ http://www.ageuk.org.uk.
The Pension Service. ℘ http://www.thepensionservice.gov.uk.

# Benefits

Many pensioners are poor. In 2008/9, there were 1.8 million pensioners in poverty (defined as below 60% of contemporary median income). Despite this, many do not claim all the benefits they are entitled to, usually because they are not aware of them, perceived stigma about 'hand-outs' (that can often be diminished by a few well-judged words from a doctor), or are daunted by application forms.

Care managers can help ensure all benefits are claimed, as can professional welfare rights advisers (working for Citizens Advice Bureau, Age UK, social services departments, etc.). Some charity volunteers will also assist with filling in forms (e.g. Age UK).

Benefits vary with changes in government, and from country to country. The following describes the situation in the UK.

## Benefits for low-income households

### Pension credits

Given to >60s, to top income up to a set amount (guarantee credit). This does not depend on NI contributions. In 2015, a single person is topped up to around £150 per week. This amount may be more in certain circumstances, e.g. severe disability.

### Housing benefit

Helps towards rent and service charges for low-income households.

### Council tax support

Allows low-income households to pay less council tax, depending on income and savings.

## The Social Fund

Provides lump sum payments, grants, and loans:

- Community care grants can be given to help with exceptional expenses such as home adaptations for disability
- Funeral payments can be made to low-income households if needed
- Cold weather payments are made to low-income households to help with heating costs when the temperature is below 0°C for a week
- Budgeting loans available to low-income households to cover one-off expenses (e.g. clothing, household equipment). Repaid (interest-free) from weekly allowance
- Crisis loans are available to all income households, if there is an immediate difficulty in paying for something in an emergency. Repaid without interest

## Attendance allowance

Given to >65s who need help with personal care because of an illness or disability (equivalent to the disability living allowance which is paid to younger people, but no account taken of mobility). Eligibility based on *need* for help or supervision, so even if a spouse is already providing this care, the benefit is still awarded.

### Carers' allowance

Paid to low-income carers of people receiving attendance allowance or disability living allowance.

### Healthcare assistance

- Free prescriptions for all over the age of 60
- Low-income households can apply for free dental treatment, wigs, travel to hospital, and eye tests, and get assistance with paying for glasses

### Travel assistance

- Free local bus travel available in most areas but has different age thresholds
- Reduced train fares with an appropriate rail card for pensioners
- Free renewal of driver's licence >70, subject to filling a medical questionnaire regarding fitness to drive every 3 years. A report from a doctor is not routinely required

### Other benefits

- Free television licence for >75s
- Winter fuel payments made to all households where there is a person >60 years; payment ↑ if >80 years

Many of these are available regardless of income and savings, to reflect the additional costs of disability. Often older people (and the professionals caring for them) assume that they will not be entitled because they are not poor.

### Further reading

Age UK. ℧ http://www.ageuk.org.uk.
Department for Work and Pensions. ℧ http://www.dwp.gov.uk.

# Peri-operative medicine

# Background

In the USA, over half of all operations are performed on patients over the age of 65; in the UK, almost a quarter of all operations are performed on over 75-year olds. This trend will ↑ exponentially over the next 30 years.

In 1999, the UK NCEPOD (National Confidential Enquiry into Patient Outcome and Death) report '*Extremes of age*' recommended sufficient daytime theatre and recovery facilities (including higher dependency units) with clinicians of seniority and experience to ensure that no older patient requiring urgent surgery waited for >24h, once fit for that operation. It is a shame to see that their follow-on report in 2010 '*An age old problem*' highlighted many of the same deficiencies. They noted that the population was older and had more comorbidities than 10 years ago. This is compounded by sarcopenia (and frailty) which results in medical, not surgical, complications and poor functional recovery. They prioritized the need for geriatricians to be involved in all older patients undergoing surgery, before and after the operation. The remaining recommendations provide a framework to ensure good geriatric care:

- Early, routine, and daily involvement by the MDT
- Assessment of comorbidity and disability by an agreed method
- Formal assessment and documentation of capacity and cognitive status
- Formal nutritional assessment and management of under-nutrition
- Medication review either by the geriatrician or senior pharmacist
- Pain management with assessment as the fifth 'vital sign'
- Temperature monitoring and management, avoiding hypothermia during surgery
- Regular audit of any delays to theatre
- Access to level 2/3 (high dependency or intensive) care when appropriate, or if less major surgery, extended recovery/high observation bays should be used

# Models of care

The UK National Emergency Laparatomy Audit (2016) found that only 10% of older adults (aged over 70 years) undergoing emergency laparotomy had input from geriatric medicine; mortality in this group was 30%. Over 98% of hospitals stated they had access to geriatric medicine—the disparity between need and availability and what is provided shows that barriers still exist in providing support and excellent care to this patient group. The methods of providing geriatric expertise to surgical inpatient areas will vary depending on resource, time, and manpower:

- *Visit on request*—the traditional, and now outdated (but common), practice of surgical juniors calling for help from the on-call medical registrar, promoting a reactive, disjointed, and non-standardized approach
- *Regular visits*—dedicated ward rounds, allowing relationships to build and knowledge of what key questions/problems will be asked of each specialist. The geriatrician will assist in management and input into the MDT and discharge planning
- *Shared care*—the geriatrician (usually) is embedded within the surgical ward, using and supervising surgical juniors. Allows early pre-operative involvement, as well as post-operative management, all the way through to discharge. Some also attend surgical pre-op clinics to provide comprehensive geriatric assessment and aid decision-making, e.g. POPS (Proactive care of Older People going to have Surgery)
- *Medically led*—patients with surgical problems admitted to a ward run by the medical/geriatric team and the surgeons come to consult. Has shown to be successful in some areas (hip fracture) but may lead to disengagement from surgical and anaesthetic colleagues over time and also does not provide support for those older patients still being admitted to the surgical wards

---

### Hip fracture—emergency surgery with an evidence base for geriatric medicine input

- The British Orthopaedic Association Standards for Trauma recommends all patients with hip fracture should have surgery on the day of admission or the next day; a geriatrician should assess them within 72h with focus on comorbidity management
- These interventions have resulted in a reduction in 30-day mortality from 10% in 2007 to just over 6% in 2015
- There has also been a reduction in length of stay and morbidity such as AKI
- This has led the way in embedding geriatricians in other areas of surgery—emergency and elective
- Continued audit through the National Hip Fracture Database allows comparison and drives improvement

# Elective surgery

In 2015, there were just over 7 million elective operations performed in England. Increasingly, this is on older and more complex patient groups. Careful consideration to the benefits of surgery over the harms and how best to prepare for surgery should be undertaken. Limiting surgery based purely on age is wrong and yet bias still exists. For example, the contribution of operative mortality in carotid endarterectomy surgery is greater with ♀ sex than being aged over 75 years. Should and would women ever be denied surgery due to their proven ↑ operative risk? In the UK, only when a man reaches 86 and a woman 89 years old is their life expectancy <5 years. Factors other than age alone should take precedence when deciding who should have surgery.

## Patient selection

- Quantify risk of complications and intended benefits; make this explicit to the patient using 'shared decision-making' tools where available (⅋ http://sdm.rightcare.nhs.uk/pda) in order to personalize options relevant to that person. Clearly document and use this to plan the level of peri-operative care required
- Use validated risk prediction tools, either surgery-specific or, if not available, general (see Table 29.1)
- Age should not be used alone; it is a poor surrogate for 'physiological age'. Better predictors of death include high Charlson comorbidity index score, dementia, dependency for ADLs, ↓ mid-arm circumference, and low albumin
- Cardiopulmonary exercise testing is a non-invasive method of measuring cardiac, pulmonary, and metabolic physiology to identify patients at risk for complications. It is gaining popularity but is time- and resource-heavy and cannot be used in people with cognitive impairment. Being able to climb a flight of stairs, performing a 6min walk test, or a timed up-and-go test may be just as enlightening
- Comprehensive geriatric assessment has been proven to reduce complications when performed pre-operatively (POPS service) and may allow traditionally 'high-risk' patients undergo surgery that previously may have been denied to them. These services often include therapy and social workers to plan discharge, even before surgery has occurred

## Pre-operative optimization

- Nurse-led pre-op clinics are safe and cost-effective at identifying those at high risk and can initiate agreed protocols for improving patient care (e.g. diabetes team input, therapist referral)
- Identification and management of anaemia (see ➲ 'HOW TO . . . Manage peri-operative anaemia', p. 691)
- 'Pre-habilitation' is designed to optimize physical and nutritional function before the insult of surgery and has been shown to be effective in orthopaedic and some cancer surgeries. Usually includes PT-guided exercise programmes and dietary supplementation

**Table 29.1** Risk prediction tools for peri-operative medicine

| Scoring system | Advantages | Disadvantages |
|---|---|---|
| ASA (American Society of Anesthesiologists) grade | Grading 1–6<br>Does not rely on investigations or specialist knowledge | Devised over 70 years ago<br>Highly subjective<br>Large physiological changes between each group<br>Does not formally provide a risk score of outcome |
| Revised Cardiac Risk Index (Lee index) | Best validated scoring system for predicting death and major cardiac outcomes<br>Incorporates type of surgery and host factors<br>Simple to use, does not require specialist tests | Only predicts risk of major cardiac events, and not other complications |
| POSSUM (physiological and operative severity score for the enumeration of mortality and morbidity) score | Can be used pre-op to estimate risk<br>Refinements available for specific types of surgery (e.g. V-POSSUM for vascular procedures) | Overpredicts mortality in low-risk groups and hip fracture patients<br>Uses 12 patient variables and six operative variables |
| Nottingham Hip Fracture Score | Simple to use<br>Predicts 30-day mortality | |

- Pre-operative tests for older patients should include FBC, electrolytes, renal function, ECG, and CXR
- Routine echocardiography does not improve 1-year survival or length of hospital stay, compared to matched controls, and should be considered only if there is suspicion of heart failure or identification of a murmur associated with chest pain, breathlessness, or syncope
- Routine coronary revascularization—no study has shown improved outcomes for non-cardiac surgery and it only adds delays in the pathway
- Implantable cardio-defibrillators (ICDs) and permanent pacemakers (PPMs) should be identified, as most necessitate the use of bipolar diathermy to minimize interference. Adjustments to implant function may be required, e.g. temporary inhibition of shocks from ICDs (can sometimes use a magnet) or suspension of 'high-rate' pacing, and so liaise with the cardiac team

### Peri-operative period

- Enhanced recovery after surgery (ERAS) programme—a multimodal package of care that starts pre-operatively and includes prehabilitation, optimal anaesthesia, and minimally invasive surgery, early mobilization, pain management, and enteral nutrition. Developed in Denmark for colorectal surgery, now used for orthopaedic, urology, and gynaecology procedures. Evidence for reduction in length of hospital stay, with no change in mortality or complications
- Minimize the duration of 'nil by mouth' by allowing solids up to 6h before anaesthesia and, in some cases, clear fluids up to 2h. Provision of high-energy liquid supplements on the day of surgery may help and post-operatively, in all cases, initiate enteral feeding as soon as possible
- Fluid management—intra-arterial BP monitoring and cardiac output monitoring (e.g. oesophageal Doppler) during surgery has been shown to improve outcomes in abdominal and proximal neck of femur surgery
- Early mobilization to reduce VTE and lung complications—adequate analgesia should be provided to allow this, including regional anaesthesia
- Delirium prevention—CGA and appropriate action (orientation boards, clocks, bowel and bladder management, glasses and hearing aids, PT) reduce the rates of delirium in orthopaedic and general abdominal surgery groups. It will likely benefit all patient groups and certainly not cause harm. Hypoxia and hypotension (especially during the anaesthetic) are associated with delirium—every 10mmHg below 100mmHg during surgery doubles the risk
- VTE—all older surgical patients are high risk and should have a risk assessment and management according to local guidelines
- AF—should be managed in the usual way with β-blockers if BP allows or digoxin
- Urinary catheters—should be avoided if possible; spinal anaesthesia greatly ↑ urinary retention risk, and so be extra vigilant in this group. If placed, aim to remove as soon as possible

### Recovery

- Patient expectations should be set prior to elective surgery and as part of the ERAS. Realistic expectations reduce the hospital length of stay
- Delivery of equipment and home adaptations should occur, so that everything is in place for discharge, e.g. a second handrail installed before knee surgery or the bed moved downstairs for the initial recovery period
- Early mobilization
- If recovery is slow, consider hypoactive delirium, electrolyte imbalance, and anaemia

## HOW TO . . . Manage peri-operative anaemia

*Pre-operative*
- Anaemia is an independent predictor of poorer outcomes in cardiac and non-cardiac surgery, including major cardiac events, longer length of stay, admission to ITU, ↑ need for blood transfusion, and ↑ mortality
- Perform FBC, iron studies, $B_{12}$, and folate to identify the type of anaemia, ideally at least 6 weeks prior to planned surgery
- Iron deficiency anaemia is the most common. It should be investigated to identify the cause of blood loss while replacing supplies with oral iron or, if not tolerated, iv iron at least 4 weeks prior to the operation date
- Trials have shown benefit of pre-operative iv iron therapy for conditions where surgery is being done to cure the blood loss (e.g. hysterectomy for menorrhagia or colectomy for cancer)
- Anaemia of chronic disease and/or CKD should be managed with nephrology colleagues, using iron supplementation and recombinant human erythropoietin

*Peri-operative anaemia*
- Minimally invasive techniques and 'no blood' loss surgery have reduced the expected blood loss in many operations
- If large blood loss is expected (>20% of volume or 1L in adults) in a clean operative field, cell salvage should be considered, e.g. in cardiac, scoliosis, urology, and vascular surgery
- Anti-fibrinolytics (e.g. tranexamic acid) at time of surgery have been shown to reduce blood loss and the need for transfusions (e.g. trauma, hip fracture surgery)
- Restrictive transfusion strategy should be used—transfuse if Hb <70g/L; consider if <80g/L and symptomatic (chest pain, congestive cardiac failure, orthostatic hypotension, or tachycardia not responding to iv fluids
- Give 1U of blood at a time and reassess

*Post-operative*
- Over 75% of patients with post-operative anaemia will have recovered their Hb levels by 30 days
- If rapidly fatigued or slower-than-expected rehab with concomitant anaemia, consider iron replacement

## Further reading

De Hert S, Imberger G, Carlisle J, et al.; Task Force on Preoperative Evaluation of the Adult Noncardiac Surgery Patient of the European Society of Anaesthesiology. Preoperative evaluation of the adult patient undergoing non-cardiac surgery: guidelines from the European Society of Anaesthesiology. *Eur J Anaesthesiol* 2011; **28**: 684–722.

Goodnough LT, Maniatis A, Earnshaw P, et al. Detection, evaluation, and management of preoperative anaemia in the elective orthopaedic surgical patient: NATA guidelines. *Br J Anaesth* 2011; **106**: 13–22.

Joint United Kingdom (UK) Blood Transfusion and Tissue Transplantation Services Professional Advisory Committee. ℜ http://www.transfusionguidelines.org.uk.

# Emergency surgery

True surgical emergencies pose a different set of questions and challenges. The benefit in these cases is usually to save life, and the risks of morbidity are high. This needs rapid and careful discussion by senior decision-makers with the patient and their family. It should be realistic—time and time again, surgeons and anaesthetists refuse to take patients to theatre based on high risk, whereas without the procedure, death is guaranteed. Some patients in these scenarios would, and should, be offered the chance to take that risk. Ceilings of care and DNACPR decisions should be discussed and set prior to surgery. For example, the older patient with severe COPD and CKD who has a hip fracture would benefit from surgery over non-operative management; care could be on intensive care for NIV and inotropic support, but not intubation or resuscitation.

Conversely, some conditions may have non-operative approaches that are sensible to try in the face of high surgical mortality, e.g. abdominal diverticular perforation treated conservatively with antibiotics, rather than colectomy.

Over 35% of patients in the 2010 NCEPOD report into emergency operations had dementia, delirium, or memory impairment. This needs acknowledgement by the surgical team, and capacity should be assessed according to the Mental Capacity Act 2005 and documented in every patient. In the absence of an LPA, best interests would apply and a consent form 4 (in England and Wales) should be completed. Basic cognitive testing on surgical wards is still sub-optimal and the geriatrician embedded within the ward can improve this.

## Pre-operative priorities

- Restore physiology as quickly as possible—temperature, fluid and oxygen management, electrolyte replacement; identify and treat infection and sepsis
- Investigations should be limited to those that will affect management and not slow down the timeliness of surgery (e.g. the Association of Anaesthetists of Great Britain and Ireland have stated that it is unacceptable to delay hip fracture surgery waiting for echocardiography)
- Medication review—see ➲ 'Peri-operative medication management', pp. 696–8
- Establish premorbid functional state, wishes, and any pre-existing advanced care plans or POAs
- Assess for delirium and put in place measures to reduce risk
- Discuss alternatives to surgery if surgical risk high

# Peri-operative delirium

Delirium occurs in up to 15% of general surgical, and up to 60% of orthopaedic, patients (higher than on general medical wards). It is the most common post-operative complication. Development of delirium increases length of stay, risk of infection, falls, discharge into long-term care, the likelihood of development of dementia, and mortality. It is preventable and treatable through application of excellent comprehensive geriatric assessment and nursing care.

## Predisposing factors

- Advanced age (as a surrogate for reduced cognitive reserve)
- Dementia (known or undiagnosed)
- Comorbidities
- Polypharmacy (>5 medications)
- Physiological stress at presentation
- Length and depth of anaesthetic
- Blood loss
- Peri-operative hypotension

## Prevention

- Non-pharmacological—orientation boards, clocks, attention to bowel and bladder function, regular PT, use of glasses and hearing aids, and attention to sleep hygiene all reduce the incidence of delirium in orthopaedic and abdominal surgical patients
- Anaesthetic—no clarity exists as to which type of anaesthetic is better at preventing delirium. The 'gentle' administration of any anaesthetic will have the best outcomes, and the Association of Anaesthestists of Great Britain and Ireland recommends measuring the depth of general anaesthetic or sedation (e.g. using Bispectral Index Monitors)
- Hypotension—defined as either a 20% drop in BP from pre-induction or <100mmHg should be avoided at all costs both during surgery and post-operatively. Studies where this is achieved report markedly reduced delirium rates within the first 72h post-operatively (in some cases to zero)
- Pharmacological—be careful not to miss drug withdrawal from alcohol and benzodiazepines. Avoid delirium-inducing drugs where possible (e.g. benzodiazepines, antihistamines, anticholinergics, opiates). Use regional blocks over opiate analgesia. If preparing for an elective procedure, calculate the Anticholinergic Burden Score of the current medication list, and try to switch to less offending medications. Pre-treatment with antipsychotics has been shown to reduce the incidence of delirium in certain groups (olanzapine in elective hip and knee surgery) or reduce the severity and duration of delirium (haloperidol in fractured neck of femur surgery), but the trials were small and so not recommended in everyone. Cholinesterase inhibitors have not shown to prevent or reduce delirium in the peri-operative setting

### Identification
- Diagnosis using validated scoring systems such as the CAM or 4AT, or within the intensive care setting, CAM-ICU
- Need to be vigilant for hypoactive delirium

### Investigations
- Observations—temperature, taking care to avoid hypothermia; BP and fluid balance; oxygen saturation (if low, is there a PE, pulmonary oedema, or infection?). Pain should be assessed as the fifth vital sign and actively managed
- FBC, electrolytes, renal function, calcium, ECG, and, if suspicious, troponin
- Septic screen
- Check for urinary retention (especially after spinal anaesthetic)
- Check for constipation
- Medication (e.g. opiates) review
- Assess for alcohol/benzodiazepine withdrawal
- Brain imaging should occur if there is a history of head trauma or localizing neurological signs and no other identifiable cause has been found

### Follow-up
- Peri-operative delirium should be documented on the patient's discharge summary with the results of a cognitive assessment (e.g. AMTS or MoCA)
- Interval cognitive testing (e.g. at 2 months) can check for resolution or the presence of a cognitive deficit, and potentially the onset of dementia

# Peri-operative medication management

## Elective surgery

- Review all prescription medications against comorbid conditions; they are meant to treat and ensure appropriate and optimal doses (STOPP/START or Beers criteria can help here)
- Review non-prescribed medications, including alcohol, over-the-counter NSAIDs, and herbal remedies
- Calculate the Anticholinergic Burden Score of current medications, and if high risk of delirium, suggest switching medication or cessation (e.g. chlorphenamine may be switched to loratadine, amitriptyline should be encouraged to stop)
- BP medications—continue up to the day of surgery, but prioritize those that should be withheld post-operatively due to inevitable post-operative hypotension. Suspend ACE inhibitors/ARB, α-blockers, and diuretics until sure BP normalizing and no AKI

## Specific medications

*Aspirin and antiplatelets*

- Aspirin can be continued for the majority of operations; some surgeons may want cessation for 7 days prior to intracranial, prostate, or posterior chamber of the eye procedures. No contraindication for regional anaesthesia
- Clopidogrel and ticagrelor ↑ risk of bleeding and also risk of complication after spinal anaesthesia. If possible, should suspend for 7 and 5 days, respectively. However, if drugs started due to cardiac event or coronary stent insertion, then cessation of dual antiplatelet therapy is associated with a 37% risk of MI or death. Surgery should be delayed for a minimum of 3–6 months. Cardiology should be consulted

*Warfarin and direct oral anticoagulants*

- Anticoagulation for AF should be withheld for 5 days prior to elective surgery and then restarted the next day, unless there are surgical reasons not to (drains in place, open wounds)
- Rivaroxaban and apixaban should be discontinued for 48h prior to elective major surgery with moderate to high risk of bleeding, and 24h prior to surgery with low risk of bleeding
- Dabigatran excretion is more renal-dependent and so timescales depend on the eGFR. If eGFR >50mL/min, then suspend as above; if eGFR <50mL/min, suspend 4 days prior to high or moderate bleeding risk surgery, and at least 48h prior to low-risk surgery
- 'Bridging therapy' is indicated in special circumstances: metallic heart valves (especially mitral or non-bileaflet aortic), VTE episode within 3 months, cardiac thrombus, and stroke/TIA due to AF. Seek haematology expertise as the method of bridging will vary depending on patient and surgery factors. For major bleeding risk and VTE, an IVC filter can be placed to cover the period of surgery

*Benzodiazepines*
- Do not suspend abruptly as can cause withdrawal delirium. Do not start in the peri-operative period as also ↑ risk of delirium and falls

*Parkinson's disease medications*
- Plans should be made to continue Parkinson's disease medications while the patient is 'nil by mouth', and this can be with either placement of an NGT or conversion of oral medications into dose-equivalent topical patches (e.g. rotigotine). Dose conversion is available on the ℜ http://www.parkinsons.org.uk website. This will reduce freezing, rigidity, pain, and swallowing difficulties. Anti-dopamine medications must be avoided (e.g. metoclopramide as an antiemetic)

*Insulin and oral hypoglycaemics*
- Each hospital will likely have its own protocol for the management of diabetes in the peri-operative period. Patients with type 2 diabetes having morning surgery can forego their oral hypoglycaemic medication on the day of surgery and restart when eating and drinking. If the procedure is in the afternoon/evening, then the morning medications can be taken with breakfast and no more until after surgery. Metformin should be suspended the day before a procedure with iv contrast and for 48h afterward. SGLT-2 inhibitors and GLP-1 agonists should be omitted for the day of surgery, irrespective of the timing of the operation. Long-acting insulins should be maintained, and the period of nil by mouth covered with iv glucose. If >1 meal is being missed, then a variable-rate insulin regimen should be used
- Patients with type 1 diabetes must continue with insulin, even while nil by mouth, and usually an iv variable-rate insulin regimen is started with supporting glucose fluids

*Anticonvulsants*
- Should be maintained through the surgical period. Most can be given either iv or pr

*Steroids*
- Should be maintained through the surgical period and doses doubled if taking >7.5mg prednisolone equivalent per day to avoid hypoadrenal crises. iv hydrocortisone can be used if prolonged periods of nil by mouth

*Beta-blockers*
- Should be continued pre- and post-operatively if already established on treatment for IHD, arrhythmia, or hypertension with other cardiac risk factors. Recent meta-analyses and a robust investigation of trial data on initiating β-blocker therapy in the immediate pre-operative period have clearly shown that this causes harm and ↑ mortality. They should not be initiated unless there is a good underlying cardiac cause for starting them and at least 4 weeks before surgery

*Statins*
- Evidence that being on a statin reduces cardiovascular complications and so should not be stopped if already on one. If having planned vascular surgery, then initiation of a statin prior to surgery is beneficial

## Emergency surgery
- Anticoagulant reversal—warfarin should be fully reversed with iv prothrombin complex concentrate (PCC) based on weight and 5–10mg iv vitamin K. Dabigatran has a monoclonal antibody that is available to some hospitals, and the other DOACs are also producing reversal agents. Otherwise, provide support with tranexamic acid, recombinant factor VIIa, factor VIII inhibitor bypass activity (FEIBA), PCC, and blood products
- Provide antibiotic prophylaxis as per local guidelines
- Provide analgesia as required, avoiding NSAIDs, and give regular laxatives if using opiates
- Suspend antihypertensives, as the risk of AKI and delirium outweighs the harm of a (moderately) high BP. The most common cause for hypertension in this setting is pain which should be actively managed

# Further information

# Dermatomes

See Fig. A.1.

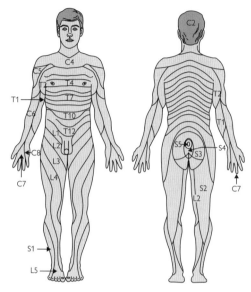

| Myotomes | Reflexes |
|---|---|
| Muscle group | Nerve supply |
| Diaphragm | C(3), 4 (5) |
| Shoulder abductors | C5 |
| Elbow flexors | C5, 6 |
| Supinators/pronators | C6 |
| Wrist extensors | C6 |
| Wrist flexors | C7 |
| Elbow extensors | C7 |
| Finger extensors | C7 |
| Finger flexors | C8 |
| Intrinsc hard muscles | T1 |
| Hip flexors | L1, 2 |
| Hip adductors | L2, 3 |
| Knee extensors | L3, 4 |
| Anide dorsiflexors | L4, 5 |
| Toe extensors | L5 |
| Knee flexors | L4, 5 S1 |
| Ankle plantar flexors | S1, 2 |
| Toe flexors | S1, 2 |
| Anal sphincter | S2, 3, 4 |

Reflexes (right column):
Biceps jerk C5, 6
Supinator jerk C6

Triceps jerk C7

Abdominal reflex T8–12

Knee jerk L3, 4

Ankle jerk S1, 2

Bulbocavernosus reflex S3, 4
Anal reflex S5
Plantar reflex

**Fig. A.1** Overview of the dermatomes, myotomes, and associated reflexes.

Reproduced from Ward I. (2009) *Oxford Handbook of Clinical Rehabilitation*, 2nd edn, Figure 20.1, p.317, with permission from OUP.

# Geriatric Depression Scale

Suitable as a screening test for depressive symptoms in the elderly. Ideal for evaluating the clinical severity of depression, and therefore for monitoring treatment. It is easy to administer, needs no prior psychiatric knowledge, and has been well validated in many environments—home and clinical.

The original GDS was a 30-item questionnaire—time-consuming and challenging for some patients (and staff). Later versions retain only the most discriminating questions; their validity approaches that of the original form. The most common version in general geriatric practice is the 15-item version.

## Instructions

The test (see Table A.1) is undertaken orally. Ask the patient to reply, indicating how they have felt over the past week. Obtain a clear yes or no reply. If necessary, repeat the question. Each depressive answer (bold) scores 1.

**Table A.1** The Geriatric Depression Scale

| | | |
|---|---|---|
| 1 | Are you basically satisfied with your life? | Yes / **No** |
| 2 | Have you dropped many of your activities and interests? | **Yes** / No |
| 3 | Do you feel that your life is empty? | **Yes** / No |
| 4 | Do you often get bored? | **Yes** / No |
| 5 | Are you in good spirits most of the time? | Yes / **No** |
| 6 | Are you afraid that something bad is going to happen to you? | **Yes** / No |
| 7 | Do you feel happy most of the time? | Yes / **No** |
| 8 | Do you often feel helpless? | **Yes** / No |
| 9 | Do you prefer to stay at home, rather than going out and doing new things? | **Yes** / No |
| 10 | Do you feel you have more problems with memory than most? | **Yes** / No |
| 11 | Do you think it is wonderful to be alive now? | Yes / **No** |
| 12 | Do you feel pretty worthless the way you are now? | **Yes** / No |
| 13 | Do you feel full of energy? | Yes / **No** |
| 14 | Do you feel that your situation is hopeless? | **Yes** / No |
| 15 | Do you think that most people are better off than you are? | **Yes** / No |

*Scoring intervals*
0–4 No depression
5–10 Mild depression
11+ Severe depression

# Barthel Index

### Bowel status

0 Incontinent
1 Occasional accident (once a week or less)
2 Continent

### Bladder status

0 Incontinent, or catheterized and unable to manage
1 Occasional accident (maximum once in 24h)
2 Continent (for >7 days)

### Grooming

0 Needs help with personal care (face, hands, teeth, shaving)
1 Independent (with equipment provided)

### Toilet use

0 Dependent
1 Can do some tasks, needs assistance
2 Independent (on/off, wiping, dressing)

### Feeding

0 Dependent
1 Can do about half, needs help with cutting, etc.
2 Independent (food within reach)

### Transfers

0 Unable (no sitting balance)
1 Major help (e.g. two people)
2 Minor help, able to sit (e.g. one person verbal or physical)
3 Independent

### Mobility

0 Immobile
1 Wheelchair independent
2 Able to walk with the help of one person
3 Independent (can use walking aids if necessary)

### Dressing

0 Unable
1 Can do about half unaided, needs some help
2 Independent

### Stairs

0 Unable
1 Needs some help (including stair lift)
2 Independent up and down

### Bathing

0 Dependent
1 Independent

TOTAL POSSIBLE SCORE = 20

- Aim to record what the patient actually does do in daily life, not what he/she can do (i.e. a poorly motivated, but capable, patient may score poorly)
- The score reflects the degree of independence from help provided by another person:
  - If supervision is required, the patient is not independent
  - If aids and devices are used but no help is required, the patient is independent
- Use the best available evidence, asking the patient or relatives, carers, nurses, and therapists, and using common sense. Observing the patient is helpful, but direct testing is not necessary
- Middle categories imply that the patient supplies over 50% of the effort
- It is useful to also ask about abilities before admission or acute illness, and to compare both the total Barthel score and elements of it to determine the magnitude and nature of the setback

## Source

Adapted from: Mahoney FI, Barthel D. (1965). Functional evaluation: the Barthel Index. *Maryland State Med J* **14**: 56–61. Used with permission.

# The Abbreviated Mental Test Score

- The AMTS is a widely applicable, well-validated, brief screening test of cognitive function
- Derived by Hodkinson from a 26-item test, by dispensing with those questions which were poor discriminators of the cognitively sound and unsound (see Table A.2)

Table A.2 The Abbreviated Mental Test

| | |
|---|---|
| Age | Must be correct (years) |
| Time | Without looking at timepiece; correct to nearest hour |
| Short-term memory | Give the address '42 West Street' <br> Check registration <br> Check memory at end of test |
| Month | Exact |
| Year | Exact, except in January when the previous year is satisfactory. Replies '206', '207', etc. in place of 2006, 2007 should be considered correct, as they confirm orientation |
| Name of place | If not in hospital, ask type of place or area of town |
| Date of birth | Exact |
| Start of World War 1 | Exact |
| Name of present monarch | Exact |
| Count from 20 to 1 (backwards) | Can prompt with 20–19–18, but no further prompts. Patient can hesitate and self-correct, but no other errors are permitted |

### Scoring intervals
8–10 Normal
7 Probably abnormal
<6 Abnormal

### Source

Reproduced from Hodkinson, HM. (1972). Evaluation of a mental test score for assessment of mental impairment in the elderly. *Age Ageing* 1: 233–8, with permission from OUP.

# MoCA test

The MoCA is a widely applicable and well-validated test. It is a 30-point test, takes 10–15min to complete, and covers a broader range of cognitive domains than the AMTS. It is therefore less useful as a brief screening test in general medical or geriatric practice, but it is very useful in confirming the nature and magnitude of deficits identified by clinical suspicion or by the AMTS and also in tracking changes (see Fig. A.2).

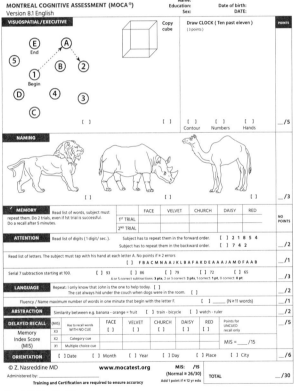

**Fig. A.2** The MoCA test.

Copyright Z. Nasreddine MD. Reproduced with permission. Copies are available at ⌕ www.mocatest.org.

# Confusion Assessment Method (CAM)

A positive test requires the presence of items 1 and 2, and 3 or 4.

The positive likelihood ratio is 5.06, and the negative likelihood ratio is 0.23.

1. Acute onset and fluctuating course. Evidence of acute change in mental status from baseline; behaviour fluctuates during the day
2. Inattention. Easily distracted, difficulty focusing attention and keeping track with conversation
3. Disorganized thinking. Irrelevant conversation, unclear flow of ideas, unpredictable switching from subject to subject
4. Any mental state, other than alert, is abnormal. Describe altered states as: (a) vigilant, (b) drowsy, (c) difficult or unable to arouse

## Source

Adapted from Inouye SK, van Dyck CH, Alessi CA, *et al.* (1990). Clarifying confusion. The Confusion Assessment Method. A new method for detection of delirium. *Ann Intern Med* **113**(12): 941–8. Confusion Assessment Method: Training Manual and Coding Guide, copyright 2003, Sharon K. Inouye, M.D., MPH.

# Clock-drawing and the Mini-Cog™

Clock-drawing tests (CDTs) are widely accepted and well-validated screening tools for dementia. Their strength is in the brisk assessment of multiple cognitive domains, including long-term memory, auditory and visual processing, motor planning and execution, etc. There are many test methods. All ask subjects to draw a clock face showing a specific time, but other details vary. Despite these differences, most appear sensitive and specific and are well tolerated. There is also evidence that non-systematic assessment—simply asking a patient to draw a clock face showing a named time and assessing it informally—has great value in ruling in or ruling out significant cognitive dysfunction.

## The Mini-Cog™

One test that has found widespread favour is the Mini-Cog™, which combines a 3-item recall test with a CDT. It takes 2–3min to administer, is sensitive and specific, and is largely uninfluenced by the level of education, language, or other cultural factors.

Administration

1. Get the patient's attention, then say three unrelated words (e.g. banana, sunrise, chair). Ask the patient to repeat the words to confirm registration. If the patient is unable to repeat the words after three attempts, move onto the next item
2. Ask the patient to draw a clock face on a blank sheet of paper. You should prompt with:
   • 'First draw a large circle'
   • 'Now put all the numbers in the circle'
   • 'Now set the hands to show ten past eleven (11.10)'

Instructions may be repeated, but no more detail/help given. If they have not completed the clock in 3min, move to the next item.

3. Ask the patient to repeat the three words

### Scoring

Give a point for each word correctly recalled after the CDT.
A normal clock scores 2; an abnormal clock scores 0 (see Fig. A.3).
The total score is therefore out of 5 points.
*Positive screen for dementia* is indicated by:
  Score of 0, 1, or 2
*Negative screen for dementia* is indicated by:
  Score of 3, 4, or 5

## Source

## Further reading

Borson S, Scanlan J, Brush M, *et al*. The mini-cog: a cognitive vital signs measure for dementia screening in multi-lingual elderly. *Int J Geriatr Psychiatry* 2000; **15**: 1021–7.

# Clock-drawing test interpretation

See Fig. A.3.

CLOCK SCORING

NORMAL CLOCK

A NORMAL CLOCK HAS ALL OF THE FOLLOWING ELEMENTS:

All numbers 1–12, each only once, are present in the correct order and direction (clockwise).

Two hands are present. One pointing to 11 and one pointing to 2.

ANY CLOCK MISSING ANY OF THESE ELEMENTS IS SCORED ABNORMAL. REFUSAL TO DRAW A CLOCK IS SCORED ABNORMAL.

SOME EXAMPLES OF ABNORMAL CLOCKS (THERE ARE MANY OTHER KINDS)

Missing number

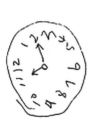

Abnormal hands

Fig. A.3 Clock-drawing test.

# 'Malnutrition Universal Screening Tool' ('MUST')

See Fig. A.4.

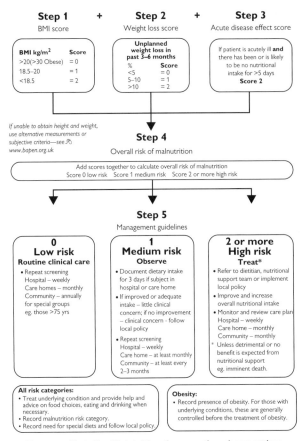

**Fig. A.4** The 'Malnutrition Universal Screening Tool'.

## Source

Reproduced here with the kind permission of BAPEN (British Association for Parenteral and Enteral Nutrition) from the 'MUST' Explanatory Booklet. For further information on 'MUST' see ℘ www.bapen.org.uk.

# Glasgow Coma Scale

The GCS provides a framework with which to describe a patient's state in terms of three elements of responsiveness: eye opening, verbal, and motor.

The GCS score is an artificial index that is obtained by adding scores for each of the three responses. The range of scores is 3–15, 3 being the worst, and 15 the best.

## Best eye response

4   Spontaneous opening
3   Open to speech
2   Open to pain
1   No eye opening

## Best verbal response

5   Orientated
4   Confused conversation
3   Inappropriate words
2   Incomprehensible sounds
1   None

## Best motor response

6   Obey commands
5   Localize pain
4   Withdrawal from pain—pull limb away
3   Abnormal flexion to pain (decorticate posture)
2   Extension to pain (decerebrate posture)
1   No motor response

Note that the term 'GCS 11' has limited meaning. It is important to state the components of the GCS, e.g. E2V2M4 = GCS 8.

Broadly, a GCS of:

- ≥13 suggests mild brain injury
- 9–12 suggests moderate injury
- ≤8 suggests severe brain injury (coma)

# Index